SALEM HEALTH
AGING

SALEM HEALTH
AGING

Second Edition

Volume 2
Hip Replacement – *You're Only Old Once!*
Appendices
Index

Editor, First Edition
Pamela Roberts, PhD
California State University, Long Beach

Editor, Second Edition
Paul Moglia, PhD
Mount Sinai South Nassau

SALEM PRESS
A Division of EBSCO Information Services, Inc.
Ipswich, Massachusetts

GREY HOUSE PUBLISHING

Copyright © 2019, by Salem Press, A Division of EBSCO Information Services, Inc., and Grey House Publishing, Inc.

Salem Health: Aging, Second Edition, published by Grey House Publishing, Inc., Amenia, NY, under exclusive license from EBSCO Information Services, Inc.

All rights reserved. No part of this work may be used or reproduced in any manner whatsoever or transmitted in any form or by any means, electronic or mechanical, including photocopy, recording, or any information storage and retrieval system, without written permission from the copyright owner. For permissions requests, contact proprietarypublishing@ebsco.com.

For information contact Grey House Publishing/Salem Press, 4919 Route 22, PO Box 56, Amenia, NY 12501.

∞ The paper used in these volumes conforms to the American National Standard for Permanence of Paper for Printed Library Materials, Z39.48 1992 (R2009).

Note to Readers
The material presented in *Salem Health: Aging*, Second Edition is intended for broad informational and educational purposes. Readers who suspect that they or someone they know has any disorder, disease, or condition described in this set should contact a physician without delay. This set should not be used as a substitute for professional medical diagnosis. Readers who are undergoing or about to undergo any treatment or procedure described in this set should refer to their physicians and other health care providers for guidance concerning preparation and possible effects. This set is not to be considered definitive on the covered topics, and readers should remember that the field of health care is characterized by a diversity of medical opinions and constant expansion in knowledge and understanding.

Publisher's Cataloging-in-Publication Data
(Prepared by The Donohue Group, Inc.)

Names: Moglia, Paul, editor.
Title: Aging / editor, Paul Moglia, Ph.D., South Nassau Communities Hospital.
Other Titles: Salem health | Salem health (Pasadena, Calif.)
Description: Second edition. | Ipswich, Massachusetts : Salem Press, a division of EBSCO Information Services, Inc.; Amenia, NY : Grey House Publishing, [2019] | Includes bibliographical references and index. | Contents: Volume I. AARP–Heart Changes and Disorders — Volume II. Hip Replacement–You're Only Old Once!, Index.
Identifiers: ISBN 9781642652956 (set) | ISBN 9781642653649 (v. 1) | ISBN 9781642653656 (v. 2)
Subjects: LCSH: Older people--Encyclopedias. | Aging--Encyclopedias. | LCGFT: Encyclopedias.
Classification: LCC HQ1061 .A42453 2019 | DDC 305.26/03--dc23

First Printing
Printed in the United States of America

Table of Contents

Volume 2

Complete List of Contents	vii
Hip Replacement	381
Home-Delivered Meals Programs	383
Homelessness	385
Home Ownership	387
Home Services	389
Hospice	392
Hospitalization	396
Housing	401
Humor	406
Hypertension	408
I Never Sang For My Father (Play)	412
Illnesses Among Older Adults	412
In Full Flower: Aging Women, Power, and Sexuality (Book)	418
Incontinence	419
Individual Retirement Accounts (IRAs)	423
Infertility	424
Influenza	428
Injuries Among Older Adults	430
Jewish Services For The Elderly	433
"Jilting of Granny Weatherall, The" (Short Story)	433
Johnson v. Mayor and City Council of Baltimore	435
King Lear (Play)	435
Kübler-Ross, Elisabeth	437
Kuhn, Maggie	438
Kyphosis	439
Laguna Woods	440
Last Rites	441
Latinx Americans	443
Leisure Activities	447
Lgbtq+	451
Life Expectancy	454
Life Insurance	457
Little Brothers—Friends of The Elderly	460
Living Wills	461
Loneliness	463
Longevity Research	465
Long-Term Care	469
Look Me in The Eye: Old Women, Aging, and Ageism (Book)	475
Macular Degeneration	476
Malnutrition	479
Mandatory Retirement	482
Marriage	485
Massachusetts Board of Retirement v. Murgia	489
Matlock (T.V. Show)	490
Maturity	490
Measure of My Days, The (Book)	491
Medicaid	492
Medicare	494
Medications	498
Memento Mori (Book)	502
Memory Loss	503
Men and Aging	507
Menopause	512
Mentoring	517
Middle Age	520
Midlife Crisis	522
Mobility Problems	525
Multiple Sclerosis	529
Murder, She Wrote (T.V. Show)	532
National Asian Pacific Center on Aging	532
National Caucus and Center on Black Aged	533
National Council on Aging	534
National Hispanic Council on Aging	535
National Institute on Aging	535
Native Americans	536
Nearsightedness	538
Neglect	540
Neugarten, Bernice	541
No Stone Unturned: The Life and Times of Maggie Kuhn (Book)	542
Nutrition	542
Obesity	547
Old Age	550
Old Man and The Sea, The (Book)	553
Older Americans Act of 1965	554
Older Workers Benefit Protection Act	554
On Golden Pond (Play)	555
Osteoporosis	556
Ourselves, Growing Older: A Book For Women Over Forty (Book)	559
Over The Hill	559
Overmedication	560
Palliative Care	564

Parenthood	565
Parkinson's Disease	568
Pensions	571
Personality Changes	575
Pets	577
Picture of Dorian Gray, The (Book)	580
Pneumonia	581
Poverty	585
Premature Aging	589
Prostate Cancer	590
Prostate Enlargement	593
Psychiatry, Geriatric	594
Reaction Time	597
Reading Glasses	598
Religion	598
Relocation	603
Remarriage	607
Reproductive Changes, Disabilities, and Dysfunctions	610
Respiratory Changes and Disorders	615
Retired and Senior Volunteer Program (RSVP)	618
Retirement	619
Retirement Communities	625
Retirement Planning	628
Rhinophyma	630
Robin and Marian (Film)	631
"Roman Fever" (Short Story)	632
Sandwich Generation	632
Sarcopenia	635
Sarton, May	638
Senior Citizen Centers	639
Sexual Dysfunction	641
Sexuality	646
Sheehy, Gail	650
Shepherd's Centers	651
Shootist, The (Film)	652
Sibling Relationships	653
Singlehood	655
Skin Cancer	657
Skin Changes and Disorders	661
Skipped-Generation Parenting	665
Sleep Changes and Disturbances	667
Smoking	670
Social Media	672
Social Security	674
Social Ties	677
Sports Participation	682
Stereotypes	684
Stones	686
Stress and Coping Skills	689
Strokes	691
Suicide	695
Sunset Boulevard (Film)	697
Tell Me A Riddle (Book)	698
Temperature Regulation and Sensitivity	699
Terminal Illness	700
This Chair Rocks: A Manifesto Against Ageism (Book)	703
Thyroid Disorders	703
Townsend Movement	705
Transportation Issues	706
Trip To Bountiful, The (Film)	708
Trusts	709
Urinary Disorders	711
Vacations and Travel	715
Vaccines	718
Vance v. Bradley	721
Varicose Veins	722
Veterans	725
Virtues of Aging, The (Book)	726
Vision Changes and Disorders	727
Vitamins and Minerals	730
Volunteering	733
Weight Loss and Gain	735
Wheelchair Use	738
When I Am An Old Woman I Shall Wear Purple (Book)	739
White House Conference on Aging	740
Why Survive? Being Old in America (Book)	741
Widows and Widowers	742
Wild Strawberries (Film)	744
Wills and Bequests	745
Wisdom	748
Woman's Tale, A (Film)	752
Women and Aging	752
"Worn Path, A" (Short Story)	757
Wrinkles	758
You're Only Old Once! (Book)	759
List of Entries by Category	761

Appendices

Bibliography: Nonfiction	767
Mediagraphy: Film, Fiction, Television & Music	775
Organizational Resources	787
Notable People in the Study or Image of Aging	799
Glossary	807
Index	815

Complete List of Contents

Volume 1

Publisher's Note ... vii	*Bless Me, Ultima* (Book) ... 107
Introduction to the Second Edition ... ix	Bone Changes and Disorders ... 108
Contributor List ... xi	Brain Changes and Disorders ... 113
Complete List of Contents ... xvii	Breast Cancer ... 118
	Breast Changes and Disorders ... 122
AARP ... 1	*Bucket List, The* (Film) ... 125
Abandonment ... 3	Bunions ... 127
Acquired Immunodeficiency Syndrome (AIDS) ... 4	Caloric Restriction ... 128
Adopted Grandparents ... 7	Cancer ... 131
Adult Education ... 7	Canes and Walkers ... 137
Adult Protective Services ... 10	Cardiovascular Disease ... 139
Advocacy ... 11	Caregiver Absenteeism ... 143
Affordable Care Act ... 15	Caregiving ... 145
African Americans ... 18	Cataracts ... 149
Age Discrimination ... 22	Centenarians ... 151
Age Discrimination Act of 1975 ... 27	Center For The Study of Aging and Human Development ... 154
Age Discrimination in Employment Act of 1967 ... 28	*Change: Women, Aging, and The Menopause, The* (Book) ... 154
Age Spots ... 29	Childlessness ... 155
Ageism ... 30	Children of Aging Parents ... 157
Aging: Biological, Psychological, and Sociocultural Perspectives ... 34	Cholesterol ... 158
Aging Experience: Diversity and Commonality Across Cultures, The (Book) ... 45	Circadian Rhythms ... 159
Aging: Historical Perspective ... 46	*Cocoon* (Film) ... 161
Aging Process ... 50	Cohabitation ... 162
Alcohol Use Disorder ... 57	Communication ... 165
All About Eve (Film) ... 61	Consumer Issues ... 167
Alzheimer's Association ... 62	Corns and Calluses ... 169
Alzheimer's Disease ... 63	Cosmetic Surgery ... 171
American Society on Aging ... 70	Creativity ... 173
Americans With Disabilities Act ... 71	Cross-Linkage Theory of Aging ... 176
Anti-Aging Treatments ... 74	Crowns and Bridges ... 177
Antioxidants ... 77	Cryonics ... 178
Arteriosclerosis ... 79	Cultural Views of Aging ... 180
Arthritis ... 82	Cysts ... 187
Asian Americans ... 86	*Darling v. Douglas* ... 188
Autobiography of Miss Jane Pittman, The (Book) ... 89	Death and Dying ... 189
Baby Boomers ... 90	Death Anxiety ... 195
Back Disorders ... 94	Death of A Child ... 198
Balance Disorders ... 98	Death of Parents ... 201
Beauty ... 99	Dementia ... 204
Behavioral and Mental Health ... 102	Dental Disorders ... 207
Best Exotic Marigold Hotel, The (Film) ... 105	Dentures ... 210
Biological Clock ... 106	Depression ... 212

Diabetes	216
Disabilities	221
Discounts	225
Divorce	228
"Dr. Heidegger's Experiment" (Short Story)	232
Driving	233
Driving Miss Daisy (Play/Film)	235
Dual-Income Couples	236
Durable Power of Attorney	239
Early Retirement	240
Elder Abuse	243
Emphysema	248
Employment	252
Empty Nest Syndrome	256
Enjoy Old Age: A Program of Self-Management (Book)	258
Epidemiology and Population Statistics	259
Erikson, Erik H.	261
Estates and Inheritance	263
Estrogen Replacement Therapy	266
Euthanasia	269
Executive Order 11141	273
Exercise and Fitness	273
Face Lifts	280
Facility and Institutional Care	283
Fallen Arches	287
Family Relationships	288
Fat Deposition	294
Filial Responsibility	294
Foot Disorders	295
Fountain of Age, The (Book)	298
401(K) Plans	299
Fractures and Broken Bones	300
Fraud Against Older Adults	303
Free Radical Theory of Aging	307
Friendship	309
Full Measure: Modern Short Stories on Aging (Book)	313
Full Nest	313
Funerals	316
Gastrointestinal Changes and Disorders	318
Genetics	323
Geriatrics and Gerontology	330
Gerontological Society of America	333
Gin Game, The (Play)	334
Glaucoma	335
Golden Girls, The (T.V. Show)	336
Gout	337
Grace and Frankie (T.V Show)	338
Grandparenthood	340
Gray Hair	344
Gray Panthers	345
Great-Grandparenthood	346
Grief	349
Growing Old in America (Book)	352
Grumpy Old Men (Film)	353
Hair Loss and Baldness	353
Hammertoes	356
Harold and Maude (Film)	357
Harry and Tonto (Film)	358
Having Our Say: The Delany Sisters' First One Hundred Years (Book)	358
Health Care	359
Health Insurance	364
Hearing Aids	368
Hearing Loss	371
Heart Attacks	374
Heart Changes and Disorders	378

Volume 2

Complete List of Contents vii

Hip Replacement 381
Home-Delivered Meals Programs 383
Homelessness 385
Home Ownership 387
Home Services 389
Hospice 392
Hospitalization 396
Housing 401
Humor 406
Hypertension 408
I Never Sang For My Father (Play) 412
Illnesses Among Older Adults 412
*In Full Flower: Aging Women, Power, and
    Sexuality* (Book) 418
Incontinence 419
Individual Retirement Accounts (IRAs) 423
Infertility 424
Influenza 428
Injuries Among Older Adults 430
Jewish Services For The Elderly 433
"Jilting of Granny Weatherall, The"
    (Short Story) 433
Johnson v. Mayor and City Council of Baltimore . . 435
King Lear (Play) 435
Kübler-Ross, Elisabeth 437
Kuhn, Maggie 438
Kyphosis 439
Laguna Woods 440
Last Rites 441
Latinx Americans 443
Leisure Activities 447
Lgbtq+ 451
Life Expectancy 454
Life Insurance 457
Little Brothers—Friends of The Elderly 460
Living Wills 461
Loneliness 463
Longevity Research 465
Long-Term Care 469
*Look Me in The Eye: Old Women, Aging,
    and Ageism* (Book) 475
Macular Degeneration 476
Malnutrition 479
Mandatory Retirement 482
Marriage 485

Massachusetts Board of Retirement v. Murgia . . . 489
Matlock (T.V. Show) 490
Maturity 490
Measure of My Days, The (Book) 491
Medicaid 492
Medicare 494
Medications 498
Memento Mori (Book) 502
Memory Loss 503
Men and Aging 507
Menopause 512
Mentoring 517
Middle Age 520
Midlife Crisis 522
Mobility Problems 525
Multiple Sclerosis 529
Murder, She Wrote (T.V. Show) 532
National Asian Pacific Center on Aging 532
National Caucus and Center on Black Aged 533
National Council on Aging 534
National Hispanic Council on Aging 535
National Institute on Aging 535
Native Americans 536
Nearsightedness 538
Neglect 540
Neugarten, Bernice 541
*No Stone Unturned: The Life and Times of
    Maggie Kuhn* (Book) 542
Nutrition 542
Obesity 547
Old Age 550
Old Man and The Sea, The (Book) 553
Older Americans Act of 1965 554
Older Workers Benefit Protection Act 554
On Golden Pond (Play) 555
Osteoporosis 556
*Ourselves, Growing Older: A Book For
    Women Over Forty* (Book) 559
Over The Hill 559
Overmedication 560
Palliative Care 564
Parenthood 565
Parkinson's Disease 568
Pensions 571
Personality Changes 575
Pets 577
Picture of Dorian Gray, The (Book) 580

Pneumonia 581
Poverty 585
Premature Aging 589
Prostate Cancer 590
Prostate Enlargement 593
Psychiatry, Geriatric 594
Reaction Time 597
Reading Glasses 598
Religion 598
Relocation 603
Remarriage 607
Reproductive Changes, Disabilities, and
  Dysfunctions 610
Respiratory Changes and Disorders 615
Retired and Senior Volunteer Program (RSVP) . . . 618
Retirement 619
Retirement Communities 625
Retirement Planning 628
Rhinophyma 630
Robin and Marian (Film) 631
"Roman Fever" (Short Story) 632
Sandwich Generation 632
Sarcopenia 635
Sarton, May 638
Senior Citizen Centers 639
Sexual Dysfunction 641
Sexuality 646
Sheehy, Gail 650
Shepherd's Centers 651
Shootist, The (Film) 652
Sibling Relationships 653
Singlehood 655
Skin Cancer 657
Skin Changes and Disorders 661
Skipped-Generation Parenting 665
Sleep Changes and Disturbances 667
Smoking 670
Social Media 672
Social Security 674
Social Ties 677
Sports Participation 682
Stereotypes 684
Stones 686
Stress and Coping Skills 689
Strokes 691
Suicide 695

Sunset Boulevard (Film) 697
Tell Me A Riddle (Book) 698
Temperature Regulation and Sensitivity 699
Terminal Illness 700
This Chair Rocks: A Manifesto Against Ageism
  (Book) 703
Thyroid Disorders 703
Townsend Movement 705
Transportation Issues 706
Trip To Bountiful, The (Film) 708
Trusts 709
Urinary Disorders 711
Vacations and Travel 715
Vaccines 718
Vance v. Bradley 721
Varicose Veins 722
Veterans 725
Virtues of Aging, The (Book) 726
Vision Changes and Disorders 727
Vitamins and Minerals 730
Volunteering 733
Weight Loss and Gain 735
Wheelchair Use 738
When I Am An Old Woman I Shall Wear Purple
  (Book) 739
White House Conference on Aging 740
Why Survive? Being Old in America (Book) 741
Widows and Widowers 742
Wild Strawberries (Film) 744
Wills and Bequests 745
Wisdom 748
Woman's Tale, A (Film) 752
Women and Aging 752
"Worn Path, A" (Short Story) 757
Wrinkles 758
You're Only Old Once! (Book) 759

List of Entries by Category 761

Appendices
Bibliography: Nonfiction 767
Mediagraphy: Film, Fiction, Television & Music . . 775
Organizational Resources 787
Notable People in the Study or Image of Aging . . 799
Glossary 807
Index 815

HIP REPLACEMENT

Relevant Issues: Health and medicine
Significance: Total hip replacement is one of the most common elective surgical procedures chosen by adults over the age of sixty-five.

Key Terms:
acetabulum: the socket of the hipbone, into which the head of the femur fits
cemented prosthesis: uses fast-drying bone cement to help affix prosthetic to the bone
cementless prosthesis: sometimes called a press-fit prosthesis, is specially textured to allow the bone to grow onto it and adhere to it over time
femoral head: the highest, globular part of the femur; it participates in the hip joint

Total hip replacement is surgery for individuals with severe hip damage. It is one of the most common surgical interventions that older adults face. The American Academy of Orthopedic Surgeons (AAOS) estimates that more than 120,000 hip replacement surgeries are performed in the United States each year. The average age of the patient who undergoes hip replacement surgery is sixty-seven years, while 67 percent of total hip replacements are performed on individuals age sixty-five or older. Approximately 60 percent of hip replacement surgeries are performed on women.

REASONS FOR HIP REPLACEMENT

The most common reason for hip replacement surgery is the decline in efficiency of the hip joint that often results from osteoarthritis. Osteoarthritis is a common form of arthritis that causes joint and bone deterioration, which may lead to the wearing down of cartilage and cause the underlying bones to rub against each other. This may result in severe pain and stiffness in the affected areas. Other conditions that may lead to the need for hip replacement include rheumatoid arthritis (a chronic inflammation of the joints), avascular necrosis (loss of bone caused by insufficient blood supply), and injury.

Generally, physicians may be more inclined to choose less invasive techniques such as physical therapy, medications including injections into the hip joint, or walking aids before resorting to surgery. In some cases, exercise programs may help reduce hip pain. In addition, if preliminary treatment does not improve the patient's condition, doctors may use corrective surgery that is not as invasive as hip replacement. However, when these efforts do not reduce pain or increase mobility, hip replacement may be the best option. In addition, the age of the patient may be an important factor in the decision to replace the hip. The majority of hip replacements are performed on individuals over the age of sixty-five. One of the reasons for this is that the activity level of older adults is lower than that of younger adults, therefore, reducing the concern that the new hip will wear out or fail. However, technological advances have improved the quality of the artificial hip, making hip replacement surgery a more likely intervention for younger adults as well.

TOTAL HIP REPLACEMENT (THR) SURGERY

Generally, a candidate for total hip replacement surgery (THR) possesses a hip that has worn out from arthritis, falls, or other conditions. The hip consists of a ball-and-socket joint where the head of the femur (thigh bone) fits into the hip socket, or acetabulum. In a normal hip, this arrangement provides for a relatively wide range of motion. For some older adults, however, deterioration caused by arthritis and other conditions reduces

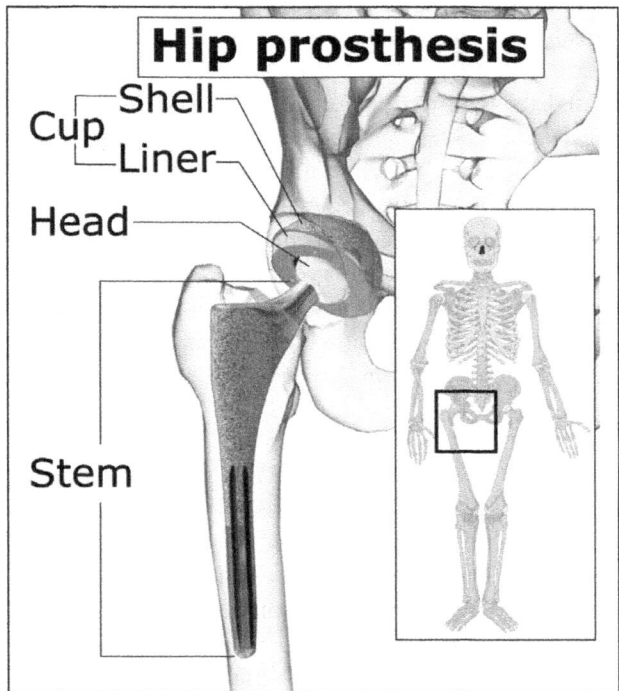

Components of a hip prosthesis. (via Wikimedia Commons)

the effectiveness of this arrangement, compromising the integrity of the hip socket or the femoral head. This state can lead to extreme discomfort.

Total hip replacement may deliver the best long-term relief for hip pain. Traditional surgery and minimally invasive surgery are the two types of hip replacement surgeries. Traditional surgery uses a 6-8-inch incision on the side of the hip through the muscles. The head of the femur and acetabulum are replaced with new, artificial parts. The hip materials allow a natural gliding motion of the joint. A minimally invasive hip replacement, or mini-incision, hip replacement provides a shorter recovery time than traditional hip replacement. It is based on the patient's age, weight, physical condition, and overall health. Replacements may be cemented or uncemented. Older, less active patients and people with weak bones usually require a special glue or cement. A cementless prosthesis has pores that allow bone to grow in to hold the replacement. Activity is limited for three months for natural bone to grow and attach. Thigh pain may occur while the bone is growing into the prosthesis. A hybrid replacement may use a cemented femur part and an uncemented acetabular component.

Both procedures have strengths and weaknesses. In general, recovery time may be shorter with cemented prostheses as one does not have to wait for bone growth to attach to the artificial prostheses. However, the potential for long-term deterioration of the replaced hip must be considered. A cemented hip generally lasts about fifteen years. With this in mind, physicians may be more likely to use a cemented prosthesis for patients over the age of seventy. Cementless hip replacement may be more advisable for younger and more active patients. Some physicians have used a combination of approaches, known as a "hybrid" or "mixed" hip. This combination relies on an uncemented socket and a cemented femoral head.

COMPLICATIONS AND RECOVERY

Total hip replacements are generally quite successful, with about 96 percent of surgeries proceeding without complications. In rare instances, however, complications occur, including blood clots and infections during surgery, and hip dislocation or bone fracture after surgery. In addition, in some cases, bone grafts may be used to assist in the restoration of bone defects. In these instances, bone may be obtained from the pelvis or the discarded head of the femur. Other postoperative complications may include some pain and stiffness.

Patients recovering from total hip replacement usually remain in the hospital for one to four days if there are no complications. However, physical therapists may initiate therapy as soon as the day after surgery. Patients with minimally invasive hip replacement may be up walking the afternoon of surgery with physical therapy support. Physical therapy involves the use of exercises that will improve recovery. Many patients are able to sit on the edge of their bed, stand, and even walk with assistance as early as the same day of surgery. Patients must remember that their artificial hip may not offer the same full range of motion as an undiseased hip. Physical therapists teach patients how to perform daily activities

---

> **SENIOR TALK:**
>
> **How Do You Feel About Hip Replacement?**
> Deciding whether to have hip replacement surgery can feel onerous. You may be conflicted between wanting to relieve your hip pain and wanting to avoid the risks and recovery time of major surgery. You may be getting conflicting advice from family and friends. To avoid an overwhelming feeling of confusion, it is best to get as much information as you can from your doctor and specialists. This way you will be in a better position to make an informed decision about what's best in your individual case. It is also possible to seek a second and even a third opinion, which can help relieve any doubts.
>
> Even once you have opted to have surgery, it is common to be concerned about the outcome and the recovery process. Know that being in a good state of general health prior to the surgery improves your chance of a relatively quick recovery. Focus on the positive goal of gaining full functionality and freedom from pain to elevate your mood and sense of well-being. Although it is normal to feel anxious about undergoing a major procedure and dealing with an extended recovery period, you may also be happy and excited knowing that hip replacement brings the possibility of greatly improved quality of life.
>
> —*Leah Jacob*

without placing an undue burden on their new hips. This may require learning a new method of sitting, standing, and performing other activities such as entering a car.

At discharge from the hospital, supportive care drugs such as pain medicine, anti-inflammatories, and laxatives may be ordered. A walker progressing to a cane is the norm. Exercises and/or follow-up physical therapy visits may be ordered. You and your physician will decide your best course of care after discharge.

Although many factors may affect recovery time, full recovery from surgery may take up to six months. At that point, many patients enjoy such activities as walking and swimming. Doctors and physical therapists may discourage patients from participating in such high-impact activities as jogging or playing tennis, which may burden the new hip. Despite these restrictions, many patients are able to perform normal activities without pain and discomfort. Nonetheless, people who have undergone hip replacement surgery are advised to consult with their doctor about proper exercise and activity levels.

—H. David Smith
Updated by Patricia Stanfill Edens, RN, PhD, FACHE

See also: Arthritis; Bone changes and disorders; Canes and walkers; Mobility problems

For Further Information

American Academy of Orthopedic Surgeons. www.aaos.org.
"Hip Replacement Surgery | Hip Arthroplasty." MedlinePlus, U.S. National Library of Medicine, 31 Aug. 2016. medlineplus.gov/hipreplacement.html. Collection of resources on hip replacement.

Harbour, John. *Diary of a Hippie: A Real-Life Journal of What to Expect during a Total Hip Replacement.* Orsorum P, 2017. A personal account of getting a total hip replacement chronicles the author's journey from diagnosis through the operation and recovery. Harbour shares his fears, hopes, joys, and information gleaned during undergoing the process himself. Combined with inspirational quotes relevant to the steps along the way, Diary of a Hippie provides invaluable insight into what to expect once you decide to have your hip replaced.

Li, Mengnai, and Andrew H. Glassman. "What's New in Hip Replacement." *The Journal of Bone and Joint Surgery*, vol. 100, no. 18, 19 Sept. 2018, pp. 1,616-24. doi:10.2106/jbjs.18.00583. Reviews studies on total hip arthroplasty published in 2017.

Miles, Troy A. *Life after Hip Replacement: A Complete Guide to Recovery and Rehabilitation.* CreateSpace Independent Publishing Platform, 2016. This practical guide reveals tips for a speedy and minimally painful recovery, bridging the gap between scientific evidence and real-world advice. Written by orthopaedic surgeon Dr. Troy A. Miles, this concise guide gives you a clear understanding of what to expect following total hip replacement surgery.

Taylor, Rob, and Wayne Moschetti. *Get Hip!: How to Prepare for and Recover from Total Hip Replacement.* Frog's Leap, 2018. Get Hip! tells the story of hip replacement, from the first pains of osteoarthritis, through medical decisions, surgery, and recovery. It is the story of retired journalist Rob Taylor and 11 other hip surgery patients, men and women, ages 30 to 88.

HOME-DELIVERED MEALS PROGRAMS

Relevant Issues: Economics, health and medicine, sociology

Significance: Home-delivered meals programs provide nutritionally balanced meals to an elderly population that is at increased risk for malnutrition.

Good nutrition is an important part of the quality of life as people age. Good nutrition means not only eating a balanced diet but also eating enough to maintain a healthy lifestyle. Older adults are at much greater risk for malnutrition than the general population because of both normal and disease-related changes that occur with aging. These changes are many and varied. For example, physiological changes can impair an individual's food absorption, or a decline in functional ability may limit an older person's capacity to go to the store and shop for food or to prepare food. Declining functional status may also make it difficult to eat a meal once it has been prepared. Most elderly people are also on fixed incomes, so the cost of food must be balanced against other demands, such as rent and utilities. Finally, eating is a social experience—most people do not choose to eat alone, although the home-bound elderly are often forced to do so by the death of a spouse or by their own limitations.

Home-delivered meals programs are designed to help meet some of the biggest challenges seniors face. This includes having access to nutritious meals, a suitable and safe living environment, and meaningful social interaction. The Meals-on-Wheels program is the oldest and largest national organization that addresses senior isolation and hunger, with more than 5,000 community-based programs. The Older Americans Act (OAA) Program has provided 38 percent of the total cost of the program for the last 50 years. The other 62 percent comes from other federal, state, local, and private donations. These programs deliver one nutritious midday meal on a daily basis to the disabled and the elderly who are homebound and unable to prepare their own meals. Individual programs differ; many deliver different kinds of meals, including regular, low-salt (2 to 3 grams of sodium), and diabetic meals. Costs vary from program to program. Home-delivered meals programs are set up to serve specific geographic areas. Each program is responsible for client intake, client assessment, and the day-to-day activities required to provide the meals to the elderly at their homes. Many rely on volunteers and recruit them from the community.

Home-delivered meals programs do not deliver only food. They provide daily social contact with a trained volunteer for the homebound elderly. Oftentimes these volunteers are the only people the seniors will interact with for the day. These volunteers establish a relationship with the seniors and help conduct safety checks of their homes to ensure they are able to live independently at home with dignity. Home-delivered meals volunteers also supply important referral information about other appropriate community resources.

Among home-delivered meals participants, 59 percent reported having three or more diagnosed, chronic illnesses or conditions. Only 46 percent of participants reported getting out of their homes at least once during the week. When poor health is compounded by low income, elders are at risk. About 6.9 million seniors in the United States live in poverty, meaning they have an income of less than $228 a week to be shared between

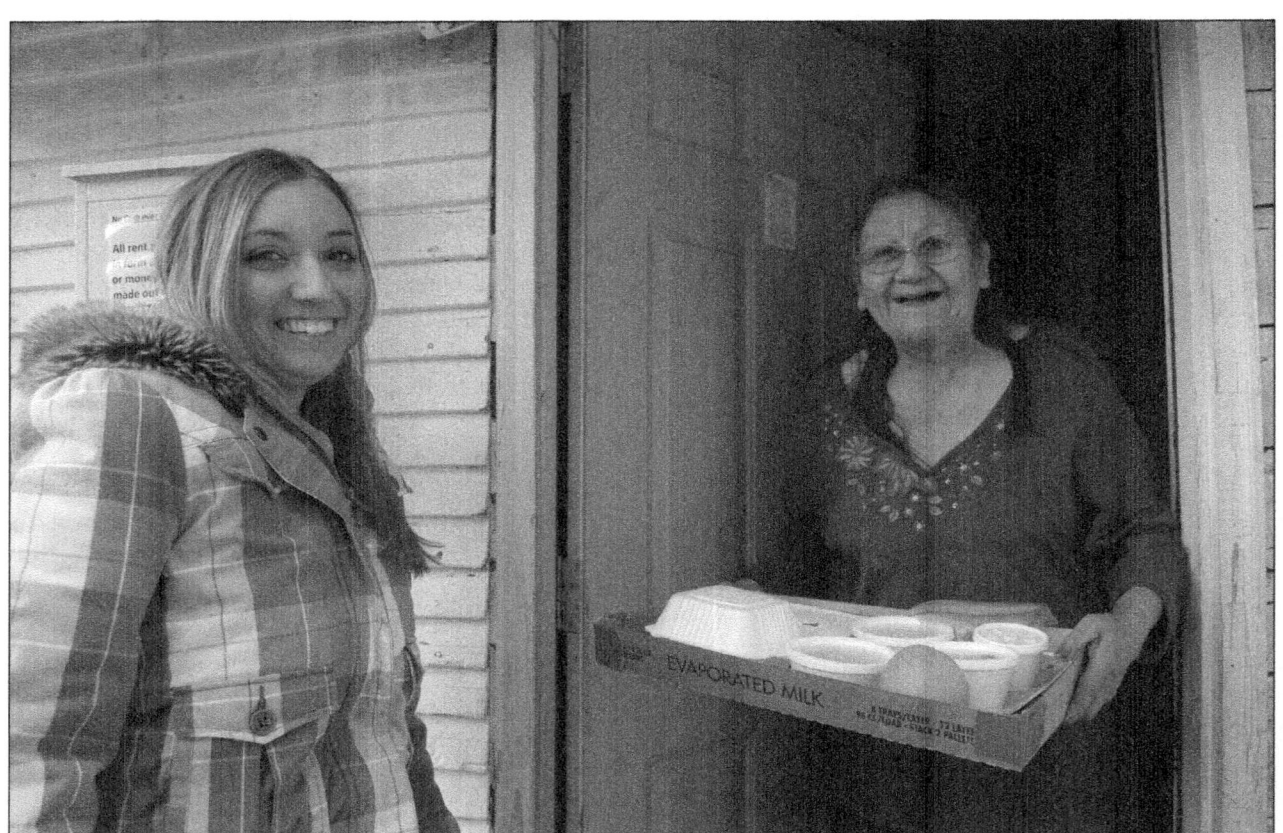

Airman 1st Class Courtney Taylor (left) delivers a Thanksgiving dinner to Clara Donney (right) in Great Falls, Montana. (via Wikimedia Commons)

housing, utility, medical, and food. Many program participants divide their midday meals in order to have something for dinner. For these elderly in particular, meals-on-wheels programs promote a better quality of life.

Two major aging trends ensure that the demand for home-delivered meals services will continue to increase. It has been estimated that the elderly population in the United States will reach 80 million people by 2050. Within this aging population, the oldest-old—those eighty-five or older—are the fastest growing group. The number of people within the oldest-old category is expected to reach 19 million by 2050. This population requires more services, such as home-delivered meals programs, to remain independent in the community.

—George F. Shuster
Updated by Shirley Kuan, RN

See also: Disabilities; Home services; Malnutrition; Mobility problems; Nutrition; Older Americans Act of 1965; Poverty; Social ties

For Further Information

Campbell, Anthony D., et al. "Does Participation in Home-Delivered Meals Programs Improve Outcomes for Older Adults? Results of a Systematic Review." *Journal of Nutrition in Gerontology and Geriatrics*, vol. 34, no. 2, 2015, pp. 124-67. doi:10.1080/21551197.2015.1038463. A comprehensive and systematic review of all studies related to home-delivered meals to shed light on the state of the science.

Hollander, Ellie. "Meals on Wheels Is Working for Everyone." *The Huffington Post*, 20 Mar. 2017. Hollander, President and CEO of Meals-on-Wheels explains the benefits the program has had on not only seniors, but taxpayers and Congress as well.

Lin, Louis. "The Impacts of Meals on Wheels for Older Adults." Wharton Public Policy Initiative, Wharton University of Pennsylvania, 23 Oct. 2018. publicpolicy.wharton.upenn.edu/live/news/2661-the-impacts-of-meals-on-wheels-for-older-adults. Describes how proposed budget cuts might affect the positive impacts Meals-on-Wheels has on the country.

Meals on Wheels America. www.mealsonwheelsamerica.org/. Homepage for the program.

HOMELESSNESS

Relevant Issues: Demographics, family, health and medicine, sociology

Significance: The growing problem of homelessness among older adults is a significant national issue, which until very recently received little attention.

Homelessness is a major concern in the United States, and indeed, the world. Although stigma, isolation and misunderstanding of the root causes of homelessness can create a sense of separation from the issue, homelessness is a reality in nearly every large city in America.

PROBLEM OF HOMELESSNESS AMONG THE ELDERLY

Many among the growing homeless population are older adults who, prior to the 1980s, have been largely ignored by public social service agencies. Gerontologists attribute this lack of attention to the problems and identification of the homeless to misconceptions and stereotypes about the older homeless as a group. Older adults are increasingly vulnerable to homelessness due to the declining availability of affordable housing as well as increased poverty among specific segments of the elderly population. Findings from a 1996 study released by the United States Department of Housing and Urban Development revealed that of the 5.3 million households experiencing "worst case housing needs," 1.2 million were headed by an elderly person. Additionally, almost half of the low-income elderly renters who receive no public assistance were identified as having the "worst case housing needs."

Accurate studies about the rate of homelessness in older populations is lacking for several reasons. First, homeless persons disproportionately die at a young age or without medical care; second, elderly homeless persons are undercounted because of their reluctance to stay in shelters. Finally, resources available to elderly homeless persons can be difficult to access or navigate without appropriate community outreach programs. Overall, the proportion of older persons among the homeless population has declined over the last twenty years, but their absolute number has grown.

CHARACTERISTICS OF THE ELDERLY HOMELESS

Many of the elderly homeless have problems common to the low-income elderly population: inability to work because of physical conditions and chronic health and dental problems, or insecurity about food or medications. Still others have experienced domestic violence or abuse, substance abuse, or suffer from mental illnesses. Many of these people do not qualify for public assistance or are unable to access resources that they do qualify for.

However, elderly homeless men are disproportionately diagnosed with substance abuse, serious mental health conditions, exposure to violence or trauma, and are more likely to suffer from malnutrition, communicable diseases such as tuberculosis, or untreated chronic conditions such as heart or kidney disease.

INATTENTION TO THE ELDERLY HOMELESS PROBLEM

In the late 1990s, older Americans occupied 21 percent of the country's 88 million residential dwellings. They also made up of two out of every five low-income households nationwide. Increasingly, the elderly are being forced to move from the cheap single rooms that they once called home. Most of these elderly are entitled to Social Security benefits, but these benefits are often inadequate to cover housing costs. Further complicating the problem is the fact that some homeless older persons are unaware of their eligibility for public assistance and face even greater difficulties getting through the bureaucratic web and acquiring their benefits. A 1990 study by the National Law Center on Homelessness and Poverty found that in some parts of the United States, less than 10 percent of eligible homeless persons receive Social Security. With less financial resources to pay for food, health care, and medical costs, the elderly are especially vulnerable to homelessness.

Moreover, older adults who are homeless often find shelters and programs inadequate to accommodate their needs. The shelters usually provide for short-term stays based on the assumption that job-training programs and other types of assistance will enable homeless patrons to leave the shelters and move on into better situations. Poor health or mental disabilities prevent most older homeless persons from qualifying for training programs. Further, the lack of stable environments or other related complications prevent the elderly from obtaining needed assistance. The homeless problem is exacerbated by the lack of social service programs available to those in their early fifties.

Several factors contributed to the lack of attention to the issues of elderly homeless in the past. First, the elderly homeless were viewed as responsible for their own condition or situation. Second, due to hearing problems, mental illnesses, and chronic health problems, older persons were viewed as difficult patients and thus received inadequate medical care. Priority for limited financial resources and assistance was often diverted to younger, single homeless persons and homeless families with children because they were perceived as being more salvageable. As the population of homeless grows, agencies that service the elderly have begun to give some significance to their needs and problems.

RESPONSE TO ELDERLY HOMELESSNESS

The housing crisis of the 1980s as well as major federal budget cuts in programs designed to assist the homeless motivated many segments of society to respond to the homeless problem. In 1993, Henry Cisneros, secretary of the Department of Housing and Urban Development (HUD), unveiled a model program to end homelessness in large cities. The program recognized that homelessness was broader than previous studies acknowledged. State and local agencies, volunteer organizations, and coalitions from private and religious sectors developed additional initiatives to combat the homeless problem.

Among the programs implemented to assist the elderly homeless were Project Rescue in New York City and the Senior Reach Program in Chicago. Project Rescue serves older homeless adults with basic needs and health, depression, and alcohol abuse problems, as well as providing legal assistance to elderly persons at risk of being evicted. The Chicago Senior Reach Program provides resettlement for older adults, many of whom are distrustful of shelters and clinics.

Elderly homeless persons face additional perils of chronic health problems and mental illnesses. To prevent more elderly persons from becoming homeless, more low-income housing, income supplements, and health-care services to support independent living must be provided. For older adults who are already homeless, comprehensive outreach health and social services must be implemented and special assistance given to help access public assistance programs. Elderly homeless persons also need sufficient incomes and affordable housing and health care to remain adequately housed.

—*Shirley Rhodes Nealy*
Updated by Patrick Richardson, MSRN

See also: Alcohol use disorder; Disabilities; Divorce; Home ownership; Housing; Malnutrition; Poverty; Singlehood; Widows and widowers

For Further Information

Brown, Rebecca T., et al. "Pathways to Homelessness among Older Homeless Adults: Results from the HOPE HOME Study." *Plos One*, vol. 11, no. 5, 10 May 2016. doi:10.1371/journal.pone.0155065. Identifies life course experiences associated with earlier versus later onset of homelessness in older homeless adults and examined current health and functional status by age at first homelessness. Uses interviews from homeless adults over 50.

"Elder Homelessness." National Coalition for the Homeless, nationalhomeless.org/issues/ elderly/. A collection of information on elder homelessness, including resources.

Kimbler, Kristopher J., et al. "Characteristics of the Old and Homeless: Identifying Distinct Service Needs." *Aging & Mental Health*, vol. 21, no. 2, 24 Sept. 2015, pp. 190-98. doi:10.1080/13607863.2015.1088512. By determining characteristics of homelessness and aging this study identifies areas that can be improved in serving this population.

Nagourney, Adam. "Old and on the Street: The Graying of America's Homeless." *The New York Times*, 31 Mar. 2016. www.nytimes.com/2016/05/31/us/americas-aging-homeless-old-and-on-the-street.html. An in-depth article using personal stories of the homeless elderly to highlight the changing nature of homelessness in America.

Pynoos, Jon. "The Future of Housing for the Elderly: Four Strategies That Can Make a Difference." *Public Policy & Aging Report*, vol. 28, no. 1, 29 Mar. 2018, pp. 35-38. doi:10.1093/ppar/pry006. Reviews a number of policies and programs that have been implemented over the years to improve housing for low-income older persons, including subsidized housing, housing vouchers, and housing connected with services.

HISPANIC AMERICANS. See LATINX AMERICANS.

HOME OWNERSHIP

Relevant Issues: Economics, family, sociology
Significance: Racial identity and life events such as change in marital status, economic success or failure, number of children, income, and employment history all may affect home ownership in the later years, as all these factors may be reflected in the equity that resides in the home.

Equity is a resource that may be managed to enable the older person to spend his or her later years in greater comfort. Home ownership enables the older citizen to provide for his or her senior years, to feel emotionally secure in a changing world, and to leave a legacy to loved ones. Psychological well-being is an important aspect of home ownership, as is economic self-sufficiency. Yet, many older citizens, who own their homes live on the edge of poverty.

BACKGROUND

If the American Dream can in any way be quantified, it must certainly be through the possibility, and for many people the reality, of owning one's own home. This dream goes back to the founding of the United States, as well as of other countries in the Western Hemisphere. The earliest immigrants to the United States and Canada often had been disenfranchised in their countries of origin, The possibility of acquiring land and a home—whether through homesteading, cash payment, or inheritance—was one of the features of New World life that promised a decent living and a secure future.

Over time, and with the gradually increasing value of real estate, new options and new burdens have accompanied the original vision of home ownership, the chief of these being the long-term mortgage. Although for many younger persons, the decision and financial obligations involved in the buying of a home are daunting at best, for the older citizen who owns a home, the advantages of owning real property are considerable. This fact is reflected in the constantly accelerating rates of home ownership for persons over sixty-five during the second half of the twentieth century, when the rate of home ownership slowly but steadily increased in spite of fluctuations in cost of living, increases in the cost of real estate, and demographic changes.

Most older people in the United States own their homes, including 76.2 percent aged over 50 and 78.7 percent of those over 65. Home ownership rates rose with age to about 80 percent of elderly aged 75 to 79 in 2016. However, almost half of people aged 60 to 70 (44 percent) had a mortgage when they retired, including 17 percent who said that they may never pay it off, according to a 2014 survey by American Financing, a national mortgage banker,

THE MONETARY ANGLE

It is a truism that owning real estate, particularly a home, is a hedge against inflation. Mortgages at a fixed interest rate, particularly a low rate, mean that housing costs remain stable, even when all other living costs may rise. For those elderly persons who purchased a home during their working years, this often means that by the time they retire, they pay much less for living in the family home than they would pay for comparable rental housing. For those persons fortunate enough to have paid off a mortgage, this cost may be limited to property tax, utilities, and maintenance. As even a modest house may represent considerable monetary value, a person living in such a situation may seem to be in an enviable position.

It is also often the case, however, that older retired workers have incomes that have been greatly reduced from that of their working lives. Therefore, retired or older citizens may live in houses that are too large, and beyond their means in terms of the overall cost of living and may find that other desires, such as travel and social expenditures, must be forgone.

Various options exist for managing this situation. One option is to sell the house, invest the proceeds, and use that money as a form of income. This option has been enhanced by changes in the capital gains taxation structure, which allow for the sheltering of profit from the sale of a principal residence from capital gains tax. The drawback of selling the home, however, is that it removes what may be the older person's greatest equity resource from any future use. On a practical level, however, many older homeowners may decide to sell a house that has suddenly become bigger than they need, purchase a smaller one, and use the profit to finance other expenditures.

Another financial stratagem that has become available to older homeowners is the reverse mortgage, which allows the older person to continue living in the family home for as long as wished while drawing down its equity over time. This financial instrument was instituted in the 1980s for homeowners over sixty-two years of age. Although repayment is not required until the homeowner no longer occupies the home, this could easily mean that no value would remain in the home at that point. Other options might include sharing the home with former family members, returning children, or acquaintances needing temporary or permanent shelter. This may be of particular benefit for older persons who require care or need help in maintenance of the homes.

THE PSYCHOLOGICAL ANGLE

The common-law tenet that "A man's home is his castle" is more than an outworn legal maxim. For many people, and particularly the elderly, the most important factor about continuing to be a homeowner is a psychological and sociological one. Although a younger person may enjoy the freedom of feeling geographically unattached, with increasing age often comes a desire for greater permanence, particularly in relation to place. The Irish poet William Butler Yeats described this as the desire for a "dear, perpetual place," a refuge that does not seem so affected by the inevitable changes that life brings.

When one adds to this preference for "aging in place" the memories that accumulate in the course of many years spent in a house, perhaps surrounded by loving family members or friends, pets, and acquaintances, the prospect of leaving to live in an alien space can be quite chilling. These are personal considerations that may outweigh some imagined financial advantage or tax break. It is not surprising then that statistical studies of home-owner attitudes reveal a decided preference for home ownership among older persons, who are understandably reluctant to uproot themselves.

A further psychological factor that affects home ownership among the elderly is simply fear of the unknown, which may be considerable for someone who has lived as a homeowner in a particular neighborhood for many years. The feeling that one is in control of his or her environment, particularly in the United States, depends to a great extent on the same factors that are also operative in home ownership: the ability to suit surroundings to one's own liking, the feeling of autonomy that comes with living in a neighborhood that has become familiar, as well as the freedom to make choices about living arrangements.

FAMILY MATTERS

It is not uncommon for American families to disperse once the children leave home. It is also not unusual, however, for children to have concerns about the housing and welfare of their parents in their later years or even to have some unexpected housing needs themselves. Concern about elderly parents is often reflected in decisions about home ownership because of problems of mobility, medical care of ailing elders, or the high costs of alternative care. All these factors enter into the consideration of whether continued home ownership is the best solution to the housing of older family members. The sheer number of older Americans in the baby-boom generation reaching retirement age and beyond guarantees that this situation will persist for the foreseeable future.

Added to this situation is the desire of many older persons with families to leave the fruits of their efforts to their loved ones. With ownership of the family home representing a large portion of the inheritable property of many older persons, this is a matter that becomes of material concern and affects the upcoming generation as well.

—Gloria Fulton
Updated by Bruce E. Johansen, PhD

See also: Caregiving; Empty nest syndrome; Estates and inheritance; Facility and institutional care; Family relationships; Full nest; Home services; Housing; Retirement planning

For Further Information

"Aging in Place: Growing Older at Home." National Institute on Aging, U.S. Department of Health and Human Services, 1 May 2017. www.nia.nih.gov/health/aging-place-growing-older-home. This site is for seniors interested in maintaining their home ownership, including risks, options, and resources.

Lawlor, Drew, and Michael A. Thomas. Residential Design for Aging in Place. Wiley, 2008. The definitive guide, endorsed by the American Society of Interior Designers (ASID), for designing homes for aging people.

Olick, Diana. "As More Older Americans 'Age in Place,' Millennials Struggle to Find Homes." CNBC, 11 Feb. 2019. www.cnbc.com/2019/02/11/as-more—americans-age-in-place-millennials-struggle-to-buy.html. This article explores a new housing crisis: as older adults age in place, fewer homes have become available for younger generations.

Power, Emma R. "Housing, Home Ownership and the Governance of Ageing." *The Geographical Journal*, vol. 183, no. 3, 2 June 2017, pp. 233-46. doi:10.1111/geoj.12213. This paper argues that housing, and specifically home purchase, is fundamental to the governance of active aging in liberal welfare states such as Australia, the United Kingdom, the United States, and Canada.

HOME SERVICES

Relevant Issues: Family, health and medicine, sociology

Significance: Home services include many things, such as home maintenance, shopping, companions, equipment, skilled nursing visits, physical therapy, and hospice care; these services are offered in a variety of ways, both public and private.

The advantages to assisting the older adult to stay in his or her own home are many. There are obvious benefits to the individual's own independence and sense of well-being. Less obvious are benefits to the community, such as the economic benefits from taxes being paid and shopping in local businesses. The older adult is usually a law-abiding person who contributes to the stability of a neighborhood. Society benefits when nursing home placement is delayed because of the expenses incurred. Often, older adults need only a few services to keep them in their own homes.

One common way older adults receive home services is from family members. This works well in an extended family arrangement, but many times this system is inadequate and the caregiver experiences fatigue and frustration. Systems to support family caregivers are slow in coming and have many needs to address. The basic maintenance and custodial supports that can assist people to meet their goal of living at home as they age are many times unavailable or unaffordable. Several volunteer programs have developed to fill the gap that older adults and their families experience.

Three such programs are the Healthy Seniors Project, Interfaith Volunteer Caregivers, and the Living at Home/Block Nurse Program. These programs were chosen because they function in several areas of the United States and each represents a slightly different approach to care of the older adult.

The Healthy Seniors Project is a neighborhood-based nurse case-management model. There are award-winning sites in Arizona, Illinois, New York, and Minnesota. This project is a partnership between community-health nurses and an established health-care facility. They work together to establish health-care services in a specific neighborhood to serve the Medicare population. The community is involved through volunteer recruitment and training. Some services are included that Medicare does not reimburse, such as wellness care, respite care, custodial and maintenance services, and friendly visits and phone calls.

The National Federation of Interfaith Volunteer Caregivers (NFIVC) coordinated the start of Interfaith Volunteer Caregivers all over the United States. A toll-free call to headquarters in Kingston, New York, will provide any "church" group (regardless of religion) with the information, support, and material needed to start its own program. Members of the church volunteer to be partnered with a person needing help. Services are provided to all age groups, without regard to insurance, religion, or specific need. The primary focus is support services (lawn work, baby-sitting, transportation, shopping), but when health-care professionals are among the volunteers, they do participate in some direct care activities.

The Living at Home/Block Nurse Program starts with a steering committee from within the community whose members discuss and define the needs and capabilities of the community. The focus is to provide the coordinated care that would meet the individual needs of each older adult in the designated "block" (community). This typically includes social support, health education, prevention-oriented intervention, support for daily living needs, and custodial and maintenance care. This essential care is provided regardless of insurance coverage or the ability to pay. Enhancing the ability of the family to meet the needs of its own members and organizing community support when the family is not available are the cornerstones of the Living at Home/Block Nurse Program. This program is funded by local fundraisers, local donations, grants, and some government funding where available.

Churches may provide some in-home services to their members. Large churches often have a person dedicated to community outreach programs. Nonmembers may find that a local church might be able to provide leads on individuals in the community who provide sitter or domestic service in homes, although reference checks are the responsibility of the person doing the hiring. If there is a college or university in the area, its social work or nursing department can be a source for temporary help (nursing or social work students could make good temporary hired help). These departments might also be able to give referrals to other area agencies.

HOME HEALTH SERVICES

Private and public home health agencies are abundant. They provide health-care services that are paid for by insurance carriers, state-funded reimbursement plans, and Medicare. To receive services, the older adult with Medicare or one of the Medicare options usually must require skilled services (a nurse with a license, physical therapy, speech or occupational therapy); require services intermittently (visits are about one hour each and usually not more than once a day, many times less often); be homebound (leave the home seldomly, only for medical purposes and with much difficulty); and have the services ordered by a physician.

The services available through a home health agency are subject to change depending upon the latest federal regulations governing reimbursement. The most common reasons for home health services include education regarding new medications or a new diagnosis, dressing changes, diabetic care, severe cardiac or respiratory problems, and physical therapy following a stroke, fracture, or joint replacement.

Depression is prevalent among older adults. Psychiatric nursing care is available through many home health agencies when the other criteria for services are met. There are home health agencies that specialize in one specific type of care, such as psychiatric, ventilator-dependent, cardiac, or acquired immunodeficiency syndrome (AIDS) patients. The nurse or therapist in the home may make a referral for a home visit from a social worker. This is usually related to financial issues or the need for services that the home health agency cannot provide. Some home health agencies, especially those affiliated with church-related institutions, will provide chaplain visits, although there would likely be no reimbursement for such a visit.

While home health care patients are receiving skilled care, they may also be eligible for a home health aide to meet personal hygiene needs. This service may include bathing, shampoo, shaving, changing linen, and tidying the bedroom, bath, and kitchen area. The aide visits average between one to two hours and may be as often as daily for a person who is confined to bed. When the skilled need (services of a nurse or therapist) no longer exists, the aide visits cease also, regardless of continued personal hygiene needs.

HOSPICE CARE

Hospice care is a Medicare benefit and is also provided by many of the health maintenance organizations (HMOs). The National Hospice Organization (NHO) has developed general guidelines that direct and explain the services provided by most reputable hospice organizations. NHO guidelines directly affecting the client include palliative care (may include comfort measures up to and including surgical procedures) to all terminally ill people and their families with a focus on keeping terminally ill persons in their homes as long as possible; coordination of trained professionals and volunteers working together to meet the physiologic, psychologic, social, spiritual, and economic needs of the patient and family through illness and bereavement (this may be intermittent or continuous care); work with the physician for an individualized plan of care (may provide patient advocates to facilitate medical care); and availability of care twenty-four hours a day, seven days a week without interruption even if the care setting changes (it is possible to be admitted to a hospital and still maintain hospice status; rules for this type of admission include no curative treatment).

Hospice care provides pain control, needed physical maintenance, and the opportunity to die at home but not alone. The family is supported during the dying process and continues to receive supportive services after the death of a loved one. Life and death are made as meaningful and humane as possible.

PUBLIC SERVICES

Most communities have an organization dedicated to the needs of older adults. The services provided vary but often include transportation, home cleaning, and meals-on-wheels. These services are provided by volunteers and paid employees with money from grants and the government. Funding may vary year to year and, therefore, affect the services provided.

The local public hospital can furnish information about the services it provides, which may include home services. Public health departments differ considerably in the services they provide. Many times, home health-care services are available, but some public health departments concentrate their efforts on women and children. Some public health departments will make home visits only in a crisis situation.

PRIVATE HOME SERVICES

There are agencies that specialize in providing home services not covered any other way; for example, all-night or all-day sitters, private duty nurses, or extended respite care. These agencies are listed in the phone book under "nurses." They may or may not be connected with a home health agency. It is wise to ask for references and check with the Better Business Bureau before hiring in-home help through such an agency. There are many well-managed, reputable agencies available.

Home delivery of goods is a service that home-bound older adults need. Many pharmacies and most medical supply companies will deliver to a home. Grocery stores are also beginning to deliver. Catalog and online shopping present other ways to receive goods at home. Beauticians, barbers, and massage therapists are available for in-home service.

IN-HOME EQUIPMENT

In many cases, all that older adults might need to maintain independence in their own home is specialized equipment. This can range from a bedside commode to supplemental oxygen obtainable from a durable medical equipment (DME) company. Needed equipment is often covered by Medicare or the HMO options. A physician's order and documented need are required. Some items require special testing. For example, to obtain oxygen for home use, the oxygen in the blood must be below a certain level before the expense will be covered. If a client is receiving home health services, that agency can facilitate obtaining needed equipment.

Besides the obvious equipment such as wheelchairs, shower chairs, walkers, and hospital beds, there are types of equipment for more specialized use. For example, sometimes a very simple alteration in eating utensils or scoop dishes can make a person able to feed himself or herself again. There are devices to enable a person to dress independently, such as a button hook, zipper pull, dressing stick, hip sock aide, and reacher.

SERVICES BY SPECIFIC ORGANIZATIONS

There are special-interest organizations that provide goods and services for in-home use. Lighthouse for the Blind will provide books on tape for the blind or when holding a book or turning pages is impossible. Many of these groups maintain websites that can be accessed easily through most search engines. The local library can assist in this referral also. The Arthritis Foundation operates chapters in many cities. They provide education, equipment, and services and can be found in the phone book. Any time there is a specific medical diagnosis, it is wise to look for an organization whose primary goal is devoted to that problem. The local library or the social worker department in the local hospital will be able to assist with a list of services specific to a given community. Many cities have published manuals of groups in the area, including the services they provide, addresses and phone numbers, and fees for service.

The challenge of finding needed services is great. If older adults do not have family members or very close friends to help in the search process, it can be overwhelming to an already compromised individual. People without families would be well advised to develop an extended family of friends within their neighborhood or "church" family before a dire need arises.

—Penny Wolfe Moore

See also: Canes and walkers; Caregiving; Communication; Disabilities; Friendship; Health care; Home delivered meals programs; Home ownership; Hospice; Housing; Medicare; Psychiatry, geriatric; Religion; Transportation issues; Wheelchair use

For Further Information

"Aging in Place: Growing Older at Home." National Institute on Aging, U.S. Department of Health and Human Services, 1 May 2017. www.nia.nih.gov/health/aging-place-growing-older-home. This article contains suggestions to help you find the in-home services you need to continue to live independently.

Boland, Laura, et al. "Impact of Home Care versus Alternative Locations of Care on Elder Health Outcomes: An Overview of Systematic Reviews." *BMC Geriatrics*, vol. 17, no. 1, 2017. doi:10.1186/s12877-016-0395-y. A summary of the evidence that examines home care compared to other care locations can inform decision-making.

Ferrini, Armeda, and Rebecca Ferrini. *Health in the Later Years*. 6th ed. McGraw-Hill, 2016. Discusses the expected changes in the aging process, possible complications, and suggested interventions, including in-home services that may be needed.

Joling, Karlijn J., et al. "Quality Indicators for Community Care for Older People: A Systematic Review." *Plos One*, vol. 13, no. 1, 2018. doi:10.1371/journal.pone.0190298. This systematic review identified existing quality indicators (Qis) for community care for older people and assessed their methodological quality.

Mason, Diana, and Judith Leavitt. *Policy and Politics in Nursing and Health Care*. 7th ed. Elsevier, 2016. Covers all the political and government issues that contribute to the in-home services that are and are not available.

"Senior Home Care Guide." SeniorLiving.org. www.seniorliving.org/home-care/. A guide for seniors on choosing in-home services.

HORMONE REPLACEMENT THERAPY. *See* ESTROGEN REPLACEMENT THERAPY.

HOSPICE

Relevant Issues: Death, family, health and medicine, sociology

Significance: Hospice care is a holistic approach to caring for the dying and their families by addressing their physical, emotional, and spiritual needs.

Hospice is a philosophy of care directed toward persons who are dying. Hospice care uses a family-oriented holistic approach to assist these individuals in making the transition from life to death in a manner that preserves their dignity and comfort. This approach, as Elisabeth Kübler-Ross would say, allows dying patients "to live until they die." Hospice care encourages patients to participate fully in determining the type of care that is most appropriate for their comfort. By creating a secure and caring community sensitive to the needs of the dying and their families and by providing care that relieves patients of the distressing symptoms of their disease, hospice care can aid the dying in preparing mentally as well as spiritually for their impending death.

Unlike traditional health care where the patient is viewed as the client, hospice care with its holistic emphasis, treats the family unit as the client. There are usually specific areas of stress for the families of the dying. In addition to the stress of caring for the physical needs of the dying, family members often feel tremendous pressure maintaining their own roles and responsibilities within the family itself. The conflict of caring for their own nuclear families while caring for dying relatives places a huge strain on everyone involved and can be a source of anxiety and guilt for the patient as well. Another area of stress experienced by family members involves concern for themselves; that is, having to put their own lives on hold, not getting physically run down, dealing with their newly acquired time constraints, and viewing themselves as isolated from friends and family. Compounding this is the guilt that many caregivers feel over not caring for the dying relative as well or as patiently as they might, or secretly wishing for the caregiving experience to reach an end.

Due to the holistic nature of the care provided, the hospice team is actually an interdisciplinary team composed of physicians, nurses, psychologists and social workers, pastoral counselors, and trained volunteers. This medically supervised team meets weekly to decide on how best to provide physical, emotional, and spiritual support for dying patients and to assist the surviving family members in the subsequent grieving process.

This type of care can be administered in three different ways. It can be home health-agency based, delivered in the patient's own home. It can be dispensed in an institution devoted solely to hospice care. It can even be administered in traditional medical facilities (such as hospitals) that allot a certain amount of space (perhaps a wing or floor, or even a certain number of beds) to this type of care. Hospice care is designed for any patient at the end stage of life. Often, people think Hospice care is just for cancer but can be for any patient facing death from any terminal disease. Heart disease, lung disease, and amyotrophic lateral sclerosis (ALS or Lou Gehrig's Disease) are others that may involve Hospice care at end of life. Hospice is available for both adults and children. A newer approach to care for patients experiencing a life-limiting condition requiring on-going medical care or a terminal disease is palliative care. Palliative care begins much earlier in the disease process and is designed to manage the problems and issues that impair quality of life and to assist the patient to a compassionate death. Palliative care occurs much in advance of the need for Hospice care.

PRINCIPLES

Hospice care uses a team-oriented approach to provide quality, compassionate care individualized to the patient and family's needs. Hospice care focuses on managing a patient's symptoms, including pain. The principles of hospice care focus on alleviating the anxieties and physical suffering that can be associated with the dying process and to ensure that the patient and family can make the most of the time that remains. The goal is to not delay the dying process by using invasive medical techniques or heroic efforts. Hospice care is also based on the assertion that dying patients have certain rights that must be respected. These rights include a right to absent themselves from social responsibilities and commitments, a right to be cared for, and the right to continued respect and status.

There are several basic components of hospice care. Hospice care provides highly personalized and holistic care of the dying, which includes treating dying patients emotionally and spiritually as well as physically. This interpersonal support, known as bonding, helps patients in their final days to live as fully and as comfortably as possible, while retaining their dignity, autonomy, and individual self-worth in a safe and secure environment. This one-on-one attention involves therapeutic communication. Knowing that someone has heard, that someone understands and is concerned can be profoundly healing.

Pain management is a critical component of Hospice care. Hospice care advocates the use of narcotics at a dosage that will alleviate suffering while still enabling patients to maintain a desired level of alertness. Efforts are made to employ the least invasive routes to administer these drugs (usually orally, if possible). In addition, pain medication is administered before the pain begins, thus alleviating the anxiety of patients waiting for pain to return. As it has been shown that fear of pain often increases the pain itself, this type of aggressive pain management gives dying patients more time and energy to respond to family members and friends and to work through the emotional and spiritual stages of dying. Use of pain medication before the pain actually occurs has historically been a controversial element in hospice care, with some critics charging that the dying are being turned into drug addicts. Given the fact that patients are not admitted into Hospice care until death is inevitable, addiction is not a factor. Hospice care generally starts no sooner than six months before predicted death. With the advent of Palliative care, entry into Hospice care is occurring later. Maintaining the comfort of the dying patient is crucial.

The participation of families in caring for the dying is a cornerstone of Hospice care. Family members are trained by Hospice nurses to care for the dying patients and dispense pain medication. The aim is to prevent the patients from suffering isolation or feeling as if they are surrounded by strangers. Participation in care also helps to sustain the patients' and the families' sense of autonomy. For patients without family support, there is an increasing attention to inpatient Hospice care in either a stand-alone facility or as part of a hospital or nursing home.

Maintaining the familiarity of surroundings is a comfort measure important to the dying patient. Whenever possible, it is the goal of hospice care to keep dying patients at home. This eliminates the necessity of the dying to spend their final days in an institutionalized setting, isolated from family and friends when they need them the most. It is estimated that close to 90 percent of all hospice care days are spent in patients' own homes. When this is not possible and patients must enter institutional settings, rules are relaxed so that their rooms can be decorated or arranged in such a way as to replicate the patients' home surroundings. Visiting rules are suspended when possible, and visits by family members, children, and pets are encouraged.

Emotional and spiritual support for the family caregivers is important to better provide for the patient. Hospice volunteers are specially trained to use listening and communicative techniques with family members and to provide them with emotional support both during and after the patient's death. Because the care is holistic, the caregivers' physical needs are attended to (for example, respite is provided for exhausted caregivers), as are the caregivers' emotional and spiritual needs. This spiritual support applies to people of all faith backgrounds. In attending to the spiritual dimension, the hospice team is respectful of all religious traditions while realizing that death and bereavement have the ability to both strengthen and weaken faith. For patients and families without a professed faith, support is provided based on their needs and wants and may focus more on counseling. Support groups are often available to address the needs of family members, including children and grandchildren of patients.

Hospice services should be available twenty-four hours a day, seven days a week. Because of its reliance on the assistance of trained volunteers, round-the-clock support is available to patients and their families.

The intervention of the Hospice team does not end with the death of the patient. Bereavement counseling is provided for the survivors. At the time of death, the hospice team is available to help families take care of tasks such as planning the funeral and probating the will. In the weeks after the death, hospice volunteers offer their support to surviving family members in dealing with their loss and grief and the various phases of the bereavement process, always aware of the fact that not all bereaved need or want formal interventions. Many Hospice organizations offer support groups for families after the death of the patient. Often, family members want to become Hospice volunteers. While this is noble, many Hospices require a period of time between the death of their family member and undergoing training to become a volunteer as an objective manner is expected of volunteers.

HISTORY

The term "hospice" comes from the Latin hospitia, meaning "places of welcome." The earliest documented example of hospice care dates to the fourth century, when a Roman woman named Fabiola apparently used her own wealth to care for the sick and dying. In medieval times, the Catholic Church established inns for poor wayfarers and pilgrims traveling to religious shrines in search of miraculous cures for their illnesses. Such "rest homes," usually run by religious orders, provided both lodging and nursing care, as the medieval view was that the sick, dying, and needy were all travelers on a journey. This attitude also reflects the medieval notion that true hospitality included care of the mind and spirit as well as of the body. During the Protestant Reformation, when monasteries were forcibly closed, the concepts of hospice and hospital became distinct. Care of the sick and dying was now considered a public duty rather than a religious or private one, and many former hospices were turned into state-run hospitals.

The first in-patient hospice establishment of modern times (specifically called "hospice") was founded by Mary Aitkenhead and the Irish Sisters of Charity under her leadership in the 1870s in Dublin, Ireland. Cicely Saunders, a physician at St. Joseph's Hospice in London, which was founded by the English Sisters of Charity in 1908, began to adapt the ancient concept of hospice to modern palliative techniques. While there, Saunders became extremely close to a Holocaust survivor who was dying of cancer. She found that she shared his dream of establishing a place that would meet the needs of the dying. Using the money he bequeathed her at his death as a starting point, Saunders raised additional funds and opened St. Christopher's Hospice in Sydenham, outside London, in 1967. Originally it housed only cancer patients, but with the financial support of contracts with the National Health Service in England and private donations, it later expanded to meet the needs of all the dying. In fact, no patient was ever refused because of inability to pay. St. Christopher's served as a model for the hospices to be built later in other parts of the world.

Even though hospice care did not originate with Cicely Saunders, she is usually credited with founding the first modern hospice, as she introduced the concept of dispensing narcotics at regular intervals to preempt the pain of the dying. She was also the first to identify the need to address other, nonphysical sources of pain for dying patients.

Two years after St. Christopher's Hospice was opened, Kübler-Ross wrote On Death and Dying, which validated the hospice movement by relating stories of the dying and their wishes as to how they would be treated. In 1974, the United States opened its first hospice, Hospice, Inc. (later called the Connecticut Hospice), in New Haven, Connecticut. Within the next twenty-five years, over three thousand hospice programs would be implemented in the United States. In Canada, the first "palliative care" unit (as hospices are referred to in Canada) was opened in 1975 by Dr. Balfour M. Mount at the Royal Victoria Hospital in Montreal. This is considered to be the first hospital-based hospice in North America.

COST

Because of hospice care's reliance on heavily trained volunteers and contributions, and because death is seen as a natural process that should not be prolonged by invasive and expensive medical techniques, hospice care is much less costly than traditional acute care facilities.

SENIOR TALK:

HOW DO YOU FEEL ABOUT HOSPICE?

With a terminal diagnosis, you might go through a period of shock and denial as you process the severity of the prognosis both emotionally and mentally. Facing the possibility of an impending end of life, or that of someone near and dear, you likely feel a myriad of emotions. These emotions may feel like a rollercoaster as you move through fear, grieving, and acceptance at various times. Before beginning hospice care, trained hospice staff are available to speak to and support you and your family in the decision-making process. You can also contact others who have experienced hospice services to learn more about it.

Many people choose a hospice as a best option for seeing out the final days of a serious and terminal illness. While there is often great sadness associated with the end of life, the facilities and care provided by the hospice often ease and heal the pain. If you are confronting your own mortality and deciding to do this in a hospice, you may feel comforted that you will be assisted in your journey by a loving and dedicated group of people. This applies, too, if you are placing a loved one into hospice. You may be nervous and concerned about aspects of dignity as you or your loved one's health deteriorates, but the hospice will ensure all measures are taken to make certain patients are treated with the utmost care and respect. As someone watching a dear family member in the months, weeks, days, and hours prior to passing, your distress may be ameliorated by the hospice staff's expertise and guidance.

—*Leah Jacob*

Because hospice care is a philosophy of care rather than a specific facility, legislation to provide monetary support for hospice patients took a great deal of time to be approved. In 1982, the U.S. Congress finally added hospice care as a Medicare benefit. In 1986, it was made a permanent benefit. Medicare requires, however, that there be a prognosis of six months or less for the patient to live. Hospice care is also reimbursable by many private insurance companies.

The National Hospice and Palliative Care Organization (NHPCO) (formerly The National Hospice Organization) originated in 1977 in the United States as a resource for the many groups across the country who needed assistance in establishing hospice programs in their own communities. The purpose of this organization is to provide information about hospice care to the public, to establish conduits so that information may be exchanged between Hospice and Palliative Care organizations, and to maintain agreed-upon standards for developing hospices around the country. The NHO publishes Guide to the Nation's Hospices on an annual basis.

—Mara Kelly-Zukowski
Updated by Patricia Stanfill Edens, RN, PhD, FACHE

See also: Death and dying; Death of a child; Death of parents; Euthanasia; Family relationships; Funerals; Grief; Health care; Hospitalization; Kübler-Ross, Elisabeth; Medicare; Palliative care; Religion; Terminal illness; Widows and widowers

For Further Information

Lima, Liliana De, and Lukas Radbruch. "The International Association for Hospice and Palliative Care: Advancing Hospice and Palliative Care Worldwide." *Journal of Pain and Symptom Management*, vol. 55, no. 2, 8 Aug. 2017. doi:10.1016/j.jpainsymman.2017.03.023. IAHPC focuses on the advancement of four areas of palliative care: education, access to medicines, health policies, and service implementation.

Edens, Pat Stanfill, et al. "Developing and Financing a Palliative Care Program." *American Journal of Hospice and Palliative Medicine®*, vol. 25, no. 5, 2008, pp. 379-84. doi:10.1177/1049909108319269. This article attempts to model a palliative care program using a cost aversion financial model to quantify benefits of a palliative care programs as one strategy to address reimbursement shortcomings.

"Hospice Care." National Hospice and Palliative Care Organization, 20 Feb. 2019. www.nhpco.org/about/hospice-care. Collects resources on hospice and palliative care, including often asked questions and advice on how to choose a hospice.

Kübler-Ross, Elisabeth. *On Death and Dying*. Macmillan, 1969. Landmark work that outlines the psychological stages of dying and the deficiencies in modern medicine's ability to care for dying patients in an appropriate manner.

Marrelli, Tina M. *Hospice & Palliative Care Handbook: Quality, Compliance, and Reimbursement.* 3rd ed., Sigma Theta Tau International, 2018. This book offers concise, focused coverage of all aspects of hospice and palliative care for clinicians, managers, and other team members who provide important care while meeting difficult multilevel regulations.

Moments of Life: Made Possible by Hospice, National Hospice and Palliative Care Organization, moments.nhpco.org/. The goal of Moments of Life: Made Possible by Hospice is to educate the public about the choices we all have when facing a life-limiting illness, and how choosing hospice is not 'giving up.'

Wrenn, Paula, and Jo Gustely. *Dying Well with Hospice: A Compassionate Guide to End of Life Care.* Amans Vitae P, 2017. Co-authored by a hospice professional and the spouse of a hospice patient, Dying Well with Hospice addresses the fears we have about death, discusses the many options available for making this a productive and loving time of transition. It also describes how to begin this dialogue for yourself and others.

HOSPITALIZATION

Relevant Issues: Health and medicine

Significance: The elderly are substantial users of inpatient hospital services. The number of hospital admissions for individuals sixty-five and over rises significantly with increasing age.

In 1996, those aged sixty-five and over accounted for 38 percent of the admissions to nonfederal, acute care hospitals. Those aged forty-five through sixty-four accounted for 20 percent of all admissions. The average length of stay (ALOS) was 5.3 days for people forty-five through sixty-four and 6.5 days for those sixty-five and over. In 2010, the ALOS was found to be 5 days for a patient aged forty-five to sixty-four, and 5.5 days for a patient sixty-five or older. Moreover, since 1996, the percentage of hospital patients aged sixty-five and over has slightly decreased. The most recent National Hospital Discharge Survey, conducted in 2007, found that although people aged sixty-five and older accounted for only 13 percent of the population, they comprised 37 percent of hospital discharges. In 2012, patients sixty-five and older accounted for 34.2 percent of inpatient stays—but patients aged forty-five to sixty-four had risen 4.7 percent. Consistently, medical stays top inpatient hospitalizations for those aged sixty-five or older, followed by surgical stays. Although the major portion of inpatient services is provided in acute care community hospitals, elderly patients may also receive inpatient services in hospitals operated by the Department of Veterans Affairs or in proprietary facilities such as psychiatric hospitals.

Approximately 96 percent of all hospital care in the United States is financed by third parties. In 2013, hospital care accounted for 38 percent of all United States health-care expenses. Only 4 percent of expenses were paid out of pocket; private insurance, Medicare, Medicaid, and other public insurances funded the majority of the costs. The vast majority of Americans over the age of sixty-five have medical insurance through the Medicare program; in 2018, Medicare insured over 43.5 million adults aged sixty-five and older—with 52 million adults aged sixty-five and older in the United States in total—from 33.4 million people in 1996. According to data compiled by the Health Care Financing Administration (HCFA), the administrative agency for the Medicare program, the largest component of national health expenditure is hospital care. Inpatient hospital care for beneficiaries resulted in costs to the Medicare program of $79.9 billion in 1996. As enrollment grows, costs to the Medicare program increase. Consequently, inpatient hospital care resulted in a cost of $146.3 billion for the Medicare program in 2018.

COST AND PAYMENTS

Medicare pays most short-stay hospitalization under a prospective payment system (PPS) in which hospitals are reimbursed for services according to the diagnosis-related group (DRG) to which the patient is assigned. The DRG system is used to classify patients based on their principal diagnosis and other patient data, such as comorbidity or coexisting conditions. Medicare has set a fixed, pre-established amount of payment for each DRG based on the average cost of resources needed to treat a patient with that particular diagnosis.

The PPS was instituted as a means of containing costs for hospital services by replacing the cost-plus payment system. Because the hospital is paid a fixed amount for each patient stay, the incentive is for the hospital to reduce the average length of stay per inpatient episode. The PPS has been effective in reducing the growth of short-stay hospitalization by providing financial incentives to shift services from inpatient to outpatient settings, to provide services in a more efficient manner, and to reduce the length of stay. These measures were effective in reducing the ALOS from 8.8 days in 1990 to 5.1 days in 2016 and reducing the portion of Medicare payments for inpatient services to 47.8 percent by 1996 (from a high of 69.7 percent in 1974). Hospital admissions have increased over 125 percent since 1946, with 35.4 million people admitted in 2013. In 2013, there were nearly 2 million deaths among persons aged sixty-five or older in the United States, and one-third of these deaths occurred in the hospital. Approximately 13.2 million adults aged sixty-five years and older were hospitalized in 2003, with an ALOS of 5.7 days. Of these 13.2 million patients, nearly 60 percent were admitted through the emergency department, with a mean charge per day of $4,350.

Before Medicare existed, only 54 percent of people aged sixty-five and over had health insurance. In 2013, it was reported that 98.4 percent of people in this age group now have health insurance. Fifty percent of Medicare holders have an income of less than $26,200, and 25 percent have an income below $15,250. Incomes among beneficiaries vary across demographic characteristics; individuals who are married or have college degrees are likely to have higher income than individuals who are divorced, widowed, or single, or individuals who have less than a high school education. Moreover, from 2010 to 2016, median per capita income rose more among White beneficiaries ($23,850 to $30,050) than Black ($14,750 to $17,350) or Latino beneficiaries ($11,450 to $13,650). In the last months of life, Medicare services, including hospital usage, intensify. About 25 percent of Medicare costs are reserved for the last year of a person's life, a policy that has not changed since first established in the 1980s. Nearly 40 percent of beneficiaries require nursing home care, and 19 percent of Medicare enrollees who have died were in hospice. On average, beneficiaries with Medicare Advantage are allotted $783 per month, and beneficiaries with traditional Medicare are allotted $699 per month.

DISEASES AND PROCEDURES
Hospitalization for an elderly individual commonly occurs because of acute illness, such as pneumonia; because of the exacerbation of a chronic illness, such as an episode of pulmonary edema caused by chronic heart failure; for a major operative procedure, such as coronary artery bypass surgery; because of injury, such as a fracture; or for complex diagnostic procedures, such as an endoscopy.

In 2002, a reported 87 percent of non-institutionalized Medicare beneficiaries were living with at least one chronic condition. The majority of Medicare expenditures are for beneficiaries with one or more chronic conditions—treating chronic diseases can cost over 75 percent of the 2.5 trillion-dollar annual healthcare budget—with 68 percent of expenditures utilized for beneficiaries with five or more chronic conditions. A study conducted in 2006 found that people being treated for multiple chronic conditions can cost up to seven times as much as people with only one chronic condition. The prevalence of chronic conditions has been identified as one of the most significant factors in the growth of Medicare spending.

The most often diagnostic category resulting in hospital admission for adults aged sixty-five and older are cardiovascular diseases. These patients made up 28.6 percent of all older adult hospitalizations and had an ALOS of 5.5 days. Related conditions include chest pain (angina), cardiac arrhythmia and conduction disorder, and coronary artery bypass surgery. Altogether, in 2011, cardiovascular diseases cost an estimated $442 billion to treat. The second most common diagnostic category was infections, accounting for 16.2 percent of all hospitalizations, with pneumonia and septicemia being the two most often occurring infections in older adult patients. Respiratory disorders were the third most often cause of hospitalization, accounting for 14.9 percent of all hospitalizations for patients ages sixty-five and older. Digestive and musculoskeletal disorders were the fourth leading cause of hospitalization, with 10.7 and 10.8 percent of all older adults hospitalized, respectively. The fifth-leading condition resulting in hospitalization was nervous system disorders, including multiple sclerosis, Alzheimer's, epilepsy, stroke, and Parkinson's accounted for 8 percent of all hospitalizations for patients aged sixty-five and older.

Currently, Alzheimer's is considered to be one of the most expensive chronic illness in the United States. In 2010, the National Institute on Aging (NIA) reported that for a person with dementia, health-care treatment for the last five years of their life will total over $287,000, compared to $173,000 for a person with cancer and $175,000 for a person with heart disease. It is expected that in 2019, an estimated $146 billion in federal Medicare funding will be spent caring for people with Alzheimer's and other dementias. On average, Medicare beneficiaries with Alzheimer's require more than three times the annual spending than those without ($24,598 for those with Alzheimer's and other dementias compared to $7,561 for those without). It is projected that by 2050, Medicare spending on people with Alzheimer's and other dementias will total $578 billion. This would mean an increase of nearly three hundred percent of current spending levels and represent an estimated 1 in every 3 dollars of future total Medicare spending.

Surgical patients aged sixty-five and older represent a significant proportion of the overall surgical population. In 2006, the National Hospital Discharge Survey reported that patients aged sixty-five and older accounted for 35.3 percent of all inpatient surgical procedures, and 32.2 percent of all outpatient procedures. Between the years 2010 and 2013, the most common procedures performed on patients aged sixty-five to sixty-nine and seventy to seventy-nine were cataract and lens procedures (11.49 percent and 17.09 percent, respectively), knee replacements (6.8 percent and 6.78 percent, respectively), partial and total hip replacements (3.29 percent and 3.54 percent, respectively), and cholecystectomies (the removal of the gallbladder) (3.27 percent and 3.06 percent, respectively). For patients aged eighty to eighty-nine, the second most often surgical procedure was treating a fractured or dislocated shoulder or femur (6.76 percent, with cataract and lens procures being the most often surgical procedure at 17.49 percent), and for patients aged ninety and older, treating a fractured or dislocated shoulder or femur was the most sought-out procedure (22.16 percent). Less than one percent of surgical patients aged sixty-five to seventy-nine experienced the following serious adverse events: major respiratory complication; major hemodynamic instability; required resuscitation; death. For patients aged eighty to eighty-nine, 1.18 percent of patients undergoing a surgical procedure experienced serious adverse events. The procedures that contributed to the largest mortality rates for patients aged sixty-five and older include exploratory laparotomy surgeries, heart valve-related surgeries, and colorectal resection.

In the years 2000-2006, the readmission rate to hospitals was 17.3 per 100 discharges of persons with noninstitutionalized beneficiaries aged sixty-five or older. In 2010, Congress enacted the Hospital Readmissions Reduction Program (HRRP), which penalized hospitals with above-average readmission rates for a select number of conditions. According to the 2018 Medicare Payment Advisory Commission—a nonpartisan panel that advises Congress—report, between 2010 and 2016, rates of readmissions declined across all conditions. These readmission rates declined without material increases in observation stays, emergency department visits, or a net adverse effect on mortality rates. In 2008, patients with heart failure were readmitted at a rate of 24.8 percent; by 2016, patients with heart failure were readmitted nearly five percent less often. Patients with heart failure, progressive lung disease, and hip and knee replacements experienced similar drops in risk-adjusted readmission rates.

ADVERSE REACTIONS
Longer and more frequent hospitalizations place the elderly patient at higher risk for iatrogenic complications (those accidentally induced by the physician), nosocomial infections (those acquired in the hospital), and falls. One of the most often encountered problems in hospitalized elderly is an adverse drug reaction. The elderly are especially prone to adverse drug reactions because of age-related changes in body composition and function, resulting in altered ability to absorb, metabolize, and excrete medications. Elderly patients often require a number of medications (polypharmacy) to control multiple health problems, and additions to and changes in the medication regimen are common during hospitalization.

Functional decline of the elderly person is a common problem leading to hospitalization, and deterioration in function can be worsened during hospitalization. For instance, one 2003 study found that one-third of patients aged sixty-five and older being treated for acute illness were discharged from the hospital with lower capacity than they were admitted with, explaining that many of these patients struggle to perform their activities of daily living. Factors that contribute to a decline in functional level are the disease process itself, medical procedures and treatments, and deconditioning caused by restricted activity. Patients most likely to experience reduced functional ability during hospitalization are those who are older, those with cognitive impairments, and those who exhibited functional losses prior to hospitalization. Early recognition and intervention can decrease the likelihood of functional losses during and after hospitalization.

Delirium or confusion develops in many hospitalized elderly patients. The development of delirium can have multiple causes, such as drug reactions, sepsis, or the disruption caused by hospitalization. Rapid identification and treatment of the cause is essential to prevent permanent impairment. Elderly patients are more likely to develop respiratory tract infections as a result of immobility, decreased immunity, and decreased respiratory function. They are also more susceptible to urinary tract infections (UTIs) caused by urinary stasis or the use of indwelling catheters. Age-related skin and circulatory changes often increase the older patient's risk of developing pressure ulcers. Pressure, or decubital, ulcers (commonly called bed sores) are more likely to develop in patients who are immobile, incontinent, febrile, or malnourished, or in those who have poor circulation. Special attention to the skin care of the hospitalized elderly is important in preventing skin breakdown.

Visitation by family members and friends plays a therapeutic role in the patient's recovery. Interacting with familiar people helps keep the patient mentally alert and oriented, decreases the sense of loneliness, and increases motivation. Because of the special needs of elderly hospitalized patients, a team approach to treatment is suggested. Involvement by physical therapists, nutritionists, pharmacists, and social workers, as well as nurses and physicians, can be beneficial in promoting rapid and maximum recovery.

ADVANCE DIRECTIVES

The federal Patient Self-Determination Act, which went into effect on December 1, 1991, dictates that all Medicare providers, including hospitals, must have policies and procedures in place that ensure that all patients receive information about advance directives at the time of admission. Advance directives, such as "do not resuscitate" orders or living wills, allow competent people to extend their right of self-determination regarding health care into the future. Such directives ensure that the patient's decisions regarding the acceptance or rejection of particular types of treatment will be respected should the patient become incompetent. At admission, patients should be asked whether they have an advance directive; and, if they do, it should be included in the medical record. Advance directives are especially important for elderly patients, because they are more prone to cognitive impairments caused by illness.

—*Roberta Tierney*
Updated by Anna Giannicchi

See also: Cancer; Cardiovascular disease; Fractures and broken bones; Health insurance; Heart attacks; Illnesses among older adults; Injuries among older adults; Living wills; Medicare; Medications; Pneumonia; Strokes; Urinary disorders

For Further Information

"2019 Annual Report of the Boards of Trustees of the Federal Hospital Insurance and Federal Supplementary Medical Insurance Trust Funds." The Centers for Medicare & Medicaid Services, 22 Apr. 2019. The Trustees Report is a detailed, lengthy document, containing a substantial amount of information on the past and estimated future financial operations of the Hospital Insurance and Supplementary Medical Insurance Trust Funds.

"5 Statistics to Know about Hospital Admission Rates." *Becker's Hospital Review*, 16 Mar. 2015. www.beckershospitalreview.com/population-health/5-statistics-to-know-about-hospital-admission-rates.html. Five statistics to know from the American Hospital Association's annual hospital statistics report from 2015.

Ayaz, Teslime, et al. "Factors Affecting Mortality in Elderly Patients Hospitalized for Nonmalignant Reasons." *Journal of Aging Research*, vol. 2014, 3 Aug. 2014. doi:10.1155/2014/584315. This study investigates the factors affecting mortality in elderly patients hospitalized for nonmalignant reasons and to determine the relation between laboratory parameters measured routinely in clinical practice and in-hospital mortality, as well as to determine the predictors of mortality.

Cire, Barbara. "Health Care Costs for Dementia Found Greater than for Any Other Disease." National Institute on Aging, 27 Oct. 2015. www.nih.gov/news-events/news-releases/health-care-costs-dementia-found-greater-any-other-disease. National Institutes of Health (NIH)-funded study examines medical care costs in last five years of life.

"Costs of Alzheimer's to Medicare and Medicaid." Alzheimer's Association, Mar. 2019. Statistics on spending related to Alzheimer's disease.

Deiner, Stacie, et al. "Patterns of Surgical Care and Complications in the Elderly." *Journal of the American Geriatrics Society*, vol. 62, no. 5, 14 Apr. 2014. doi:10.1111/jgs.12794. This article reports the pattern of surgical procedures, complications, and mortality found in the National Anesthesia Clinical Outcomes Registry (NACOR), which is one of the few data sets that contains data from community hospitals and individuals with all types of insurance.

Erdem, Erkan, et al. "Medicare Payments: How Much Do Chronic Conditions Matter?" *Medicare & Medicaid Research Review*, vol. 13, no. 2, 13 June 2018. doi:10.5600/mmrr.003.02.b02. The authors analyze differences in Medicare Fee-for-Service utilization (i.e., program payments) by beneficiary characteristics, such as gender, age, and prevalence of chronic conditions.

Gorina, Yelena A., et al. "Hospitalization, Readmission, and Death Experience of Noninstitutionalized Medicare Fee-for-Service Beneficiaries Aged 65 and Over." *National Health Statistics Reports*, vol. 84, 28 Sept. 2015. This report provides descriptive measures of hospitalization, readmission, and death among the noninstitutionalized population aged 65 and over using data from a national survey of the noninstitutionalized population linked to Medicare data and the National Death Index.

Hall, Margaret Jean, et al. "National Hospital Discharge Survey: 2007 Survey." *National Health Statistics Reports*, vol. 29, 26 Oct. 2010. The NHDS was conducted annually from 1965 to 2010 by the National Center for Health Statistics. This survey collected medical and demographic information from a sample of discharge records selected from a national sample of non-Federal, short-stay hospitals.

"Health Care Spending and the Medicare Program." Medicare Payment Advisory Commission, June 2018. The MedPAC Data Book provides information on national health care and Medicare spending as well as Medicare beneficiary demographics, dual-eligible beneficiaries, quality of care in the Medicare program, and Medicare beneficiary and other payer liability.

Hogan, Christopher, et al. "Medicare Beneficiaries' Costs of Care in the Last Year of Life." *Health Affairs (Project Hope)*, vol. 20, no. 4, 2001, pp. 188-95. doi:10.1377/hlthaff.20.4.188. This paper profiles Medicare beneficiaries' costs for care in the last year of life.

"Infographic—US Health Care Spending: Who Pays?" California Health Care Foundation, 22 May 2019. www.chcf.org/publication/us-health-care-spending-who-pays/. This interactive graphic uses data from the Centers for Medicare & Medicaid Services (CMS) to show national spending on personal health care from 1960 to 2017 for health care by payer and spending category.

Mattison, Melissa. "Hospital Management of Older Adults." *UpToDate*, 5 Mar. 2019. This article discusses common issues related to the management of older hospitalized patients.

Russo, C Allison, and Anne Elixhauser. "Hospitalizations in the Elderly Population, 2003." *Healthcare Cost and Utilization Project (HCUP) Statistical Briefs*, May 2006. Agency for Healthcare Research and Quality. This Statistical Brief presents data from the Healthcare Cost and Utilization Project (HCUP) on patterns of hospital utilization and expense for the treatment of individuals age 65 and older in 2003.

Weiss, Audrey J, and Anne Elixhauser. "Overview of Hospital Stays in the United States, 2012." Agency for Healthcare Research and Quality, Oct. 2014. This Statistical Brief presents data from the Healthcare Cost and Utilization Project (HCUP) on characteristics of inpatient stays in U.S. community hospitals in 2012.

HOUSING

Relevant Issues: Demographics, economics, family, sociology

Significance: Housing becomes a critical part of self-identity with increasing age, as it not only reflects career success, life choices, and familial circumstance but also has implications for future security, physical and mental health, and well-being. Persons entering retirement or older persons who have suddenly found themselves on their own due to loss or absence of family, economic difficulties, or physical hardship may find themselves making housing decisions that help them to cope with, or at least minimize, changed circumstances.

A TIME OF CHOICE

Housing needs change with increasing age and not always in expected ways. A family group may be formed, endure years of economic, social, and personal crisis, and then, seemingly without warning, disband, leaving the elderly family founders alone in a house echoing with memories. The years of retirement that had been anticipated as a time of personal exploration, freedom, and leisure may become encumbered by unexpected illness or disability. Lives lived at the brink of economic hardship may be suddenly imploded—by job loss, forced early retirement, or physical incapacity—leaving the older worker with no nest egg beyond a Social Security pension inadequate for more than the most austere living style. Persons who have faced adversity or discrimination during their working years may find that this situation does not change, and may even worsen, with increasing age. Altered family circumstances such as illness, divorce, and death may also dictate choices in housing arrangements.

On the other hand, housing needs may change in very positive ways. Seniors released from daily familial obligations may experience the exhilaration of being able to choose new housing options from numerous possibilities: caravanning with groups of like-minded enthusiasts in a variety of mobile shelters, establishment in retirement communities designed with the needs of the older person in mind, or adventurous experiments in multigenerational living. Other options might include turning the family home into a home-based business enterprise, opening up a bed and breakfast inn, sharing living quarters with family members or other relatives, or even hitting the road, gypsy-style, leaving behind "no known address." Perhaps the feeling of having earned a well-deserved retirement offers a chance to take up new hobbies and ventures in familiar territory. All these new or changed circumstances bring up a host of choices to be made.

The housing challenges that confront the older citizen may be considered as threats or opportunities, depending partly on how they are viewed but also on the ability of the persons involved to respond to them. For many older persons who have achieved economic independence, the decision about where, with whom, and how to live may offer liberation from former responsibilities. On the other hand, for many persons facing old age, housing choices may seem to confine the older person to a restricted universe in which there is little choice. A number of factors affect how these choices are made, including health, physical and emotional makeup, family support systems, financial condition, intellectual interests, and general outlook on life.

Issues that emerge for seniors contemplating housing possibilities after retirement and into old age have a great deal to do with earlier life choices. The older person who already has a home, who has raised a family and made lifelong friends, may prefer to stay in the home as he or she grows older, welcoming returning family members, hosting visiting friends, and enjoying the fruits of economic security and success. This is not an infrequent choice. Numerous studies reveal that the majority of older persons would actually prefer to stay in the family home. In many cases, this is a viable option. If the home is paid for, the expense of maintaining it may be significantly less than finding a smaller house or apartment to rent, because these are costs that are constantly rising. Even for those who have ongoing house payments, options such as renting living space to students, younger workers, family members, or other older persons may make economic sense. Such financial instruments as refinancing to lower mortgage payments or taking out a reverse mortgage to recoup home equity are additional options. Here, the personal preference of the person affected, and his or her ability to make flexible decisions, is a crucial factor.

LIFESTYLES

Just as there is no typical child, teenager, young worker, or middle-aged person, older persons, too, have a wide variety of lifestyles and housing preferences. The choice of what kind of housing is the best fit for an aging person should reflect the lifestyle that seems most in keeping with that individual's own preference and physical adaptability. Most older persons would prefer a housing choice that enables them to continue the lifestyle they have developed over time. On the other hand, some might prefer to try a different housing option.

Such variables as health, family ties, marital status, financial condition, economic resources, and even political persuasion all enter into the decision about housing. Although the majority of older persons might prefer to remain in the family home, even they might not want to spend the remainder of their lives at home alone. Women, in particular, often find themselves alone in later life, having raised their children and lost their husbands through divorce or death, and perhaps have insufficient financial resources to continue the upkeep on a house that may suddenly seem too large. Such persons often decide to sell the house and make other arrangements. Some decide to live with children or other relatives, while others might prefer a footloose life of travel and independence. Still others might want to join a social organization and perhaps find another life partner. Older couples often decide to see the world together, perhaps in a motor home or other recreational vehicle (RV). A variety of options, from RV campers to mobile home parks, might meet the needs of the newly peripatetic. Still others decide to have the best of both worlds, spending part of the year in the family home and the remainder of the year in a vacation or second home in another location.

SNOWBIRDS

Older people from the northern regions often migrate to milder climates in the south for the winter. Florida, for example, has based a great deal of its statewide social and economic decision-making on its ability to lure the "snowbirds" of the northern states to its warm shores. Many smaller and medium-sized cities in Florida cater to the needs of the aging, with social organizations, churches, clubs, and community services designed with the older resident in mind. In planning for a future in which the number of older citizens will be much greater than at present, it is instructive to consider how Florida, where more than 25 percent of the population is over sixty, has addressed this situation. On the one hand, the influx of large numbers of wealthy retirees has brought unprecedented affluence to the state, while on the other, the increasing needs of the elderly for health and other services have caused social inequities to develop. For some older persons, Florida seems to be the ideal solution to their housing problems, as the sunny climate, social ambiance, and tax structure are all designed to attract the elderly. For others, however, the social setting that caters to the elderly does not provide the variety that they feel is essential.

Among older people who want to retire in a place where their money will go as far as possible, many consider spending their postretirement years abroad. Americans flock to Mexico and other of the less-affluent countries, where they often find the combination of lower living expenses, cheaper housing, and a more relaxed social environment attractive. Some popular periodicals feature articles on places that promise great benefits to the leisure class of senior citizens who are in the market for new living accommodations. Such features as climate, a favorable tax structure, easy availability of transportation, abundance of social and community programs, and varied cultural offerings can be important to older citizens who may live on a fixed income, need to use public transportation, or want to become involved in community life. For these people, a number of housing choices exist, from bringing a mobile home or RV to staying in a pension, renting a villa, or buying a house. Often older persons in these locations seek out others of their own nationality to feel more at home in unfamiliar surroundings.

HOUSING ALTERNATIVES

For many persons, the later years become an ideal time to try out social experiments that interested them in their youth. The concepts of communal living and cohousing, for example, have a great deal of appeal to many aging baby boomers who have always believed in various types of social experimentation and who want in their later years to take advantage of their greater maturity and life experience to try new ways of sharing lifestyles with others of similar interest. A number of highly successful communal efforts of this kind have been made, often seeking to create a utopian social milieu in which persons of all ages feel welcome and secure. Notable examples of such intentional communities include the Findhorn community in Scotland, with its tradition of ecological and spiritual self-sustenance, the Twin Oaks community in rural Virginia, and the New Age Sirius community in Amherst, Massachusetts. Typical of a great number of these large intentional communities is the philosophy of making all age groups equally welcome. In many ways, these "new" communities replicate an earlier age, in which the extended family lived together on shared property and was responsible for the wellbeing of all its members. In other areas of the world, the multigenerational family model is looked upon as the normal pattern for housing the elderly in a rural setting. In many agricultural communities in Europe and elsewhere, the older and younger generations all live together, with the younger members of the family providing the farm labor, while the older family members provide cooking, childcare, and knowledge.

Other successful examples of multigenerational living accommodations are afforded by numerous nonprofit organizations, particularly in medium and large urban areas. The object of these housing ventures is to create an environment that is friendly to the elderly, but that takes advantage of support that can be provided by other age groups, college students, for example.

Older persons in city settings also often share housing on a private or independent basis, either out of economic necessity or to alleviate feelings of loneliness or alienation. The popular television program The Golden Girls featured one variation on this theme, but many other possibilities exist. A frequent occurrence in university and college communities, for example, is the renting of rooms in houses owned by older citizens to students, a form of small business that is profitable to the homeowners and helpful to the student population. This can be of particular benefit to older people who want to maintain some connection with the upcoming generation after their own children are grown. If supplemental income is not the primary objective, living space may be traded for home and garden maintenance, food preparation, transportation, or other services.

Some older persons may prefer to spend their later years with other senior citizens who are similar to themselves in interests, socioeconomic status, age, sex, or educational level. For many of these people, a retirement community that is planned and marketed to their age or income group might be the preferred housing choice. These can range from retirement communities that are designed to appeal to older persons who prefer to live with their peers but who are able to take care of most of their needs, to congregate housing projects, often called life care facilities, which are designed to provide health care assistance to elderly residents, including those who are less able to look after themselves.

The latter may become of increasing importance as projections of population growth into the twenty-first century prove to be accurate. According to these projections, the percentage of persons over sixty-five will nearly double between 1995 and 2050, while the percentage of persons aged eighty-five and over will nearly quadruple, and those over one hundred will become a measurable statistic for the first time in history. This fact, in conjunction with the increasing number of householders living alone, will have great implications for the managed care facilities of the short- to long-term future. In the course of the twentieth century, the life expectancy at birth in the United States nearly doubled. Although it is questionable whether a similar increase in longevity will characterize the twenty-first century, the results of this dramatic change in life span will inevitably have major social implications for housing far into the twenty-first century.

Some housing facilities are designed with the needs of the very frail elderly in mind, in order that the elderly needing assistance with daily tasks be able to get help in a positive living environment. The style of accommodation for this type of housing can range from modest to quite luxurious, depending on the economic status of the occupants. Managed care options vary greatly in quality and cost, as do the capabilities of the elderly that inhabit them. Although many very elderly people require only assistance on occasion, elderly Alzheimer's disease patients and other invalids require almost constant attention.

THE ECONOMIC IMPERATIVE

Some housing alternatives are driven more by economic necessity than choice. Many older workers, for a variety of reasons, have only meager economic resources in their later years. These people often subsist on inadequate Social Security income. Many of them can expect little or no assistance from family and have little in the way of savings. In most cases, these persons are not homeowners, or, if so, they have little equity in their homes. Often, these older persons would need to seek rental housing.

For these senior citizens, some kind of government-subsidized housing is a frequent recourse, because the portion of the rent that the tenant pays is dependent on income, with the government supplying the balance. Public housing was begun as the U.S. Housing Act of 1937 and was designed to serve as temporary housing for the unemployed, but it has instead been viewed by many, including many older citizens, as a permanent solution to their housing needs. This type of housing is often located in inner cities or rural areas, which may not be the ideal locations for older citizens. For example, 12 percent of public housing in the United States is in New York City. Funding for public housing, and whether it should be centrally or locally administered, is a further issue affecting housing resources for the elderly, as many of the poorest frail elderly have virtually no income. The benefits of this type of housing include low cost, proximity to city centers, and convenience. Availability is a further issue, however, since there is seldom enough housing of this type to meet demand. In some of the larger cities, safety may also be a concern. The quality of subsidized housing ranges from excellent to minimal but is usually better than the substandard housing that may be the only other option for the economically disadvantaged.

For those homeowners who do have substantial equity in their homes but insufficient cash flow to meet their monthly expenses, investigating reverse mortgage options might be advisable. Free information and referrals on these mortgages, in which equity is gradually deducted from the house in return for access to money, with the repayment delayed until after the present owner dies or sells the home, are available from the Housing and Urban Development (HUD) Administration. There is also a list of HUD-approved counseling agencies on the Internet at www.hud.gov.

Many housing issues become matters of public policy, with legislation introduced to protect the interest of older citizens. For example, legislators voiced many concerns about the lack of public housing options for older Americans following the Reagan administration of the 1980s, during which market-driven considerations dominated. For example, many lending institutions that specialized in reverse mortgages charged fees in excess of those charged for other types of lending instruments for real estate. This resulted in legislation being introduced to modify this practice. Unfortunately, such legislative remedies often become foci of partisan politics, which may delay much-needed housing legislation in being passed. Other public policy issues relate to welfare reform, which attempts to address one problem, that of welfare for unemployed people of working age, but which then might militate against the aged, many of whom live in subsidized housing but are too old or frail to work.

ELDERLY MINORITIES

The American Housing Survey, conducted by the United States Census Bureau, and studies by other agencies have shown that, statistically, elderly African Americans and Latinos, whether renters or homeowners, are more likely to live in substandard housing than are other Americans, with African Americans faring worse in that regard than Latinos. Many elderly American Indians also live in substandard housing, although this problem is associated with the wider problem of housing for American Indians on government reservations.

The issue of minority housing and its deficiencies brings up a host of social and health issues, as older persons are more likely to suffer from discrimination and extreme poverty than younger persons and are less able to adjust to it. Demographic data project a relative increase in the numbers of African American and Latino elderly into the future, which makes addressing their housing needs of primary importance in planning public policy. Complicating factors for this population include frequency of health problems, less stable societal and family structures, and fewer cultural opportunities.

INTERNATIONAL ASPECTS

Housing of the elderly is an issue that is international in dimension, because changes in social structure, demographics, and even economics are an increasingly worldwide phenomenon. Just as the selection of a place to live for older people is not restricted to their country of origin, solutions to the housing problem are also not restricted geographically. A number of countries have devised answers to the elderly housing dilemma, including some that can be adopted on a global level.

An often concern of the aging is that they not become a burden to their children or families. However, some assisted-living housing options are quite expensive and beyond the means of the individual. An option that some families are increasingly choosing originated in Australia and is known there by the name "granny flat." This is a type of detached dwelling that can be quickly assembled and then removed if no longer needed. It may resemble a mobile home or may be attached to the main house. This type of housing is called echo housing in some communities, while others call this type of subsidiary housing a mother-in-law unit. Increasingly, forward-looking communities are modifying zoning laws in order to permit construction of this type of housing in residential neighborhoods. It has the virtue of permitting independent living while allowing caring family members to be available in case assistance or simply proximity is desired.

Among the most forward-looking Europeans in the matter of housing the elderly have been the Scandinavians. Sweden, in particular, has been a pioneer in building communities for a mixture of older and younger citizens at public expense. In these communities, cooking is centralized, household chores and the upkeep of the community is shared, but each resident has private space as well. Germany, on the other hand, has instigated some programs that promote the exchange of large homes owned by older citizens for smaller apartments, with the government paying the moving costs.

Worldwide, women have been among the greatest leaders and innovators in the movement to make housing for the elderly more humane and individual. Perhaps this is in part due to the greater longevity of women, but it may also be attributed to women's greater empathy for the discomforts of age. Women in particular have been among the most active in establishing communities for shared living for the elderly that are comfortable, affordable, and appealing.

A key factor in the study of the housing preferences of elderly people that is sometimes overlooked is the intense emotional attachment to a particular place that can develop over a lifetime. The concept of "aging in place" recognizes the importance of sentimental values in planning and providing housing for older citizens. The psychological dimension of housing is perhaps more significant for the elderly than for any other group, as a lifetime of memories associated with a place may be among their most prized possessions.

—*Gloria Fulton*

See also: African Americans; Home ownership; Home services; Laguna Woods, California; Latinx Americans; Older Americans Act of 1965; Relocation; Retirement communities; Vacations and travel; Women and aging

For Further Information

Fox, Siobhan, et al. "Exploring the Housing Needs of Older People in Standard and Sheltered Social Housing." *Gerontology and Geriatric Medicine*, vol. 3, 2017. doi:10.1177/2333721417702349. This research describes a survey of older adults living in two forms of social housing ("standard" or "sheltered"), asking them what they feel are their current and anticipated housing needs.

Frederick, Ryan. "How Will Housing for Older Adults Change?" *Forbes*, 9 Mar. 2016. www.forbes.com/sites/nextavenue/2016/03/09/how-will-housing-for-older-adults-change/#6d79614048ba. Details a panel on housing for seniors that discussed three major changes: changing demographics and related psychographics, a shift in health care from fee-for-service to more values-based models and accelerating advances in technology.

"Housing Help." USA.Gov, Official Guide to Government Information and Services. www.usa.gov/housing-help-audiences#item-36852. Resources for seniors looking for advice on housing issues.

"Programs." National Center for Healthy Housing (NCHH), 2016. nchh.org/program/healthy-housing-for-older-adults/. Describes the characteristics of healthy housing for older adults.

HUMOR

Relevant Issues: Health and medicine, psychology, sociology

Significance: The relationship between humor and aging well is being explored by professionals interested in the aging process.

The benefits of humor for all people, and especially the elderly, have increasingly become a topic of research in medicine and psychology. The results confirm that laughter makes people healthier and helps them control pain and manage stress.

Much has been written concerning the benefits of laughter and having a sense of humor. In his 1979 best-seller Anatomy of an Illness, Norman Cousins proclaimed that laughter had helped speed his recovery from a serious disease. William F. Fry, professor emeritus of psychiatry at Stanford University, studied humor and its effect on the human body. He noted that laughter increases heart rate and hormone production, improves muscle tone and circulation, and helps move nutrients and oxygen along to the body's tissues. According to Fry, a good laugh is similar to an aerobic workout. Other researchers have indicated that a sense of humor is a significant characteristic of executives and those in leadership roles in business, while others have espoused the power of a sense of humor in enhancing a person's mental well-being and social status. All suggest that a sense of humor is one of the most important characteristics that a person can possess.

THE HISTORY OF HUMOR

The English word "humor" stems from a Latin word meaning "liquid," "fluid," or "moisture." In ancient Greece, a person's temperament was thought to be controlled by four humors (fluids). When in proper balance, a person was in good humor. Too much of one of the fluids produced moods: irritable if yellow bile was disproportionate, gloomy if black bile predominated, sluggish if phlegm was too abundant, and sanguine if an individual had an oversupply of blood. A person possessing an excess of one of the fluids came to be known as a "humorist." The prescription for controlling bad temperament caused by excessive "humors" was laughter.

Throughout history, scholars and philosophers have studied humor and why people laugh, with philosophers being the first laughter critics. Plato described laughter as something to be avoided, and Aristotle believed that people laughed too much. Christians during the Middle Ages believed that laughter and play contradicted their values, and the Pilgrims in America thought that humor and laughter were low forms of behavior that contradicted Christian sobriety. The Bible, however, refers to laughter and humor. The Old Testament has twenty-nine references to humor, many in the book of Proverbs. An often-quoted passage from Ecclesiastes 3:4 is, "To everything there is a season, and a time to every purpose under heaven; a time to weep, a time to laugh; a time to mourn, and a time to dance."

Over the centuries, views of humor and what makes people laugh have changed. These views have included everything from wit and buffoonery to mocking and jesting. Another view—using humor appropriately in social situations and using it creatively in thinking and writing—examines a more cognitive aspect of what makes people laugh. Through it all seems to have remained the idea that humor is something that is ludicrous, incongruous, abnormal, and out of the ordinary. A contemporary view of humor is that whereas humor is characterized by making people laugh, it is not necessarily jokes, stories, and anecdotes but rather an attitude.

STRATEGIES FOR PEOPLE WORKING WITH THE ELDERLY

Professionals in medicine, health care, education, nutrition, social work, religion, and fitness/wellness who work with the elderly have long understood the benefits of laughter for this population. Many elderly find themselves with chronic pain and chronic stressors related to aging. Humor and laughter can help control pain by distracting attention from pain, reducing tension, changing one's expectations and outlook on a situation, and increasing the production of endorphins, the body's natural painkillers. Laughter also has the ability to cause muscles suddenly to go limp, a great value in the treatment of stress.

Those who work with older people can employ simple strategies to make humor a part of their own lives and their caring attitude toward the elderly. They can adopt a playful frame of mind and not take themselves too seriously. They can look for the lighter, brighter side of situations. They can laugh at themselves, thus enabling others to laugh with them. They can make a humor first-aid kit containing stories, anecdotes, cartoons, and jokes to be shared on bulletin boards, in newsletters, in presentations, and on a one-on-one basis. They can laugh with others, not at them. They also can make others laugh by letting one's own natural sense of humor emerge. They can listen and look for humor in their surroundings: in church bulletins, in newsletters, on television, in magazines and journals, and in daily life experiences. They can build a humor support group by gathering together people who share the same sense of humor, especially in the workplace. They also can use a sense of humor to get them through embarrassing moments and enable them to accept problems that have no immediate solutions. Finally, they can get the "maximum requirement" of humor; the average person laughs fifteen times per day.

For professionals who want to get serious about laughing, an organization founded by Joel Goodman is available. The Humor Project at 110 Spring Street, Saratoga Springs, NY 12866 (518-587-8770. www.humorproject.com) provides workshops, a speakers' bureau, an e-mail newsletter, and podcasts, as well as seminars for people who wish to use humor as a positive force in their work. It also supplies a free information packet on the positive power of humor. A sampling comes from humor in medical situations on the organization's homepage: "Serious illness is not a laughing matter, but sometimes you stumble across unintentional humor, such as the medical record that stated: 'Patient has been married twice, but denies any other serious illnesses.'"

SOURCES OF HUMOR AND INSPIRATION FOR OLDER PEOPLE

Sources of humor abound in society. Humor appears in almost every facet of daily living. Popular publications such as Reader's Digest are resources of humor on numerous topics. Television supplies many weekly series of situation comedies. Books such as those by Erma Bombeck and Dave Barry portray American life in a humorous fashion. Comments from comedians George Burns, Andy Rooney, Phyllis Diller, and Joan Rivers often brought laughter to the older generation, as much of their humor is about growing old. Technology provides sources of humor through the Internet and electronic mail. Newspaper cartoons are an excellent source of humor about growing old and life situations related to the aging process. Some comic strips appreciated by older readers are Peanuts, Pickles, Garfield, Frank and Ernest, Dennis the Menace, Crankshaft, Shoe, and Family Circle. Films are also sources of humor, information, and inspiration. For example, the 1998 film Patch Adams, starring Robin Williams, tells the true story of a doctor who used laughter as a healing force with his patients.

The elderly are bombarded with information concerning exercise as a key factor and positive lifestyle change that can help combat and slow down many chronic disabilities of aging. Yet, many elderly find adhering to an exercise program difficult. Humorous one-liners, used appropriately, can make light of health and exercise situations that elders might prefer to ignore. Some examples of short quips are as follows: Erma Bombeck on exercise—"The only reason I would take up jogging is so I could hear heavy breathing again"; Joan Rivers on exercise—"If God wanted us to bend over, He would put diamonds on the floor"; and George Burns on nutrition—"I want nothing to do with natural foods. At my age, I need all the preservatives I can get." Burns created a "Don't List" of things that may not make people live longer but that make life seem longer: "Don't smoke, don't drink, don't gamble, don't eat salt, don't eat sugar, don't overeat, don't under eat, don't play around."

CONCLUSION

The relationship between humor and the healing process and other health benefits is well documented. The relationship between humor and aging well is being explored by professionals interested in the aging process. One area of interest is the role of humor in assisting the elderly in their perceived control of life situations or in their personal control. Simply understanding the multidimensional nature of humor, however, is a challenge. Whereas humor is associated with creativity, social cohesion, and relief from stress, it can also be hostile, aggressive, or demeaning. Training and encouraging older people to use positive humor in their lives may allow them to remain involved in society and in relationships with family and friends. Perhaps it can enable them to take advantage of the possibilities and choices that exist and thus promote and facilitate aging well.

—*Gail Clark*
Updated by Bruce E. Johansen, PhD

See also: Communication; Depression; Friendship; Golden Girls, The; Grumpy Old Men; Harold and Maude; Social ties; Stereotypes; Stress and coping skills; Successful aging; You're Only Old Once!

For Further Information

Bolton, Martha. *Forgettable Jokes about Older Folks.* BroadStreet Publishing Group, 2018. A book of jokes focused on aging and older adults.

Cousins, Norman. *Anatomy of an Illness as Perceived by the Patient.* Twentieth Anniversary ed., W. W. Norton, 2005. Anatomy of an Illness was the first book by a patient that spoke to our current interest in taking charge of our own health. It started the revolution in patients working with their doctors and using humor to boost their bodies' capacity for healing.

Fischer, Ed. *What's So Funny about Getting Old?* Running P Adult, 2014. A collection of cartoons, quips, and insights about aging.

Lurie, Abraham, and Kathleen Monahan. "Humor, Aging, and Life Review: Survival Through the Use of Humor." *Social Work in Mental Health*, vol. 13, no. 1, 13 Dec. 2014, pp. 82-91. doi:10.1080/15332985.2014.884519. Addresses the end stage of life through the lens of humor.

Papousek, Ilona, et al. "The Use of Bright and Dark Types of Humour Is Rooted in the Brain." *Scientific Reports*, vol. 7, no. 1, 17 Feb. 2017. doi:10.1038/srep42967. Studies how neural functions are affected by auditory displays of happy and sad emotion and how they predict people's typical use of humor in social interactions.

Tse, Mimi M. Y., et al. "Humor Therapy: Relieving Chronic Pain and Enhancing Happiness for Older Adults." *Journal of Aging Research*, vol. 2010, 2010, pp. 1-9. doi:10.4061/2010/343574. Examines the effectiveness of a humor therapy program in relieving chronic pain, increasing life satisfaction, and reducing loneliness.

HUNDRED-YEAR-OLDS. *See* **CENTENARIANS.**

HYPERTENSION

Relevant Issues: Health and medicine
Significance: The incidence of high blood pressure, or hypertension, increases with age; it is known as the "silent killer" because it has no obvious symptoms.
Key Terms:
artery: any of the muscular-walled tubes forming part of the circulation system by which blood (mainly that which has been oxygenated) is conveyed from the heart to all parts of the body
diastolic: relating to the phase of the heartbeat when the heart muscle relaxes and allows the chambers to fill with blood
systolic: relating to the phase of the heartbeat when the heart muscle contracts and pumps blood from the chambers into the arteries

In 2013, it was estimated that 75 million Americans had hypertension. This number represented nearly 32 percent of the American population. A major concern for the prevalence of hypertension is its relationship to other serious diseases, such as stroke, coronary artery disease, congestive heart failure, renal (kidney) failure, and peripheral vascular disease.

High blood pressure that is not controlled by medication or lifestyle can damage the body. The higher the blood pressure, the harder the heart must work to pump blood throughout the body. When the heart has to work harder, the heart muscle gets larger. An enlarged heart will eventually not function efficiently and begin to fail. Additionally, arteries get harder and less elastic with age. Having high blood pressure accelerates this process, resulting in further degradations in heart function.

A serious concern of high blood pressure is the increased potential for a stroke, which has been the leading cause of disability in the United States. A stroke occurs when a blood vessel in the brain becomes clogged or bursts. The brain tissue that gets its blood from the affected vessel is deprived of oxygen and begins to die within minutes. The death of the brain tissue can cause paralysis, loss of vision, difficulty talking or hearing, or, in extreme cases, death.

Another complication of hypertension is related to the kidneys. When systolic pressures get high, small blood vessels in the kidneys can rupture and bleed. Over time, this can destroy kidney cells, resulting in impaired function and higher blood pressure. In order to make the kidneys filter blood effectively after the damage, the body must increase the blood pressure, further complicating the health of the whole body. In extreme cases, this process results in the need for kidney dialysis. Blood vessel ruptures can cause complications with the eyes as well. High pressures can damage the eye's retina tissues. In many cases, it can cause blindness.

When left untreated, hypertension can complicate and contribute to many other health problems. There-

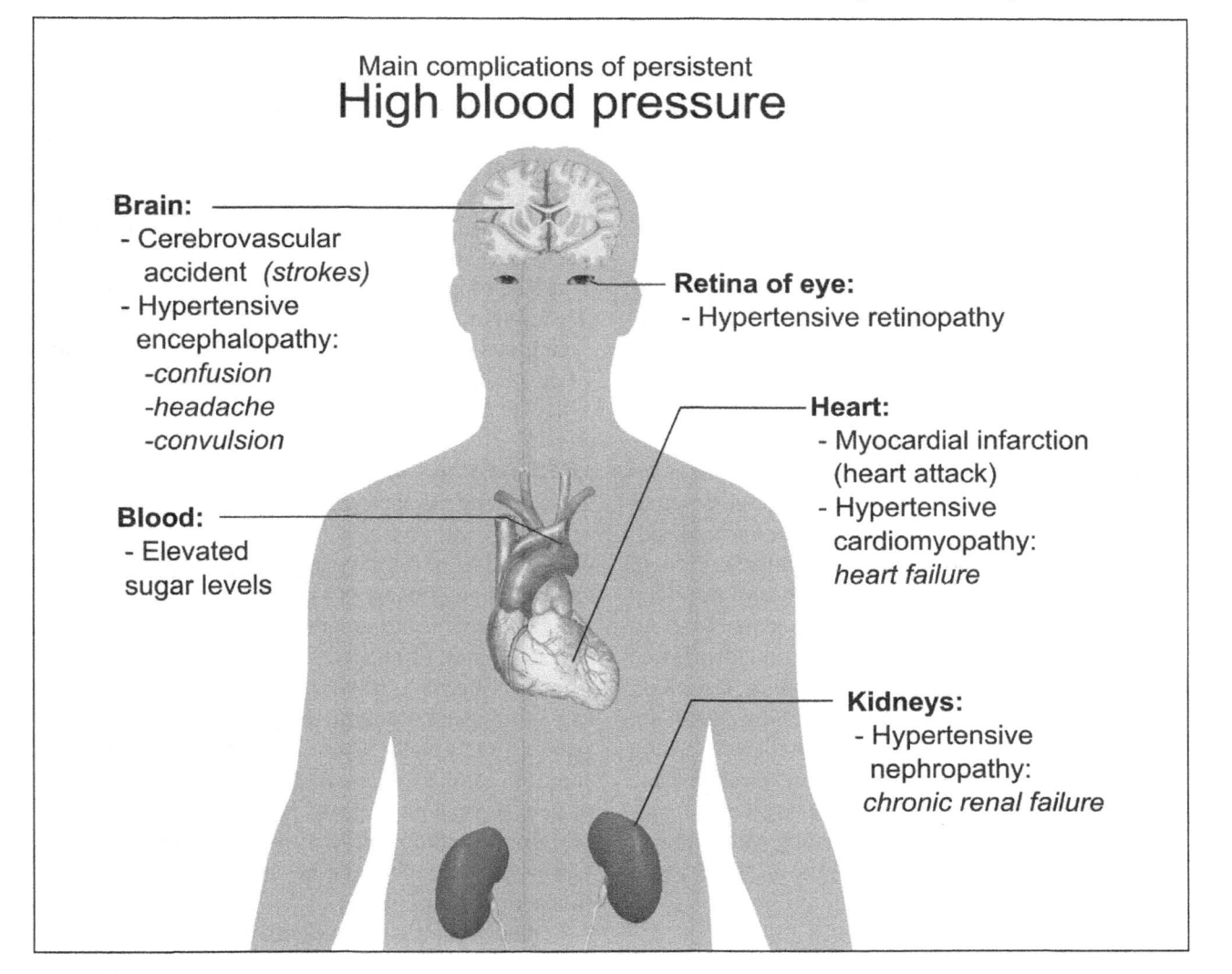

Main complications of persistent
High blood pressure

Brain:
- Cerebrovascular accident *(strokes)*
- Hypertensive encephalopathy:
  -confusion
  -headache
  -convulsion

Blood:
- Elevated sugar levels

Retina of eye:
- Hypertensive retinopathy

Heart:
- Myocardial infarction (heart attack)
- Hypertensive cardiomyopathy: *heart failure*

Kidneys:
- Hypertensive nephropathy: *chronic renal failure*

fore, individuals should be screened periodically and make the necessary lifestyle modifications to minimize their risk of this disease.

DIAGNOSIS OF HYPERTENSION

Because no symptoms are felt by individuals with hypertension, it is important to have one's blood pressure checked periodically by a qualified person. Blood pressure is measured by a sphygmomanometer (blood pressure cuff) and a stethoscope. The cuff is wrapped around the upper arm and filled with air to compress the brachial artery. The pressure is slowly released while the health practitioner listens for blood flow through the stethoscope. When the pulsating blood is first heard, the systolic blood pressure is recorded. After the pulsating sound stops, the diastolic blood pressure is recorded. All values are measured in millimeters of mercury. Systolic blood pressure indicates the pressure the blood exerts against the blood vessel walls when the heart is contracting. A value of 140 millimeters or higher would be considered high blood pressure. In general, the greater the value is over 140, the more severe the hypertension. Diastolic blood pressure is the pressure the blood exerts against the blood vessel walls when the heart is at rest (between beats). A value of 90 millimeters or higher denotes high blood pressure. As with the systolic blood pressure, the greater the value is over 90, the more severe the hypertension.

Although both systolic and diastolic pressures are measured, only one of them has to be elevated to be diagnosed as hypertension. Both blood pressure values are correlated with cardiovascular disease when considered alone and when combined. Generally, the risks of complications are higher for elevated systolic blood pressure than for elevated diastolic blood pressure. An important factor to understand is that blood pressure fluctuates greatly over the course of a day. Therefore, one random reading that happens to be high should not immediately be used to diagnose hypertension. High values at rest on two or more days are required to make an accurate diagnosis. An accurate blood pressure reading also requires the patient to be resting with both feet on the floor, and not talking during the measurement.

RISK FACTORS FOR HYPERTENSION

Conditions that increase an individual's likelihood of having a disease are called risk factors. There are several risk factors for high blood pressure. Some risk factors are controllable, while others are uncontrollable. Uncontrollable risk factors include genetics, age, and ethnic background. Men, people over age 35, African Americans, Puerto Ricans, Mexican Americans, and Cuban Americans are more likely to have high blood pressure than other groups.

Fortunately, there are several risk factors that can be controlled. Individuals who are overweight are more likely to have high blood pressure. Also, individuals who consume more than one alcoholic drink per day are at a higher risk. Some individuals are sensitive to sodium (a major component of table salt). These individuals are more likely to have hypertension if they consume too much salt or other sodium-containing products. It has also been found that women who use some types of birth control pills are more likely to develop high blood pressure. Lack of exercise is another risk factor that can be controlled. Proper aerobic exercise has been found to decrease blood pressure.

A lack of risk factors is no guarantee of good health. Therefore, medical experts urge all individuals to have their blood pressure checked at least annually (and more often if risk factors are present) to be sure the "silent killer" is not present.

LIFESTYLE MANAGEMENT OF HYPERTENSION

Based on the risk factors identified for high blood pressure, there are several activities that can decrease the likelihood of having hypertension. It is recommended that individuals maintain a proper weight and that overweight individuals implement a reduced-calorie diet. All individuals can benefit from regular exercise. Continuous, vigorous activities are best. Besides developing a stronger cardiovascular system, it can also help people lose weight. These exercises should be done three to four days per week. Long, steady walks can be as good as running for many people. Other controllable activities include decreasing or discontinuing the consumption of alcoholic beverages and reducing the intake of sodium.

For individuals who have been diagnosed with hypertension, strict adherence to the medication regimen is

> **SENIOR TALK:**
>
> **How Do You Feel About Blood Pressure Medication?**
>
> Physically, you may not feel any indication that you have hypertension and have no obvious symptoms. Otherwise, you might feel out of breath even when doing only light physical activity, or you may have experienced more serious symptoms and related conditions like eye disorders, heart disease, kidney failure, or stroke. Oftentimes, psychological stress goes hand in hand with hypertension, so you may feel heightened stress, pressure, frustration, or lack of control over anger or outbursts.
>
> Once you have been diagnosed with hypertension and are prescribed medications, you may experience emotions ranging from relief to anxiety. It can be stressful to know you have a potentially dangerous condition or that the medication itself brings risks of negative drug interactions. You may also find it frustrating that it can take time to identify the best medication for you or that you have to remember to take your medication, check your own blood pressure, or schedule doctor's visits. On the other hand, being informed can often make us feel more at ease. Gaining control over how we choose to address our health concerns as we age can bring a sense of empowerment. Discussions with a health care provider can go a long way in easing worries.
>
> *—Leah Jacob*

critical. High blood pressure medication works by getting rid of excess body fluids and sodium, opening up narrowed blood vessels, or preventing blood vessels from narrowing or constricting. It can lower the pressures substantially if taken as directed by a physician. A major problem exists with individuals forgetting or skipping doses and trading medicines with family and friends. It is critical that blood pressure medications be taken exactly as directed, and other lifestyle modification recommendations are followed.

Another lifestyle habit that affects hypertension is smoking. Smoking has also been shown to increase the risk of coronary artery disease and stroke. Both of these major health problems are related to and complicated by hypertension.

Hypertension can have serious negative effects on health. This disease can affect individuals at any age, but its incidence increases with age. Fortunately, proper lifestyle habits can significantly improve the chances of avoiding hypertension. As with many chronic conditions, early detection of hypertension can result in better long-term outcomes on patient health.

—Bradley R. A. Wilson
Updated by Patrick Richardson, MSN

See also: Alcohol use disorder; Cardiovascular disease; Exercise and fitness; Heart attacks; Heart changes and disorders; Illnesses among older adults; Nutrition; Smoking; Strokes

For Further Information

Anker, Daniela, et al. "Screening and Treatment of Hypertension in Older Adults: Less Is More?" *Public Health Reviews*, vol. 39, no. 1, 3 Sept. 2018. doi:10.1186/s40985-018-0101-z. Reviews current practices of screening and treating hypertension.

Benetos, Athanase, et al. "Hypertension Management in Older and Frail Older Patients." *Circulation Research*, vol. 124, no. 7, 28 Mar. 2019, pp. 1,045-60. doi:10.1161/circresaha.118.313236. This article proposes adapting the antihypertensive treatment using an easy-to-apply visual numeric scale allowing the identification of three different patient profiles according to the functional status and autonomy for activities of daily living.

Lionakis, Nikolaos. "Hypertension in the Elderly." *World Journal of Cardiology*, vol. 4, no. 5, 26 May 2012, p. 135. doi:10.4330/wjc.v4.i5.135. This review article highlights the importance of treating hypertension in the aging population to improve their quality of life and lower the incidence of the cardiovascular complications.

Patel, Aneet, and B. Fendley Stewart. "On Hypertension in the Elderly: An Epidemiologic Shift." American College of Cardiology, 20 Feb. 2015. www.acc.org/latest-in-cardiology/articles/2015/02/19/14/55/on-hypertension-in-the-elderly. The authors suggest changes in the diagnosis and treatment of hypertension in the elderly due to the rise of the population.

Sun, Zhongjie. "Aging, Arterial Stiffness, and Hypertension." *Hypertension*, vol. 65, no. 2, 3 Nov. 2014, pp. 252-56. doi:10.1161/hypertensionaha.114.03617. This review updates the recent advances in the mechanism of aging-related arterial stiffening and hypertension based on the articles published on hypertension in the past 2 to 3 years.

I NEVER SANG FOR MY FATHER (PLAY)

Author: Robert Anderson
Date: Produced and published in 1968
Relevant Issues: Culture, family, sociology, values
Significance: This play addresses the problem of how children must come to terms with how to relate to their aging parents.

Robert Anderson's best-known play, *Tea and Sympathy* (1953), analyzes the relationship between an older woman and a young troubled student. *I Never Sang for My Father*, which was made into a film in 1970 and a television drama in 1984, is also a play about an intergenerational relationship, this time a strained attempt at understanding between a son and his aging father.

The opening scene clearly establishes the loving attachment of the mother and son, Gene, and the love-hate connection between the father and son. Tom Garrison, the father, is a self-made and self-centered man who, although eighty years old and failing in health, still insists on being in control. When Mrs. Garrison dies, Gene attempts to connect with his father and at one point admits that he feels more open toward his father than ever before. His father, in turn, remembers that Gene used to sing to his mother but never sang for his father—he always seemed to finish just as his father entered the room. Gene's offer to find a place for his father near him and his future wife in California, however, is met with obstinate resistance, and the two relapse into their strained relationship.

Tom is hospitalized while visiting Gene, slowly lapses into senility, and dies. Gene never discovers whether he loved his father, or his father loved him. Although advised that he should accept the sadness of the situation, Gene's last words in the play are "still, when I hear the word father.... It matters."

—*Robert L. Patterson*

See also: Death and dying; Death of parents; Family relationships; Grief; Parenthood

ILLNESSES AMONG OLDER ADULTS

Relevant Issues: Biology, health and medicine
Significance: Many diseases appear with greater frequency, greater severity, and greater resultant functional impairment in older individuals than in younger groups.

Physical and intellectual performance reach their peaks between the ages of twenty and thirty, followed by more or less rapid deterioration during the life span of the individual. Substantial reserve potentials are built into human physiological functions, including the cardiovascular, pulmonary, and musculoskeletal systems. These reserves decrease with time. Illnesses and diseases may subtract from these functions; the lesser reserves of older individuals may result in a greater lessening of the ability to perform than would have occurred at an earlier age. The problems of older individuals can be compounded by the occurrence of multiple disorders, by atypical presentations, and by the withholding of important complaints and information, making diagnosis and treatment more difficult. What may be tolerated in youth may be lethal in old age.

INFECTIOUS DISEASES

Older individuals are particularly vulnerable to attacks by the influenza viruses and by the pneumococcus, an organism associated with pneumonia. Although symptoms may vary, influenza is characterized by fever, aches, pains, and prostration. Susceptibility to secondary infections, particularly of the lungs, is greatly increased. Both influenza and pneumococcal infections can, to a substantial degree, be prevented through the timely administration of vaccines that, unfortunately, do not provide complete immunity. Influenza vaccines are designed each year to protect against the most prevalent strains. These vary from year to year so that administration of the vaccine must be done yearly. Pneumococcal vaccines protect against only twenty-three of the most prevalent serotypes (there are more than eighty). The effectiveness of the vaccines is limited in older individuals because the immune responses tend to diminish with age. Influenza vaccine is recommended for all adults. Pneumococcal vaccine is strongly recommended for all people age sixty-five and over, with a repeat every five years. This has become particularly important because of the emergence of pneumococcal strains resistant to most of the usual antibiotics.

Although the incidence of tuberculosis declined markedly during the twentieth century, the disease remains a threat to older individuals, particularly to those with diminished immune responses. Fatigue, chronic cough, low-grade fever, and anemia are among the signs of tuberculosis. Early diagnosis can make a cure possible, but here again the emergence of resistant strains makes appropriate treatment more difficult. Legionnaires' disease, a relatively recently recognized pulmonary disease, is another significant threat to older individuals. Many so-called childhood diseases are now preventable with vaccines, but the immune response achieved in childhood is not always maintained. Emergence of these diseases in later life has occurred.

The increased mobility of older generations, be it by automobile, cruise ship, or airplane, can bring them into areas that are the habitat of the pathogens for malaria, Rocky Mountain spotted fever, babesiosis, ehrlichiosis, tularemia, yellow fever, cholera, Lyme disease, and the plague. Vaccines or chemoprophylaxis are available for some. Avoidance may be the only available protection for others. Physicians and public health authorities should be consulted, particularly if travel is contemplated to areas of infestation by pathogen vectors, such as ticks or to the tropics.

THE CARDIOVASCULAR SYSTEM

Some individuals maintain essentially normal, although diminished, cardiac function as they age and as their cardiac reserve diminishes. Others, less fortunate, develop disorders of the heart's rhythm or an inability to maintain a level of activity satisfactory for an enjoyable life. In still others, musculoskeletal problems may limit their physical activities so that declining cardiac function is not noticed.

Among the more frequent problems of rate and rhythm are bradycardia (reduction of pulse to below sixty beats per minute) and skipped beats. Their appearance should be brought to the attention of a physician, as should other irregularities of rhythm. Shortness of breath on exertion, a change in exercise tolerance, feelings of heaviness or oppression, and precordial pain are frequent signals of cardiac problems mediated by inadequacy of the blood supply to heart muscle.

Both large and small blood vessels can show changes with age. Atherosclerosis, the deposition of fatty substances on the interior walls of blood vessels, spares neither. The aorta, the main blood vessel from the heart, may be so damaged by atherosclerosis that the strength of its wall decreases, causing it to enlarge and form an aneurysm, or a saccular distension. Blood may leak into its wall and beyond, and it may suddenly rupture, causing a massive loss of blood, or it may compress arteries vital to organs, such as the kidneys. Decrease of the effective cross section of blood vessels can be caused by deposition of cholesterol, growth of plaques and calcification, and, not infrequently, occlusion by formation of clots on the plaques. This sequence can occur in the carotid arteries, which are major routes for bringing blood to the brain. Occasionally, small clots can detach and lodge in the brain, causing transient ischemic attacks (TIAs), essentially miniature strokes. Decreased pulsations of the carotid arteries can be felt but tested only one side at a time, and murmurs can often be heard through a stethoscope. In such an event, a physician's attention should be sought. Similar changes can occur in the arteries to the kidneys, but such changes are reflected by the development of hypertension and the accumulation of waste products in the blood.

The coronary vessels supply the blood required by the heart. If they are diseased, the blood flow through them may be adequate at rest but inadequate during exertion. Atherosclerosis of these vessels, occasionally found in young individuals, increases markedly with age. The gradual decrease of the cross section of these vessels by cholesterol deposition causes the breakdown of the continuity of the cellular lining (the endothelium), offering the opportunity for the formation of clots, which may completely block the circulation to an important part of the heart. The precordial sensations of heaviness or the dull ache felt with limitation of blood flow may eventually become severe pain and suggest the death of some muscle tissue, which, if extensive enough, can cause sudden death. When the changes in the blood vessels are more gradual, heart function deteriorates more slowly and, depending on which chamber of the heart is more affected, can lead to different symptoms. The right ventricle pumps blood through the lungs to the left side of the heart. The more dominant features of right-sided failure are swellings of the ankles and legs, sometimes extending to the abdomen because of fluid retention. In left ventricular failure, shortness of breath on exertion or on lying flat (orthopnea) are more prominent symptoms.

Small-vessel disease from atherosclerosis is frequent in diabetes mellitus and can also occur from the deposition of protein-like materials, as in amyloid disease. The decrease of the lumen of the vessels results in increases of blood flow inadequate to meet the demands of exercise. The result is pain in the muscles and the need to rest before continuing the exercise (intermittent claudication). Severe blood flow restriction can result in the death of tissue, gangrene, and the need for amputation. Early and appropriate attention may arrest this deterioration.

Underlying much of these and other cardio-circulatory problems is the tendency for more and more cholesterol to be deposited in the walls of arteries as individuals age. Paying earlier attention to reducing cholesterol intake from the diet and, if necessary, reducing cholesterol synthesis by the liver will increase the chances of reducing the levels of cholesterol in the blood. Those with a family history of early cardiac problems or elevated cholesterol levels may particularly benefit from such preventive measures.

THE GASTROINTESTINAL SYSTEM

One of the more common disorders of gastrointestinal function in the aging process is difficulty in swallowing food and, in some instances, even liquids. This may result from neurological problems with a decreased motility of the esophagus, from obstruction because of scarring from an old injury, from a growth or malignancy, or from psychological problems. In the latter case, the swallowing difficulty is apt to be episodic, while the others are more likely to be unremitting and to increase in severity with time. Ulcers in the stomach, at the pylorus, and in the duodenum are common and may bleed. This can be marked by regurgitation of blood or by black stools. Benign ulcers are often caused by the microorganism Helicobacter pylori (H. pylori), which can be eradicated by appropriate antibiotics, resulting in the cure of the ulcer. In the stomach in particular, malignancies may present as ulcers; in such cases, direct examination of the lesion and a biopsy are essential. More benign disorders can also occur, such as the decrease in acid production and resultant poor digestion. Such disorders may signal the presence of an underlying pernicious anemia.

The gallbladder, which stores bile produced by the liver and discharges it into the gastrointestinal tract and thus aids digestion, can be the site of infections, of stone formation, and, more rarely, of malignancies. Gallbladder attacks, as in acute cholecystitis (inflammation and infection of the gallbladder), more frequent in women but not sparing of men, occur about midlife and later. Symptoms include tenderness and severe pain in the region of the liver that may radiate to the back, chills and fever, and jaundice (if stones have blocked the ducts leading from the gallbladder to the duodenum). Fever suggests an infection. In younger individuals, such symptoms can lead to early diagnosis and intervention. In older individuals, the symptoms and signs may be lacking, and diagnosis may be delayed. Many individuals have stones in their gallbladders and manifest neither symptoms nor disease.

The pancreas, which discharges insulin and bile by way of a common duct into the duodenum, plays an essential role in digestion. Lack of insulin results in diabetes mellitus. The latter disorder occurs frequently in older individuals as adult-onset diabetes (type II) and may require dietary control, the use of agents to lower the blood glucose, or the administration of insulin. Diabetes is often accompanied by circulatory problems because of associated small-vessel disease.

Inflammatory diseases of the small intestine include regional enteritis (Crohn's disease), which occurs mainly in younger people but has significant persistent residual effects from scarring. The large bowel (the colon) can be the site of similar inflammatory changes often referred to as ulcerative colitis, more usual in younger individuals but sometimes requiring colostomies, which can be a problem as the patients age. Quite common in older individuals is diverticulosis, outpocketings of the colon that can become infected and cause diverticulitis, which is occasionally accompanied by perforation and infection of the abdominal cavity. Large-bowel polyps are more frequent with age and may be the site of malignancies. Colon cancer often presents with rectal bleeding in men and obstruction in women. If detected early, the prognosis is excellent.

However, hemorrhoids are probably the most common cause of rectal bleeding.

RESPIRATORY, KIDNEY, AND URINARY PROBLEMS

Cigarette smoking is a major risk factor in diseases of the respiratory tract. Smoking is a major cause of cancers in the nasopharyngeal passages and lungs, usually after many years so that the incidence increases greatly with aging. In addition, the natural decline in respiratory functions from age twenty on is accelerated in smokers and is often associated with chronic obstructive pulmonary disease (COPD) and emphysema. Susceptible individuals who smoke cigarettes may become oxygen-dependent respiratory cripples by age sixty and die within a few years, while nonsmokers may live comfortably to eighty and beyond. Malignancies unrelated to smoking can also occur as individuals age. Periodic medical checkups with respect to pulmonary functions are appropriate, but chest X-rays have not been found to be very effective because their resolution is not sufficient to detect the earliest stages of malignancies. However, new, more effective technologies are being developed.

Kidney function declines with age so that, despite a substantial reserve in youth, the capacity of the kidneys to excrete waste and other products decreases. Adjustments must be made in the dosages of medications excreted by the kidneys, and the blood levels may have to be monitored closely. Excretion of urine, which is mostly water, is not affected unless there is disease of the heart, liver, kidneys, or lower urinary tract. Hypertrophy (enlargement) of the prostate can markedly affect the process of urination (dribbling, decrease in the force of the stream, or urinary retention). The hypertrophy may be benign or the result of a malignancy. Prostate cancer may occur in nearly 80 percent of the male population by the time the age of eighty has been reached. Systematic and regular rectal examinations, along with the prostate-specific antigen (PSA) test, provide the basis for early detection. Surgical procedures, local radiation, and, in case of spread, chemotherapeutic agents can be used, in most cases quite successfully.

Both sexes can develop renal (kidney) stones (calculi), which often produce extraordinary flank pain, requiring narcotics for control. The stones may pass spontaneously or may need to be broken up by ultrasonic radiation (lithotripsy). Surgical intervention is sometimes necessary. The stones can result from metabolic abnormalities or, more usually, from infection; the latter is often not suspected, particularly in older women. The frequency of stones and of urinary tract infections, whether of the bladder or of the kidneys, increases with age, as does urinary incontinence, a cause of major embarrassment to many older individuals.

Chronic infection of the kidneys (pyelonephritis) is often unsuspected but frequent in those who have had lower urinary tract infections (UTIs), incompetent sphincters, or obstruction to the flow of urine, as occurs in prostate enlargement. Small-vessel disease, such as occurs in diabetes mellitus and in lupus, is often associated with hypertension and the appearance of red cells and protein in the urine.

THE CENTRAL NERVOUS SYSTEM

The brain also suffers declines of function with aging. These are often related to a decrease in brain tissue, which can result in a condition called normal-pressure hydrocephalus, in which loss of brain tissue allows more water to accumulate in the brain. The blood flow to the brain may decrease or may not increase during stimulation to the extent seen in younger individuals. Symptoms include memory loss, attention lapses, increased caution in voluntary movements, and prolonged reaction times (of concern while driving). These individuals, in general, continue most of their mental and physical activities, which may serve to maintain the essential blood flow to the brain. Continuation of intellectual activity after retirement may be helpful in slowing the natural decay process.

More disturbing, more profound, and more rapidly progressing are the changes seen in Alzheimer's disease, which causes defects in memory (both recent and remote), difficulty in recognizing errors, reduction in attention span, decrease of coordination, limitations in abilities of self-care and, distressing to all, nonrecognition of close family members. The patient's awareness of the deterioration is not always lost. One estimate is that about one-half of the population over eighty-five has Alzheimer's disease and that a total of nearly 2 million Americans are so affected. The disease occurs more frequently in women than in men and often manifests itself at a younger age. A family history of the disease puts the individual at higher risk than those who do not have such a history. The disease is associated with the occurrence in the brain of neurofibrillary tangles and the deposition of the protein beta amyloid. These abnormalities are under intensive study, and some means have been proposed that may prevent or even reverse their occurrence. Alzheimer's disease, a major problem for its victims, is also a major problem for society because of the costs of the care that must be provided by families or in nursing homes or other institutions.

Among the other major abnormalities of the brain that occur with increasing frequency with age is, in addition to the damage related to carotid artery changes, blockage of blood vessels by clots that form in the brain or that are brought there by the circulation. These produce infarcts, areas without blood flow in which the tissue is dead. Similar damage can be produced by rupture of blood vessels and hemorrhage into the brain substance. Small defects in the walls of cerebral arteries produce aneurysms, which may rupture, particularly when there is hypertension, and become a source of hemorrhages. Small infarcts and hemorrhages may have mainly transient effects, while large ones may lead to strokes, which often cause major losses of control (paralyses), speech (aphasia), or cognition. Death may occur.

Other losses of central nervous system function that occur with age include those of hearing and smell (more common in males). Loss of vision may occur because of cataracts, macular degeneration, and retinal detachment or hemorrhages. The latter frequently occur with uncontrolled hypertension. Parkinson's disease, manifested by uncontrollable tremors and a peculiar, rigid gait, imposes further limitations on physical activities.

MUSCULOSKELETAL PROBLEMS AND OTHER THREATS

Some degree of osteoarthritis occurs in practically all older and aging individuals. Fingers and toes, as well as major joints (such as knees and hips), may be affected. Pain and limitation of motion are common, and analgesics (painkillers) are often necessary. The deformities often limit activities and motion, sometimes severely. Medications and surgical procedures can provide relief from pain and a return to full activity. Osteoporosis (bone loss), which can lead to fractures of long bones and collapse of vertebrae, is most common in postmenopausal women and is largely preventable.

Breast cancer in women and prostate cancer in men remain major problems, in spite of earlier detection and improvements in treatment. Lung cancers in women are increasing in relation to the increase in cigarette smoking. Liver malignancies associated with hepatitis C infections are on the increase and are likely to be a major problem later in life because of the long latent period. Brain tumors, as well as pancreatic and renal carcinomas, increase with increasing life spans, as do skin cancers and leukemias.

Menopause in women and the decrease in sexual performance in men are indicators of decreases of endocrine functions in aging. The thyroid may provide fewer hormones than needed. Because of declines in activity, possibly related to blood flow changes, the endocrine responses to stresses may be blunted, and older individuals may become more vulnerable to environmental stresses. Limited physical abilities may be accompanied by mental impairment and an underlying chronic disease. The need to escape from an overheated environment may not be recognized, and heat stroke may result. Cold, with a drop of body temperature, blunts mentation and slows physical activity. Unprotected older individuals may not recognize and respond to environmental extremes and may not survive situations that are easily tolerated by younger people.

—*Francis P. Chinard*

See also: Alzheimer's disease; Arteriosclerosis; Arthritis; Bone changes and disorders; Brain changes and disorders; Breast cancer; Breast changes and disorders; Cancer; Dementia; Dental disorders; Diabetes; Emphysema; Gastrointestinal changes and disorders; Glaucoma; Gout; Health care; Heart attacks; Heart changes and disorders; Heart disease; Hypertension; Immunizations and boosters; Influenza; Macular degeneration; Medications; Memory loss; Menopause; Multiple sclerosis; Osteoporosis; Parkinson's disease; Pneumonia; Prostate cancer; Prostate enlargement; Respiratory changes and disorders; Sarcopenia; Stones; Strokes; Temperature regulation and sensitivity; Terminal illness; Thyroid disorders; Urinary disorders; Varicose veins; Vision changes and disorders; Weight loss and gain

HOW TO TALK TO SENIORS ABOUT ACCEPTING A DIAGNOSIS

How Do They Feel?

When someone of any age receives a serious diagnosis, it is distressing. For older adults in particular, negative feelings may be exacerbated by preexisting concerns about losing independence, who will take care of them, and being a burden to others. They may be fearful of potential pain or the side effects of treatment. Those with a terminal diagnosis may especially be terrified to face their own mortality. Feeling anxious and alone is common, as is feeling helpless, powerless, shocked, and stressed. Many people are simply overwhelmed by a rollercoaster of emotions that may also include grief, denial, bargaining, anger, and sadness.

Often those diagnosed with a serious illness avoid speaking about it. This may be intended to protect those around them from stress and worry, but it is also a way to avoid coping with the diagnosis themselves. Fear and anxiety may make them avoid seeing a specialist or pursuing medical treatment. A bleak diagnosis might lead them to feel that nothing can be done. On the other hand, it may make them more determined to do everything necessary to have the best chance of recovery.

Sometimes seniors are not in a position to fully understand the extent of the diagnosis. This can be the case when cognitive decline has already progressed. They may express confusion or go through alternating periods of awareness. They might direct angry outbursts at you, the doctor, or others as they lose their sense of control. In some instances, seniors may not be told the full diagnosis if it's determined that it will cause excessive distress. The complexities of their mental and physical health will determine what is shared and how.

How Do I Start The Conversation?

Once you have come to terms with your own emotions and reached a level of acceptance about the diagnosis, you can begin to discuss it with your senior. It remains important that you do your best to not let your understandable fear, sadness, and other negative emotions further overwhelm them. Your conversation requires a framework of love, caring, and support, while providing appropriate information. Your timing will need to be sensitively considered, both in bringing up the diagnosis, in general, and dealing with future plans or lifestyle changes that may be necessary. Take things one step at a time, without bombarding the senior with too many details or suggestions.

It can be helpful to mention further ways to cope with the diagnosis:
- Gain emotional and practical support through consultations with a counselor, therapist, or social worker.
- Ask the doctor any questions that will help gain clarity or comfort.
- Make time for pleasurable activities and relaxation.
- Clear any commitments that might be causing undue stress.
- Socialize with positive people (and eliminate contact with unsupportive or negative people).

It may also be necessary to discuss health-care guidelines provided by the doctor. Let them know you will be there to provide or arrange for help as needed. Be sure that they understand what steps might be necessary to manage the illness:
- Medical treatments
- Physical therapy
- Dietary changes
- Lifestyle changes

Research indicates that people who are able to confront their diagnosis will be in a far better position to devise coping strategies and a plan of action. Conversely, people who are unable to face the emotions associated with finding out about chronic or terminal illness are less likely to develop helpful strategies. By calmly introducing the topic, and perhaps by giving examples of individuals who faced similar circumstances, you can give hope and encouragement. Even in cases of terminal illness, comfort and solace may be offered through examples of how people have reached calmness and a sense of inner peace. Stories about people who have raised awareness of an illness, started foundations, or raised money for research can also be uplifting.

Continued on following page...

> *...continued from previous page*
>
> When talking to your senior about a diagnosis that may already be fraught with emotion, always take care to remain as calm as possible. Do not react aggressively or judgmentally if they are stubborn, angry, or displaying emotions or behaviors you feel to be irrational. Allow their grief to be processed in their own way while providing empathy and support. Let conversations be discussions, not lectures, to encourage positive thinking and healthy coping. Reach out for your own sources of emotional and practical support as you help your senior accept the diagnosis and move forward with treatment.
>
> —*Leah Jacob*

For Further Information

Abrams, W. B., et al., eds. *The Merck Manual of Geriatrics.* 3rd ed. Merck Research Laboratories, 2014. A convenient repository of useful information in an easily handheld format. Accurate and concise.

Bennett, J. C., and F. Plum, eds. *Cecil Textbook of Medicine.* 22nd ed. Elsevier, 2004. One of the several standard textbooks of medicine with excellent sections on geriatric medicine.

Brocklehurst, J. C., et al. *Brocklehurst's Textbook of Geriatric Medicine and Gerontology.* 8th ed., Elsevier, 2017. A thoroughly revised textbook with comprehensive presentations.

Cassel, C. K., et al., eds. *Geriatric Medicine.* 4th ed. Springer, 2003. Easier to read, but not as extensive as most specialized texts on the subject.

Dale, D. C., and D. D. Federman. Scientific American Medicine. *Scientific American*, 2014. A loose-leaf, frequently updated textbook of medicine with several useful, clearly written sections on aging and geriatrics; includes information on dosages of medications in relation to age.

Fauci, A. S., et al., eds. *Harrison's Principles of Internal Medicine.* 20th ed. McGraw-Hill, 2018. Contains several well-documented chapters on aging and associated illnesses.

Hazzard, W. R., et al., eds. *Principles of Geriatric Medicine and Gerontology.* 5th ed. McGraw-Hill, 2003. An excellent and in-depth text.

Wallace, R. B., et al., eds. *Maxcy-Rosenau-Last Public Health and Preventive Medicine.* 15th ed. Appleton & Lange, 2008. Contains several chapters that deal with preventive and public health aspects of geriatrics and aging.

IMMUNIZATIONS. See VACCINES.

IN FULL FLOWER: AGING WOMEN, POWER, AND SEXUALITY (BOOK)

Author: Lois W. Banner

Date: Published in 1992

Relevant Issues: Demographics, economics, marriage and dating, values

Significance: Banner's book examines the ways in which women's sexuality and power have been interconnected with aging from ancient times to the twentieth century.

In Full Flower: Aging Women, Power, and Sexuality was Lois W. Banner's fourth published work. In the introduction, she acknowledges that her inspiration for the book came from her own personal experience with aging and relationships. This inspiration was nurtured by her interest in feminist spirituality and prepatriarchal goddesses. The work's strength and relevance to the present come from her involvement in the fields of women's studies and history. She describes her purpose in writing the book as that of celebrating aging and unconventionality. Throughout *In Full Flower*, Banner examines changes in the way that aging women have viewed themselves and in the way that aging women have been viewed by others from ancient Greek and Roman times to the twentieth century.

The book's title suggests a variation on the typical use of flower imagery to describe women's beauty. Banner suggests an image of aging more aligned with abundance, richness of color and texture, and continued blooming rather than with the loss of beauty or decay, as in the seventeenth century description of menopause as the "end of flowers."

Two topics are interconnected throughout *In Full Flower*: repeating cycles of attitudes toward aging woman, and the incidence of age-disparate relationships or associations between older women and young men. Banner contends that repeating cycles of attitudes toward aging women can be grouped in such a way that periods of freedom are usually followed by periods of repression.

According to Banner, age-disparate relationships and society's attitude toward them are influenced by demographics, economics, beliefs about physiology, and understanding of psychology. To support the demographic argument, she contends that when there are more men than women, younger men seek relationships with older women. From the economic perspective, Banner argues that, historically, young men seem more likely to seek relationships with older women when older women have an increased possibility for accumulated wealth and higher social status. She claims that this was true during the medieval period and suggests that it may have been true again during the last decades of the twentieth century.

Banner discusses the menopause as one of the physiological factors influencing how women are viewed by society. She explains that the menopause has been viewed as providing positive attributes at some times in history, while at other times it has been viewed as providing negative attributes. The impact of psychology on the lives of older women is illustrated by several examples throughout the book, including gender equivalency resulting from widowhood during the late medieval period and the nineteenth century view of older women as being more spiritual than sexual.

Banner acknowledges that most of *In Full Flower* is viewed from the European American perspective. However, she does suggest that exploration of experiences of women of other ethnicities might create new levels of understanding, awareness, and power for all aging women in the United States.

—Janet C. Benavente

See also: Beauty; Menopause; Sexuality; Women and aging

INCONTINENCE

Relevant Issues: Health and medicine
Significance: Incontinence, the inability to control evacuative functions, affects 30 percent of community-dwelling elderly and 53 percent of the home-bound elderly; the condition has important physical, psychological, social, and economic consequences.

Key Terms:
diverticulitis: inflammation of a diverticulum, especially in the colon, causing pain and disturbance of bowel function

prostate enlargement: a common condition as men get older; can cause uncomfortable urinary symptoms, such as blocking the flow of urine out of the bladder; can also cause bladder, urinary tract or kidney problems

sacrum: a triangular bone in the lower back formed from fused vertebrae and situated between the two hipbones of the pelvis; supports the weight of the upper body as it is spread across the pelvis and into the leg

urinalysis: analysis of urine by physical, chemical, and microscopic testing for the presence of disease, drugs, etc.

urinary tract infection: an infection of the kidney, ureter, bladder, or urethra; common symptoms include a frequent urge to urinate and pain or burning when urinating

Urinary incontinence is the second-leading cause of early institutionalization of the elderly and is twice as common in women as in men. According to researchers in 2017, the annual cost in the United States of providing care for community dwelling urinary incontinence sufferers was estimated to be $14 billion, while the cost of providing care for those of the nursing home population was another $6 billion. In 2009, the Society of Urologic Nurses and Associates estimated that 13 million Americans were suffering from urinary incontinence, 85 percent of them female.

A TREATABLE PROBLEM

Less than one-half of the 13 million Americans with urinary incontinence have been evaluated or treated. One of the unanswered questions about urinary incontinence is why, given the high prevalence of incontinence, so few people report it and seek treatment. One reason may be that individuals, believing that incontinence is a normal aging-related condition, believe that they can manage urinary incontinence effectively on their own.

When a person reports such symptoms as urgent, painful, and frequent urination, along with frequent night toileting, many health professionals fail to evaluate the problem because of the myths associated with urinary incontinence and the lack of knowledge regarding solutions. A persistent myth is that urinary incontinence is a normal occurrence of aging often associated with mental incompetence. Inability to control urine is unpleasant and distressing. One major consequence is that untreated incontinence often becomes progressively worse. Secondary problems, such as rashes, decubitus ulcers, and skin and urinary tract infections (UTIs), also may occur. Psychological consequences are common, including embarrassment, loss of self-esteem, social isolation, and even depression.

Studies have demonstrated that as many as 80 percent of urinary incontinent patients can be cured or significantly improved. Even incurable problems can be effectively managed to reduce complications, anxiety, and stress. When treatment is not completely successful, management can help make the problem more livable.

The urinary tract begins with the two kidneys, one on each side of the spinal column, midway in the back. They filter chemical wastes and excess water from the blood. Tiny tubes called ureters connect the kidneys to the bladder, which is located under the pelvic bone. The bladder is like a muscular holding tank that is capable of storing 8 to 16 ounces of urine and, in some cases, much more. The bladder empties to the outside of the body through the urethra. This muscle has sturdy internal and external sphincters that keep the bladder tightly closed until it reaches capacity. When the bladder is full, it sends a signal to the brain. This signal is translated as an urge to urinate. When a cognitively alert person reaches an appropriate place to void, the sphincter muscle is relaxed, the bladder contracts, and urine is released into the urethra.

TYPES OF INCONTINENCE

Urinary incontinence has many definitions. The American Heritage Dictionary defines it as being "incapable of controlling the excretory functions." Taber's Cyclopedic Medical Dictionary (1997) defines it as "the inability to retain urine, semen, or feces because of a loss of sphincter control, or cerebral or spinal lesions." The Agency for Health Care Policy and Research (AHCPR) guidelines define urinary incontinence as an "involuntary loss of urine which is sufficient to be a problem." The four basic types of urinary incontinence are: stress, urge, overflow, and functional.

Stress incontinence is apparent by the involuntary loss of small to moderate amounts of urine when pressure is placed on the pelvic floor, as when one coughs, sneezes, or laughs. It is caused by weak supporting pelvic muscles, estrogen deficiency, and obesity. This form of incontinence is common in women as they age, particularly those who have had several pregnancies, and men who have had prostrate surgery. It may be caused by congenital weakness of the sphincter or acquired after exposure to radiation, trauma, or a sacral cord lesion. It is common to leak continuously or with minimal exertion. Behavioral approaches, such as habit training and pelvic muscle exercises, are useful in improving some stress incontinence; surgery may be needed in some instances.

A sudden loss of moderate to large amounts of urine is characteristic of urge incontinence. Urge incontinence is the most common type, affecting an estimated 65 percent of all cases. It results from irritation or spasms of the bladder wall because of UTIs, prostate enlargement, diverticulitis, or tumors of the bladder or pelvic region. Urge incontinence also may be caused by bladder stones, fecal impaction, stroke, dementia, suprasacral injury, and Parkinson's disease. Highly spiced foods, artificial sweeteners, coffee (including decaffeinated), tea, cola, wine, chocolate, and medicines that contain caffeine may cause bladder irritation. Treatment of infections can correct the problem in some people with this form of incontinence. As the person notes a sudden urge to urinate but is unable to reach the toilet in time, behavioral approaches, such as habit training, prompted voiding, and bladder retraining, can improve continence for some cases.

A failure of the bladder muscles to contract or of the muscles around the urethra to relax causes retention of an excessive amount of urine in the bladder and, consequently, overflow incontinence. The main symptom of overflow incontinence is frequent or constant leaking (dribbling) of small amounts of urine. Bladder neck obstructions from an enlarged prostate, fecal impaction, or urethral stricture can be associated with overflow incontinence. Habit training can be used to completely empty the bladder.

Functional incontinence is caused by factors outside the urinary tract. This occurs when the function of the lower urinary tract is intact but other factors, such as impaired mobility, impaired cognition, and environmental barriers, may result in incontinence. This may be as simple as being unable to get to the bathroom in time because of arthritis. People with cognitive impairments, such as Alzheimer's disease, may be unable to understand the need to void, may be unfamiliar with the location of the bathroom, or may no longer remember the function of the toilet itself.

A THREE-PART EXAMINATION

In order to determine the type of urinary incontinence from which the patient suffers, a comprehensive examination is necessary. The basic evaluation includes three parts: a patient history, a physical examination, and urinalysis. The use of both prescription and nonprescription medications, herbs, and vitamin supplements also may be considered. Close attention is paid to the patient's symptoms and such characteristics as the frequency and timing of continent and incontinent episodes, as well as the amount voided during each episode. These questions can be answered with the help of a voiding diary that is kept for several days, preferably one to two weeks. This diary can provide useful clues to the underlying cause of urinary incontinence and helps gauge the severity of the problem and what treatment options are best.

A complete physical examination often includes an evaluation of the environment and social factors. Important considerations include how far the individual must walk to the toilet or whether he or she understands instructions or has the physical ability to undress well enough to go to the bathroom unassisted. These types of considerations would help with a diagnosis of functional urinary incontinence.

The third part of the examination is the laboratory study of the urine itself. Analysis of the different cells, sediment, color, specific gravity, and presence or absence of bacteria are suggestive of the cause of urinary incontinence. Older adults may have an infection without experiencing the fever, chills, and pain that are common among younger patients. The amount of post-void urine or residual in the bladder is also important to know. This can be tested either by scanning the bladder with a noninvasive pelvic ultrasound or by catheterization, in which a sterile tube is inserted into the bladder to drain it.

MANAGING INCONTINENCE

AHCPR guidelines designate three treatment categories for urinary incontinence: behavioral, pharmacologic, and surgical. The least invasive and least dangerous technique, the behavioral one, is usually tried first. A number of behavioral techniques are available. Habit training is used for urge incontinence. The goal is to get the person to ignore the urge to void and to train the bladder to tolerate larger volumes of urine without urgency. The person is encouraged to gradually and consciously extend the time between voidings. This approach can sometimes be used with cognitively impaired people as well. Like habit training, bladder training also emphasizes scheduled voiding, but it also involves a substantial retraining effort through education and positive reinforcement, using booklets and other teaching aids.

Using exercise to strengthen the pelvic muscles, which are often weakened by childbirth, extreme obesity, or the menopause, is another behavioral technique that can work for women. Kegel exercises involve squeezing and relaxing the pelvic muscles. Squeezing the muscles helps keep the urethra closed until it is time to void. Upon reaching the toilet, a woman can relax the muscles surrounding the urethra and allow it to open. At that point, the bladder contracts and forces urine out through the urethra. Sixty to eighty Kegel exercises daily, done properly, can reduce significantly or even eliminate stress incontinence. Improvement can occur within three weeks to nine months, with most women noting some progress by the end of the eighth week. To make sure women are contracting the right muscle, they are told to constrict the anus as if holding back stool or to try to stop and start the stream while urinating in the toilet. However, doing Kegel exercises routinely during urination can damage the urethra.

Biofeedback helps ensure that the woman is doing the contractions correctly and is a good complement to Kegel exercises. The perineometer, a device used for biofeedback, has a manometer attached to a probe that can be inserted into the vagina. Vaginal cones can also help strengthen the pelvic floor. When one is inserted, wide end first, and it begins to slip out, the pelvic floor contracts to retain it. The woman holds the cone in place for fifteen minutes, twice per day. In time, she will be able to progress to heavier cones. In several studies, approximately 70 percent of the women using the cones reported significant improvement in their stress incontinence. Although the cones work faster than Kegel exercises, some women may be reluctant to use them.

Depending on the type of urinary incontinence, behavioral techniques are not always successful, and the person may need to be referred for pharmacologic treatment. Urge incontinence caused by detrusor muscle instability and stress incontinence caused by urethral sphincter insufficiency may both be helped with medications. In post-hysterectomy or post-menopausal women, stress incontinence may be treated with estrogen replacement therapy.

If pharmacologic treatment is not appropriate, or if it fails, surgery may be recommended. Guidelines state that surgery may be necessary to return the bladder neck to its proper position in women with stress incontinence, to remove tissue that is causing a blockage, to support or replace severely weakened pelvic muscles, or to enlarge a patient with a small bladder to hold more urine. Before undergoing surgery to correct urinary incontinence, the patient should understand the procedure, its risks and benefits, and the expected outcome.

SUPPORTIVE DEVICES
Once all the alternative approaches to resolving incontinence have been explored and exhausted, supportive devices—including intermittent, indwelling, and external (condom) catheters; penile clamps; pessaries; and absorbent pads and undergarments—may be considered.

Performing self-catheterization intermittently may help people with overflow incontinence caused by an inoperable obstruction or other detrusor muscle problems. The caregivers and the involved individual must be both physically and psychologically able to insert a clean catheter tube into the bladder every three to six hours. When done properly, this procedure can be performed at home without any increased risk of infection. Only those with untreatable urinary retention should leave the catheter in place. Using an indwelling catheter for longer than two to four weeks greatly increases the risk of chronic bacteria in the urine and urinary tract infections.

Men may be able to use external collection systems, or condom catheters, which are best for short-term use because of skin irritation. Men with chronic obstruction are advised not to use condom catheters. Urine-collecting devices are also available for women but are not as satisfactory, causing redness and perineal itching. As a temporary solution for males with stress incontinence that is caused by inadequate sphincter contraction, a penile clamp may be an option. The clamp must be removed every three hours to empty the bladder. Improper use can lead to penile and urethral erosion, penile swelling, pain, and obstruction.

Women who have pelvic prolapse with or without urinary incontinence can obtain temporary relief by means of a pessary, a doughnut-shaped rubber or silicone device that is inserted into the vagina. The pessary may help frail, elderly women who have no other treatment options. A specially trained physician or nurse fits and inserts the pessary, then monitors it frequently. A misused or neglected pessary can lead to ulceration of the vagina and fistulas.

There is a growing trend to make use of absorbent pads and pants, largely because urinary incontinence is so often dismissed rather than treated. Although absorbent garments help people feel more secure about their incontinence, the AHCPR recommends that the person's level of disability, preference, gender, and type and severity of incontinence be considered before absorbent products are used. Before choosing a product, the person and caregivers must consider the amount of urine voided per incontinent episode, the type of clothing the person usually wears, manual dexterity, and financial means. Regardless of which absorbent products are chosen, people are advised that they must maintain proper hygiene and change the garment or pad frequently to prevent UTIs and skin problems.

Urinary incontinence affects people of all age groups, especially those in the geriatric population. An overwhelming number are women. In fact, it has been estimated that one-half of all adult women suffer from loss of bladder control at some time in their lives. Yet the number of women and men who fail to seek treatment for urinary incontinence is surprisingly high. Many people think loss of bladder control is a normal part of growing old. Still others think urinary incontinence is just something one must live with. The truth is that urinary incontinence is not caused by aging. Usually, it is brought on by specific changes in the body function that result from infection, hormonal changes, diseases, pregnancy, or the use of certain medications. In most cases, it can be controlled or cured. Left untreated, however, urinary incontinence can make life miserable. It can increase the chance of skin irritation and the risk of developing bedsores, and it often leads to social isolation and personal frustration.

—*Maxine M. McCue*
Updated by Bruce E. Johansen, PhD

See also: Men and aging; Prostate enlargement; Urinary disorders; Women and aging

For Further Information

Emmons, Kevin R., and Joanne P. Robinson. "The Impact of Urinary Incontinence on Older Adults and Their Caregivers." *Journal of Aging Life Care*, Spring 2014. www.aginglifecarejournal.org/the-impact-of-urinary-incontinence-on-older-adults-and-their-caregivers/. This paper reviews the impact of urinary incontinence on the quality of life of older adults and caregivers. Assessment and care considerations are addressed.

Kassai, Kathryn, and Kim Perelli. *The Bathroom Key: Put an End to Incontinence.* Demos Health, 2012. A treatment plan for women to cure their own incontinence issues. It allows women to identify with other women through anecdotal stories that echo feelings of isolation and embarrassment. Written in easy-to-understand language, this book is a genuine teaching tool, guiding the reader to a better understanding of her body and effective remedies.

MacLachlan, Lara S., and Eric S. Rovner. "New Treatments for Incontinence." *Advances in Chronic Kidney Disease*, vol. 22, no. 4, July 2015, pp. 279-88. doi:10.1053/j.ackd.2015.03.003. This review highlights the existing treatment of stress, urge, mixed, and overflow urinary incontinence in adult men and women and discusses many of the novel treatments including potential future or emerging therapies.

Thirugnanasothy, S. "Managing Urinary Incontinence in Older People." *BMJ*, vol. 341, 9 Aug. 2010, p. c3835. doi:10.1136/bmj.c3835. Discusses different management and prevention techniques to avoid incontinence.

"Urinary Incontinence." MedlinePlus, U.S. National Library of Medicine, 9 Aug. 2016. medlineplus.gov/urinaryincontinence.html. The National Library of Medicine's collection of information on urinary incontinence, treatments, clinical trials, resources, and so on.

"Urinary Incontinence in Older Adults." National Institute on Aging, U.S. Department of Health and Human Services, 16 May 2017. www.nia.nih.gov/health/urinary-incontinence-older-adults. Explains types and causes of urinary incontinence, treatment and management of the disorder, as well as the link between Alzheimer's disease and urinary incontinence.

INDIVIDUAL RETIREMENT ACCOUNTS (IRAs)

Relevant Issues: Economics, work

Significance: Individual retirement accounts (IRAs) can help provide a more comfortable and secure financial future for aging Americans.

The Employee Retirement Income Security Act (ERISA) of 1974 was enacted to protect employee pension rights. It specified certain conditions that a pension plan in the private sector must meet and also made some provision for workers whose employers did not have pension plans. These individuals were encouraged to save for retirement by opening individual retirement accounts (IRAs), which provided tax-sheltered retirement savings. For federal tax purposes, taxpayers could deduct the annual amount deposited to the IRA from their gross incomes for the year. Income tax would be deferred on the deposit and on the earnings of the account until withdrawal. The popularity of this retirement vehicle lies in its simplicity and its benefits.

Under President Ronald Reagan's 1981 tax revisions, the rules were changed to allow any person to open an IRA. Withdrawals before the age of fifty-nine years and six months became generally subject to a penalty tax of 10 percent, and withdrawals had to begin when the account holder reached the age of seventy years and six months. The Tax Reform Act of 1986 limited tax deferrals on IRA contributions to those whose incomes fell below $25,000 for single people and $40,000 for married couples filing joint income-tax returns.

Individuals may establish an IRA account with tax-deferred contributions of $2,000 annually. For an individual with a nonworking spouse who files a joint return, $2,250 may be contributed to an IRA, and this money can be split into two different IRA accounts, one for each spouse. The only stipulation is that the amount contributed to any one account may not exceed $2,000. Any individual covered under another retirement plan is not permitted tax deferrals on the contributions. However, all earnings in the IRA are tax-deferred.

Almost any debt or equity security can be held by the IRA. However, investment brokers and firms typically do not recommend investment in speculative stocks, bonds, or aggressive mutual funds. IRA contributions may not be invested in collectibles, including coins, stamps, rugs, or artwork, with the exception of new gold and silver coins that are issued by the United States government. If any part of an IRA is used to purchase collectibles, that amount is immediately taxed as a premature distribution.

If after reaching the age of seventy years and six months, an individual does not withdraw a sufficient amount annually from an IRA, the Internal Revenue Service (IRS) levies a 50 percent tax on the insufficient withdrawal. The IRS does not want older people leaving their money in an IRA that earns tax-deferred savings. As at the age of seventy years and six months a man has a life expectancy of twelve years, the IRS requires that one-twelfth of the IRA be withdrawn.

When it comes time for payout, there are two choices. The one almost always chosen is a monthly payout. The individual only pays tax on the annual IRA payout, which is taxed as ordinary income. The alternative is a lump sum payout. However, the IRS taxes the entire lump sum distribution at that time as ordinary income.

In 1998, the federal government introduced a new form of IRA, the Roth IRA. This variant allowed individuals to make contributions out of after tax dollars (rather than having taxes deferred, as in conventional IRAs), but with all distributions from the accounts being free of taxation; that is, all earnings would be tax-free even though the initial contribution had been taxed. In addition, these accounts have no minimum required distribution and no maximum age at which contributions can be made. Individuals can make a total of $2,000 in qualified contributions to the two types of IRA in each calendar year. The law allowed for "rollovers" of traditional IRAs into the new Roth IRAs.

—*Alvin K. Benson*

See also: Employment; 401(k) plans; Pensions; Retirement; Retirement planning

For Further Information

Anspach, Dana. "IRA Withdrawal Rules." *Balance*, July 2019. This e-periodical reviews the rules for withdrawals that apply before you reach retirement age, and others for when you're ready to retire.

Daugherty, Greg. "Converting Traditional IRA Savings to a Roth IRA." *Investopedia*, June 2019. This e-periodical explores the advantages of Roth IRAs versus traditional IRAs, and when you should consider converting from one to the other.

Maeda, Martha. *The Complete Guide to IRAs & IRA Investing.* Atlantic Publishing Group, 2014. As more and more baby boomers reach retirement age, and because retirement seems to come at an earlier age, this book provides information about the importance of saving for your nonworking years, which has become increasingly apparent.

———. *The Complete Guide to IRAs & IRA Investing: Wealth Building Strategies Revealed.* Atlantic Publishing Group, 2013. Many people find themselves worrying that they will not be able to maintain their current life style once they retire. Strategies provided in this book will help you turn your IRA into a wealth-building tool. It also outlines how to take control of your investment future and make sure your investments are performing for you.

INFERTILITY

Relevant Issues: Biology, health and medicine, marriage and dating

Significance: Aging is accompanied by a progressive decline in the reproductive production of gametes, particularly in women during menopause, but also in men because of various physiological processes.

Key Terms:

diploid cells: cells that contain two sets of chromosomes

haploid cells: cells that have half the usual number of chromosomes

meiosis: a type of cell division that results in four daughter cells each with half the number of chromosomes of the parent cell, as in the production of gametes

oogenesis: the production or development of an ovum

spermatogenesis: the production or development of mature spermatozoa

As people age, their cells accumulate damage. Although reproductive cells receive greater protection, at least for a time, these germ-line cells ultimately succumb to age-related damage as well, thereby contributing to infertility. The term "infertility" refers to the inability of a couple to conceive a child after at least one year of frequent, unprotected sexual activity together. The lack of fertility can exist in the reproductive physiology of the man, the woman, or both.

Infertility is often confused with the term "impotence," the failure of the male penis to achieve or maintain erection for sexual intercourse. Whereas impotence certainly contributes to infertility and is caused by many of the same factors, infertility may involve many different problems with the male and female reproductive physiologies or anatomies that ultimately prevent the fusion of sperm and egg to form a new individual.

GAMETOGENESIS
Eggs in the female ovaries and sperm in the male testicles are formed by a common process called meiosis, or reduction division. Adult somatic cells (all of the cells of the body except the germ-line cells) are diploid, meaning that they have two copies of each chromosome per cell. Germ-line cells (sperm and egg cells) are haploid, meaning that they have one copy of each chromosome per cell. In humans, the diploid chromosome number in the somatic cells is forty-six, or a pair for each of twenty-three chromosomes. Prior to meiosis in germ-line cells, the deoxyribonucleic acid (DNA) of every chromosome is copied, doubling the chromosome number to ninety-two. When meiosis occurs, this single cell proceeds through a series of two meiotic divisions to yield four haploid cells, each containing twenty-three chromosomes.

In the female ovary, one of every four haploid cells produced by meiosis actually becomes an egg. The other three cells degenerate. Egg-producing meiosis is called oogenesis, and through this process an average woman produces about five hundred mature eggs in her lifetime. A woman's eggs begin meiosis in her ovaries while she is still a fetus. The eggs are maintained in a suspended, meiotic state for several decades. Then, beginning at puberty, one meiotic cycle is completed and one egg becomes ready for possible fertilization during each lunar cycle (about twenty-eight days). These monthly cycles, which include menstruation, continue until menopause (usually by the age of fifty to fifty-five), when the cycles stop permanently.

In the male testicle, sperm are produced continuously throughout the man's life, beginning at puberty. All four haploid cells from each cycle of meiosis become fully functional sperm by a process called spermatogenesis. Beyond meiosis, this process compacts each cell, which grows a mitochondrion-rich midpiece for energy production and a long flagellum for propulsion of the sperm. A man's two testicles can produce over one hundred million sperm in just a few days. Sperm production can be maintained at relatively high levels even into later life, although the numbers of sperm decline steadily past age fifty. Furthermore, average worldwide male sperm production across the life span appears to have declined since the 1950s, likely due to environmental exposure to industrial chemicals.

The meiotic halving of the chromosome number from forty-six to twenty-three in oogenesis and in spermatogenesis has one critical goal: sexual reproduction, in which one haploid sperm carrying twenty-three chromosomes fuses with one haploid egg carrying twenty-three chromosomes. The resulting diploid cell, called a zygote, with forty-six chromosomes, will give rise to all the adult somatic cells of a new individual person.

FEMALE PHYSIOLOGY AND INFERTILITY
Among the major contributors to female infertility are tumors of the reproductive tract, hormonal imbalances, reproductive tract inflammation (pelvic inflammatory disease, PID), ovulation irregularities, increased cervical mucus, persistent infections and sexually transmitted diseases, menopause, and exposure to certain drugs and environmental chemicals.

The woman's reproductive tract contains two ovaries, each surrounded by an ovarian follicle where one egg completes meiosis about halfway through each menstrual cycle. Under the influence of hormones secreted by the pituitary gland, the follicle completes an egg's oogenesis and then ruptures to release the mature egg into the Fallopian tube. The egg is moved slowly down the few inches of the Fallopian tube by tiny hair-like cilia over the course of several days. The egg has a life span of about two days, after which it will die if it is not fertilized. If sexual intercourse occurs and a sperm fertilizes the egg in the Fallopian tube, the resulting zygote begins dividing and implants itself in the endometrium, the nerve- and blood-rich lining of the uterus. The early embryo then releases human chorionic gonadotropin (hCG), a hormone that stimulates the mother's ovaries to produce the steroid hormone progesterone, whose critical function is to maintain the thick endometrial lining to support the embryo and to maintain the pregnancy. If the egg is not fertilized or if the ovaries do not produce enough progesterone, the endometrium and its contents will be discharged out of the woman's vagina; she will experience menstrual bleeding, and her body will then reset a new cycle to prepare another egg.

Tumors, including both benign cysts and malignant cancers, of the Fallopian tubes and uterus can block both egg and sperm transport, thus causing infertility. Such blockages can be detected by a special X-ray analysis called uterosalpingography (HSG).

Hormonal imbalances in the woman's endocrine glands, particularly the pituitary gland and the hypothalamus in the brain, can cause infertility. The pituitary gland releases follicle-stimulating hormone (FSH) and luteinizing hormone (LH), which are essential for egg preparation and release during the menstrual cycle. The hypothalamus controls bodily rhythms and many endocrine glands, including the pituitary. The ovaries produce the steroid hormones estrogen and progesterone, which make a pregnancy possible by building and maintaining the endometrium. Imbalances in any of these hormones would make conception or the maintenance of a pregnancy impossible.

Inflammation of the endometrium, Fallopian tubes, or the presence of pelvic inflammatory disease (PID), a condition characterized by pain and severe discomfort in the lower abdominal-pelvic region of the body, can impede both egg and sperm movement. Ovulation irregularities can disrupt or inhibit egg release and can result from a variety of factors, including psychological stress, hormonal imbalances, and exposure to certain drugs and environmental chemicals. Increased mucus and acidic secretions in the cervix and vagina can slow or kill many sperm, decreasing the probability of conception.

Infections of the female reproductive tract, especially sexually transmitted diseases, can cause infertility and even permanent sterility. Bacteria (such as Escherichia coli, a normal inhabitant of the large intestine) and yeast (such as Candida albicans) can irritate and inflame the vagina and other parts of the female reproductive tract. Both of the sexually transmitted bacteria Chlamydia trachomatis and Neisseria gonorrhoeae can cause PID. Both chlamydia and gonorrhea can inflame the Fallopian tubes, creating difficulty in achieving conception. Untreated gonorrhea can cause severe accumulation of fallopian scar tissue (mimicking PID) that may permanently block the tubes, resulting in sterility. Among sexually transmitted viruses, herpes simplex II, or genital herpes, affects about one out of every five Americans and may contribute to both cervical cancer and sterility. Many individuals infected with genital herpes are unaware of their infection, and the sores in the reproductive tract are highly contagious.

Menopause is the permanent shutdown of the ovaries, usually occurring between ages fifty and fifty-five in most women. This follows several years of perimenopause during which menstrual cycles become irregular and egg production may be skipped, making conception not possible during those months. Decreasing bodily estrogen levels following menopause can cause loss of sexual desire in many, but not all, women (in some it may actually increase, leading to added anxiety about fertility). The menstrual cycles eventually end altogether, and the linings of the uterus and vagina become drier, shrinking because of the lack of hormonal stimulation from the pituitary gland and the ovaries. Menopause can sometimes occur prematurely before the age of forty, but this is a fairly rare cause of infertility. Surgical menopause—the removal of the ovaries for any reason—will cause immediate infertility because there are no eggs for ovulation.

A somewhat lesser known area of infertility understanding is the link between prior elective abortions and infertility. It is well established that women who have had multiple voluntary abortions (perhaps as a means of birth control) have a significantly higher incidence of later infertility, likely due to scarring of the endometrial tissue caused by the abortion procedure. There does not appear to be such a link for those with multiple spontaneous miscarriages, although the cause of those miscarriages may also be an underlying cause for later infertility.

Finally, drugs and environmental chemicals that can cause infertility include organic solvents, such as benzene, toluene, and xylene; pharmaceuticals, such as alkylating agents, cimetidine, diethylstilbestrol, and salicylazosulfapyridine; metals, such as boron, cadmium, lead, and mercury; marijuana; methamphetamines; alcohol; and tobacco. The heavy use of insecticides on food crops, exposure to chemicals in the daily environment, and improper use of medications can increase the chances of infertility. These drugs and chemicals have similar effects upon the male reproductive system.

MALE PHYSIOLOGY AND INFERTILITY

Major contributors to female infertility that also contribute to male infertility include hormonal imbalances of the hypothalamus and pituitary glands, tumors of the reproductive tract, drugs and environmental chemicals, and infectious and sexually transmitted diseases. Infertility factors that are unique to male physiology include abnormal sperm development, autoimmune diseases, damage to the testicles, and the effect of wearing tight-fitting clothing around the scrotum.

A major feature of the male reproductive system is the descent of the two testicles out of the pelvic cavity into the scrotum, a pouch of skin located immediately posterior to the man's penis. This anatomical arrangement is critical to sperm survival because the scrotum keeps the sperm at a temperature about 3 to 4 degrees Celsius cooler than body temperature (37 degrees Celsius), which would kill the sperm. Surrounding each testicle is the epididymis, a follicle-like structure that can store hundreds of millions of sperm. Within the epididymis, specialized nurse cells surround and protect the sperm from attack by the man's own immune system cells.

During sexual intercourse and ejaculation, over one hundred million sperm are rapidly forced from the two epididymi into the vas deferens, two tubes several inches long that coil up into the pelvic cavity and then down to meet at the urethra. In this region, the seminal vesicle, the bulbourethral gland, and the prostate gland release sugar-rich semen to the sperm. The semen protects the sperm and supplies sugar to the sperm mitochondria for propulsion of their flagella (tail). The sperm-semen ejaculate exits the man's erect penis through the urethra.

Hormonal imbalances in the hypothalamus or in the pituitary gland hormones can lead to underdeveloped testicles or low sperm count. Simultaneously, low testosterone production by the testicles would inhibit sperm production as well. Tumors, both benign and malignant, can block sperm flow or affect critical production sites. Testicular cancer severely reduces sperm production. Likewise, prostate cancer affects semen production, shutting off the supply of energy for the sperm. Surgery for prostate cancer can also lead to erectile dysfunction, also known as male impotence. Furthermore, chemotherapy and radiation therapy kill sperm.

Drugs and environmental chemicals that generate infertility in the female reproductive system also can make men infertile. Sexually transmitted gonorrhea can make men sterile. The herpes simplex II virus can produce pus in the urethral tract, which comes from painful sores in the tract. These sores, which can spread the virus to a sexual partner, make urination and erection difficult.

Abnormal sperm development, termed germ-cell dysplasia, in the testicle can produce sperm that are too large, have abnormal heads, have abnormal flagella, or have multiple flagella. Such sperm have considerable motility problems and never reach the egg during intercourse. Autoimmune disorders can damage and destroy many sperm when hyperactive immune-system cells penetrate the protective nurse cells and attack the sperm. Injuries to the testicles caused by severe blows, disease, or surgery can seriously impair the production of sperm. Also, wearing tight clothing can hold the testicles closer to body temperature, thus killing many sperm.

In all men, sperm production decreases with age, up to 3.3 percent per year according to some studies. As sperm concentrations decline, the probability of sperm reaching the point of conception in the Fallopian tube decreases, leading to increased incidences of infertility.

Finally, new studies on the effect of alcohol consumption in males indicate interference with functioning of the hypothalamus and pituitary, as well as with the testes, leading to infertility, impotence, and reduced sexual characteristics.

TREATING INFERTILITY

Infertility can be a serious emotional issue for couples desiring to have children. A variety of unpredictable, uncontrollable factors in either or both partners may cause infertility. Facing the reality of infertility involves each partner working with the other and with a fertility specialist, who may suggest several techniques for addressing the condition. Older couples may find discussing sexual matters with a physician to be difficult. However, the basic human sexual drive is important to humans, and most physicians are prepared to work with couples facing infertility.

Several assisted reproduction techniques may be used to help couples conceive. When a woman is infertile, a willing surrogate mother can be artificially inseminated with her mate's donated sperm, carry the child to birth, and then give up the child to the couple. There are occasional legal problems with this approach when the surrogate mother wishes to keep the child. With improving technology, an embryo transfer procedure from the surrogate mother to the infertile woman's uterus may help to alleviate these problems in the future.

When the man is infertile, the woman can be artificially inseminated with sperm from an anonymous donor male. This widespread procedure relies upon the ease of freezing donated sperm in sperm banks for long periods of time. In the case of male impotence, certain medications, such as Viagra, are promising treatments for erectile dysfunction.

A difficult but increasingly popular procedure is in vitro fertilization (IVF), in which injected hormones are used to hyperstimulate a woman's ovaries to develop and release eggs. The eggs are collected from the woman's ovary by an instrument called a laparoscope, fertilized by the man's sperm in a culture dish, allowed to grow and divide, and then surgically implanted into the woman's uterus. A modification of this procedure called gamete intrafallopian transfer (GIFT) involves using the laparoscope to reinsert the artificially fertilized eggs into the Fallopian tube for natural passage and implantation into the uterus.

Finally, many infertile couples choose adoption. Even with the strict confidentiality involved in this approach, legal cases exist in which the biological parents have wished to reclaim the children that they had previously put up for adoption. Nevertheless, adoption is a humane, popular option that has been chosen by tens of thousands of infertile couples.

—*David W. Hollar, Jr.*
Updated by Kerry Cheesman, PhD and Maryann Cheesman, RN

See also: Biological clock; Childlessness; Men and aging; Menopause; Parenthood; Prostate cancer; Reproductive changes, disabilities, and dysfunctions; Sexual dysfunction; Sexuality; Women and aging

For Further Information

Domar, Alice. *Conquering Infertility.* Penguin Books, 2002. Tools you need to stay positive and avoid depression and anxiety.

Russell, Shane T. *Male Infertility Guide for Couples.* Male Fertility P, LLC, 2015. How to manage low sperm counts, unexplained infertility, and IVF failure.

Starr, Cecie, and Ralph Taggart. *Biology: The Unity and Diversity of Life.* 15th ed. Wadsworth, 2018. This popular, comprehensive introductory biology textbook includes two chapters on reproduction and development, as well as detailed information on sexually transmitted diseases and agents that affect fertility.

Weschler, Toni. *Taking Charge of Your Fertility, 20th Anniversary Edition.* Harper Collins, 2015. How fertility works and how to gain control over your body. Written by a female educator.

INFLUENZA

Relevant Issues: Health and medicine

Significance: Influenza is a common illness that annually causes a significant number of deaths among the elderly; effective prevention and treatment methods are underutilized.

Influenza is a respiratory infection caused by the influenza virus. Although many viral illnesses are commonly referred to as influenza, or "the flu," true influenza has a characteristic set of symptoms. Influenza is characterized by muscle aches (myalgias), fever (up to 39.4 degrees Celsius or 103 degrees Fahrenheit), cough, pain behind the eyes, sore throat, and headache. Gastrointestinal symptoms such as nausea or diarrhea are generally not associated with true influenza. Periods of weakness and depression may be associated with influenza, and bacterial pneumonia may follow it. Influenza usually lasts from three to seven days, and most cases in the United States occur from late December through March.

CAUSE AND SPREAD

The term "influenza" was derived four hundred years ago from an Italian word for "influenced by the stars." This term was coined because of the seasonality of influenza; it was thought that influenza epidemics were influenced by the alignments of certain stars and planets. The influenza virus is spread via exhaled droplets or hand-to-hand contact. There are three strains of influenza viruses: A, B, and C. Strains A and B account for the majority of cases of severe influenza; strain C usually produces a mild form of the disease. Influenza can be deadly. It causes thousands of deaths annually in the United States, primarily among the elderly and people with chronic illnesses.

A drastic change in the structure of the influenza virus can cause a widespread outbreak, called a pandemic. The most-famous influenza pandemic was the Spanish flu of 1918-1919, which killed about twenty-two million people worldwide. Other worldwide influenza outbreaks include the Asian flu of 1957 and the Hong Kong flu of 1968. Influenza can also be found in other animals, including birds and pigs. In 1976, an outbreak of a virus found in pigs which was similar to the deadly Spanish flu virus caused U.S. health officials to vaccinate people against the "swine flu" virus. After several vaccine recipients contracted a rare nerve disorder called Guillain-Barré syndrome, the 1976 vaccine program was canceled and the feared "swine flu" pandemic never materialized. More recently in 2009, however, a strain of influenza known as H1N1 did become pandemic and resulted in approximately 12,000 deaths and nearly 300,000 hospitalizations in the United States alone. This strain, also stylized by media as "swine flu," was a new version of the same virus that led to the 1918 outbreak and constituted a major public health emergency.

PREVENTION AND TREATMENT

Prevention of influenza includes appropriate use of an influenza vaccine, good handwashing techniques, and cough control to prevent the spread of the virus via aerosol droplets. A bout of influenza confers temporary immunity, but only against the specific virus that caused the infection. An influenza vaccine is usually effective in providing immunity for six months or longer. However, the A and B strains of the influenza viruses undergo periodic changes in their genetic structure, which leads to variability in seasonal effectiveness and requires annual updates to the influenza vaccine (flu shot).

Annually, manufacturers develop vaccines to protect against the three types of influenza most likely to be found during the current "flu season." The vaccine is routinely recommended for all individuals at least 6 months old who are medically able to receive the vaccine. In the case of emergency shortage, further emphasis is placed on the vaccination of those at greatest risk of death during an influenza outbreak. These high-risk groups include the elderly (50 years), the young (years), women who may become

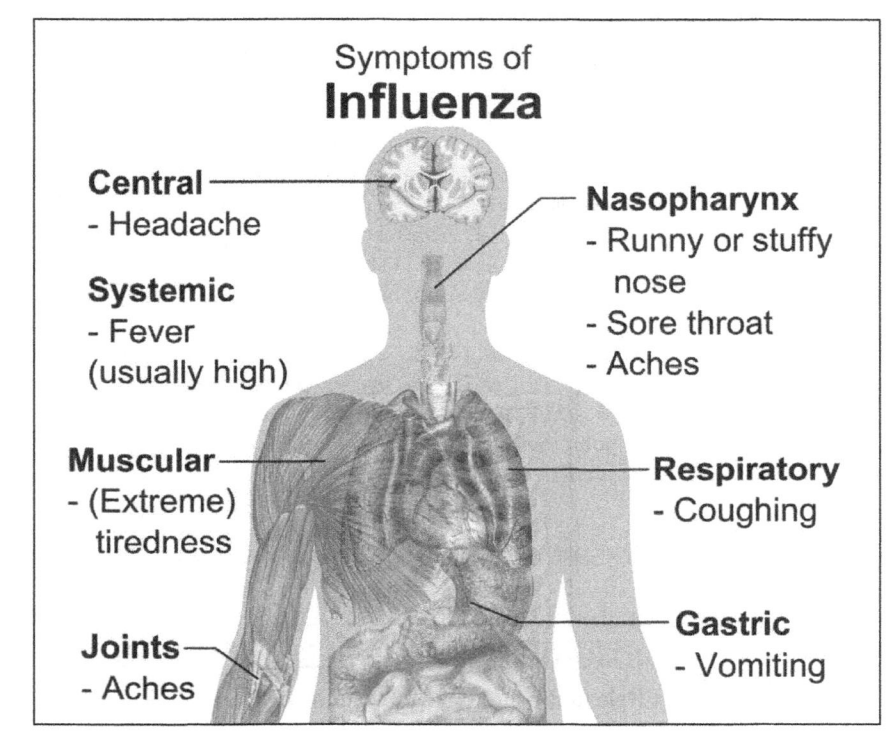

Symptoms of Influenza

Central
- Headache

Systemic
- Fever (usually high)

Muscular
- (Extreme) tiredness

Joints
- Aches

Nasopharynx
- Runny or stuffy nose
- Sore throat
- Aches

Respiratory
- Coughing

Gastric
- Vomiting

pregnant during flu season, residents of long-term care facilities, individuals who are immunocompromised, health-care providers, and emergency medical responders such as police, fire, and EMS personnel.

Influenza vaccine generally becomes available in every October or November, confers immunity within two weeks, and can be given any time during the flu season. Side effects, which are relatively uncommon, are usually mild fever and mild muscle aches. Even though the influenza vaccine and associated medications could prevent hundreds or thousands of deaths in the United States each year, it is estimated that fewer than 50 percent of the susceptible population is protected by either vaccine or medication.

For individuals with flu symptoms or "influenza-like illness" treatment includes proper amounts of fluids, analgesics for pain relief, and bed rest. For those with confirmed cases of influenza or known exposure, some antivirals, including oseltamivir, may be used within the first 48 hours for treatment or prevention. While antivirals including oseltamivir have been shown to reduce severity and duration of illness in some individuals, administration may be associated with side effects including nausea, vomiting, or headache.

In some cases, individuals may develop a secondary bacterial pneumonia after resolution of the original influenza infection. In the most severe cases, individuals may develop acute respiratory distress syndrome or other complications that may necessitate inpatient or critical care management in the hospital.

—*Paul M. Paulman*
Updated by Thomas J. Martin, MS II

See also: Health care; Hospitalization; Illnesses among older adults; Vaccines

For Further Information

"2009 H1N1 Flu ('Swine Flu') and You." CDC, Centers for Disease Control and Prevention, 10 Feb. 2010. www.cdc.gov/h1n1flu/qa.htm. The CDC's collected information on the 2009 H1N1 pandemic.

Andrew, Melissa K, et al. "The Importance of Frailty in the Assessment of Influenza Vaccine Effectiveness against Influenza-Related Hospitalization in Elderly People." *The Journal of Infectious Diseases*, vol. 216, no. 4, 2017, pp. 405-14. doi:10.1093/infdis/jix282. Studies vaccine effectiveness against influenza hospitalization in older adults, focusing on the impact of frailty.

Dunkle, Lisa M., et al. "Efficacy of Recombinant Influenza Vaccine in Adults 50 Years of Age or Older." *New England Journal of Medicine*, vol. 376, no. 25, 22 June 2017, pp. 2,427—436. doi:10.1056/nejmoa1608862. This trial compares the protective efficacy in older adults of a quadrivalent, recombinant influenza vaccine (RIV4) with a standard-dose, egg-grown, quadrivalent, inactivated influenza vaccine (IIV4).

Grohskopf, Lisa A., et al. "Prevention and Control of Seasonal Influenza with Vaccines: Recommendations of the Advisory Committee on Immunization Practices-United States, 2018-19 Influenza Season." *MMWR. Recommendations and Reports: Morbidity and Mortality Weekly Report.* Recommendations and Reports / Centers for Disease Control, vol. 67, no. 3, Aug. 2018, pp. 1-20. These updated guidelines provide current recommendations for vaccination against influenza in the United States and include guidance on special issues including egg allergy.

"People 65 Years and Older & Influenza." CDC, Centers for Disease Control and Prevention, 21 Feb. 2019. www.cdc.gov/flu/highrisk/65over.htm. A collection of information for seniors about influenza, including causes, symptoms, and vaccine information.

Shobugawa, Yugo, et al. "Social Participation and Risk of Influenza Infection in Older Adults: a Cross-Sectional Study." *BMJ Open*, vol. 8, no. 1, Jan. 2018. doi:10.1136/bmjopen-2017-016876. This study examines the association between social participation and influenza infection in Japanese adults aged 65 years or older.

Uyeki, Timothy M., et al. "Clinical Practice Guidelines by the Infectious Diseases Society of America: 2018 Update on Diagnosis, Treatment, Chemoprophylaxis, and Institutional Outbreak Management of Seasonal Influenza." *Clinical Infectious Diseases: An Official Publication of the Infectious Diseases Society of America*, vol. 68, no. 6, Mar. 2019, pp. e1-47. This resource provides updated guidelines from the Infectious Diseases Society of America (IDSA) on the diagnosis, treatment, and chemoprophylaxis of influenza.

Van Hartesveldt, Fred R., ed. *The 1918-1919 Pandemic of Influenza: The Urban Impact on the Western World.* E. Mellen P, 1992. This resource provides a historical viewpoint on the impact of the 1918-1919 "Spanish Flu" pandemic.

INHERITANCE. *See* ESTATES AND INHERITANCE

INJURIES AMONG OLDER ADULTS

Relevant Issues: Health and medicine

Significance: As people age, they tend to become more prone to injuries; such injuries often constitute a threat to the elderly person's health and functional abilities.

Accidents are the seventh leading cause of death in people over the age of sixty-five and the fifth leading cause of death in those over the age of eighty-five. When such accidents do not result in death, they may lead to serious threats to the person's health and functional abilities. Because elderly people often fear a recurrence of injury, accidents may cause a decrease in physical and social activity, as well as a loss of confidence.

INJURIES FROM FALLING

Falls are the most frequent cause of injury among the elderly. Those people over eighty years of age have a mortality rate from falls eight times greater than people sixty years of age. Falls are the major risk factor for hip fractures; elderly people who suffer from osteoporosis have a greater chance of sustaining fractures of the hips, wrist, pelvis, lumbar vertebra, and ribs. Approximately 200,000 hip fractures occur each year in the United States, 12 to 20 percent of which lead to death. Only one-fourth of older adults who sustain a hip fracture fully recover. Following hip fracture, the elderly often face decreased mobility secondary to primary injury or operative management. The resultant immobility alone or in combination with concomitant rib fracture often predispose the elderly to decreased inspiratory volumes, atelectasis, and development of pneumonia. The presence of these factors greatly contributes to increased mortality following falls. The loss of skin elasticity and subcutaneous tissue that generally accompanies aging can also lead to bruising and skin tears, and contribute to development of pressure ulcers with prolonged downtime following falls.

Although most falls occur when a person is descending a stairway, they may be caused by numerous factors in the home, including unstable furniture, loose floor coverings, poor lighting in hallways and bathrooms, clutter, pets, and slick substances on the floor, such as polish, ice, water, or grease. The use of certain medications may also cause the elderly to fall. Some diuretics, sedatives, antibiotics, antidepressants, and antipsychotics can cause drowsiness, confusion, or dizziness. Physical changes that accompany the aging process can also make people more susceptible to sustaining injuries from falls. Vision and hearing may become impaired, leading to changes in perception. Reflexes may become slower. Vertigo and syncope episodes may cause falls. Mental changes, such as depression and inattention, can also cause falls in the elderly.

Medical experts advise elderly people to take precautions against falls. People who do not have good balance are often advised to wear shoes with a soft sole and a low, broad heel. High heels, loose-fitting slippers, or socks without shoes on stairs or waxed floors should be avoided. In addition, tennis shoes that have good traction can cause people to trip. Elderly people with poor night vision can use bedside lamps or night-lights in case they have to get up in the middle of the night. Those prone to dizziness are advised to stand up slowly to avoid vertigo. Keeping the thermostat at 65 degrees Fahrenheit or above at night can help people avoid the drowsiness that tends to accompany prolonged exposure to cold temperatures.

Another way to prevent falls is to keep walkways free of clutter and to keep electrical and phone cords out of the way. Low furniture can be positioned so it is not an obstacle to people when walking. White paint or white strips on the edges of steps can help elderly people see them better. The risk of falls in the kitchen can be minimized by placing frequently used items in accessible cupboards to avoid reaching, bending, or stooping, and by covering tile or linoleum floors with nonskid wax. In the bathroom, grab bars can be installed on the wall by the tub, shower, and toilet, while nonskid mats or adhesive strips can be placed on all surfaces that can get wet and slippery.

Exercise can also help minimize the risk of injury from falls. Such activities as walking, gardening, and housework can improve gait, posture, and balance. Weight-bearing exercise, such as walking, helps prevent loss of bone mass, as well as stiffness and loss of muscle tone. Lifting small weights can prevent loss of muscle tone and help strengthen hand grip, both of which are important for holding on to railings and properly executing such tasks as getting up from chairs.

Elderly people who fear falling may decrease their activity level, which causes their muscles to deteriorate even more. The fear of falling can also make them clinically depressed, which often shortens their attention span and makes them more likely to fall. This is especially true if they have fallen before and have sustained an injury or fracture.

POISONING AND CHOKING
Decreases in visual acuity may make some elderly people susceptible to taking poison that might be on a shelf or in the medicine cabinet, especially the wrong medication. Because of the poor eyesight, they may use something in their eyes for eye drop medication when in reality it is some other type of fluid that can damage the eyes or cause blindness.

Decreases in the sense of smell and taste may lead people to eat spoiled food or inhale toxic fumes from substances in the home. Decreased gag and swallowing reflex may lead to choking, which can be fatal for someone who lives alone and dies before help arrives. Poorly fitted dentures, poor dental hygiene, or other factors that make chewing difficult may also increase the risk of choking.

BURNS AND INJURIES FROM EXTREME HEAT AND COLD
Burns account for 8 percent of the accidental deaths among the elderly. Burn injuries are most commonly caused by scalds from hot baths, showers, or fluids on the stove; flames from the ignition of clothing or flammable liquids; and house fires. A large percentage of fires started by elderly people are caused by the use of electrical equipment for cooking and heating and by careless smoking. The danger posed by fire is even greater among those elderly people who have a decreased sense of smell and, therefore, cannot detect smoke or the odor of leaking gas.

Elderly people are often susceptible to temperature extremes. Those without air conditioning may be overcome by heat during the summer months. Diminished sense of thirst may lead to dehydration. In the winter, some elderly people may not be able to afford to heat their homes properly. Low body temperatures can lead to hypothermia, particularly among those who do not eat well enough to provide the energy necessary for the body to stay warm. The problem is exacerbated by the fact that aging reduces the body's percentage of subcutaneous tissue, which helps keep the body warm.

TRAFFIC ACCIDENTS AND CRIME
Approximately 25 percent of accidental deaths in people over sixty-five years of age are from motor vehicle accidents. Among the physiological changes that increase the risk of accidents are poor depth perception, decreased response time, sensory impairment, and alterations in musculoskeletal, nervous, and cardiovascular systems. Despite these changes, many elderly people continue to drive in order to maintain a certain degree of independence. Traffic injuries may also be sustained by pedestrians who step off the curb into traffic, often because they do not see well or hear the cars. Declining perceptions may decrease a person's ability to judge the speed and distance of approaching traffic.

The elderly are more likely to be attacked by strangers than other age groups. The reason is their vulnerability. Many poor elderly people depend on public transportation and live in high-crime neighborhoods. Many lack the physical strength to defend themselves, while others suffer from poor eyesight and may not be able to identify their attacker. An attack can cause physical damage—such as broken bones, heart and respiratory failure, or head injuries—and can also cause serious damage to pride and self-esteem. Victims may become so fearful of another attack that they will not leave their homes, even to buy food or get medical care.

—*Mitzie L. Bryant*
Updated by Thomas J. Martin, MS II

See also: Back disorders; Balance disorders; Bunions; Canes and walkers; Disabilities; Driving; Exercise and fitness; Fallen arches; Foot disorders; Fractures and broken bones; Hammertoes; Hip replacement; Hospitalization; Medications; Mobility problems; Osteoporosis; Reaction time; Sports participation; Temperature regulation and sensitivity; Vision changes and disorders; Wheelchair use

For Further Information
"Falls Prevention Facts." NCOA, National Council on Aging, 4 June 2018. www.ncoa.org/news/resources-for-reporters/get-the-facts/falls-prevention-facts/. Statistics on falls among the elderly and explanations of programs that NCOA has created for fall prevention.

Lee, Hyeji, et al. "Severe Injuries from Low-Height Falls in the Elderly Population." *Journal of Korean Medical Science*, vol. 33, no. 36, 2018. doi:10.3346/jkms.

2018.33.e221. This study was conducted to determine characteristics of injuries from low-height falls.

Lenartowicz, Magda. "Prevention of Injuries in the Elderly—Geriatrics." *Merck Manuals Professional Edition*, Merck & Co., Inc., Jan. 2018. www.merckmanuals.com/professional/geriatrics/prevention-of-disease-and-disability-in-the-elderly/prevention-of-injuries-in-the-elderly. Information for caregiving professionals on how to prevent falls and injuries.

Martin, Thomas J., et al. "Clinical Management of Rib Fractures and Methods for Prevention of Pulmonary Complications: A Review." *Injury*, vol. 50, no. 6, June 2019, pp. 1,159-65. This review provides an overview of the development of pulmonary complications following rib fractures and highlights specific factors associated with increased mortality among the elderly.

IRAs. *See* INDIVIDUAL RETIREMENT ACCOUNTS (IRAs).

JEWISH SERVICES FOR THE ELDERLY

Relevant Issues: Culture, demographics, religion

Significance: Providing support and service for the elderly within the context of the Jewish religion has become an increasingly important component in the care of an aging population.

Caring for the elderly is considered among the most important components of tzedakah, in literal context meaning an obligation within the Jewish religion. Services are provided not only to help the elderly survive but also to promote independence and maintenance of health in their senior years. There are few formal national organizations whose sole purpose is providing service for the elderly. Instead, most regions with a significant Jewish population provide programs under one of two umbrella organizations: the Jewish Community Center (JCC), providing mainly social programs, and Jewish Family Services (JFS), which provides a wide variety of counseling, care, and management programs.

The JCC generally provides a means for seniors to interact. It is often the site of lectures, informal academic courses, free films, and social gatherings. The JFS generally offers more comprehensive programming to aid the elderly in facing the challenges of aging. It provides support groups, advice in long-term care or planning, and outreach and ElderLink programs. If necessary, the organization may provide home-care management, such as help with cleaning or shopping. Programs may include emergency assistance, emergency or periodic transportation, and day-to-day management, such as paying bills, depositing checks, or helping to decipher medical claims or solve problems. Help in contacting physicians if illness develops is also provided.

The JCC is often associated with the local synagogues, providing programs for a range of demographic categories, such as teenagers, local college students, and even infants. Officers are either elected or appointed by a governing board. In contrast, JFS is generally overseen by geriatric professionals, whose purpose and training is in the care of the aged.

—*Richard Adler*

See also: Cultural views of aging; Home services; Religion; Social ties

For Further Information

Association of Jewish Aging Services, ajas.org/. AJAS is a unique association of not-for-profit community-based organizations, rooted in Jewish values, which promotes and supports the delivery of services to an aging population.

Friedman, Dayle A., et al. Jewish Visions for Aging: a Professional Guide for Fostering Wholeness. Jewish Lights, 2008. This rich resource probes Jewish texts, spirituality and observance, uncovering a deep approach to responding to the challenges of aging with a refreshing and inspiring vitality.

Glicksman, A., and T. Koropeckyj-Cox. "Aging Among Jewish Americans: Implications for Understanding Religion, Ethnicity, and Service Needs." *The Gerontologist*, vol. 49, no. 6, 2009, pp. 816-27. doi:10.1093/geront/gnp070. This article challenges popular conceptions of the nature of ethnicity and religiousness in the gerontological literature.

"Jewish Assisted Living Organizations: Jewish Senior Living & Care." SeniorLiving.org, 16 Aug. 2018. www.seniorliving.org/care/faith/jewish/. General information on Jewish care organizations, including a list of Jewish senior living organizations.

"JILTING OF GRANNY WEATHERALL, THE" (SHORT STORY)

Author: Katherine Anne Porter

Date: Published in 1930 in the collection Flowering Judas

Relevant Issues: Death, family, marriage and dating, religion

Significance: This short story presents the universal themes that all people consider as they face death.

SUMMARY

At the age of eighty, Granny Weatherall, the central character of Katherine Anne Porter's short story "The Jilting of Granny Weatherall," had faced all of life's challenges except one, death. As she lay in her bed, on the eve of this final challenge, she considered all the things that her life had meant and what the costs have been. Throughout her life, she had served God; at the moment of death, she hoped for a sign from Him of what was to be, but no sign came.

God's failure to offer a sign was especially bitter to Granny Weatherall because by her bed stood God's emissary, her own priest. For the second time in her life, Granny Weatherall found herself in the presence of a priest without a bridegroom. As a young woman, she had been jilted by George, whom she had refused to think about for years. Now, at the moment of her death, the thought of George returned to her; she would have liked to have made him believe his betrayal had not mattered. She wanted George to know that although he had left her at the altar, she still had a good husband, a family, and a nice house. Unfortunately, at that moment, she also had to admit that George's betrayal had cost her a part of her soul. God offered no sign that that part of her soul would be returned to her; for this reason, Granny Weatherall felt a final betrayal. She was twice jilted.

ANALYSIS

Despite the twenty years of preparation for death that Granny Weatherall has experienced, she continues, to her last moment, to think of "tomorrow." As human beings fade into sleep, they often consider the events of tomorrow, and they fully expect to wake up in the morning. Granny's denial, or at least lack of acceptance, that death will indeed come is a common technique to relieve death anxiety from those nearing the end of their lives.

Though Granny is reluctant to give up the future, she also finds comfort in death. She begins to see her daughter Hapsy in the room, whom the reader can conclude has already died. Instead of feeling fear of a supernatural presence in the room, Granny finds comfort in seeing her lost daughter. Hapsy helps Granny believe that death will reunite her with loved ones. That the afterlife holds joyous reunions is a belief shared by many, especially those who practice a religion. This consolation can help ease the time of passing.

The story shows the aged that it is normal to tally up one's triumphs and tragedies when contemplating the end of life. It also reveals that it is human to doubt God and to blame Him for failing to provide an easy answer to prayers, requests, and hopes. Though George's betrayal happened to Granny years ago, though she did eventually marry and have children, she cannot help but to focus on that part of her life. Her desire to push the betrayal out of thought and forget it has, in the long run, not been successful. It has become unfinished business that plagues her on her deathbed and even her final moments are spent thinking about George and God.

—*Annita Marie Ward*

See also: Death and dying; Death anxiety; Religion

For Further Information

Als, Hilton. Enameled Lady: How Katherine Anne Porter Perfected Herself. *The New Yorker*, 13 Apr. 2009. www.newyorker.com/magazine/2009/04/20/enameled-lady. A biography of Katherine Anne Porter and interpretation of her work.

Britton, Eleanore M. "An Approach to 'The Jilting of Granny Weatherall.'" *The English Journal*, vol. 76, no. 4, Apr. 1987, pp. 35-39. doi:10.2307/818446. Presents an approach to Literature teachers in teaching "The Jilting of Granny Weatherall."

Keeley, Maureen. "Family Communication at the End of Life." *Behavioral Sciences*, vol. 7, no. 3, Sept. 2017, p. 45. doi:10.3390/bs7030045. Scholars contributing to this special issue on "Family Communication at the End of Life" have provided evidence that communication is important between and for terminally ill individuals, family members, and healthcare/palliative care specialists.

Sauls, Roger. "Katherine Anne Porter and 'The Jilting of Granny Weatherall.'" PorterBriggs.com, 4 May 2015. www.porterbriggs.com/katherine-anne-porters-the-jilting-of-granny-weatherall/. An article analyzing "The Jilting of Granny Weatherall" through the lens of Porter's own biography.

JOBS. *See* **EMPLOYMENT.**

Johnson v. Mayor and City Council of Baltimore

Date: Decided on June 17, 1985
Relevant Issues: Economics, law, work
Significance: This United States Supreme Court decision established that state governments may not violate the Age Discrimination in Employment Act of 1967 even when federal government employment practices differ.

Under the Age Discrimination in Employment Act (ADEA) of 1967, employers are prohibited from discriminating on the basis of age against employees who are between the ages of forty and seventy. Thus, employers may not establish a mandatory retirement age of less than seventy, except when they can show that age is a "bona fide occupational qualification" (BFOQ) for the work. A BFOQ is granted only if the employer can show that age as such is relevant to the duties of the employee and that testable health and fitness standards are impractical. The ADEA was amended in 1974 and 1978 to bring federal employees under its coverage, but the amendments excluded federal firefighters, for whom the mandatory retirement age was fifty-five. The city of Baltimore attempted to establish a mandatory retirement age of less than seventy for its own firefighters. Baltimore argued that the federal mandatory retirement practices had established a general BFOQ for firefighters. The petitioners, six Baltimore firefighters who were being involuntarily retired under the Baltimore law, sued under the provisions of the ADEA. The United States District Court held against the firefighters, but the Court of Appeals reversed the decision, and the firefighters appealed to the Supreme Court.

The Supreme Court held unanimously for the firefighters. The opinion, which was written by Justice Thurgood Marshall, argued that neither the ADEA nor the federal civil service law that determined the mandatory retirement age for federal firefighters showed congressional intent to establish a BFOQ of fifty-five years. In fact, Marshall argued, there was evidence in the legislative history of the civil service law suggesting that Congress's motive was to make employment as a federal firefighter more attractive by making early retirement attractive and maintaining the image of a youthful workforce. According to the Court, neither of these justifications allowed Baltimore to override the provisions of the ADEA. If Baltimore wished to retire its firefighters automatically at age fifty-five, it would have to show evidence that age as such is relevant to the performance of the firefighter's duties and that physical examinations and fitness testing would not serve the city's interest in having competent firefighters.

Although the Supreme Court's ruling in this case is technically narrow, the case stands for a more significant proposition, which is that federal rules doing away with mandatory retirement before age seventy for all employers may be constitutionally applied not just to private employers but also to state and local governmental employers such as the city of Baltimore.

—*Robert Jacobs*

See also: Age discrimination; Age Discrimination Act of 1975; Age Discrimination in Employment Act of 1967; Employment; Mandatory retirement; Massachusetts Board of Retirement v. Murgia; Retirement; Vance v. Bradley

KING LEAR (PLAY)

Author: William Shakespeare
Date: Produced c. 1605-1606, published 1608
Relevant Issues: Death, family, values, violence
Significance: Shakespeare's only tragedy of old age dramatizes its dangers and humiliations; the play warns that love must replace any loss of dignity and authority.

SUMMARY

In William Shakespeare's tragic play of old age and its indignities, King Lear, an aged king in pre-Christian Britain rashly announces his plan to divide the kingdom into three parts. Under his foolish scheme, each of his three daughters is to receive her share in exchange for a proclamation of love for the old king. Lear is enraged when his youngest and most faithful daughter, Cordelia, refuses to conform to this charade.

When the two professedly loyal daughters soon humiliate him, Lear vows revenge and wanders off onto the bare heath. There, he grasps a basic truth: A human is only a "poor, bare, fork'd animal." Lear is last seen embracing the body of Cordelia, who has been hanged, and he dies pitifully, tormented by a false hope that his daughter might still be breathing. The play's subplot, involving Lear's loyal supporter, the duke of Gloucester, confirms the universality of Lear's painful situation. Gloucester is deceived into disinheriting his loyal son, Edgar, and he is viciously punished for aiding Lear by having his eyes plucked out. He grimly concludes, "As flies to wanton boys are we to th' gods./ They kill us for their sport."

A self-confessed "foolish fond old man," Lear dies with a glimmer of hope that Cordelia still lives, while Gloucester dies of a broken heart, despite the comfort of Edgar. The play seems to endorse Edgar's insistence that people must endure the harshness of life with fortitude: "Ripeness is all." King Lear is Shakespeare's only mature tragedy to focus on the decline of self-awareness that can accompany old age.

ANALYSIS

In King Lear, Shakespeare explores the fundamental anxieties humans have towards old age and death. Many readers of the play consider Lear's decline into insanity as a natural part of the aging process, but Shakespeare suggests that the degradation of Lear by his younger daughters and courtiers is the true cause of his madness. Lear does not abdicate the throne because of any mental impairment, but because he would like to enjoy the rest of his life "unburdened." His disloyal daughters and their husbands are the ones who push Lear into his confused state, pitting him against his loving daughter Cordelia and making him question his thoughts, motives, and actions.

These villains take advantage of Lear's old age, especially his desire to "retire," to claim some measure of power and wealth for themselves. Here, age has become political. Shakespeare illustrates the fact that the transition of power from one generation to the next often comes with serious consequences, most usually death. A man like Lear, having reached his eighties and still king, is obviously not a frail or powerless man at the start of the play. He had been able to keep control for decades, and only when the younger generation gets involved do things become treacherous. The fact that Cordelia is only one of three daughters who respects her father could suggest that Shakespeare felt that the majority of

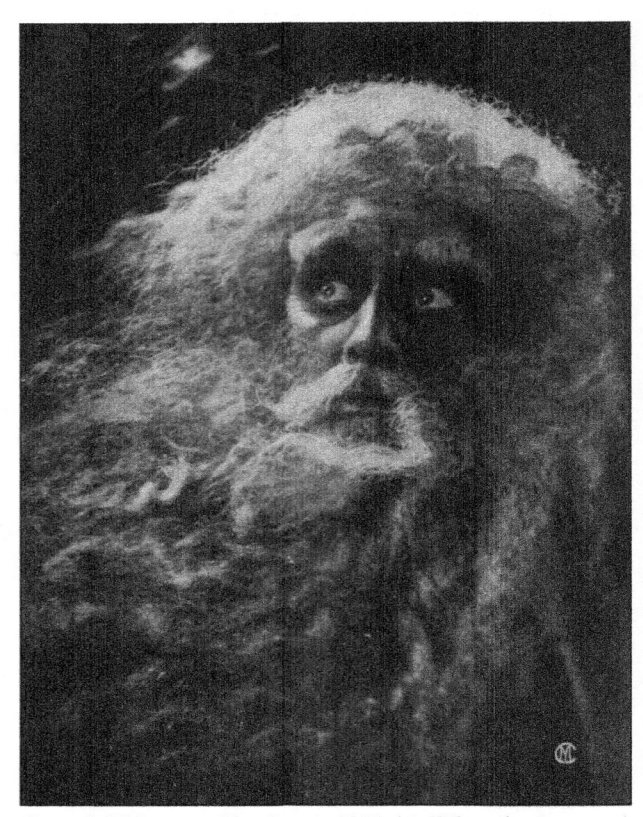

Cavendish Morton as King Lear in 1909. (via Wikimedia Commons)

contemporary youth were disrespectful of their elders, hoping to exploit them for money, land, and power.

The play relies heavily on contemporary inheritance and estate law. British nobility was, and still is, hereditary. Shakespeare drew on real life incidents of scandal, corruption and murder within the aristocracy as they attempted to secure their place in an inheritance. Younger sons and distant relatives have motive for removing members of the family that are closer to the crown, title, estate, and so on. Goneril and Regan, Lear's disloyal daughters flatter their father insincerely to gain their shares of the kingdom and to appease his vanity. As soon as they are given any measure of power, they immediately show their falseness, plotting against their father and treating him like a dotard and a burden. Cordelia is unique in that she speaks honestly, apparently not coveting her third of the kingdom, resulting in her disownment. Lear unwisely succumbs to flattery and does not realize until too late that Cordelia was the most deserving of the three. Here, Shakespeare seems to be critiquing the system of inheritance, suggesting riches and property should go to those who are worthy, not those who are "next-in-line."

King Lear explores the vulnerability of old age from several perspectives, setting it within the highest echelons of nobility. Familial fighting over inheritance is not uncommon, even among those very far removed from any type of aristocracy. It is disheartening to think that as we age we must become more suspicious, even of our own family. Lear wanted only to enjoy his last few years; and instead his family is destroyed, and he is thrown into destitution and madness, an unfortunate fate for many heads of households. King Lear teaches us that a long life can lead to an abundance of wealth and power but also a retinue of enemies and conspirators ready to take it all away.

—Byron Nelson

See also: Death anxiety; Family relationships; Fraud against the elderly; Literature; Old age

For Further Information

Bate, Jonathan, and Ian McKellen. "Discussing Ageing in 'King Lear' with Sir Ian McKellen." FutureLearn, University of Warwick, 15 Feb. 2016. www.futurelearn.com/courses/literature/0/steps/12622. Jonathan Bate and Sir Ian McKellen discuss McKellen's experience with his role as King Lear, and how it relates to and enriches his own aging experience.

Harkins, Matthew. "The Politics of Old Age in Shakespeare's King Lear." *Journal for Early Modern Cultural Studies*, vol. 18, no. 1, 2018, pp. 1-28. doi:10.1353/jem.2018.0000. The essay claims that King Lear—along with a handful of other plays by Shakespeare from the late 1590s to the early 1600s—reveals how vulnerable patriarchal authority could be in early modern England when older men were defined and classified in ways that disempowered them.

Hess, Noel. "King Lear and Some Anxieties of Old Age." *British Journal of Medical Psychology*, vol. 60, no. 3, Sept. 1987, pp. 209-15. doi:10.1111/j.2044-8341.1987.tb02733.x. This paper draws on two sources, literary (Shakespeare's King Lear) and clinical (consultations with elderly patients in primary care) to highlight a fundamental anxiety of old age: the dread of being abandoned to a state of utter helplessness.

Minton, Eric. "King Lear and the Nihilism of Being Old." Shakespeareances, 26 Oct. 2012. www.shakespeareances.com/dialogues/commentary/Lear_Aging-121017.html. Minton visits his father four times a year in a nursing home, surrounded by "Lears." He argues that old age is Lear's fatal flaw and compares and contrasts the story with present-day issues of abuse of the elderly.

KÜBLER-ROSS, ELISABETH

Born: July 8, 1926, in Zurich, Switzerland
Died: August 24, 2004, in Scottsdale, Arizona.
Relevant Issues: Death and dying, health and medicine, psychology, sociology.
Significance: Elisabeth Kübler-Ross is considered by many to be the preemptive scientist who studied, researched, and published in the field of death and dying. She is most known for her stages of dying, first described in her classic text *On Death and Dying* (1969).

Born and educated in Switzerland, Kübler-Ross rose to prominence during her tenure as a professor of psychiatry at the University of Chicago's Billings Memorial Hospital. Though she worked with patients diagnosed with schizophrenia, that patient population served as a launching pad for her research on death, dying, and bereavement. Her approach involved asking her patients about the nature of the treatment they received, and how psychological treatments could be improved upon. After hearing about her person-centered approach to treatment, she was contacted by university students studying theology. The students were seeking guidance on how to counsel the terminally ill. Kübler-Ross developed and implemented a series of seminars during which she would discuss the needs and wishes of dying patients. Students and health-care providers were present for these interviews, which ultimately became the basis of her research on the process of death and dying.

In 1969, Kübler-Ross published *On Death and Dying*, which became a national best-seller and a classic in the field. *On Death and Dying* proposed her theory of the five stages experienced by the terminally ill or those suffering from significant loss: denial, anger, bargaining, grieving, and acceptance. Offering straightforward yet compassionate advice, the book became a classic in the field, and her work spawned countless additional works on the subject. Though not without controversy, including the order of the steps as well as absence of possible additional stages, Kübler-Ross's philosophy of terminal care and the five-stage theory continues to be studied and utilized by students, researchers, caregivers, and the bereaved.

—*Irene N. Gillum*
Updated by Robert S. Cavera, PsyD

See also: Caregiving; Death and dying; Death of a child; Death of parents; Family relationships; Grief; Hospice; Psychiatry, geriatric; Religion; Terminal illness; Widows and widowers

For Further Information

"Coping with Grief." National Institutes of Health, U.S. Department of Health and Human Services, 1 Nov. 2017. newsinhealth.nih.gov/2017/10/coping-grief. A collection of tips on how to cope with loss.

Gordon, Steve, and Irene Kacandes. *Let's Talk About Death: Asking the Questions that Profoundly Change the Way We Live and Die.* Prometheus Books, 2015. The coauthors take up challenging questions about pain, caregiving, grief, and what comes after death.

Kübler-Ross, Elisabeth. *On Death and Dying.* New York: The Macmillan Company, 1969. Through sample interviews and conversations, Dr. Kübler-Ross gives readers a better understanding of how imminent death affects the patient, the professionals who serve that patient, and the patient's family, bringing hope to all who are involved.

KUHN, MAGGIE

Born: August 3, 1905; Buffalo, N.Y.
Died: April 22, 1995; Philadelphia, Pa.
Relevant Issues: Law, media, sociology
Significance: Kuhn founded the Gray Panthers, an advocacy and educational organization that works for social change for aging people.

Maggie Kuhn was one of the leading opponents of discrimination based on age. After graduating from Case Western Reserve University in 1926, she worked for the General Alliance of Unitarian Women and the United Presbyterian Church of the United States, serving as editor of Social Progress magazine and as an alternative observer at the United Nations (UN). In 1970, forced to retire from her career with the Presbyterian Church at age sixty-five, Kuhn and a group of her friends founded the Gray Panthers.

Kuhn's primary goal in creating the Gray Panthers was to establish an organization that worked on the issues that concern the elderly, including pension rights and age discrimination, and that also concerned itself with broader public issues, such as the Vietnam War and a variety of social problems. The core of Kuhn's message was that older people need to be in control of their lives and should be active in working for issues that they support. Her candor, charisma, and lively approach to the needs and problems of the aging drew major media attention and painted an image in the public mind that the elderly can make a difference in society.

Kuhn, who remained active in the Gray Panthers until her death at age eighty-nine, redefined the meaning of age and the importance of young and old working together to produce a better society. She and the Gray Panthers were directly instrumental in nursing home reforms, ending forced retirement provisions, and fighting fraud against the elderly in health care. She wrote several books, including Get Out There and Do Something About Justice (1972), Maggie Kuhn on Aging (1977), and No Stone Unturned: The Life and Times of Maggie Kuhn (1991).

—*Alvin K. Benson*

See also: Advocacy; Gray Panthers; No Stone Unturned: The Life and Times of Maggie Kuhn

For Further Information

Attie, Barbara, and Janet Goldwater, directors. Maggie Growls. *Women Make Movies*, 2003. This short documentary combines commentary, interviews, and secondary sources (including black and white photos and descriptive cartoon sequences commissioned for the film) to tell the life story of Kuhn.

Estes, Carroll, and Elena Portacolone. "Maggie Kuhn: Social Theorist of Radical Gerontology." *International Journal of Sociology and Social Policy*, vol. 29, no. 1/2, 2009, pp. 15-26. doi:10.1108/01443330910934682. Explores Maggie Kuhn's theoretical and analytical contributions to social gerontology and more broadly to the advancement of critical and public sociology.

Kuhn, Maggie, et al. *No Stone Unturned: The Life and Times of Maggie Kuhn.* Ballantine Books, 1991. The founder of the Gray Panthers recounts her life as a social reformer, from her early days in the United Services Organization (USO) and the Young Women's Christian Association (YWCA) to nursing home reform.

———. *Get out There and Do Something about Injustice.* Friendship P, 1972. Kuhn uses her own experience in the church ministry to argue that the church should "launch a massive attack on ageism in all its oppressive and constraining forms."

———. *Maggie Kuhn on Aging: A Dialogue.* Edited by Dieter T. Hessel, Westminster P, 1977. The outspoken founder of the Gray Panthers speaks with students in the San Francisco Theological Seminary's Advanced Pastoral Studies Program about opportunities for older persons in the church and the community.

Sanjek, Roger. *Gray Panthers.* U of Pennsylvania P, 2009. Traces the roots of Maggie Kuhn's social justice agenda to her years as a YWCA and Presbyterian Church staff member. It tells the nearly forty-year story of the intergenerational grassroots movement that Kuhn founded and its scores of local groups.

Thomas, Robert Mcg., Jr. "Maggie Kuhn, 89, the Founder of the Gray Panthers, Is Dead." *The New York Times*, 23 Apr. 1995. www.nytimes.com/1995/04/23/obituaries/maggie-kuhn-89-the-founder-of-the-gray-panthers-is-dead.html. Kuhn's obituary in *The New York Times* gives a biographical account of her life and works.

KYPHOSIS

Relevant Issues: Biology, health and medicine

Significance: Kyphosis, a marked increase of the normal curvature of the thoracic vertebrae or upper back, is sometimes referred to as dowager's hump because of its prevalence in elderly women. Kyphosis may be more prevalent in the older population but can occur at any point throughout the life span. Although not an uncommon condition, there is no standard diagnostic criteria to diagnose a person, especially throughout the life span.

Key Terms:

thoracic vertebrae: twelve vertebral bodies that make up the mid-region of the spine; this section of the spine has a kyphotic curve

Patients with kyphosis appear to be looking down with their shoulders markedly bent forward. They are unable to straighten their backs, their body height is reduced, and their arms, therefore, appear to be disproportionately long. The increased curvature of the thoracic vertebrae tilts the head forward, and the patient has to raise her head and hyperextend her neck in order to look forward. This posture increases the strain on the neck muscles and leads to discomfort in the neck, shoulders, and upper back. It limits the field of vision and increases the patient's chances of tripping over an object not directly in the line of vision. It also shifts forward the body's center of gravity and increases the chances of falling.

In severe cases, kyphosis limits chest expansion during breathing, which may cause difficulty breathing. As a result, less air gets into the lungs, which become underventilated and prone to infections. Pneumonia is a common cause of death in these patients. Those with kyphosis may also present with acid reflux due to the abnormal position of the stomach pushing upward towards the head. In very severe cases, the curvature of the thoracic vertebrae is so pronounced that the lower ribs lie over the pelvic cavity. Patients with severe kyphosis are not able to lie flat on their backs, and many spend most of their time sitting up in a chair or in bed, propped by a number of pillows. Unless the patient changes positions frequently, the pressure exerted by the vertebrae on the skin and subcutaneous tissue may

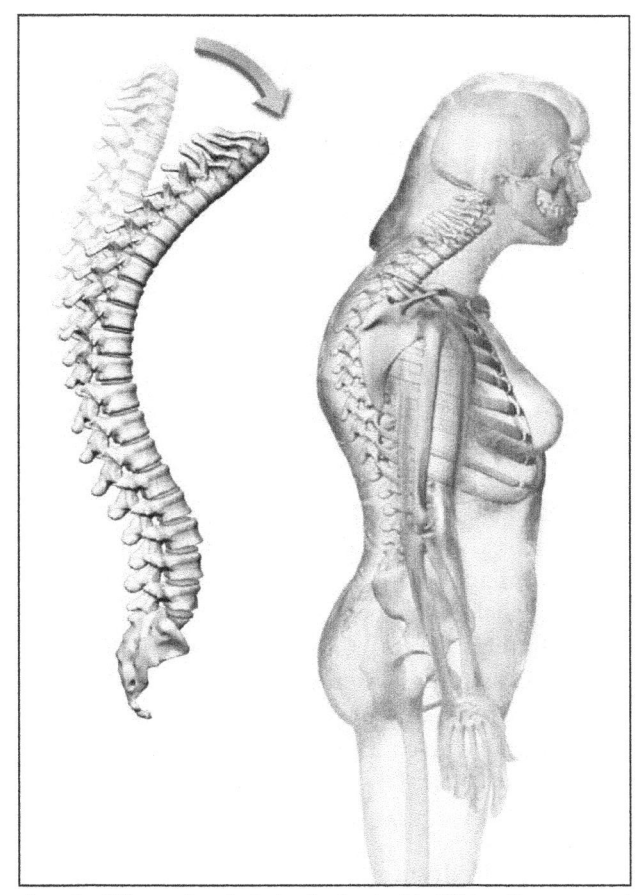

A medical illustration depicting kyphosis. (via Wikimedia commons)

precipitate pressure sores (bed sores) on the upper back that may worsen over time deeper into their tissue, exposing muscle and bone if not properly treated. Pressure sores may also develop on the buttocks. The sores often become infected, especially when not properly cared for, and the infection may spread to the blood, leading to septicemia and death.

The most common cause of kyphosis is osteoporosis, a disease in which the bone mass is reduced. As a result, the bones become mechanically weak and are unable to sustain the pressure of the body weight. The vertebrae gradually become wedged and partially collapsed, more so in the front (anteriorly) than in the back (posteriorly), thus increasing the forward curvature of the thoracic vertebrae. Sometimes, the compression of a vertebra is associated with sudden, very severe, and incapacitating pain that is usually relieved spontaneously after about four weeks. In most cases, however, the compression is a gradual process associated with slowly worsening back discomfort. The discomfort is caused by the strain imposed on the muscles on either side of the vertebrae. In rare instances, the nerves exiting the spinal cord become trapped by the wedged or collapsed vertebrae, and the patient experiences severe pain that tends to radiate to the area supplied by the entrapped nerve. The availability of medications to treat and prevent osteoporosis should significantly reduce the prevalence of both that disease and kyphosis. There are also stretches and strengthening exercises that may help with this condition as well as surgical options reserved for extreme cases.

Less common causes of kyphosis include the compression of a vertebra as a result of tumors or infections. In these cases, the angulation of the thoracic curvature is very prominent. Other conditions that can cause kyphosis include endocrine diseases, other vertebrae diseases such as scoliosis, and infection. Genetic conditions such as Ehlers-Danlos Syndrome, Marfans syndrome, and osteogenesis imperfecta may cause kyphosis in the juvenile ages.

—*Ronald C. Hamdy*
Updated by Stephanie Marie Ong, RN

See also: Back disorders; Bone changes and disorders; Mobility problems; Osteoporosis; Pneumonia; Women and aging

For Further Information

Jang, Hyun-Jeong, et al. "Effects of Corrective Exercise for Thoracic Hyperkyphosis on Posture, Balance, and Well-Being in Older Women." *Journal of Geriatric Physical Therapy*, vol. 42, no. 3, 2019. doi:10.1519/jpt.0000000000000146. The purpose of this study was to identify the effects of a corrective exercise for thoracic hyperkyphosis on posture, balance, and well-being in Korean community-dwelling older women.

Katzman, Wendy B., et al. "Physical Function in Older Men with Hyperkyphosis." *The Journals of Gerontology Series A*, vol. 70, no. 5, May 2015, pp. 635-40. doi:10.1093/gerona/glu213. A cross-sectional study that evaluates the association of hyperkyphosis and physical function in men, aged 71-98 from the Osteoporotic Fractures in Men Study.

"Kyphosis (Roundback) of the Spine." *OrthoInfo*, American Academy of Orthopaedic Surgeons, Aug. 2016. orthoinfo.aaos.org/en/diseases—conditions/kyphosis-roundback-of-the-spine/. General information on kyphosis.

Lorbergs, Amanda L., et al. "Severity of Kyphosis and Decline in Lung Function: The Framingham Study." *The Journals of Gerontology Series A: Biological Sciences and Medical Sciences*, vol. 72, no. 5, May 2017, pp. 689-94. doi:10.1093/gerona/glw124. A longitudinal study to quantify the impact of kyphosis severity on decline in pulmonary function over 16 years in women and men.

Roghani, Tayebeh, et al. "Age-Related Hyperkyphosis: Update of Its Potential Causes and Clinical Impacts—Narrative Review." *Aging Clinical and Experimental Research*, vol. 29, no. 4, 18 Aug. 2016, pp. 567-77. doi:10.1007/s40520-016-0617-3. A narrative review of observational and cohort studies describing the risk factors and epidemiology of hyperkyphosis from 1955 to 2016 using key words.

LAGUNA WOODS

Date: Leisure World built in 1964; Laguna Woods incorporated on March 2, 1999
Relevant Issues: Culture, recreation, sociology, values
Significance: Laguna Woods is a community conceived and built to serve the needs, desires, and interests of active elderly people.

In the late 1950s, Ross Cortese, a nationally recognized builder and developer in Southern California, conceived the idea of building a community for the elderly. Because of advances in health care and better living conditions, more people were surviving to old age. Observing the rapid growth in the elderly population, Cortese thought that major housing programs should be undertaken for this group; when no one else launched a program, he decided that he would. Cortese felt that elderly people would like to have their own housing, to live independently, to be near people of their own age group, to have nice recreational and religious facilities, and to be spared the details of maintenance of their homes and yards.

Early in 1961, Cortese built an adult community project in Seal Beach, California, that contained 3,472 dwellings for the elderly on 1,200 acres. It became the prototype for Leisure World (now Laguna Woods). In order to determine exactly what mature, elderly people needed and wanted, Cortese collaborated with the University of Southern California to obtain research results on what the elderly looked for in environmental conditions, social and recreational activities, and health and medical requirements. Based upon this information, Cortese purchased several sites across the United States, including 3,500 rural acres of the Moulton Ranch, located in the Saddleback Valley of southern Orange County, California. This site, which became his primary retirement housing development, was initially named Leisure World.

The goal of the Leisure World project was to provide the basic needs of life for people fifty-five years of age and older by creating a place of serene beauty, security, and recreation, with religious facilities. Following negotiations with city, county, and federal agencies, as well as the military administration of the nearby El Toro Marine Corps Air Force Base, construction of Leisure World began in the spring of 1963, with an initial phase of 530 dwelling units. On September 10, 1964, the first ten homeowners moved into Leisure World. In 1982, the final phase of Leisure World was completed, providing 12,500 dwellings on 2,100 acres.

One of the landmarks of the city is the clock tower at Clubhouse One that bears the crest of its founder, Ross Cortese. By 1999, there were eighteen thousand residents living in the gated community. Management and maintenance became the task of Professional Community Management, one of the nation's most respected community management organizations.

On March 2, 1999, the residents of Leisure World voted to change the name of their community to Laguna Woods and incorporate it as the thirty-second city of Orange County, California. Nearly 67 percent of the 15,498 registered voters cast ballots in the special election, and incorporation passed by a slim margin of 342 votes. The voters also elected five city council members from a field of sixteen candidates. Laguna Woods became the only municipality whose entire population was made up of elderly people.

—*Alvin K. Benson*

See also: Advocacy; Housing; Leisure activities; Relocation; Retirement communities; Social ties

LAST RITES

Relevant Issues: culture, death, family, psychology, religion, sociology

Significance: As people age, they think about death more often as their contemporaries die, and they know their own death is approaching. For those with religious affiliations, the church can offer comfort through rituals that mark the transition between life and death.

In the Roman Catholic Church, last rites are administered to people of faith just before death. The last rites are a blessing that gives the dying person a plenary indulgence (a remission of the temporal punishment due to sin). The words of the blessing are "Through the holy mysteries of our redemption may almighty God release you from all punishments in this life and in the life to come. May He open to you the gates of paradise and welcome you to everlasting joy" Or "By the authority which the Apostolic See has given me, I grant you a full pardon and the remission of all your sins in the name of the Father, and of the Son, and of the Holy Spirit." It is termed "last rites" as it likely the final blessing a person will receive.

This blessing normally follows the sacraments of Penance (if the ill person is capable of making a confession), Communion (this final Eucharist is called viaticum, meaning the provision for a journey), and the Anointing of the Sick. Some people use the term "last rites" to include not only the final blessing, but also the administration of the three sacraments for the last time.

If the ill person is not capable of confessing, the Anointing of the Sick can also grant forgiveness of sins.

LAST RITES VS. ANOINTING OF THE SICK

Many people confuse last rites with the sacrament of The Anointing of the Sick. Although last rites typically include the Anointing of the Sick, the two are not the same thing. A person who receives the Anointing of the Sick is ill, but not necessarily dying. The purpose of this sacrament is to strengthen the person who is seriously ill. The Anointing of the Sick bestows upon the person who receives it a gift of grace from the Holy Spirit that gives strength, peace, and courage. The person is encouraged to face their illness or even upcoming death and receive healing of the soul, and, if it is God's will, the body.

The Anointing of the Sick was initiated by Christ who used touch to heal, and it is also referred to in the writings of the apostles Mark and James. Over time, it became the custom to administer this sacrament only when someone was close to death. At that point, it became known as "Extreme Unction" which reinforced the idea that it is a sacrament administered only to the dying. More recently, there has been a shift back to the original use of the sacrament at times of illness. In modern times, if the sacrament is administered to a person who is close to dying, it may be referred to as sacramentum exeuntium (the sacrament of those departing). In this case, the sacrament completes the anointings that began with baptism and were reinforced by Confirmation. However, the sacrament is not only for the dying. To limit the Anointing of the Sick in this way means that many Catholics might miss out on this blessing during other times of need.

The Second Vatican Council (1962—1965) noted that, "The sacrament of the Anointing of the Sick is given to those who are seriously ill by anointing them on the forehead and hands with duly blessed oil—pressed from olives or from other plants—saying, only once: 'Through this holy anointing may the Lord in his love and mercy help you with the grace of the Holy Spirit. May the Lord who frees you from sin save you and raise you up.'" It is appropriate to receive this sacrament prior to a major surgery or when one is seriously ill. Furthermore, a person may receive the Anointing of the Sick multiple times when facing different illnesses across the life-span, when an illness becomes more serious, or when a person becomes frail due to advanced age. This sacrament is administered by a priest or bishop, and it is customary to have loved ones present along with the person who is ill. The sacrament may take place in a variety of locations including churches, homes, or hospitals.

Finally, the Anointing of the Sick is only administered to the living. If the person has already died, this sacrament is not appropriate.

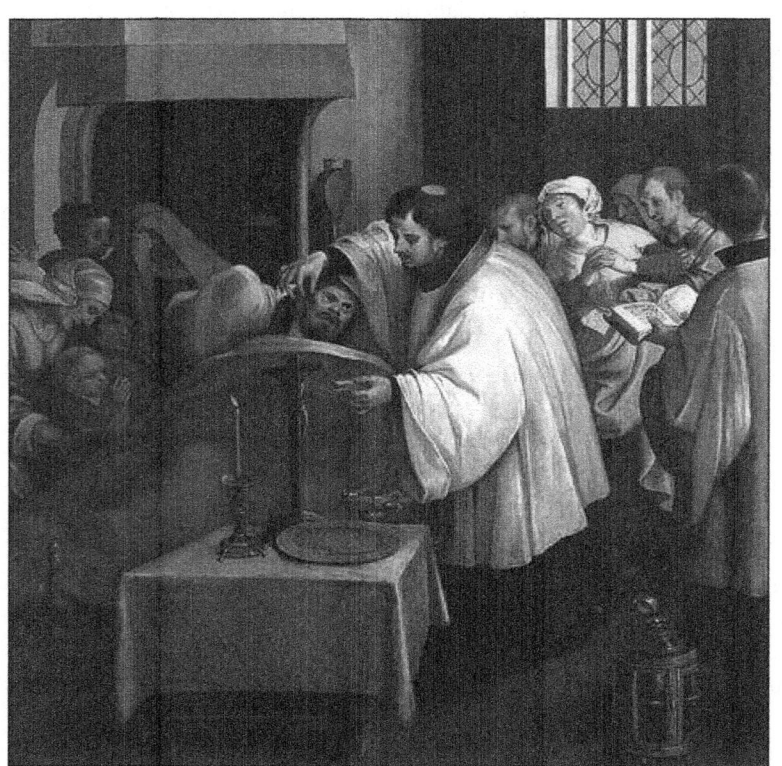

A Dutch School painting c. 1600 depicting a Catholic priest administering last rites. (via Wikimedia commons)

LAST RITES OUTSIDE OF CATHOLICISM

A number of non-Catholic Christian denominations also make use of the term last rites. Some follow practices very similar to that of the Catholics. For example, the Episcopal Church also recommends that people who are close to death should make a confession, receive communion, and be anointed. They also include a Prayer for a Person Near Death and a Litany at the Time of Death.

Other Christian Denominations, like the United Methodists, do not have sacraments that are related to dying, but they have instructions for ministering to people who are dying. For instance, within The United Methodist Book of Worship there is a section entitled "Ministry with the Dying" that includes prayers for the dying person along with a commendation. Methodist ministers are also encouraged to have the person who is dying reaffirm their Baptismal Covenant and receive Communion.

—*Monica L. McCoy, PhD*

See also: Death and dying; Death anxiety; Funerals; Grief; Jewish services for the elderly; Religion; Terminal illness

For Further Information

Catholic Church. "Article 5: The Anointing of the Sick." *Catechism of the Catholic Church*. 2nd ed. Libreria Editrice Vaticana, 1994, 417-26. Defines the purpose of the sacrament as "the conferral of a special grace on the Christian experiencing the difficulties inherent in the condition of grave illness or old age."

Episcopal Church. "Ministration at the Time of Death." *The (Online) Book of Common Prayer*, The Church Hymnal Corporation. www.bcponline.org/PastoralOffices/death.html.

Iovino, Joe. "God Is with Us: Blessing the Dying and Those Who Grieve." UMC.org, The United Methodist Church, 11 Jan. 2016. www.umc.org/what-we-believe/god-is-with-us-blessing-the-dying-and-those-who-grieve. Explains the practices for blessing the dying.

Vitelli, Romeo. "Can Rituals Help Us Deal with Grief?" *Psychology Today*, Sussex Publishers, 31 Mar. 2014. www.psychologytoday.com/us/blog/media-spotlight/201403/can-rituals-help-us-deal-grief. Analyzes a study that asked participants to describe the rituals, if any, they used to cope with a loss. Rituals were both religious and secular, but those who used ritual felt a stronger sense of control over their grief.

"What Is the Difference?—Anointing of the Sick\Last Rites." St. Luke the Evangelist, Catholic Church Houston, stlukescatholic.com/what-is-the-difference-anointing-of-the-sicklast-rites. Explains the difference between last rites and Anointing the Sick.

LATINX AMERICANS

Relevant Issues: Culture, family, race, and ethnicity
Significance: At the beginning of the twenty-first century, Latinx elders were one of the fastest growing groups in the United States.

In 2018, according to the U.S. Census, Latinx elders in the United States made up about 7 percent of the Latinx population, or about 4 million people out of 59 million, about 18.1 percent of U.S. population of 327 million. It was estimated that by 2050, this sixty-five and older group would represent 10.4 percent of the Latinx population. This growth will bring with it much diversity because of the variety of countries from which these elders come and their different cultures. Early in the twenty-first century, roughly 47 percent of Latinx elders were of Mexican origin, 15 percent were Cuban, 13 percent were Puerto Rican, and 25 percent were from other Hispanic subgroups. There were seventy-one men for every one hundred women in this population, and nearly twice as many Latinx men as women aged sixty-five and older were married and living with their spouses. Only 58 percent of this population had been born in the United States, and, in 2018, about 80 percent were United States citizens. By 2018, "Latinx" was widely used rather than "Latino," which is gendered, and "Hispanic," which denotes only Spanish origin. Many Latinx people have indigenous roots as well as Spanish. Some also have European heritages other than Spanish; others have African blood as well.

WHO IS LATINX?

The U.S. Census Bureau identifies the word "Hispanic" and "Latino/a" to describe persons of Mexican, Puerto Rican, Cuban, Caribbean, Latin/Central American, or other Spanish origin. This definition looks at the spoken language to define "Hispanics" or "Latinos" Some people find the Hispanic label uncomfortable and prefer to be called Latinos or Latinx. "Latino" or "Latinx" implies a connection with cultural similarities in addition to language. This overarching term also includes Chicanos and Mexican Americans, Cuban Americans, and so on. "Chicanos" is a term used by some Latinos or Latinx (usually Mexican Americans) who are activists from the 1960s. Use of the term "American" after another nationality, as in "Cuban American," denotes that the person was born in the United States. Many Latinx prefer this method of self-identification, as it represents the country of origin of their ancestors and distinguishes them from other Latinos or Latinx.

Older Latinx vary both within and between specific groups. The differences within a group are evident if one looks at the number of generations that a given family has been in the United States, as well as the reasons for immigrating and where the members live. A Mexican American elder may have a long family history in the United States and, therefore, may be more acculturated. More recent Mexican American immigrants, on the other hand, may be less acculturated. They often depend on their children to translate information from Spanish to English for them and are more fearful of dealing with mainstream service providers and government agencies. There are also differences stemming from the reason for coming to the United States. For example, Latinx from El Salvador and other countries in Central America may have left to escape regimes of terror. They may have come as illegal immigrants and now shy away from being noticed by "outsiders" and government agencies. This fear and the need to go unnoticed permeates how they live from day to day and how they teach their children to survive. There may be a mistrust of any person or agent who represents the majority culture. Their interactions with almost everyone are guarded.

The differences between groups are based on cultural differences, history, and the reason for coming to the United States. For example, many Cuban American elders are extremely different from other immigrants. The first group of Cubans fleeing the communist government under Fidel Castro were enthusiastically welcomed into the United States. This was the only Latinx group to have this experience, which also differed from that of later Cuban refugees. This first group of Cuban refugees were, for the most part, well educated, wealthy, and eager to learn about being Americans. This is in sharp contrast to Latinx who come from other countries and hope not to be discovered. These early Cuban refugees, who currently are the elders, were provided information about how to access services and no-interest loans to begin businesses. They were welcomed as a political statement to demonstrate the superiority of a capitalist system over a communist one.

Therefore, the degree of willingness to assimilate varies among Latinx elders. Many of the differences between groups are also due to their geographic area of origin, the cultural norms that they bring with them, and how they view the government systems both in their countries of origin and in the United States.

In 2018, a large majority of Latinx elders lived in metropolitan areas. However, large numbers also live in small towns where major industries are agricultural or draw families to meatpacking. Some of these are far from the Mexican border. Several small towns in the Yakima Valley of Washington State are majority Latinx; Dennison, Iowa, near Omaha (population 8,000) is half Latinx. Also, the vast majority of Latinx elderly lived in four states, each with different concentrations of Latinx groups: The majority of the Latino population in California and Texas were from Mexico and Central America, Florida attracted the Cuban population, and New York received a large number of immigrants from Puerto Rico and the Caribbean islands.

EDUCATION

Of all minority elderly, those of Latinx background are the least educated. This is particularly significant because education greatly influences other aspects of people's lives. In the United States, a higher educational level also allows individuals to have access to resources provided within their communities.

The proportion of Latinx elders with no formal schooling is nine times as great as for whites. Of Latinx sixty-five and older in 1999, 10 percent had no education and only 20 percent had graduated from high school. In addition, 33 percent had less than five years of education.

In comparing the three largest Latinx groups (Mexican American, Cuban American, and Puerto Rican), Cubans have the highest educational levels of the three and Mexican Americans have the lowest. More specifically, in 1999, Cuban Americans had a mean of 8.11 years of education, Puerto Ricans had a mean of 5.23 years, and Mexican Americans had a mean of 5.21 years of formal education. There is also some variance by gender, with the men in all three groups having more years of formal education in comparison to the women.

By 2014, however, educational attainments of Latinx aged 65 and older had advanced dramatically. By that time, more than half had completed high school. About 12 percent held bachelor's degrees or higher, according to the American Council on Education.

SOCIOECONOMIC STATUS

At the end of the twentieth century, the percentage of Latinx elders with incomes below the poverty level was twice as large (22.5 percent) as among elderly non-Hispanic whites (10 percent). Poverty rates were higher in nonmetropolitan than in urban areas and higher among women than among men. Thus, nonmetropolitan women were the most impoverished group of all. For example, among the Latinx elderly, 22.7 percent of nonmetropolitan women had a below-poverty income, as compared to 15.7 percent of white nonmetropolitan women. Generally, elderly Latinos have lower incomes than their white counterparts. For example, in 1995 the median personal income for elderly Latinos was $6,411 while the median income for white elders was $10,767. In addition, in many cases, elderly Latinos may retire from work earlier than the retirement age. These elders are more likely to become impoverished because of lower benefit levels throughout the rest of their lives.

In comparing late 1990s income levels among the three largest groups of Latinos, Cuban Americans had the highest annual income ($11,950), followed by Mexican Americans ($10,650) and then Puerto Ricans ($9,649). Again, in all three groups, the men earned higher incomes than the women, which meant that Puerto Rican women were the most likely to be poor. In 2018, the median income for Latinx Medicare beneficiaries was $12,800.

Private pensions and incomes from interest-bearing accounts are uncommon among elderly Latinx because the majority of them worked in jobs with little access to retirement benefits. Another issue that contributes to low socioeconomic status is that Latinx do not access Social Security at the same rates as their white counterparts. In 1988, a mere 77 percent of Latinx elders received Social Security, compared to 93 percent of white elders. Those who do receive Social Security are more likely to receive lower benefits as a result of their history of working in low-paying jobs such as laborers, farm or migrant workers, and in the service industry. The combination of these facts makes Latino elders more impoverished as well as more likely to depend on family for financial support. Those who do receive Social Security are more likely to depend on it for a greater amount of their subsistence.

Another resource that is not used to the extent that it could be is Supplemental Security Income (SSI). It has been estimated that only 44 percent of eligible Latino elders receive this benefit. This benefit is for those who are near poverty even after receiving Social Security. This statistic illustrates the low rate of benefit utilization among Latinos even though these elders may be very poor.

HEALTH

Many individuals in all groups who are sixty-five and older and who do not live in nursing homes report at least one chronic ailment and some limitation in performing day-to-day activities. Latinx elderly have somewhat higher rates of activity limitation and have more days per year in bed because of illness. Latinx suffer from relatively high rates of hypertension, and additional health concerns include high cholesterol, diabetes, and arthritis. Latinx have a higher incidence of cardiovascular disease than whites, which is the leading cause of mortality in this group. Cancer is the second-highest cause of mortality; while Latinx have lower rates of cancer than their white counterparts, the incidence is increasing. Non-insulin-dependent (type II) diabetes mellitus is a significant cause of morbidity and mortality that affects 25 percent of adult Puerto Ricans and Mexican Americans.

Health is an area that sometimes may be perceived differently by diverse people. Among elderly Mexican Americans, Cuban Americans, and Puerto Ricans, only 11.4 percent said that their health was poor. However, 41.9 percent said that their health status was fair. In looking at how the same elders perceived their limitations by activities of daily living (ADLs), 16.3 percent had three or more ADLs. Similarly, 17.7 percent said that they had three or more limitations in instrumental activities of daily living (IADLs). ADLs and IADLs are a prevalent evaluation tool for assessing an individual's ability to remain independent and out of nursing homes or other care facilities. Usually, the assessment is based on a combination of limitations, with a final decision based on the overall health of the individual as well as the ability to remain at home with informal and formal support systems playing a significant role. One of the ADLs that is highly correlated with one's ability to remain independent and in one's own home is mobility. This activity is usually assessed by the ability of an elder to walk and to get in and out of bed or chairs. In looking at the three groups of Latinx elders in 1999, 27.3 percent had problems with walking and 21 percent had problems with getting in and out of bed or chairs. Therefore, although only 11.4 percent said that their health was poor, it is likely that the family or informal support system is keeping them out of long-term care facilities.

In spite of higher activity limitations, in 1989, 33 percent of all Latinos had no health insurance. By 2018, the proportion without health insurance had fallen to about 20 percent, due in part to higher educational levels, with increased access to jobs with these benefits, as well as access under the Affordable Care Act (ACA) ("Obamacare"). Much of the lack of insurance is attributable to the fact that in their working years, many elderly Latinx held jobs that simply did not offer health or retirement benefits. The impact of this situation is far-reaching in the older years. With a history of lacking insurance, there has been little preventive care. As a result, when Latinx elders do go in for health care, they usually need more intense levels of care; and their diseases are more complicated and, therefore, more costly to treat. As in other arenas, there are differences among the Latino groups on rates of health-care insurance. In the late 1990s, it was estimated that 38 percent of Mexican American elders, 16 percent of Puerto Rican elders, and 24 percent of Cuban American elders were not insured. Puerto Rican elders were more likely to have Medicaid coverage, which plays a role in decreasing the numbers of these elders who are not insured.

Mental health issues in old age are exacerbated by years of poverty or near poverty, low educational levels, substandard housing, and a lack of opportunity. Generally, Latinx have larger families, which is a resource for them in their old age. As more and more families are influenced by mainstream society, however, more adult children move away to seek jobs or to improve their economic status. In these situations, elders are left to deal with health and mental health issues with the help of established community resources such as priests, friends, and extended family members. In many cases, this amounts to few formal services being accessed by these elders. Studies that looked at psychological distress in Mexican American populations found a lower incidence of psychological distress than in the White non-Hispanic population that was studied.

Puerto Rican-born and Cuban-born older men have higher rates of suicide than other groups. In contrast, all Latino women have a lower rate of suicide. At issue is the ability to discern when a Latinx elder is depressed or experiencing psychological problems. An important variable is whether psychometric tests are applicable to these populations. Another variable that has to be considered is whether the language and interpretation of the test are valid. There is a high probability that with these variables, there may be an underdiagnosis of psychological distress in this population.

EXTENDED FAMILY SYSTEMS

Latinx families are noted for being tightly connected and supportive of their family members. Generally, among the elders, the family and not the individuals make decisions. Functionally, this implies that decisions are a result of familial cooperation, interdependence, and affiliation. While this process may be on the decline due to the relocation of younger families away from their parents, this is still a common occurrence. Mexican American families tend to be larger, with a mean of 4.15 persons per family in the late 1990s. Next were Puerto Rican families, with a mean number of 3.62 persons per family. Cuban Americans had the smallest mean number of persons per family, with 3.13.

In essence, these family members and their children become the most important informal support for these elders. In many cases, the family support system works so well that agencies tend to forget to plan services for Latinx elders. Yet, given that even the younger family members are also likely to be in poverty or have limited resources, caring for elderly family members becomes a serious burden to families. Outreach services to provide information about services and about eligibility guidelines need to be aggressive in Latino communities. Otherwise, Latino elders and their adult children will carry an inordinate portion of the care and responsibility of these elders.

Another component is that by the time Latino elders receive services, be they health or other, they are more frail, and their needs are more complicated. By this time, they have exhausted all or most of the family's resources, both financial and emotional. This family dynamic is responsible for lower utilization rates of all services among Latinos.

—Sara Alemán
Updated by Bruce E. Johansen, PhD

See also: Bless Me, Ultima; Cultural views of aging; Family relationships; Health care; National Hispanic Council on Aging; Old Man and the Sea, The; Poverty

For Further Information

Angel, Jacqueline. "Aging in America: The Latino Perspective." UT News, The University of Texas at Austin, 28 Apr. 2011. news.utexas.edu/2011/04/28/aging-in-america-the-latino-perspective/. Professor Jacqueline Angel discusses her research on the economic and cultural aspects of caring for the growing population of older Latinos.

———. "Changing Latinx Family Dynamics Beg the Question: Who Will Care for Us When We Are Viejitos?" *Latina Lista*, 28 Oct. 2017. latinalista.com/columns/guestvoz/changing-latinx-family-dynamics-beg-the-question-who-will-care-for-us-when-we-are-viejitos. Professor Angel discusses how the increased longevity of the Latinx community could present issues in caring for the aging Latinx population.

Angel, Ronald, and Jacqueline Lowe Angel. *Latinos in an Aging World: Social, Psychological, and Economic Perspectives.* Routledge, Taylor & Francis Group, 2015. This textbook fosters a deeper understanding of the growing Latino elderly population and the implications on society. It examines post-WWII demographic and social changes and summarizes research from sociology, psychology, economics, and public health to shed light on the economic, physical, and mental well-being of older Latinos.

Fox-Grage, Wendy. "The Growing Racial and Ethnic Diversity of Older Adults." AARP, American Association of Retired Persons, 18 Apr. 2016. blog.aarp.org/thinking-policy/the-growing-racial-and-ethnic-diversity-of-older-adults. Explores how the growing ethnic and racial diversity of the older population has enormous implications for meeting diverse personal and family caregiver preferences, providing services with cultural sensitivity, and training the paid health-care workforce in cultural competence.

National Hispanic Council on Aging. www.nhcoa.org/. The National Hispanic Council on Aging (NHCOA) is the leading national organization working to improve the lives of Hispanic older adults, their families, and their caregivers.

Schmidt, Elaine. "Latinos Age Slower than Other Ethnicities, UCLA Study Shows." UCLA Newsroom, University of California, Los Angeles, 16 Aug. 2016. newsroom.ucla.edu/releases/latinos-age-slower-than-other-ethnicities-ucla-study-shows. Discusses a recent UCLA study that showed that Latinx DNA aged slower than other ethnic groups. The UCLA research team next plan to study the aging rate of other human tissues and to identify the molecular mechanism that protects Latinos from aging.

U.S. Bureau of the Census. *Statistical Abstract of the United States: 2010.* 129th ed. U.S. Department of Commerce, Economics and Statistics Administration, Bureau of the Census, 2010. www.census.gov/library/publications/2009/compendia/statab/129ed.html. The 2010 Statistical Abstract of the United States contains 30 sections, 926 pages and over 1300 individual tables covering over 200 topics including income and wealth, imports/exports, agriculture, energy production and consumption, natural resources, and some international comparisons.

LEISURE ACTIVITIES

Relevant Issues: Culture, recreation, values

Significance: Leisure roles may be undertaken on the initiative of the older individual, who has complete latitude as to when, where, how much, and whether such roles will actually be performed.

Aging is the outcome of living. Longevity is a matter of genetics and other environmental factors that permit long life, but whether an individual merely survives or has a quality of life that is satisfying and enjoyable depends on many variables, not the least of which is the positive use of leisure. If one is to hold off the vicissitudes of life and the vulnerabilities that the normal aging process brings, it appears that that life is best which contributes to the common good and fosters participation, in the sense of focus, involvement, and enjoyment. These values can be obtained when two fundamental needs are met. The first is interpersonal behavior or social contact, and the second is physical capacity to perform. The commingling of these experiences leads to the good life.

The older adult has many needs; the impingements to which the human organism is vulnerable as it ages is a prime factor. If a person has an educational preparation suitable for all aspects of life, then it is probable that leisure used in a variety of activities will have been acquired. Where this assumption is invalid, the individual may have a lack of interests and be forced to be passive or vegetate. While a number of agencies may be able to stimulate the learning of leisure skills and other socializing experiences, too often the older adult does not know about the opportunities at his or her disposal, or the agencies that should be concerned are not aware of the older person's existence. When this occurs, no service is given or received.

For the most part, recreational activity is defined as enjoyable, voluntary, socially acceptable, and occurring in leisure. All four aspects must be operational at the same time. The physical activity or motor skill and interpersonal relationships justify each other and contribute to the overall pleasure and satisfaction that a person needs throughout life generally and intensely during later life.

Financial status, condition of health, cognitive ability, sensory acuity, personal loss, residence, transportation availability, and other factors are involved to an increasingly significant extent in an older person's leisure. Leisure in abundance is the experience of the older adult, especially for the retired person, and may be viewed as either a reward or a punishment. Depending upon the perception of the individual and the preparation that has been garnered in preceding years, leisure may be the enrichment of old age or it can be poor, drab, and a time of boredom.

RECREATIONAL SERVICES FOR THE AGING

The aging process and its implications for the recreational service field (primarily leisure-based) and other related services may be analyzed in terms of the responsibilities of social agencies that sponsor programs for older adults (public recreational service departments, age-oriented agencies, sectarian agencies, and other voluntary organizations), treatment centers (convalescent homes, rehabilitation centers, skilled nursing facilities, and other such organizations), and opportunities for private marketing enterprise. Increasingly, older adults who are able want to be involved and active during their leisure. The varied experiences available to aging individuals present challenges and opportunities to use cognitive ability, knowledge, appreciation, proficiency, and physical capacity to perform. The spectrum of opportunities available during leisure includes a surprising variety of organizations and individual initiatives to which the older person may apply insofar as recreational engagement is concerned.

Recreational programs for the elderly sponsored by social agencies (public, quasi-public, or private) need to combine enjoyable activities with emphasis on social service programming to meet the entire range of needs of the aging person. Whenever feasible, recreational programs should incorporate the possibility of having older persons provide meaningful service for others. This strengthens the volunteer's sense of self-esteem, maintains his or her interest, and furthers involvement.

It is worthwhile to promote intergenerational activities and break down the barriers of age segregation. The recruitment of elderly people as volunteers to work with children or adolescents is one of the effective means to increase personal growth, development, and satisfaction.

An important area of leisure opportunity is touring for older adults. There is growing commercial interest in providing travel experiences for elderly people, and it is obvious that many older adults (even those with disabilities) are interested. Different approaches in terms of accommodations, arrangements, security, comfort, and destinations may be required, but this seems to be a significant sector of growth for tour operators and other organizations in the travel industry.

Only about 6 percent of persons over the age of sixty-five are institutionalized in any one year. This means that 94 percent continue to reside in the community. While not all within the community are able to participate in leisure experiences outside the home, for any number of health or disability reasons, the greater proportion of older persons are not dependent and have the capacity to do whatever they want to do, if they have the means and the information, concerning leisure use.

Even when the older adult is disabled, to the extent that institutionalization is necessary, leisure experiences can be extended through a variety of recreational experiences that can assist the dependent adult in reclaiming a sense of purpose and control in an environment that tends to undermine individuality and choice. Special care facilities can arrange for a comprehensive series of recreational activities that will accommodate whatever limitation the older person has due to a pathological condition or other debilitation that accrues as a result of advanced age. Many older adults confined to treatment centers of various types have much free time on their hands. Adroit programming dedicated to the psychosocial needs of these residents can do much to overcome the tendency to withdraw from social contact and become isolated. It is particularly important to assess individual needs and thereby determine the interests, based upon past performance, that might stimulate participation on the part of these confined and sometimes non-ambulatory persons.

Many elderly persons are in good health, vigorous, extroverted, financially secure, and actively involved in a variety of activities. Some of these individuals are still fully employed because they receive a sense of identity and purpose from their position. Others work on a part-time basis to obtain additional money for discretionary use or for the social contact that such employment offers. In many instances, volunteering in service organizations does much to satisfy the need for socialization as well as to achieve personal enjoyment and satisfaction when assistance is given to others. Older persons continue to be active in sports and fitness activities, engage in sexual relationships, are active within their communities, and continue to be creative and innovative and to seek satisfactions in ways that are a natural outgrowth of typical life experiences. Moreover, these people tend to be independent.

The number of agencies devoted to the provision of recreational activities for elderly people runs the gamut from senior centers and "golden age" clubs to retirement communities and age-oriented organizations that operate travel and study opportunities. Intergenerational experiences and other leisure-based activities designed to take advantage of the individual's talents, skills, interests, and vital capacities are also served by these kinds of organizations.

LEISURE ACTIVITIES AND SERVICES

Vigorous physical activity is important for life maintenance as well as personal enjoyment and high-quality living. It would be extremely beneficial if everyone developed the habit of exercise at a young age and engaged in it throughout their lives, but there are individuals to whom any physical activity is an anathema. They must be convinced of the enjoyment and health benefits that can accrue during such participation. These persons need to be persuaded to participate in vigorous physical activity not only for the beneficial outcomes that are gained but also for the pure pleasure of putting one's body through its paces. Maintaining strength is a fundamental factor for staying active into the later years. It is tremendously important for older adults, so that they can sustain their daily living activities as well as their recreational activities. Essential skills, such as getting up from chairs, beds, and toilets, depend on muscle strength. The core of strength training is that one obtains high functional capacity so as to be better able to carry out activities of daily living. By keeping muscles stronger, one can postpone and, to some degree, prevent the inevitable muscle weakness that usually accompanies old age.

Strength is a benefit at any age and at any level of fitness. People who participate in some physical activity that requires skill, flexibility, or stamina will only improve their performance if they become stronger. In order to become stronger, people need to engage in strength-building activities. These activities do not have to be daunting, nor do they have to be competitive. The range of physical experiences can include everything from simply walking to cross-country skiing. Most experts indicate that at least twenty minutes of walking (or any activity that uses large muscles of the lower body), at least three times a week, will dramatically increase fitness with that first step from nonactivity to activity. The keyword is moderation. People can be accommodated for participation in physical activity of almost any kind that requires a modicum of regular time investment and moderate energy output.

The entire orientation of physical activity in successful aging should be in terms of fun or enjoyment. Integrating enjoyable recreational activity into a person's life can stimulate participation for fitness. Although some older adults may be attracted to competitive experiences, for the majority a variety of activities, moderately undertaken and balanced between aerobics and resistance activities, helps to develop strength and flexibility. Such activity should become an integral part of life. Positive leisure experiences are typically performed because the individual anticipates enjoyment in the performance. There usually is no ulterior motive. It is fortuitous that this kind of activity can also contribute to a healthy and attractive life condition.

SOCIAL EXPERIENCES

Recreational activities performed during leisure exalts the individual participant with a sense of purpose and an augmented physical capacity to perform. There is a concomitant upgrade in self-esteem, a feeling of mastery or being in control of one's self, and the ability to achieve whatever objectives have been set. Yet these activities are not done in isolation. Older people realize and appreciate the need for social interaction. There is much to be said for single-participant activity. However, it is much more enjoyable to be with others and to contribute to some cooperative enterprise or to take part in an activity that requires coordination and teamwork to achieve satisfaction. For this reason, most older adults choose activities that require the presence of one or more others for the experience to be successful. Walking by oneself may be pleasurable, but walking within a group is much more enjoyable because of the opportunity for commentary and conversation while walking. The same holds true for exercise classes, dance, cross-country skiing, craft activities, and nature-oriented activities such as camping, rock climbing, fishing, or bird watching. The social aspect of being within a group enhances the activity. Therefore, older people enjoy participating in a wide variety of group activities—some with a physical orientation.

Essentially, physical recreational activity within the social context stimulates a desire for further similar experiences and supplies the motivation for continued participation. The result is an exhilarating feeling of well-being and personal fulfillment. Whether the activity is racquet sports, soft-ball, marathon running, bowling, dancing, or volleyball, the give and take of social intercourse, as much as the activity itself, creates an atmosphere of satisfaction and high morale.

Older adults tend to be retired from active employment and, therefore, have free time, which offers opportunity to reinvest themselves in a personally profitable and valuable experience. Moreover, the loss at retirement of social contact that the work life provides can be compensated for through the highly social context of recreational activity. Coupling these two elements, free time or leisure and social interaction, with the third facet of physical activity brings the disparate pieces of existence into an integrated whole. This mosaic represents a situation of voluntary, wholesome participation during leisure in a totally enjoyable setting. A salubrious outcome encourages further experimentation so that the participants become more enthusiastic about their potential. In this way, attention is future focused, and there is a tendency to look ahead to the next possibility.

Midlife preparation for the inevitable process of aging as well as retirement from the workforce should be emphasized by employing organizations and other agencies that operate preretirement seminars or other educational programs. These workshops need to stress that leisure will loom large in the later years and that recreational activity is an integral element of the entire process. In fact, public agencies whose responsibility it is to serve the needs of all citizens should be closely involved with the development of comprehensive planning for the aging.

SUMMARY

Recreational activity, set in leisure, creates an environment in which the individual can take pleasure in the fact that he or she has lived to the fullest. The twin requisites for the aging person, fitness and socialization, need to be founded early on, but they can be embarked upon profitably at any age. If individuals can be persuaded to perform, they will soon find such activity is an antidote to the average problems that typically confront the older person.

Positive leisure activity is not an elixir, and it may not add years to life, but it does make a difference in the kind of lives led by those who participate. From the interconnection between group-supported recreational activity comes integration of character and the certainty of function. Whether or not an individual who is fit will live longer is not the question. Rather, the question is concerned with the condition of the individual when the aging process really begins and the period between that onset and death. Those years, whether few or many, can be successful in terms of high-quality living. To be able, to be involved, and to extend oneself to the maximum offers the performer the actuality of achievement and a heightened sense of contentment.

—*Jay S. Shivers*

See also: Creativity; Disabilities; Exercise and fitness; Friendship; Retirement communities; Retirement planning; Senior citizen centers; Social ties; Sports participation; Successful aging; Vacations and travel; Volunteering

For Further Information

Chang, Po-Ju, et al. "Social Relationships, Leisure Activity, and Health in Older Adults." *Health Psychology*, vol. 33, no. 6, 2014, pp. 516-23. doi:10.1037/hea0000051. This study examines how leisure influences the link between social relationships and health in older age.

Leitner, Michael J., and Sara F. Leitner. *Leisure in Later Life: A Source Book for the Provision of Recreational Services for Elders*. 4th ed. Sagamore Publishing, 2016. This book discusses the provision of recreational activities for older adults. A basic review of program components includes planning, implementation, and evaluation of recreational programs in institutional and community settings. Recreational activity suggestions incorporate therapeutic modalities and diversionary activities into a number of comprehensive programs, designed to address a variety of physical and psychosocial needs of older adults.

Shivers, Jay Sanford. *Recreational Services for Older Adults*. Fairleigh Dickinson U P, 2002. The first three chapters of this book contain gerontological information concerning the aging process, demographics, changes in the style of living and aging persons, and vulnerabilities encountered. This volume explicates fundamental beliefs in the need for active engagement including social, physical, cognitive, and emotional.

Weisberg, Naida, and Rosilyn Wilder. *Expressive Arts with Elders: A Resource*. Jessica Kingsley Publishers, 2nd ed. 2001. This engaging and practical book shows how older people who are disoriented or depressed by the process of aging can experience a renewed sense of connectedness and life affirmation through the expressive arts and art therapies. The contributors combine an analysis of theoretical considerations around themes of aging, society, and dementia.

LGBTQ+

Relevant Issues: Culture, demographics, family, marriage and dating, values

Significance: The older gay and lesbian population is often ignored or stereotyped; more research is needed on this segment of older adults.

GROWING DIVERSITY

As the population of older adults increases, so does the diversity of individuals in late life. An often-ignored group of older individuals is those in the lesbian, gay, bisexual, transgender and queer (or questioning) and others (LGBTQ+) community. There are several reasons that this group has been termed by some academics as the "invisible elderly." Homosexuality is an issue that makes some people in all age groups uncomfortable to consider or discuss, though this opinion has changed dramatically in recent years due to higher visibility of homosexuality in the media and several pieces of legislation giving more rights to the LGBTQ+ community. Older adults do suffer from many damaging stereotypes, especially about their sexual desires and behaviors. Therefore, older adults who are LGBTQ+ have the combined disadvantage of being a member of a sexual minority in later life. The outcome is that this group can be ignored and discounted by both younger cohorts of LGBTQ+ individuals and the overall social culture.

Just as the older population in general is diverse, so is the population of LGBTQ+ individuals. Even though both men and women are lumped together here, the experience of either gender may be very different from the other. And those that make up the transgender community typically experience more discrimination and derision from society at large. In older lesbian couples, there may be a dual economic disadvantage compared to gay men, as women's wages tend to be lower across the life span. Conversely, men tend to have shorter life expectancies than women, which may create critical issues for male partners if both are in poor health in late life.

Other aspects of diversity are found within the older LGBTQ+ population. One is the point in life at which the individual determined that she or he is not heterosexual. Some older adults may have lived their entire lives being openly LGBTQ+. Others may have come to this realization during their adulthood years. Some of these individuals chose to continue a heterosexual lifestyle for various reasons—from a desire to preserve their marriage, for the sake of their children, or out of fear of abandonment by their families. Therefore, even within this group, the experience of being LGBTQ+ can be vastly different for various individuals.

DISCRIMINATION

Approximately 2.7 million of adults over 50 are LGBTQ+, 1.1 million of whom are older than 65. One third of LGBTQ+ older adults live below 200 percent of the federal poverty line, with higher rates for minorities, bisexual women and transgender adults. As a group, LGBTQ+ older adults experience unique economic and health disparities. In a Center of American Progress (CAP) 2017 study, 7 percent of LGBQ respondents said they did not tell their doctors about their sexual orientation or gender identity out of fear of being turned away. For transgender people, that number rises to 18 percent who avoided doctor's visits. This withholding of information can negatively affect treatment and prevents discussion about sexual health.

For decades, it was not only socially unacceptable to express sexuality other than heterosexuality, it was also illegal. Employers and health-care professionals were not prevented from discriminating against LGBTQ+ employees or patients. While much has changed for the better in recent years, the University of Washington's study revealed that 21 percent reported being fired from a job for their perceived sexual orientation or gender identity. Eighty percent reported being victimized, either physically or verbally, at least once during their lifetimes.

Years of this kind of discrimination may cause older LGBTQ+ adults to be more concerned about "coming out." Social isolation is also a concern because LGBTQ+ older adults are more likely to live alone, more likely to be single and less likely to have children than their heterosexual counterparts. This can cause serious financial stress if a single-income is not sufficient to get by. They also experience higher rates of loneliness and depression and less access to mental health services.

As a cohort, the LGBTQ+ population experiences higher rates of disability, physical and mental distress, and a lack of access to services. By 2060, the elderly

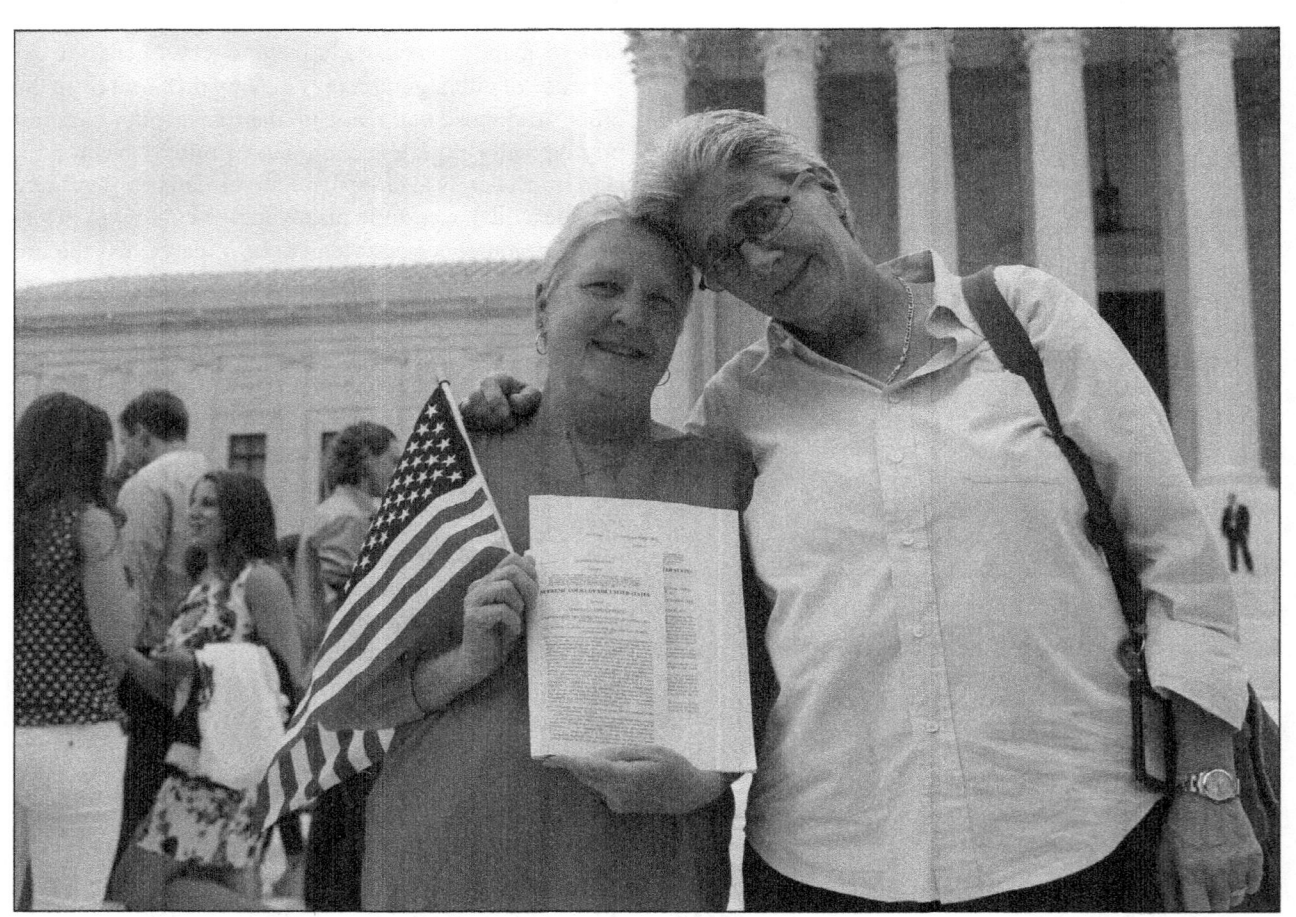

A couple stands outside of the Supreme Court, holding the decision of Obergefell v. Hodges, *which legalized same-sex marriage nation-wide. (via Wikimedia Commons)*

LGBTQ+ population is predicted to number over 5 million, revealing a dire need for more services, including housing, transportation, social support, and legal services.

A HOPEFUL FUTURE

Hope can be found in the fact that older LGBTQ+ people are beginning to build their own support systems and that several pieces of legislation have reduced the stigma around sexual orientation and gender identity. In 2015, Services & Advocacy for Gay, Lesbian, Bisexual & Transgender Elders (SAGE) launched the National LGBT Elder Housing Initiative to address the housing crisis faced by the community. SAGE is working to open senior housing developments specifically designed to provide affordable, discrimination-free living spaces for older LGBTQ+ adults. The Ingersoll Senior Residence is meant to open in the Fort Greene neighborhood in Brooklyn, and the Crotana Senior Residences will open in the Bronx. These housing developments will join others that are LGBTQ+-welcoming in Los Angeles, Philadelphia, Chicago, and Minneapolis.

Several other organizations exist to support the aging LGBTQ+ community. SAGE developed the National Resource Center on LGBT Aging that was the United States' first resource center designed to improve the quality of services and support offered to LGBTQ+ older adults. The Old Lesbians Organizing for Change (OLOC) group promotes visibility of this often unseen group, providing financial support and disability services to those who need them. Gay Reunion In Our Time (GRIOT), focuses on LGBTQ+ people of color to eliminate ageism, racism, sexism, transphobia, poverty and their intersections. The National Center for Transgender Equality (NCTE) advocates for changes in policies to increase the understanding and acceptance of transgender people. They sponsor several projects, including the Trans Legal Services Network (TLSN) that provides legal support for issues specific to the transgender community, including name changes and discrimination.

In 2010, Congress passed the Don't Ask, Don't Tell Repeal Act, officially allowing lesbian, gay, and bisexual people to serve openly in the military. Previous policy allowed them to serve, but under the condition that their sexual orientation was not discovered. The majority of troops already serving were in favor of repealing Don't Ask, Don't Tell, according to a pre-repeal survey. The 2010 Act allowed service members to live a more honest and dignified life, both for current service members and veterans. Studies done after the repeal have noted no negative effects.

In 2015, the Supreme Court made a decision in Obergefell v. Hodges, ruling that the fundamental right to marry is guaranteed to same-sex couples, repealing the Defense of Marriage Act (DOMA) of 1996. The ruling required all 50 states as well as the District of Columbia to perform and recognize marriages of same-sex couples on the same terms as opposite-sex couples. The named plaintiff in the case, James Obergefell, sought to put his name on his husband's death certificate as a surviving spouse. The ruling was mostly met with jubilant support, though several conservatives rejected it. Several counties in Alabama and Texas still do not issue marriage certificates to same-sex couples as of 2019. The impact of the ruling was profound for older LGBTQ+ people. Many had lived with a partner for decades, but because they could not receive a marriage license, they were not entitled to the many benefits of marriage, including tax, Social Security, inheritance, insurance, and emotional benefits. In the year following the Obergefell v. Hodges decision, LGBTQ+ marriages rose by 22 percent.

—*Nancy P. Kropf*

See also: American Society on Aging; Cohabitation; Friendship; Look Me in the Eye: Old Women, Aging, and Ageism; Marriage; Sexuality; Single parenthood; Singlehood

For Further Information

Cannon, Sophie M., et al. "Addressing the Healthcare Needs of Older Lesbian, Gay, Bisexual, and Transgender Patients in Medical School Curricula: a Call to Action." *Medical Education Online*, vol. 22, no. 1, 2017. doi:10.1080/10872981.2017.1320933. This article addresses some of the unique health-care needs of the aging LGBT population with an emphasis on social concerns and healthcare disparities. It supplies additional curricular recommendations to aid in the progressive augmentation of medical school curricula.

Driscoll, Mercedes Y., and Kyle J. Gray. "Special Considerations in the Mental Health Evaluation of LGBT Elders." *American Journal of Psychiatry Residents' Journal*, vol.

12, no. 5, 2017, pp. 4-6. doi:10.1176/appi.ajp-rj.2017.120503. This article shed light on some of the history of the LGBTQ+ population and the health disparities that they face. Appropriate clinical considerations are also discussed.

Fredriksen-Goldsen, Karen I. "The Future of LGBT+ Aging: A Blueprint for Action in Services, Policies, and Research." *Generations*, vol. 40, no. 2, 31 Mar. 2017, pp. 6-15. This article shares personal reflections on the future of LGBT aging, informed by findings from two landmark studies: Aging with Pride: National Health, Aging, Sexuality and Gender Study (2009 to present) and Caring and Aging with Pride.

Joshi, Yuvraj. "The Respectable Dignity of Obergefell v. Hodges." *California Law Review*, vol. 6, 12 Feb. 2016. papers.ssrn.com/sol3/papers.cfm?abstract_id=2731020. This essay demonstrates how Obergefell shifts dignity's focus from respect for the freedom to choose toward the respectability of choices and choice makers.

"Lesbian, Gay, Bisexual and Transgender Aging." APA, American Psychological Association. www.apa.org/pi/lgbt/resources/aging. A collection of information and resources on the specific issues of the LGBTQ+ population.

Mirza, Shabab Ahmed, and Caitlin Rooney. "Discrimination Prevents LGBTQ People from Accessing Health Care." Center for American Progress, 18 Jan. 2018. www.americanprogress.org/issues/lgbt/news/2018/01/18/445130/discrimination-prevents-lgbtq-people-accessing-health-care/. Distillation of survey results on LGBTQ individuals' access and avoidance of health-care visits.

National Resource Center on LGBT Aging. Services and Advocacy for LGBT Elders. SAGE. www.lgbtagingcenter.org.

Orel, Nancy A., and Christine A. Fruhauf. *The Lives of LGBT Older Adults: Understanding Challenges and Resilience*. American Psychological Association, 2015. This book uses a life course perspective to investigate how LGBT older adults have been shaped by social stigma and systematic discrimination.

SAGE, Services & Advocacy for LGBT Elders, 22 Aug. 2019. www.sageusa.org/.

Singleton, Dave. "Does It Get Better for LGBT Seniors?" *HuffPost*, 23 June 2017. www.huffpost.com/entry/does-it-get-better-for-lgbt-seniors_b_594d7569e4b0f078 efd98179. A look at services and housing for this at-risk community.

University of Washington. "New Findings Reveal Health, Aging Experiences of LGBT Older Adults across Nation." ScienceDaily, 13 Feb. 2017. www.sciencedaily.com/releases/2017/02/170213171414.htm. In a first-of-its-kind study, researchers have released new findings on the health and aging of lesbian, gay, bisexual and transgender older adults in the United States.

Wheeler, David R. "LGBT Seniors Are Being Pushed Back Into the Closet." *The Atlantic*, Atlantic Media Company, 26 Aug. 2016. www.theatlantic.com/health/archive/2016/08/lgbt-seniors/497324/. To curb harassment in care facilities, one woman is teaching staff members to respect their elders' sexual orientations.

LIFE EXPECTANCY

Relevant Issues: Death, demographics, health and medicine, race and ethnicity

Significance: Life expectancy at birth is a measure of longevity that has been increasing steadily, though disparities remain between males and females and among people of different ethnic and socioeconomic backgrounds.

Key Terms:

demographics: the number and characteristics of people who live in a particular area or form a particular group, especially in relation to their age, economic status, and race

dependency ratio: the number of dependents in a population divided by the number of working age people; dependents are defined as those aged zero to 14 and those aged 65 and older; working age is from 15 to 64

longevity: a long duration of individual life

In an attempt to maximize profits, life insurance companies devised a method for estimating the amount of time a person will live, given his or her current age. This demographic measure, known as life expectancy (e_x), is based on prevailing death rates and is expressed as the average number of additional years a person of age x can expect to live. By collecting statistics on the age at death in a particular population (compiling what is known as a static life table), it is possible to determine the current probability of surviving infancy, childhood, young adulthood, middle age, and old age. Using these patterns of survival, one can project how much longer a given person is likely to live (an actuarial prediction of the mean expectation of life for someone alive at beginning of age x based on a hazard model applied to each age and sex group).

Because some age groups experience lower survival rates than others, life expectancy changes with age. For example, once a person has made it past a particularly difficult stage of life (such as surviving infancy in the early twentieth century), the chances of living a long life actually increase. Although life expectancy at birth may be seventy, it can easily jump to seventy-six years when the person reaches age one. Populations with high infant mortality have a smaller proportion of the population living to old age, but the population will still comprise the entire range of ages.

Although the demographic measure "life expectancy" is formally calculated for a specific age class, the term is commonly used to refer to e0, or "life expectancy at birth." This figure estimates the average length of time a baby born that year is expected to live (based on the death rates of the population). It serves as an important summary measure of longevity and an indicator of the health of a population.

INCREASES IN LIFE EXPECTANCY

Among wealthier populations, life expectancy has shown extraordinary increases. For example, in 1900, the average American could not expect to live more than fifty years. By 1999, however, U.S. life expectancy at birth had climbed to seventy-six years. This increase in life span can be attributed to increases in the survivorship of infants and to decreases in both death during childbirth and the spread of infectious childhood diseases. Slowing of the onset of and decreasing of the mortality associated with a variety of diseases has further extended longevity. In North America and elsewhere, gains have been made through immunization programs, decreases in teenage motherhood, declines in the incidence of smoking, and improved medicines and technologies for combating heart disease and cancer (the two largest killers in the United States).

By 2017, however, reports from the Centers for Disease Control (CDC) indicated that average life expectancy in the United States had begun to decline for the second time in three years. This decline was most notable in middle-aged white men, and was largely due to rising rates of suicide and drug overdoses, especially opioids and their derivatives, more than 70,000 of which were reported in 2017 alone. This comprised the longest decline in U.S. life spans in a century, since 1915 to 1918, which included World War I and an influenza pandemic that killed at least 675,000 people in the United States and roughly 50 million worldwide. Life expectancy at birth in the United States stagnated in the upper 1970s in 2018.

THE CONSEQUENCES OF LONGER LIFE

Gains in life expectancy have spawned a debate regarding the upper limit of the human life span. Some project a practical upper limit of eighty-five years, pointing to the slowing decrease in mortality in the 1980s as evidence that most of the "easy" gains in longevity have already been made. Studies of the influence of genetic makeup on longevity, and the observation that the number of people in the oldest age groups is increasing rapidly, lead others to speculate that the natural human life span may be in excess of 120 years. In fact, in 1997, people one hundred and older were the fastest-growing age class in the U.S. population.

The combination of longer life span and lower birthrates means that the U.S. population is aging. This changing demographic makeup raises some difficult social and political issues. Some fear that aging baby boomers (those people born between 1945 and 1964) will create a financial burden on society, as the ratio of workers to retirees (the dependency ratio) was projected to shift from sixteen to one in 1950 to two to one in 2030. The "graying of America" means that the wealth span of the population is also increasing, with less years being spent in the (pre-retirement) accumulation stage of life and more years spent in the (post-retirement) expenditure stage. Questions were raised as to whether various assistance programs (Social Security, Medicare, and Medicaid) could remain viable, since the "pay-as-you-go" (rather than investment) structure of these programs requires that the number of people working be larger than the number collecting benefits. Socially, increased longevity also means that most families now include three generations. This situation has the potential to "sandwich" the middle aged between financially dependent teenagers and older parents. Financial gerontologists predict a shift in financial burden away from children (since families are increasingly smaller) toward longer-lived elder parents, with a growing need for intergenerational transfers of finances.

Not everyone has predicted economic stagnation as a result of the graying of the U.S. population. Some see the potential for growth in "silver industries" (those geared toward the senior or "mature" market). They also point to the large investment capital created by the pension funds of this swelling age group. It is also clear that retirement need no longer be age-dependent, as improved health in later life means improved ability for people to work into their sixties, reducing the strain on the retirement system.

THE QUALITY OF LONGER LIFE

Another concern associated with longer life is the question of adding quality as well as quantity to the extension of life. Although the concept of quality is elusive, most agree that an increase in disability-free years (years in which the individual is still able to perform routine activities) is desirable. Fears associated with a longer life include concerns about failing health, insufficient funds, loss of mental acuity, and loss of independence. Fortunately, advances in health care and an increased awareness of the role of lifestyle in preventing disability mean that old age has become less unpleasant and expensive. For women, moderate hormone replacement (estrogen) therapy, taken for less than ten years or in a "designer estrogen" form, increases life span by adding bone density and protecting against heart disease. A diet high in fruits and vegetables and low in meat also adds years, as does having a physically and mentally active lifestyle. Companionship and an optimistic view of life also appear to increase the human life span.

Almost all the years added to the life span between 1980 and 1990 were disability-free years, with the average age of nursing home residents increasing from sixty-five in 1950 to eighty-one in 1999. The increase in the proportion of life spent free of disability is known as the compression of morbidity. The prevention of chronic health problems means that people are able either to "live longer and die faster" or to "die young at an old age."

DISPARITIES IN LIFE EXPECTANCY

Despite improved public health practices and advances in technology, not everyone has benefited equally from increases in life expectancy at birth. By the late 1990s, the continuing acquired immunodeficiency syndrome (AIDS) epidemic prompted some reduced longevity in Central and South Africa between 1990 and 2018. However, high birthrates in the same areas tended to mitigate this trend. Life expectancies had also dropped to 1980 levels in former Soviet bloc nations of Eastern Europe as a result of economic and social changes that accompanied the breakup of the Soviet Union.

While those born in the most-industrialized nations in 2017 could expect to live to about eighty, those in the least-developed countries could expect to live only to the age of about forty-five. Life expectancy at age sixty-five is much more similar from one country to another, yet inferior public-health conditions in poorer nations may mean poor quality of life for the elderly. Average life expectancy using 2016 and 2017 figures ranged from 84 in Japan and 83 in Switzerland to 65 in India, 55 in South Africa, and 50 in the Central African Republic.

Probably most striking are the disparities within the U.S. population itself. The United States has a bigger spread in longevity than any other high-income nation. A 1997 study by Christopher Murray of Harvard University revealed that some residents of inner cities, Native American reservations, and the South had life spans comparable to those in less-developed countries. He reported that a Native American male in South Dakota could expect to live only 56.5 years and that an African American male in Washington, DC, could expect to live just 57.6 years—the same life expectancy as a male in Bangladesh or Senegal. Even within the city of Chicago, longevity varies up to twenty years from one neighborhood to another, a gap that doubled between 1980 and 1999. These disparities are based on sex, race, ethnicity, income, and educational differences. In general, the poor and less-educated die younger, with increased mortality at all ages and from all causes. Those with less than a high school education have a shorter overall life span as well as a decrease in active life. By 2017, life expectancy among U.S. minority groups had increased modestly since the Murray study, but so had life spans in most low-income nations around the world. All remained well below averages in high-income nations.

Women in the United States outlive men by an average of six to eight years, although this gap appears to be narrowing with time. While women live more years, they also have a higher proportion of disabled years than their male counterparts. Similarly, African Americans and American Indians are more likely to have chronic health problems, leading to racial inequalities in the active life span. These differences may be attributable to lower socioeconomic status. As a group, African Americans and young Latinos experience more risk of death from homicide and human immunodeficiency virus (HIV) infection than the population at large, and American Indians experience increased risk from suicide. Because of their mixed European, African, and American Indian ancestry, however, Latinos (or Hispanics) have been inconsistently reported in mortality reports, with many vital statistics for Latinos available only after 1989. In general, factors other than ethnicity, per se, are the main determinants of longevity. Differences in risk factors (smoking and obesity), genetic predisposition for certain diseases, access to health care (as a result of insurance, financial, or immigrant status), preventive care, nutrition, and health consciousness (which is tied to educational and cultural differences) all contribute to differences in life span.

—Lee Anne Martínez
Updated by Bruce E. Johansen, PhD

See also: African Americans; Aging: Historical perspective; Anti-aging treatments; Asian Americans; Baby boomers; Centenarians; Death and dying; Demographics; Latinx Americans; Longevity research; Middle age; Old age

For Further Information

Beltrán-Sánchez, Hiram, et al. "Past, Present, and Future of Healthy Life Expectancy." *Cold Spring Harbor Perspectives in Medicine*, vol. 5, no. 11, Nov. 2015. doi:10.1101/cshperspect.a025957. Explores past, present, and future prospects of healthy life expectancy and examines whether increases in average length of life associated with delayed aging link with additional years lived disability-free at older ages.

Bernstein, Lenny. "U.S. Life Expectancy Declines Again, a Dismal Trend Not Seen Since World War I." *Washington Post*, 29 Nov. 2018. www.washingtonpost.com/national/health-science/us-life-expectancy-declines-again-a-dismal-trend-not-seen-since-world-war-i/2018/11/28/ae58bc8c-f28c-11e8-bc79-68604ed88993_story.html. Reports on the declining life expectancy of the U.S. population as reported by the Centers for Disease Control and Prevention.

Crimmins, Eileen M. "Lifespan and Healthspan: Past, Present, and Promise." *The Gerontologist*, vol. 55, no. 6, 10 Nov. 2015. pp. 901-11. doi:10.1093/geront/gnv130. Explores how significant improvements in health and increases in life expectancy in the United States could be achieved with behavioral, life style, and policy changes.

Gratton, Lynda, and Andrew Scott. *The 100-Year Life*. Bloomsbury, 2016. Describes what to expect and considers the choices and options that the aging population will face.

Jones, Julia A. Barthold, et al. "Complexity of the Relationship between Life Expectancy and Overlap of Lifespans." *Plos One*, vol. 13, no. 7, 12 July 2018. doi:10.1371/journal.pone.0197985. Develops formal demographic measures to study the complex relationships between shared life expectancy of two birth cohort peers, the proportion of their lives that they can expect to overlap, and longevity.

Lubitz, James, et al. "Health, Life Expectancy, and Health Care Spending among the Elderly." *New England Journal of Medicine*, vol. 349, no. 11, 11 Sept. 2003, pp. 1,048-55. doi:10.1056/nejmsa020614. Estimates the relation of health status at 70 years of age to life expectancy and to cumulative health-care expenditures from the age of 70 until death.

Silvertown, Jonathan W. *The Long and the Short of It: the Science of Life Span and Aging*. The U of Chicago P, 2013. A witty and fascinating tour through the scientific study of longevity and aging.

LIFE INSURANCE

Relevant Issues: Death, economics, family

Significance: People purchase life insurance so that their beneficiaries can receive money to pay off debts and final expenses and to create an estate for survivors, but many people also think of life insurance as an investment for their retirement years.

People have been purchasing life insurance policies since the colonial period in America. Until relatively recently, almost all policies sold were whole-life policies, which included level premiums for the life of the policy, guaranteed death benefits, and cash values that accumulated gradually in older policies. Many insurance companies have also begun to offer term-life policies that provide less expensive pure life insurance coverage but do not contain cash values.

Agents selling term policies normally encourage their customers to invest the difference in price between less expensive term policies and more expensive whole-life policies. Customers who are averse to risk prefer whole-life policies that contain guaranteed cash values, whereas those who believe that they can do better by investing in mutual funds or stocks tend to prefer term policies. There are also combinations of whole-life and term policies such as universal life policies, which contain a guaranteed death benefits with cash values and death benefits that can vary depending on the performance of the investments selected by customers for their individual investments.

REASONS FOR PURCHASING LIFE INSURANCE

Life insurance companies rely on actuarial tables to determine premium rates for customers. Premiums are more expensive for older people than for younger customers because companies assume that younger customers will live longer. Health factors also influence premium rates. Smokers pay more than nonsmokers of the same age, and people with certain health problems or those who work in dangerous professions may either be denied coverage or be rated and offered life insurance coverage only at higher premiums. As the premiums for life insurance policies are determined largely by the customer's age when he or she purchases a policy, life insurance agents frequently encourage clients to purchase as much insurance as they can afford when they are young and healthy because similar policies will definitely cost more in the future and may be unavailable if the customer develops health problems.

Licensed life insurance agents and financial planners need to explain carefully to customers that life insurance needs will vary greatly for people as they age. Parents with young children clearly need a large amount of life insurance because the surviving spouse requires a significant immediate estate to replace the deceased person's income so that there will be enough money to raise and educate the children. Parents of young children have not yet had enough time to accumulate sufficient assets by investing in mutual funds or the stock market, and they need to purchase life insurance policies in amounts equal to between six and ten times their annual income. An insurance agent also needs to take into account the specific needs of individual clients. A single person with no children will need less insurance than married people with young children, but an experienced agent must not lose contact with his or her client because the client's insurance needs may change if there are new children or if there is a marriage or divorce. The owner of an insurance policy has a right to designate and change beneficiaries. Following a divorce, for example, the owner of a policy may very well want to change his or her beneficiary.

Financial planners agree that life insurance plays an essential role in financial planning, but there is serious disagreement about the type of life insurance policy that people should purchase. Traditionally, life insurance policies were presented to customers as ideal investments that combined income replacement protection with retirement planning. Life insurance agents who sell whole-life policies explain to their clients that such policies can provide them with income protection while they are working and can also be used for retirement income if they choose to turn in their policies for the cash values once they retire. Owners of whole-life policies can also borrow from their cash values and pay back these loans at either guaranteed or variable rates.

The problem with whole-life policies is that the return on cash values is often quite low, perhaps as low as 1 to 3 percent. Whole-life policies are very profitable for insurance companies because they can invest these cash values in the stock market or mutual funds and receive a return on this money that is much greater than that given to policyholders. Many retired people who purchased whole-life policies when they were much younger discover to their displeasure that the cash values in these policies are insufficient to meet their present needs. The life insurance company will pay life insurance benefits once it receives a death certificate for the person insured under a life insurance policy, but the money invested in whole-life insurance policies does not produce returns comparable to what people could have earned by investing similar amounts in mutual funds or the stock market.

Many senior citizens find themselves with much more insurance coverage than they need, but if they turn in their policies, they will receive a very poor return on their premium investments. They find themselves in a difficult situation. They may want their children or the surviving spouse to receive the life insurance benefits, but they need the money now, and the cash values are not sufficient to meet their present needs.

TYPES OF LIFE INSURANCE POLICIES

There are advantages and disadvantages to both whole-life and term policies. Clients who believe that they lack the discipline to invest regularly for their retirement may conclude that it is wiser for them to purchase whole-life policies so that they will at least have something for their retirement years. Some whole-life policies can be fully paid after twenty years or at a certain age, normally sixty-five. Whenever the annual interest paid exceeds the annual premium, the premium will be paid from this interest. The client will then have a paid policy. Many clients like the absolute guarantee provided by whole-life policies, but they should not think of life insurance policies as investments that will produce enough money for them to live on during their retirement years.

Life insurance agents from whole-life insurance companies continue, however, to present such policies not only for income protection but also as investment vehicles. They are correct in stressing both aspects of whole-life policies, but they also should explain to their clients that they need to have investments separate from their whole-life policies so that they can afford to send their children to college and to maintain the lifestyle to which they have become accustomed during their retirement years. Whole-life agents tend not to educate clients on the poor return on cash values because such information would discourage people from purchasing whole-life policies. During the last two decades of the twentieth century, however, more and more people learned about the differences between whole-life and term-life policies. As a result, the percentage of whole-life policies purchased decreased significantly as the percentage of term-life policies purchased increased.

Term-life policies have become more popular in recent years largely because they enable people to purchase for the same monthly or annual premium significantly more coverage than they could obtain with whole-life policies, but many clients do not fully understand how term policies work. As the very expression "term life" indicates, benefits for a term-life policy will be paid only if the person covered by this policy dies while the coverage is in effect. Such policies build no cash values, and, therefore, people cannot borrow from them. Many different types of term-life policies exist, including annual renewal policies, in which the policies increase every year, and level-term policies, in which the same premium is paid each year for a guaranteed numbers of years (normally ten, twenty, or twenty-five years). Some term policies can be converted to whole-life policies at certain times during the life of the policy, if the client chooses to do so. Many clients combine relatively inexpensive term-life coverage with regular investments in mutual funds that generally produce a better return than whole-life policies. Many clients, however, simply purchase term policies and do not commit themselves to a regular investment plan by contributing a set amount of money each month for their retirement. Then they are left with neither life insurance coverage nor significant investments to live on during their retirement years.

Several term-life insurance companies have developed a marketing strategy to encourage people to buy term policies and to invest the difference between the less expensive term policy premiums and more expensive whole-life policy premiums. Frequently such a strategy is referred to as "buy term and invest the difference." Some clients choose to purchase both whole-life and term policies. They may purchase a relatively small whole-life policy of perhaps $25,000, to cover final expenses and to pay certain debts, and a large term policy for income replacement during their working years when their responsibilities to their children are the highest. They also begin to make regular investments during their working years so that they can accumulate enough money for their retirement years.

Many senior citizens find themselves in difficult circumstances during their retirement years largely because they did not receive effective financial planning while they were much younger. Until the 1980s, most people thought that only wealthy people needed financial planning. This was not the case, but financial planning was relatively expensive and people believed that they did not need to plan for their retirements because they could rely on Social Security and employee pensions. People trusted their local life insurance agents who sold them reliable whole-life policies and gave them some financial advice. Life insurance agents were often licensed securities agents as well, and they would often offer their clients one or two mutual funds sold by their companies, but the choices of mutual funds were often severely limited. When the high inflation of the 1970s and the early 1980s began to significantly decrease the actual value of pensions and the cash values in whole-life policies, people suddenly began to realize that they could no longer rely on Social Security and company pensions for their retirements. Throughout the 1980s, many companies made it more and more difficult for people to qualify for meaningful pensions. As most employees now change jobs at least seven times during their working years, they never accumulate enough years with a single company to receive a meaningful pension.

THE ROLE OF LIFE INSURANCE FOR RETIRED PEOPLE

Senior citizens do not want to be a burden to their children. For this reason, many retired people set aside enough money to pay for their funerals or prepay their final expenses by means of a life insurance policy paid for in full through just one payment at a funeral home. Such "single-pay" policies were marketed very successfully by funeral home directors starting in the 1980s because they met a definite need. People who purchase such policies normally designate the funeral home as the beneficiary. In most states, funeral home directors commit themselves to accepting the benefits paid from such policies as full payment for funeral expenses, as long as the survivors do not change the original funeral arrangement by choosing, for example, a more expensive coffin.

Senior citizens who received effective financial planning during their working years do not need much life insurance during their retirement years because their responsibilities are then much lower. For example, they no longer have to pay for the education of their children. If they began investing regularly when they were younger, they now have enough money on which to live. Their insurance needs are now very different. As people age, nursing home insurance becomes more important for their financial planning than life insurance. Such policies normally cover the first two or three years of residence in a nursing home, after a specified waiting period. By their very nature, nursing homes are labor-intensive and very expensive to live in. Many elderly people each year have debilitating strokes or are diagnosed with illnesses such as Alzheimer's disease, which may make it necessary for the spouse or the adult children to place the person in a nursing home, largely because no other choices remain. Life insurance plays an important role in people's lives during their working years, but other forms of insurance become more important for people during their retirement years.

—*Edmund J. Campion*

See also: Death and dying; Facility and institutional care; Fraud against the elderly; Funerals; Life expectancy; Pensions; Retirement; Retirement planning; Smoking

For Further Information

Black, Kenneth, Jr., and Harold D. Skipper, Jr. *Life Insurance*. 15th ed. Lucretian, LL C. 2015. A college textbook that explains clearly the nature of life insurance policies and the investment strategies of life insurance companies.

Bloom, Bryan S. *Confessions of a CPA Why What I Was Taught to Be True Has Turned Out Not to Be*. Infinity Publishing, 2011. This book is a compilation of eight commonly held financial "truths" that are generally accepted as hallmarks of a sound financial plan.

Peters, Daniel A, and Douglas A. Mckay. "Life Insurance: Ownership and Investment Considerations." *Plastic Surgery*, vol. 21, no. 1, 2014. doi:10.4172/plastic-surgery.1000847. Describes factors involved in purchasing life insurance.

Steuer, Anthony. *Questions and Answers on Life Insurance: The Life Insurance Toolbook*. 4th ed., Sage P, 2015. This book is a valuable resource for anyone involved with a life insurance policy. It helps makes a complex financial product understandable for consumers as well as financial advisors.

Thompson, Jake. *Money. Wealth. Life Insurance: How the Wealthy Use Life Insurance as a Tax-Free Personal Bank to Supercharge Their Savings*. CreateSpace, 2013. This book is designed to simplify some of the concepts surrounding cash value life insurance, such as Infinite Banking and Bank on Yourself, and make them easier to understand, stripping them down to the core benefits of cash value life insurance.

LITTLE BROTHERS—FRIENDS OF THE ELDERLY

Date: Founded in 1946
Relevant Issues: Economics, sociology
Significance: This organization supplies food and attention to isolated elderly people; volunteers offer medical transportation, advocacy skills, entertainment

outings, and regular visits that promote mutual friendships.

After World War II in Paris, nobleman Armand Marquiset began a Catholic lay brotherhood whose mission was to deliver hot meals, accompanied by a bouquet of flowers, to the elderly poor. Called Les Petits Frères des Pauvres (Little Brothers of the Poor), Marquiset's organization spread to the United States in 1959 when he sent Michael Salmon to Chicago, where he founded a branch of the Little Brothers.

In 1967, Salmon married, and Little Brothers opened its volunteer opportunities to men and women of all faiths and ages. In 1983, the United States branch of the Little Brothers of the Poor was renamed Little Brothers-Friends of the Elderly. By the late 2010s, Little Brothers had eight member countries: Canada, France, Germany, Ireland, Mexico, Morocco, Spain, and the United States. Offices in the United States exist in Boston, Chicago, Cincinnati, Hancock (Michigan), Minneapolis, Philadelphia, San Francisco, and Omaha. Smaller affiliates, called Friends of Little Brothers, consist of groups of volunteers in other cities who extend services to the elderly under the auspices of the national organization.

Volunteers are usually matched with an elderly friend to offer companionship and any services that are needed, such as providing transportation to a doctor, delivering hot meals, writing letters, reading, shopping for food, and running other errands. Little Brothers also provides group outings, such as holiday parties, summer picnics, and travel to tourist attractions, thus supporting the Little Brothers' credo, Flowers Before Bread. In 2019 the organization had 21,000 volunteers serving over 52,000 elderly across the world.

—*Rose Secrest*

See also: Friendship; Home services; Leisure activities; Loneliness; Social ties

---

LIVING TOGETHER. *See* COHABITATION.

LIVING WILLS

Relevant Issues: Family, health and medicine, law

Significance: A living will is a directive to physicians giving directions as to what methods of life-prolonging medical treatment should or should not be used when individuals have a terminal condition and become unable to make their wishes known.

Living wills are not wills in the traditional sense. Traditional wills do not take effect until after persons die. Living wills come into effect while individuals are still alive but are unable to make their wishes known (for example, if they are in a coma) or when they do not have the mental ability to legally make their wishes known (for example, if they have Alzheimer's disease or dementia). Living wills are also known as medical directives, advance directives, medical orders for life-sustaining treatment, or directives to physicians. Living wills are directives to physicians and other health-care personnel to perform or not to perform certain life-sustaining medical treatments that artificially prolong life, such as resuscitation, force feeding, or breathing assistance. Persons may also indicate their wishes for drug therapy to alleviate pain. Living wills are valid only in the case of terminal illnesses in most states, and in some states doctors are permitted only to withhold treatment.

Over the years the right to die with dignity and without the expense of large medical bills has been discussed by federal and state legislators. The U.S. Supreme Court in Cruzan v. Director, Missouri Department of Health (1990) decided that individuals have the right to control their medical treatment. Indi-

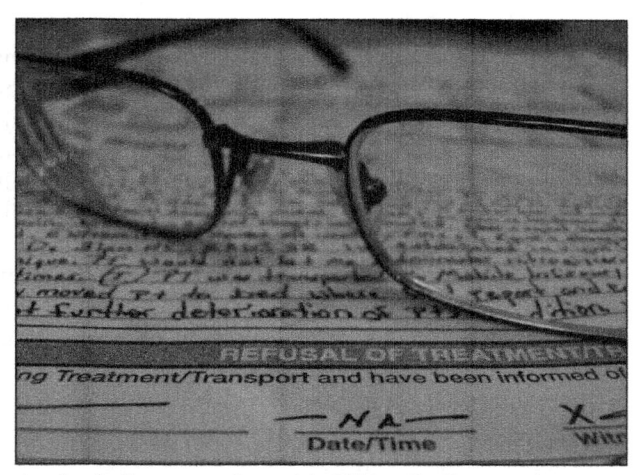

A refusal of treatment form. (via Wikimedia Commons)

viduals' desires come first, even if they choose to forgo life-prolonging medical treatment while family members or physicians want to prolong life. Sometimes individuals can make such decisions themselves. For example, they can ask to be discharged from the hospital and return home. However, when persons are near the end of an illness or are involved in severe accidents, they are often no longer capable of making their wishes known.

It is in such circumstances that living wills take effect, directing physicians to take or not to take action. Physicians who are not willing to abide by individuals' wishes must turn such cases over to other physicians.

Because accidents can happen to persons of all ages, living wills are not just for the elderly. It is easy to make a living will. Most hospitals and physicians have standard forms that have been approved by the state. When

---

HOW TO TALK TO SENIORS ABOUT LIVING WILLS

How Do They Feel?

Considering and planning for the end of one's life can feel distressing. People often avoid thinking about it as it raises a high level of discomfort. Writing a living will can feel overwhelming for a senior. Thinking about what types of treatment they would want and visualizing scenarios of being hospitalized can trigger emotions of fear and panic. Feelings of nervousness and uncertainty may arise as they consider major decisions. Many seniors worry that they will change their mind about a decision after it has been written on the will. Once they find out that they are able to change their will, this anxiety can be alleviated.

The idea of having some control over their end-of-life care can also feel empowering and reassuring. Drawing up a living will can help seniors feel proactive about making significant life decisions. By planning ahead, many seniors feel a sense of relief knowing that others will not be deciding on their behalf and that their wishes will be honored.

Some seniors may be concerned and uncomfortable about designating authority to a particular family member. They may wish to avoid hurt feelings by choosing one family member over another. On the other hand, they may be comforted knowing that their loved ones will not be placed in the difficult position of trying to decide what their wishes would be during a medical emergency. This can help their family members avoid conflict and accept their end of life with less stress and greater certainty.

How Do I Start The Conversation?

Discussing end-of-life preparations and a living will can be difficult. This does not mean that the subject should be avoided, but you should approach the topic with tact and sensitivity. You may choose to address the topic by indicating that you have drawn up such a document for yourself and sharing your experience. Alternatively, you might mention that you had family members who wrote a living will and discuss aspects of the process as well as the benefits. By engaging the senior in the conversation, you can begin to draw out his or her thoughts on the matter. If you are the adult child of an aging parent, you may assess your family dynamics to determine whether it would be best for you or another family member to raise the topic.

You may want to discuss how planning for end-of-life care will provide peace of mind. Instead of being concerned about what will happen in the future, you can suggest that writing a living will can help to alleviate these worries. Moreover, you can speak about how a living will ensure that their wishes be honored. You can also reassure the senior that they will be able to change details of the living will if there are any changes to their health, if new details or treatments become available, or if they change their mind regarding the specifications of the document.

During an emergency medical situation when crucial decisions need to be made, emotions often run high. Family disputes are more likely to occur. One adult child may believe the parent would have wanted a particular treatment, and another may believe the parent would have preferred a less aggressive intervention. A living will can dissipate some of that tension by indicating, in a legal document, the parent's decision. Make sure that the senior informs his or her family members of the location of the living will so that it is accessible if needed. Seniors may also want to give a copy of the living will to their primary care physician or lawyer. This will facilitate a speedy response in the event that medical decisions need to be made without delay.

—Leah Jacob

people are admitted to the hospital, they are usually asked if they have a living will. If not, they will be given the opportunity to make one. If they have specific wishes, they may decide to have attorneys draw up a living will.

One of the problems with living wills is that persons must decide their wishes for end-of-life care in advance, without having the opportunity to take future circumstances into account. Another problem with them is that they only take effect when a patient's condition is terminal. Persons in the early stages of Alzheimer's disease, although not terminally ill, may not be mentally fit to make health-care decisions. A durable power of attorney for health care or health-care proxies allows individuals to deal with all these problems.

—Celia Ray Hayhoe
Updated by Thomas J. Martin, MS II

See also: Alzheimer's disease; Caregiving; Death and dying; Durable power of attorney; Facility and institutional care; Health care; Hospice; Hospitalization; Terminal illness; Wills and bequests

For Further Information

Lum, Hillary D., et al. "Advance Care Planning in the Elderly." *The Medical Clinics of North America*, vol. 99, no. 2, Mar. 2015, pp. 391-403. ResearchGate. www.researchgate.net/publication/272624967_Advance_Care_Planning_in_the_Elderly. This review provides an informative background on the process of advanced care planning within the elderly population by identifying key components and barriers.

Mayo Clinic Staff. "Living Wills and Advance Directives for Medical Decisions." Mayo Clinic, Mayo Foundation for Medical Education and Research, 15 Dec. 2018. www.mayoclinic.org/healthy-lifestyle/consumer-health/in-depth/living-wills/art-20046303. A guide to advance directives including a section on living wills.

Miller, Bianca. "Nurses in the Know: The History and Future of Advance Directives." *The Online Journal of Issues in Nursing*, vol. 22, no. 3, Sept. 2017. doi:10.3912/OJIN.Vol22No03PPT57. This article defines advanced directives and discusses the evolution of patient self-determination as a concept and the Patient Self-Determination Act (PSDA).

LONELINESS

Relevant Issues: Death, health and medicine, psychology

Significance: Loneliness has profound effects on physical and mental health in all age groups; however, elderly people may be particularly susceptible to its effects.

Human beings are social animals. Most people are reared in families, and most develop significant and important relationships during their lifetimes in their many different roles: spouse, significant other, parent, child, friend, colleague, or fellow member of religious or civic group. Interpersonal relationships are central to people's sense of self and to their lives. In later life, virtually all people experience changes in their personal relationships because of retirement from paid employment, divorce, illness, death of friends and loved ones, relocation to a new community, or the move of children to their own homes. These changes can lead to a sense of isolation and loneliness or, after a period of grieving for the loss of the original relationships, to new and different, but equally rewarding, relationships.

DEFINING LONELINESS

Loneliness is largely a matter of perception. Some people are not lonely when they are by themselves, while others experience loneliness even when they are with other people. Loneliness can be defined as an uncomfortable sense of being isolated from others. It is a sense of not having anyone to rely on, even if living with others. Some researchers divide loneliness into two categories: external and internal. External loneliness occurs because of life circumstances, such as loss of a spouse; internal loneliness, on the other hand, is more a product of the personality of the person who feels alone.

Researchers who have examined loneliness in the elderly have found that about two-thirds of older people describe themselves as rarely or never lonely, about one-fifth as sometimes lonely, and one-tenth as frequently lonely. An AARP study in 2000 found that 27 percent of seniors ages 50-80 reported they sometimes or often felt isolated while a third responded they sometimes felt a lack of companionship. The National Poll on Healthy Aging reported that one in three are lonely. People over 60 years in the United States number about 50 million or about 16 percent of the population. By 2035, it is estimated that adults 65 years and older will grow to 78 million in number.

Elderly people who are chronically ill or homebound because of disability are particularly susceptible to loneliness. Others who are more likely to describe themselves as lonely include the oldest seniors, people who have lost a spouse, and those who care for a chronically ill person. The Pew Research Center found that adults sixty years and older spend over 10 hours a day alone (compared with adults ages 40 to 50 who spend less than five hours alone each day) and can be an indicator of social isolation that is associated with health risks. Poverty, inadequate financial resources, and city dwelling are also associated with loneliness. People least likely to describe themselves as lonely are those who have a strong sense of community and a good social support system. Good health and adequate financial support are other important factors.

EFFECTS OF LONELINESS ON HEALTH

Studies of heart health have demonstrated that people with strong social support systems have lower blood pressure and other evidence of good cardiac functioning. In addition, people undergoing stressful situations have lower heart rates in the presence of a familiar person than in the presence of a stranger. In addition, people who live alone are more likely to die following a heart attack. One study showed that a far greater proportion of people with good social support who had a heart attack were still alive five years later than those who were socially isolated. The death rate from all causes is two to four times higher in people who are socially isolated.

Some cardiac changes in socially isolated people may be caused by poor health habits. Lonely people may have increased difficulty buying or preparing food for themselves or even feeling like eating. They may also have difficulty getting sufficient exercise. They have no one to remind them to take their medications. These lifestyle factors may contribute to heart disease and other health problems, such as osteoporosis. However, most researchers believe that the explanation for the effects of social support or isolation on the heart are more complex than changes in health habits that come with isolation. Social support and isolation seem to affect the complex interactions of the nervous system, hormones, cells, and tissues.

The hypothalamus and pituitary gland regulate body functions by releasing stimulating hormones that cause responses in target organs elsewhere in the body. These target organs, in turn, release hormones that supply feedback to the hypothalamus and pituitary, telling them when to shut off the flow of stimulating hormones. When a person is under stress (including the stress of loneliness), the hypothalamus and pituitary activate the adrenal glands. The adrenals then produce a number of hormones, including norepinephrine, which stimulates the sympathetic nervous system. The sympathetic nervous system, in turn, causes the blood flow and heart rate to increase and breathing to be more rapid. Although these changes are valuable in an emergency, they are detrimental when they continue for long periods of time, as in the chronic stress of loneliness, and may ultimately lead to heart attack or other cardiac problems.

Other studies have shown that the immune systems of older people with good social support function better than those of lonely people. For example, people with close personal relationships have a better response to immunizations. People who are lonely have fewer antibodies against pneumococcal disease, a common cause of pneumonia in older people. Levels of natural killer cells that fight infection are lower in lonely people, and white blood cells respond more slowly.

Loneliness is thought to be at the root of much of the anxiety and depression seen in older people. In addition, some people may increase their alcohol or other drug intake to deal with the psychological pain associated with loneliness, leading to alcoholism or addiction. Loneliness also contributes to suicide. Factors strongly associated with suicide include widowed or divorced states, retirement or unemployment, solitary living conditions, isolation, recent moves, poor health, depression, alcoholism, loneliness, and feelings of rejection or of being unloved.

RECOGNIZING AND OVERCOMING LONELINESS

Older people often do not reveal their feeling of loneliness to others. Health-care workers, friends, and family may have to recognize loneliness through other clues. Psychologists have identified many behaviors that may indicate loneliness, including clutching at a visitor's arm or hand, talking excessively, sitting with tightly crossed arms or legs, wearing drab clothing, or lack of motivation. People who are deaf or depressed or who have urinary incontinence may be reluctant to interact with others, increasing their isolation and loneliness.

The key to overcoming loneliness is often as simple as increasing contact with other people. Senior centers serve group meals, offer classes, facilitate "foster grandparent" programs, and arrange for transportation to various places. Volunteering at a hospital, child care center, library, church, or school is another way of making contact with people. Pets may also supply needed companionship. Moving out of a house and into a retirement center is a solution for some. These centers allow people to live in the privacy of their own apartments but give them access to communal dining, group activities, opportunities for social and cultural events, and medical care.

Friends and relatives can visit or otherwise communicate with the homebound on a regular basis. In addition to the more traditional telephone call or letter, newer technologies, such as interactive television, the Internet, and social media such as Facebook offer interesting possibilities for maintaining contact with loved ones who are far away. Some city planners have designed neighborhoods and buildings that make it more likely for people to interact formally and informally with others. Local, state, and federal governments can assist with appropriate housing and safety policies that support the elderly.

Psychotherapy may also be useful in helping people deal with loneliness. One study indicated that blood pressure improved among elderly people who described themselves as lonely after small-group discussions. Support groups may be helpful both for individuals with chronic illness and for their caregivers. Individual counseling to guide and encourage lonely people in their interactions with others, as well as antidepressant medications, may also be useful.

—Rebecca Lovell Scott
Updated by Marylane Wade Koch, MSN, RN

See also: Alcohol use disorder; Communication; Depression; Family relationships; Friendship; Heart attacks; Heart changes and disorders; Illnesses among older adults; Pets; Psychiatry, geriatric; Senior citizen centers; Social ties; Stress and coping skills; Suicide; Volunteering

For Further Information

Ducharme, Jamie. "One in Three Seniors Are Lonely: Here's How It's Hurting Their Health." *Time Magazine*, 4 Mar. 2019. time.com/5541166/loneliness-old-age/. Presents information on how loneliness in seniors can increase the risk strokes, anxiety, depression, and heart attacks but also shorten life expectancy as much as smoking and more than being sedentary or overweight. However, loneliness can be addressed on an individual basis for improved outcomes.

Grieco, Elizabeth. "On Average Older Adults Spend Over Half Their Time Alone." *Pew Research Center: FactTank*, 3 July 2019. www.pewresearch.org/fact-tank/2019/07/03/on-average-older-adults-spend-over-half-their-waking-hours-alone/. Looks at data of non-institutionalized seniors over 60 years old from the Pew Research Center 2014-2017 American Time Use Survey.

"If You're Feeling Lonely: How to Stay Connected in Older Age." Independent Age: Advice and Support for Older Age (Operating name of the Royal United Kingdom Beneficent Association) May 2019. www.independentage.org/information/ advice-guides-factsheets-leaflets/if-youre-feeling-lonely. Includes a forty-page downloadable booklet written from the perspective of the United Kingdom but contains useful information for seniors anywhere. Can also be ordered in print copy for free.

Kamiel, Anita. "A Hot Trend: The Internet, Social Media & the Elderly" *HuffPost*, 7 Mar.2017. Updated 8 Mar. 2017. w6w.huffpost.com/entry/older-people-social-media_b_9191178?guccounter=1. Addresses how older adults are embracing technology such as social media to stay connected with family and friends, which can decrease isolation and loneliness.

"Loneliness is Bad for the Heart." *ScienceDaily.* 9 June 2018. www.sciencedaily.com/releases/2018/06/180609124652.htm. Discussion of a study presented at EuroHeartCare 2018, the European Society of Cardiology nursing congress about the relationship of loneliness to heart disease but also as a predictor of premature death.

LONGEVITY RESEARCH

Relevant Issues: Biology, demographics, economics, health and medicine

Significance: Life expectancy improved dramatically in industrialized countries throughout the world in the twentieth century as a result of advances in nutrition and medicine.

With many of the declines associated with aging having been eliminated or their onsets delayed, humans now live longer, more healthy lives. Nevertheless, the search for better understanding and control over the aging process continues. Although most aging factors are unknown, many medical treatments have been explored to prevent the process. Dietary modification, exercise, antioxidants, and hormone treatments have all been suggested as avenues to slow aging. Unfortunately, due to the close interrelationship between disease and aging, there are practical limitations in life extension research. It is often impossible to ascertain which developmental phenomena are caused by natural aging and which are disease-related. More research is necessary to assess the ethics, safety, and effectiveness of many life extension strategies.

THEORIES OF AGING

Why do humans age? Evolutionary biologist Richard Dawkins has suggested aging is part of humanity's natural evolution. Successful evolution is dependent on reproductive fitness, literally the efficiency of a species to reproduce. Yet, reproductive fitness has little to do with longevity. Humans do not need to live past the age of thirty (two human generations); in terms of evolution, any extra time alive after reproduction is superfluous. Humans need only to live long enough to pass on their genes to the next generation and ensure that generation's survival. Because long life is not important in engendering the next generation, some researchers believe that a trait for longevity is not something that can evolve.

Aging appears to be programmed into human cells from birth. Two pieces of data support this statement. First, it was once thought that human cells grown in tissue culture were immortal and could be grown indefinitely. Stanford University researcher Leonard Hayflick demonstrated that animal cells in culture could only be grown for a limited time as they were passed from one petri dish to the next. Eventually the cells died. The number of times the cells could be passed between petri dishes in the laboratory was called the Hayflick limit. This strongly supports the idea that death is programmed into the cells themselves. The second piece of data supporting this hypothesis is that telomeres, the deoxyribonucleic acid (DNA) sequences at the ends of chromosomes, seem to act like molecular clocks in aging. As cells age, telomeres shorten with each division, like tiny timekeepers keeping track of each cell multiplication.

Cancer cells do not have shortening telomeres, nor do they have Hayflick limits. These virtually immortal cells may be the key to understanding aging. Woodring Wright, a University of Texas researcher, took the enzyme telomerase, which lengthens telomeres in cancerous cells, and introduced the gene into normal cells. He examined the possibility that normal cells with telomerase can be made immortal without becoming cancerous. He hoped that if telomere shortening acts as the biological clock, he could bypass its effects.

Another theory suggests that aging occurs due to accumulated errors in DNA. Many factors damage cells and DNA. The buildup of errors over time may lead to aging as the enzymatic systems that repair DNA can no longer cope. Although ultraviolet and gamma radiation contribute to combined genetic errors, researchers suggest that cells and DNA are primarily damaged by dangerously modified molecules of oxygen. When oxygen becomes a charged, "free radical" molecule, it can easily damage DNA and proteins. Over the long term, this increasing damage presumably becomes irreparable. Substances that tend to inhibit this oxidative damage are known as antioxidants. It has been proposed that antioxidants may extend life by inhibiting the accumulation of DNA damage.

Related hypotheses suggest other ways aging damage might occur. Researcher Donald Morse proposed that cellular damage is caused by a buildup of "age pigments" that choke off and inhibit metabolic activity. Another theory suggests that thermal damage over a lifetime of heat exposure causes loss of enzymatic functions. Some researchers have suggested that lysosomal enzymes, used in cells to degrade waste, are released as bodies age and produce cellular corruption. A fourth theory states that errors accumulate in DNA as the damage repair systems decay over time. Researcher Harold Rabinowitz proposed that aging may be the result of lowered oxygen levels in critical areas of the body. One final speculation submits that aging is a result of the immune system self-destructing and attacking the body's cells. These hypotheses have little or no experimental support.

Cynthia Kenyon, a University of California researcher, believed that aging may be dependent on the activity of just a few genes. She isolated a flatworm longevity gene, called abnormal Dauer Formation (daf-16). Kenyon demonstrated that when the gene is activated, the life span of a normal adult flatworm is doubled. The gene acts through a central signaling mechanism and may function analogously to a system in human beings.

Related to Kenyon's work is that of researcher Huber Werner. Werner isolated the human mutant gene "WRN." A mutation in the single WRN gene causes Werner's syndrome, a disease characterized by rapid, premature aging in youngsters. The existence of this disease supports the hypothesis that human aging may be precipitated by just a few genes. Although it is not known how a single gene could cause premature aging, studies continue.

PHYSICAL APPROACHES TO LIFE EXTENSION

Body weight was once thought the most important factor in longevity. Much of this evidence came from the Framingham Heart Study performed over several decades in Massachusetts with a group of 5,209 men and women. The Framingham study suggested that men overweight by as little as 20 percent had significantly higher mortality—but surprisingly, the mortality of underweight men was also greatly increased. Other studies by Harvard researchers I-Min Lee and Ralph Paffenbarger suggested that body weight, within 15 percent of optimal, is unrelated to mortality and that weight fluctuations contribute more to mortality by enhancing coronary stress. The Framingham data were reanalyzed by Yale researcher Kelly Brownell to examine fluctuations of body mass over time, and results were found to support the conclusions of Lee and Paffenbarger; changes in the body mass of both men and women were positively associated with increases in mortality. The data do not advise staying obese or underweight to avoid changes in body mass, but suggest that the link between weight and longevity is complex.

Evidence from the classic work of Granville Nolen suggests that body mass is less important than caloric intake in increasing life span. In Nolen's study, one group of rats was allowed to eat freely while a second group was limited from an early age (thirty-five days) in their caloric intake to 60 to 80 percent of the control group. The life span of the restricted-diet group increased on average from about seven hundred days (in controls) to about nine hundred days. Also, caloric restriction extended life when mice started their restrictive diets at an older age of one hundred eighty days. It is still unclear whether caloric intake can be used to extend human life. The magnitude of the caloric restriction as well as the timing of it in humans is still being explored.

The amount and calories of the food eaten are not the only factors that affect longevity. Since early times one's diet has been said to contribute to longevity. The Romans and Greeks believed eating ambrosia, the "food of the gods," could grant immortality. Ambrosia is believed by ethnologist James Arthur to be a species of mushroom. In the 1800s, cod-liver oil was believed to be a life-extending agent. In the 1960s, eating oysters was said to increase virility and male potency in the elderly. In the 1970s, marketers insinuated that villages of Russian centenarians existed whose yogurt eating had brought them well into their second century of life. In the 1980s, bran, garlic, and olive oil were all proposed to lengthen life. In the 1990s, ginseng and tomatoes were touted as life extenders.

The negative aspects of foods have been stressed as well. "Age gurus" such as Karlis Ullis exhort that consuming white sugar and bleached flour may increase mortality, though this belief has little scientific support. Eating red meat is believed by many to contribute to the aging process; some even believe all meat introduces age-inducing "poisons" into the human body.

Although it seems likely that in balanced diets specific foods do not have an adverse effect upon life duration, specific nutrients of those foods may have a great impact upon mortality. Researchers Mary DeMarte and Hildegard Enesco gave one group of mice a balanced diet and a diet without the amino acid tryptophan. Both groups received the same number of calories. The tryptophan-deficient group lived seventy days longer on average than the control. The mechanism by which this dietary restriction extends life is unknown; it may be by encouraging weight loss or caloric restriction or by reducing protein levels.

The least-understood strategy to increased longevity is physical exercise. In the 1800s, extreme physical exercise was said to damage the body, although this belief is no longer credited. Long-term studies of professional athletes suggest no adverse associations between athletic competition and longevity. However, it is still not clear whether physical exercise increases human life span. John Holloszy of Washington University studied the effects of exercise on laboratory rats and found they have a longer life expectancy on average than the sedentary controls (approximately one thousand days versus approximately nine hundred days). Both groups were given as much food as they desired, but the active mice ate less food. This makes interpretation of the data complex. Did the experimental group have a longer life expectancy due to increased exercise, decreased caloric intake, other metabolic effects of the physical stress, or a combination of the three? It is not clear whether physical activity acts as a disease modifier or a true life extender.

PHARMACOLOGIC APPROACHES TO LIFE EXTENSION

Many strategies using hormones or medications to produce life extension have been tested successfully in animal systems, but these treatments have not been appraised with humans. Care must be taken in applying the results of animal testing to humans.

Antioxidant treatments may be one path to life extension. Antioxidants are dietary supplements that destroy free radicals or prevent their production in the body. Several antioxidants have been administered to rats and humans in an attempt to lengthen life. Researchers Marc Bernarducci and Norma Owens reported that vitamin E treatments increased longevity in rats and flatworms by 10 to 15 percent. This seems promising for humans, but studies by Linus Pauling suggest that "megadosing" vitamin E may actually reduce life expectancy in men and women. Animal studies have also been performed with vitamin C, but Bernarducci and Owens reported that vitamin C treatments alone had no significant effect on life span. It may be that antioxidant chemicals such as vitamins A, E, and C do not lengthen life by themselves but prevent the onset of cardiovascular and neoplastic diseases.

Spanish researcher Gustavo Barja suggested that enhanced production of antioxidant enzymes may be more effective than antioxidant dietary supplements. Barja treated frogs with aminothiazole known to induce the synthesis of an antioxidant enzyme called superoxide dismutase (SOD). The enzyme is able to degrade and nullify free radicals. Frogs receiving aminothiazole demonstrated increased longevity over untreated frogs. Clinical applicability in humans is being examined; long-term effects of chemicals like aminothiazole in humans has not yet been determined.

In addition to experiments with chemicals or dietary supplements, longevity studies have been performed using various human hormones. There may be a connection between aging and the levels of many hormones that decline during aging. It is believed by many that hormone replacement therapy (HRT) may be a route to extending human life. Human growth hormone (HGH), made in the adrenal glands, is important in maintaining skeletal and muscle strength. University of Florida researcher David Lowenthal observed that as humans age, HGH levels are reduced and, in the elderly, become deficient. Lowenthal administered HGH to elderly men and found benefits such as reduced body fat and increased muscle mass. There are several drawbacks with HGH, such as high cost, repeated need for injections, adverse physical effects such as carpal tunnel syndrome, and no evidence that it extends life.

Use of male hormones (androgens) in HRT have been documented since 1889 when Charles Édouard Brown-Séquard, the founder of modern endocrinology, self-administered canine testicular extract. The elderly Brown-Séquard claimed that the treatment increased his strength and mental clarity and gave him more energy. Although use of androgens as longevity agents has not been actively pursued, chemical precursors of androgens have been used to treat the aged.

In elderly men, there is a reduction in testosterone levels associated with a decline in its chemical precursor dehydroepiandrosterone (DHEA) made in the pituitary. Blood levels of DHEA are quite high in infancy but diminish as an individual ages. Researchers Perti Ebeling and Veikko Koivisto found that in individuals over seventy, DHEA is virtually not detectable. Long-term DHEA treatment in mice reduces weight, lengthens life, and delays the onset of immune dysfunction. The DHEA hormone may act to increase life span through a mechanism similar to caloric restriction. According to studies by University of California researcher Samuel Yen, humans do benefit from DHEA treatment. Men and women taking fifty milligrams of DHEA a day for three months felt significant increases in physical and psychological wellbeing. Long-term effects of DHEA treatment are still being analyzed. There are concerns that, with extended use, DHEA may increase risks for cancer and other diseases.

Melatonin is a hormone produced by the pineal gland. It has been implicated in a range of activities including modulation of aging, sleep, sexual maturation, and fertility. Melatonin production is circadian with maximal synthesis occurring at night. Like HGH and DHEA, melatonin production decreases with advancing age. Bernarducci and Owens report that reduced melatonin levels in adult humans have been associated with cancer and chronic insomnia. Experiments have examined whether melatonin treatments can extend life. Swiss researcher Walter Pierpaoli gave mice drinking water treated with ten milligrams of melatonin per milliliter. Mean survival was increased significantly in the melatonin-treated versus control group (930 days versus 752 days). Treated mice were more vigorous and active and had better posture.

There is evidence that part of the life-extending mechanism of melatonin may be its activity as an antioxidant. Finnish researcher Seppo Saarela suggested that melatonin is a free radical scavenger and the most powerful antioxidant known. The hormone can significantly reduce tissue damage caused by free radical generation in sunlight. Additionally, melatonin appears to be nontoxic in high, prolonged dosages. Humans who take mega doses of melatonin (300 milligrams per day) for up to five years have demonstrated few ill effects.

Despite how benign and promising melatonin appears, questions have been raised about the hormone's physiological effects. It is still not clear if melatonin functions in the same way in humans as in mice. As the hormone is normally produced in a well-defined cycle, it is not clear what administration schedules and dosages may be best for humans. Bernarducci and Owens also report worries that artificially high levels of melatonin in humans may alter levels of other hormones, such as thyroid hormone or testosterone. As with many of the treatments described, more study is required before all the risks of melatonin are understood.

—*James J. Campanella*

See also: Aging process; Anti-aging treatments; Antioxidants; Caloric restriction; Cancer; Cross-linkage theory of aging; Estrogen replacement therapy; Free radical theory of aging; Life expectancy; Nutrition; Vitamins and minerals; Weight loss and gain

For Further Information

Bernarducci, Marc P., and Norma J. Owens. "Is There a Fountain of Youth?: A Review of Current Life Extension Strategies." *Pharmacotherapy*, vol. 16, no. 2, Mar./Apr. 1996. Review covering the major paths of longevity research.

Cox, Harold. *Later Life: The Realities of Aging*. Routledge: 2017. This book provides an interdisciplinary introduction to the aging process, using symbolic interactionism as the main theoretical perspective. Chapters cover a variety of subject matters including psychology, economics, sociology and political science, biology and religion.

Heinerman, John. *Dr. Heinerman's Encyclopedia of Anti-Aging Remedies*. Prentice Hall, 1997. Compilation of anti-aging remedies from around the world.

Lee, I-Min, and Ralph Paffenbarger. "Change in Body Weight and Longevity." *JAMA: The Journal of the American Medical Association*, 268, no. 15, 21 Oct. 1992. jamanetwork.com/journals/jama/article-abstract/400626. Study examining the importance of weight fluctuation in longevity.

Nolen, Granville. "Effect of Various Restricted Dietary Regimens on the Growth, Health, and Longevity of Albino Rats." *The Journal of Nutrition*, vol. 102, no. 11, Nov. 1972, pp. 1,477-93, doi.org/10.1093/jn/102.11.1477. Study examining the effects of restricting the caloric intake on longevity of rats.

Ptacek, Greg, with Karlis Ullis. *Age Right: Turn Back the Clock with a Proven, Personalized Antiaging Program*. Touchstone, 2014. This book welcomes you to a new age of anti-aging therapy, which involves reducing your body fat, increasing your strength and energy, and boosting your sex drive, all while adding years to your life. This new revolutionary approach provides you with the latest methods for stopping and even reversing the aging process.

Weindruch, Richard. "Caloric Restriction and Aging." *Scientific American*, vol. 274, no. 1 Jan. 1996, pp. 46-52. JSTOR, www.jstor.org/stable/24989354. Review of recent research into caloric restriction and aging.

LONG-TERM CARE

Relevant Issues: Biology, family, health and medicine, psychology

Significance: The management of the health, personal care, and social needs of elderly or older adults is crucial as they experience decreases in physical, mental, and/or emotional abilities.

The process of aging can bring both joys and challenges. In the earlier stages of life, aging involves the acquisition and development of new skills and abilities, facilitated by the guidance and assistance of others. Later, the middle stages involve the challenges of maintaining and applying those skills and abilities in a manner that is primarily self-sufficient. Finally, in the later stages of life, aging involves the consolidation of and reflection on past experiences, gradual slowing of functional abilities, and may involve becoming somewhat dependent on the assistance of others.

Many individuals may experience minimal loss of their abilities to function and are able to live independently for many years and even up to the time of their passing away. Others, however, endure more extended stages of later life and may require greater care and assistance from caregivers. For these individuals, losses in physical, emotional, and/or cognitive functioning (mental processes such as awareness, knowing, reasoning, problem-solving, judging, and imagining) often result in a need for specialized care. Such care involves whatever is necessary so that these individuals may live as comfortably, productively, and independently as possible.

THE NEEDS OF ELDERS

The conditions leading to a need for long-term care are as varied as the elderly are themselves. Special needs for older adults requiring extended care often include the management of physical, health, emotional, and cognitive problems. Physical problems dictating lifestyle adjustments include decreased speed, dexterity, and strength, as well as increased frailty.

Sensory changes are common with aging. Visual changes include the development of hyperopia (farsightedness), myopia (nearsightedness) and sometimes decreased visual acuity. Hearing loss is also common, such that softer sounds cannot be heard when background noise is present, or sounds need to be louder to be perceived. Visual and hearing impairments can result in paranoia, depression, and social isolation in older adults; these are not always signs of mental deterioration. Similarly, one's sense of touch may be affected, such that the nerves are either sensitive to changes in temperatures or textures. Consequently, injuries attributable to a lack of awareness of potential hazards or super-sensitivity to temperature or texture may result. One example would be an older lady overdressing or underdressing for the weather because of inability to judge the outside temperature properly. Another example would be an older man cutting or wounding himself due to lack of awareness of an object's sharpness. Finally, both taste and smell may change, creating a situation in which subtle tastes and odors become imperceptible or in which tastes and smells that were once pleasant become either bland or unpleasant.

Health problems among older adults often lead to a need for increased attention to care coordination. Case management is an interdisciplinary approach to medical care characterized by the inclusion of physical, psychological, social, emotional, familial, financial, and historical data in patient treatment. Coordination of drug therapies and other medical interventions by a case manager is critical, as a result of increasing sensitivities in older adults to physical interventions. Typical health conditions that contribute to older adults' moving into long-term care settings may include multiple medical conditions such as heart disease, strokes, hypertension, diabetes mellitus, arthritis, osteoporosis, chronic pain, prostate disease, and different types of cancers. Estimates are that approximately 80 percent of older adults are affected by one chronic illness and about 70 percent of older adults are affected by at least two chronic diseases. Long-term care addresses both the medical management of these chronic illnesses and their impact on the individual's functioning.

An issue related to health and physical problems in older adults is malnutrition, which is defined as a physical state characterized by an imbalance of dietary proteins, carbohydrates, fats, vitamins, and minerals, given an individual's physical activity and health needs. For a variety of reasons, older adults often develop malnutrition, which can contribute to additional health problems. For example, calcium deficiency can increase the likelihood of osteoporosis. Many factors contribute to malnutrition in older adults. These factors include poverty, social isolation, decreased taste sensitivity, and poor dental health combine with lifelong dietary habits that can sometimes predispose certain individuals to malnutrition. As such, attention towards the maintenance of healthy dietary habits in older adults is critical to successful long-term care, regardless of the type of setting in which the care is provided.

Along with these physical aspects of aging come emotional and cognitive changes. Depression, anxiety, and paranoia over health concerns, for example, are common. Additionally, concerns about the threat of losing one's independence, friends, and former lifestyle may also contribute to acute or chronic mood disorders. Suicide is a danger with the older adults when mood disorders such as depression are present. Older adults are one of the fastest growing groups among those who commit suicide. The stresses accompanying losing a spouse or enduring a chronic health problem can often become triggers to suicide for depressed individuals. One should note, however, that older adults are not particularly prone to depression or suicide because of their age but that they are more likely to experience significant stressors that lead to depression.

Other symptoms associated with conditions such as depression, anxiety, and paranoia are weight change, insomnia, and other sleep problems. Distractibility decreased ability to maintain attention and concentration, and rumination over distressing concerns are also common. Finally, some older adults may become socially isolated. As a result, some individuals may become functionally incapacitated because of distressing emotions.

Some older adults may not describe their problems as emotional, even though that is the primary cause of their discomfort. Individual differences in how people express themselves must be considered. Thus, while some individuals may report being depressed or anxious, others may instead report feeling tired. Reports of low-level health problems that are vague in nature, such as aches and pains, are also common in individuals who are depressed. It is not uncommon for emotional problems to be expressed or described indirectly as physical complaints.

Decreased cognitive functioning may also result from organic brain syndromes, which are clusters of behavioral and psychological symptoms involving impaired brain function. These typically include problems such as dementias from Alzheimer's disease, Pick's disease, Huntington's chorea, alcohol-related deterioration, or stroke-related problems. With all dementias, the typical hallmark signs include a deterioration of intellectual function and emotional response. Memory, judgment, understanding, and the experience and control of emotional responses are affected. Functionally, these conditions reveal themselves as a combination of symptoms, including increased forgetfulness, decreased ability to plan and complete tasks, difficulties finding names or words, decreased abilities for abstract thinking, impaired judgment, inappropriate sexual behavior, and sometimes severe personality changes. In some cases, affected individuals are aware of these difficulties, usually in the earlier stages of the disease processes. Later, however, even though their behavior and abilities are quite disturbed, they may be completely unaware of the severity of their problems. In these cases, long-term care often begins as a result of outside intervention by concerned family members and friends.

OPTIONS FOR LONG-TERM CARE

Extended care for the older adult requires an interdisciplinary effort that usually involves a team of physicians, psychologists, nurses, social workers, and other rehabilitation specialists. Depending on the nature of the problems requiring care and management, any of these professionals may take part in the care process. Additionally, the involvement of concerned individuals who are close to the individual needing care is critical. Family members (including the spouse, children, and extended family) and close friends are invaluable sources of information and of emotional and instrumental support. Their ability to assist an individual with instrumental tasks such as cooking, house cleaning, shopping, and management of money and medication is crucial to the successful implementation of a long-term care plan.

In all cases, long-term care for the individual involves the design of a comprehensive plan to address the multiple needs of the individual. Just as younger persons have psychological, social, intellectual, and physical needs, so do older adults. As such, a comprehensive assessment of an individual's abilities, goals, expectations, and functioning in each of these areas is required. The primary methods of evaluation usually include a thorough history taking, physical examination and a mental status examination, which is a comprehensive evaluation assessing general health, appearance, mood, speech, sociability, cooperativeness, motor activity, orientation to time and reality, memory, general intelligence, and other cognitive functioning. Once needs are identified, a plan can then be designed by the team of health-care professionals, family and friends assisting with care, and, whenever possible, the older adult. In general, the overarching goal is to design a case management plan that maximizes the independent functioning of the older adult, given certain medical, physical, psychiatric, social, and other needs.

Specific management strategies are designed for the problems that need to be addressed. Physical, health, nutritional, emotional, and cognitive problems all require different management settings and strategies. Additionally, care settings may vary depending on the type and severity of the problems that are identified. In general, individuals who require more functional assistance and care provision require a more structured long-term care setting.

For those with less care needs, adequate management settings may include the elder's own home, the home of a family member or friend, a shared housing setting, or a seniors' apartment complex. There is also the option of adult day care centers for older adults who live in their homes but spend a few hours per day in the center. Shared housing is sometimes called group-shared, supportive, or matched housing. Typically, it refers to residences organized by agencies where up to twenty people share a house and its expenses, chores, and management. Ideal candidates for this type of setting include older adults who want some daily assistance or companionship but who are still basically independent. Senior apartments, also called retirement housing, are usually "older adults only" complexes that range from garden-style apartments to high-rises. Ideal candidates for this type of setting include nearly independent individuals who want privacy, but who no longer desire or can manage a single-family home. In either of these types of settings, the use of periodic or regular at-home nursing assistance for medical problems, or caregivers for more instrumental tasks, might be a successful adjunct to regular consultation with a case manager or physician.

Individuals with more complex medical or care provision requirements may need a more structured setting or a setting in which help is more readily available. Such settings might include continuing care retirement communities or assisted-living facilities. Continuing care retirement communities, also called life care facilities or communities, are large complexes offering lifelong care. Residents are healthy, live independently in an apartment, and can use cafeteria services as necessary. Additionally, residents have the option of being moved to an assisted-living unit or an infirmary as health needs dictate. Assisted-living facilities—also called board-and-care facilities or residential care facilities for the elderly—offer care that is less intense than that received in a medical setting or nursing home (skilled nursing facility). These facilities may be as small as a home where one person cares for a small group of elders or large enough with several caregivers, a nurse, and shared dining facilities. Such settings are ideal for older adults who need care for instrumental activities of daily living (iADLs) but not round-the-clock 24/7 assistance in basic activities of daily living (ADLs) such as those provided in skilled nursing facilities (SNFs) or nursing homes. The Katz ADL screening tool assesses an individual's functional status and ability to perform the ADLs without assistance. The ADLs include the functions of bathing, dressing, toileting, transferring, continence, and feeding.

For those individuals who have more severe conditions such as incontinence and dementia, or need assistance with ADLs, skilled nursing facilities, convalescent homes, or nursing homes are appropriate settings. Intense attention is delivered in a hospital-like setting where all medical and functional needs are addressed. Typical nursing homes or skilled nursing facilities serve many residents (sometimes up to 100 residents or more), utilizing semi-private rooms for personal living space and providing community areas for social, community, and family activities. Often, the decision to place an older adult in this type of facility is difficult to make. The decision, however, is usually based on the knowledge that these types of facilities provide the best possible setting for the overall care and safety of the individual's medical, health, and social needs. In fact, appropriate use of these facilities discourages the overtaxing of the elder's emotional and familial resources, allowing the elder to gain maximum benefit and prevent caregivers' burnout. An individual's placement into this type of facility does not mean that the family's job is over; rather, it simply changes shape. Incorporation of family resources into long-term care in a nursing home setting is critical to the adjustment of the individual and family members to the individual's increased need for care and attention. Visits and other family involvement in the individual's daily activities remain quite valuable.

Regardless of the management setting, some basic caveats exist with regard to determining management strategies. First and foremost is that the individual should, whenever possible, be encouraged to maintain independent functioning. For example, even though physical deterioration such as visual or hearing impairments may be present, there is no need to take decision-making authority away from the individual. Decreased abilities of hearing or seeing do not necessarily mean a decreased ability to make decisions or to think for themselves. Second, it is crucial to ask individuals to identify their needs and how they might desire assistance. Some individuals may need help with acquiring basic living supplies from outside the home, such as foods and toiletries, but desire privacy and no assistance within the home. In contrast, others may desire independence outside the home regarding social matters but need more assistance within the home for instrumental ADLs (e.g., housekeeping, cooking, doing laundry, driving/ transportation, shopping, taking medications, using telephone, managing money).

Finally, it is important to recognize that at times even the smallest amount of assistance can make a significant difference in the individual's lifestyle. A prime example is availability of transportation. The loss of a driver's license or independent transportation signifies a major loss of independence for any individual. Similarly, the challenges posed by public transit may seem insurmountable because of a lack of familiarity or experience. As such, simple and small interventions such as a ride to a store or a doctor's office may provide great relief for individuals by assisting their efforts to meet their own needs.

Special management strategies may be required for specific problem areas. For physical deterioration, adequate assessment of strengths and weaknesses is important, as are referrals to medical, rehabilitative, and home-help professionals. Hearing and visual or other devices to make lifting, mobility, and day-to-day tasks easier are helpful. Similarly, assisting the older adults with developing alternative strategies for dealing with diminished sensory abilities can be valuable. Examples would be checking a thermometer for outdoor temperature to determine proper dress, rather than relying purely on sensory information, or having a telephone that lights up when it rings. Health conditions also demand particular management strategies, varying greatly with the type of problem experienced. In all cases, however, medical intervention, drug therapies, and behavior modification therapies are commonly employed. Dietary problems (such as malnutrition or diabetes), cardiovascular problems (such as heart attacks), and emotional problems (such as depression) often require all three approaches. Finally, cognitive problems, particularly those related to depression, are sometimes alleviated with drug therapies. Others related to organic brain syndromes or organic mental disorders, which are mental and emotional disturbances from transient or permanent brain dysfunction (including drugs or alcohol ingestion, infection, trauma, and cardiovascular disease) with known organic etiology, require both medical interventions and significant behavior modification therapies and/or psychosocial interventions for older adults and their families.

PERSPECTIVE AND PROSPECTS

Advances in modern medicine are continually extending the human life span. Cures for diseases, improved management of chronic health problems, and new technologies replacing diseased organs are facilitating this evolution. For many, these advances translate into greater longevity, the maintenance of a high quality of life, and fewer obstacles related to ageism, or discrimination against individuals based on their age or the overlooking of individuals' abilities to make positive contributions to society because of their age. For others, however, the trade-off for longevity is some loss of independence and a need for extended care and management. Thus, the medical field is also affected by the trade-off of extending life, while experiencing an increasing need to improve strategies for long-term care for those who can live longer despite health conditions.

As a result of this evolution, long-term care for the older adults presents special challenges to the medical field. Over time, medicine has been a field specializing in the understanding of organ systems and the treatment

> ## HOW TO TALK TO SENIORS ABOUT PLANNING AHEAD FOR LONG-TERM CARE OPTIONS
>
> ### How Do They Feel?
>
> Many seniors resist planning for long-term care, preferring to avoid thinking about the possibility or refusing to believe that they will ever require such services. When faced with transitioning to long-term care, they will likely experience a complex range of emotions. This will, in all likelihood, be an extremely difficult time for them. They may feel deeply distressed as their day-to-day lives and health status changes considerably. The loss of independence and the ability to care for themselves, coupled with the other effects of medical conditions, can cause intense grief. Even speaking about the topic may trigger emotions of fear and impending loss.
>
> Many seniors feel uncomfortable about having to consider what type of long-term care option will be suitable for them. They may feel overwhelmed at having to make this type of major decision. Planning for long-term care can cause feelings of stress and worry. Some seniors may feel calmer planning ahead before care actually becomes necessary. Having a role in the decision-making process can be empowering and reassuring. Planning for long-term care before it is needed is also important to ensure the senior is eligible for appropriate insurance plans.
>
> Getting ill or experiencing a decline in physical or cognitive ability can be demoralizing. Disorientation, confusion, frustration, or even anger are common emotions. Seniors may feel lost as they try to understand their long-term care options. Many seniors want to hold onto their independence for as long as possible, and this can make them reluctant or resistant to entering long-term care, especially if it requires moving. A move is often distressing and traumatic, and they may feel that so many changes are too much to handle emotionally or practically. Financing long-term care is also a major source of stress.
>
> ### How Do I Start The Conversation?
>
> If possible, it is recommended to discuss long-term care options and plan for its cost before such care becomes necessary. Insurance coverage for long-term care is more affordable the earlier it is purchased. Most insurers will not provide long-term-care coverage for individuals who have already been diagnosed with serious health problems. Therefore, it can be critical to plan for such care before health problems develop later in life. Seniors who are in good health may be persuaded to buy long-term-care insurance when they realize the long-term cost savings of doing so as early as possible.
>
> Before initiating the conversation about long-term care, be aware of the emotional complexity of the topic. It is up to you to keep cool, calm, and centered, even if the senior is reluctant to plan for long-term care. Let them know that you want to act as their advocate when they might be feeling afraid and unsure. Speak in a calm manner and listen attentively to their concerns. Seniors need to feel that they are part of the discussion and decision-making process, not that someone else is forcing their preferences upon them.
>
> If the senior's health has declined and long-term care is necessary, you might begin the conversation by gently asking them if they've considered whether their current situation is still beneficial or sustainable for them or whether they're aware of other options. Hear their input and reflect on what they suggest. If they don't know what options are available in their area or for their medical condition, offer to help them research. When they feel that they are a partner in the discussion and the decision-making process, they will be more open to the prospect of transitioning to long-term care. If they remain resistant, understand that the process may take time. Continue to bring up the subject, emphasizing the positive aspects of long-term care, but avoid becoming angry, nagging, or forceful.
>
> —*Leah Jacob*

of related diseases. While an understanding of how each system impacts the functioning of the whole body is necessary, health-care providers must struggle to understand the complexities in the case management required for high-quality, long-term care for older adults. Care must be interdisciplinary, addressing the physical, mental, emotional, social, and family needs of the individual. Failure to address any of these areas may not result in successful long-term management of elderly individuals and of their problems. In this way, medical, psychiatric, social work, and rehabilitative specialists need to work together with individuals and their families for the best possible results.

Integrated case management with a team leader is increasingly the trend so that a variety of services can be provided in a well-orchestrated manner. Although specialty providers still play a role, managers, usually a primary care physician, ensure that complementary drug therapies, psychiatric, and other medical treatments are administered. Additionally, they are key in bringing forth family resources for emotional and instrumental support whenever possible, as well as community and social services when needed.

What was once viewed as helping a person to die with dignity is now viewed as helping a person to live as long and as productive a life as possible. Increasing awareness that old age is not simply a dying time has facilitated an integrated approach to long-term care. The news that older adults can be as social, physical, sexual, intellectual, and productive as their younger counterparts has greatly stimulated improved long-term care strategies. No longer is old age seen as a time for casting older adults aside or as a time when nursing home is an inescapable solution in the face of health problems affecting the elderly. Alternatives to care exist and are improving continually, with improved outcomes for both patients and care providers.

—*Nancy A. Piotrowski*
Updated by Carolyn Minter, MD
and Miriam E. Schwartz, MD, PhD

See also: Abandonment; Adult Protective Services; Caregiving; Death and dying; Dementia; Disabilities; Euthanasia; Facility and institutional care; Family relationships; Filial responsibility; Geriatrics and gerontology; Health care; Home services; Hospice; Hospitalization; Housing; Neglect; Retirement communities

For Further Information

Diagnostic and Statistical Manual of Mental Disorders: DSM-IV. 5th ed. American Psychiatric Association, 2013. This manual presents detailed descriptions of the behavior symptoms used to diagnose psychiatric disorders, such as organic brain syndromes and affective disorders. Written by mental health professionals, this manual covers issues related to psychiatry, psychology, and social work.

Kane, Robert L. "The Long and the Short Term of Long-Term Care." *Geriatric Medicine,* edited by Christine K. Cassel. 4th ed. Springer-Verlag, 2003. This article describes trends in long-term care in the United States. Target populations, special risk factors, alternatives to long-term care, and case management issues are discussed.

Kübler-Ross, Elisabeth. *On Death and Dying.* New York: Collier Books, 1970. A classic in the study of grief. The nature of the grief process is outlined, and common emotional experiences related to grief and loss are described. Highly recommended for persons wanting to understand their own grief processes or the perspective of others who are experiencing loss.

Mace, Nancy L., and Peter V. Rabins. *The Thirty-Six-Hour Day: A Family Guide to Caring for Persons with Alzheimer Disease, Other Dementias, and Memory Loss* (A Johns Hopkins Press Health Book). 6th ed. The Johns Hopkins U P, 2017. An excellent reference for anyone dealing with dementia. It is appropriate both for individuals who are interested in learning about dementia because of personal concerns and for individuals who are concerned about managing a friend or relative. Symptoms, accompanying problems, management issues, and strategies for solutions are outlined.

Matthews, Joseph L. *Long-Term Care: How to Plan & Pay for It.* 12th ed. Nolo P, 2018. A practical guide on planning for long-term care. This book includes useful topics such as different long-term care facilities, nursing home care, hospice care, caring for elders with Alzheimer's Disease, Medicare, and Medicaid.

Viorst, Judith. *Necessary Losses.* Simon & Schuster, 1986. This classic book on losses, written by a mental health specialist, focuses on clarifying losses that are common to all people at different times in the life cycle. An excellent and easy-to-read general resource for individuals experiencing losses caused by age and other factors or for those concerned about elders who are experiencing losses.

LOOK ME IN THE EYE: OLD WOMEN, AGING, AND AGEISM (BOOK)

Author: Barbara Macdonald, with Cynthia Rich
Date: Published in 1983
Relevant Issues: Culture, psychology, sociology
Significance: Macdonald's collection of essays addresses the impact of both internalized and externalized biases against aging and the aged on older women.

Over a five-year period, Barbara Macdonald wrote a series of essays concerning her experience with aging and ageism—the bias against older adults. Together with two articles written by her lesbian partner, Cynthia Rich, these writings were published as *Look Me in the Eye: Old Women, Aging, and Ageism*.

Macdonald begins by writing about her life as a lesbian and her early experiences with prejudice and discrimination. She quickly shifts, however, to her new struggles with the experience and stigma of aging. She begins describing her own sense of disconnection with her aging body and ends the book by discussing the realities of dying. Between the two, the reader is presented with an intimate glimpse into the emotional and physical realities of age and the impact of ageism on an older woman.

Macdonald's essays reflect her personal experiences with ageism. She describes the emotional impact of people's failure to look her in the eye simply because of her gray hair and wrinkles. Often her essays reveal great personal anger, pain, and frustration in the face of diminishment caused by age. In one essay, Macdonald describes her treatment during a women's march. Event organizers were afraid that she would not be able to keep pace with the march. They based this concern simply on her appearance as an older woman. To compound the problem, organizers pulled her younger lover aside to ask if she thought Macdonald's age would be a problem. Macdonald's intimate essay chronicles her emotions, from the initial exhilaration at being part of the crowd to helplessness and fury.

Macdonald highlights the presence of ageism in the women's community. She describes a community that prides itself on inclusiveness and openness to diversity. Yet she attends women's events and sees few older women. She refers to this bias as the "invisibility of age." Additionally, Macdonald challenges the stereotypic view of older women as isolated, lonely, depressed, and ill. This is most notable in a letter Macdonald addresses to the women's community in response to a program questionnaire she received. The new program being developed was based on the stereotypic assumptions already described. As part of this letter, Macdonald outlines suggestions for combating ageism within the women's community.

Throughout her work, Macdonald provides a window into the private world of physical aging. Whether she is discussing thinning hair, wrinkles, or cataracts, the description is frank and personal. She exhorts older women to break the silence imposed on them to not talk about physical aging and the process of dying. She views this form of silencing as innately political and, like much of ageism, the result of patriarchy.

Rich's articles are written for a professional audience and provide a nice complement to Macdonald's essays. Rich's contributions include a book review and newspaper article analysis. The latter provides an excellent example and commentary on ageist language in the media.

—*Linda M. Woolf*

See also: Ageism; LGBTQ+; Women and aging

LUNG DISEASE. *See* **RESPIRATORY CHANGES AND DISORDERS.**

MACULAR DEGENERATION

Relevant Issues: Health and medicine

Significance: Age-related macular degeneration (AMD), a degenerative condition of the macula or central retina affecting more than 10 million individuals in the United States, more than glaucoma and cataracts combined. It is the leading cause of vision loss and is considered incurable.

Key Terms:

macula: an irregularly oval, yellow-pigmented area on the central retina, containing color-sensitive rods and the central point of sharpest vision

retina: a layer at the back of the eyeball containing cells that are sensitive to light and that trigger nerve impulses that pass via the optic nerve to the brain, where a visual image is formed

visual acuity: sharpness of vision, measured by the ability to discern letters or numbers at a given distance according to a fixed standard

The macula is the tiny central region of the retina in the eye. It is made up of millions of light-sensing cells that help to produce central vision and provide maximum visual acuity. The inside back portion of the eye captures the images seen and sends them to the brain via the optic nerve. When the macula is damaged, a blind spot called drusen, made up of tiny yellow drops, develops in the central field of vision, and central vision becomes blurred or distorted. Central vision is needed to see clearly and to perform everyday activities such as reading, writing, driving, and recognizing people and things. Macular degeneration does not cause complete blindness since peripheral (side) vision is not affected.

As the cells of the macula degenerate, images are not seen correctly. Over time, wavy or blurred vision may occur. Central vision may ultimately be lost completely. In its most severe form, individuals with advanced macular degeneration are considered legally blind.

There are two forms of AMD: dry and wet. The dry form involves thinning of the macular tissues and disturbances in its pigmentation. About 85-90 percent of patients have the dry form. The remaining 10-15 percent have the wet or exudative form, which can involve bleeding within and beneath the retina, opaque deposits, and eventually scar tissue. The wet form accounts for 90 percent of all cases of legal blindness in macular degeneration patients. Stargardt disease (also called Stargardt macular dystrophy), caused by a recessive gene, is a form of macular degeneration found in young people.

RISK FACTORS, SYMPTOMS, AND CAUSES

Aging is the single most important risk factor. Age-related macular degeneration (AMD) most often occurs in individuals 55 years of age and older. Individuals with a family history of AMD are at higher risk. African Americans or Hispanics/Latinos are less likely than Caucasians to develop the disease. The older the patient, the higher the risk. Studies have shown that having a family with a history of macular degeneration raises the risk factor. Because macular degeneration affects most patients later in life, however, it has proven difficult to study cases in successive generations of a family. Heavy smoking, at least a pack of cigarettes a day, can double a person's risk of developing AMD. The more a person smokes, the higher the risk of macular degeneration. Moreover, the adverse effects of smoking persist, even fifteen to twenty years after quitting.

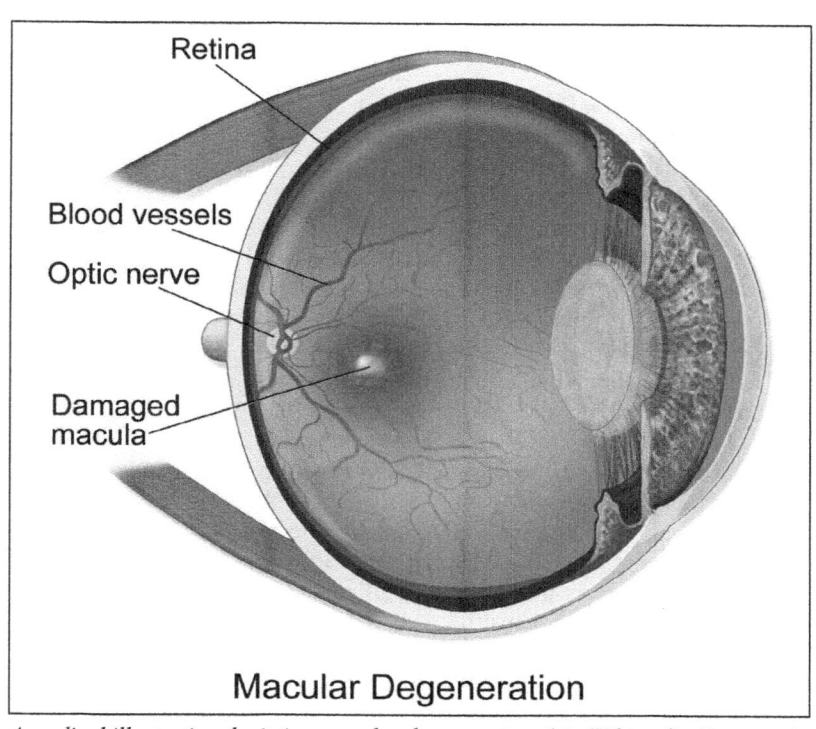

A medical illustration depicting macular degeneration. (via Wikimedia Commons)

Early AMD often does not cause problems with vision, which is why regular eye examinations are important. Diagnosis comes from the Optometrist or Ophthalmologist seeing medium size drusen on examination. With intermediate AMD, there may be no evident symptoms, or there may be mild vision loss. Late AMD demonstrates noticeable vision loss. Neither dry nor wet macular degeneration causes pain. The most common early sign of dry macular degeneration is blurring vision that prevents people from seeing details less clearly in front of them, such as faces or words in a book. In the early stages of wet macular degeneration, straight lines appear wavy or crooked. This is the result of fluid leaking from blood vessels and lifting the macula, distorting vision.

The root causes of macular degeneration are still unknown, but medical authorities consider a number of factors as probable factors. Heredity and environmental factors including aging, nutrition, smoking, and sunlight exposure all play a role. Stargardt disease is genetic in nature and is not as a result of environmental factors.

> **SENIOR TALK:**
>
> **How Do You Feel About Age-Related Macular Degeneration?**
>
> If you have been diagnosed with AMD, you likely feel deeply concerned or afraid about how AMD will affect your daily life. You may be worried that the condition will rapidly worsen and that you will someday not be able to see. It is also common for people with AMD to feel depressed because of the loss of vision, especially if it is making it difficult to do things you enjoy and interfering with your daily activities.
>
> Finding a support system in family and friends, as well as a good medical and ophthalmology team, will help considerably in managing the challenges presented by AMD. Speaking to another person who has AMD can offer a framework for how to tackle these challenges and maintain a sense of positivity. Being well informed about AMD's progression and management can help considerably in maintaining a sense of comfort and control. If you are afraid that AMD will progress to complete blindness, you may be reassured to discover this is not indicated.
>
> Developing AMD is more common in people who have a family history of AMD. If you know you have a family history of AMD, you may be more likely to take steps to reduce your risk and identify AMD's preliminary signs. While knowing you are at increased risk of developing AMD may cause you to feel apprehensive, it also gives you the opportunity to be proactive at an early stage. One of the most useful actions that can be performed is developing a healthy lifestyle to reduce the chance of developing AMD or vision loss. For many, this helps us to feel like we are doing something constructive in taking care of our eyes and general health. People who exercise, avoid or quit smoking, eat a healthy diet with a high intake of vegetables and fish, and have regular eye exams can reduce their chances of developing advanced AMD.
>
> —*Leah Jacob*

Poor dietary habits contribute as well. A diet high in saturated fats may clog the vessels leading to the eyes, thus reducing the flow of nutrient-rich blood. Excess fat may deposit itself directly in the membrane behind the retina. In this case, nutrients might not be able to pass through the "fat wall" to reach the cells that nourish the retina. There is evidence that eating fresh fruits and dark green leafy vegetables (such as spinach and collard greens) may delay or reduce the severity of age-related macular degeneration.

Some studies indicate that the mineral zinc might affect the development of macular degeneration. Zinc is important to chemical reactions in the retina. It is highly concentrated in the eye, particularly in the retina and the tissues surrounding the macula. Older people may have low levels of zinc because of poor diet or poor absorption from food. Some doctors believe that zinc supplements may slow down the progress of macular degeneration. Studies are not complete, however, and there are some adverse side effects of zinc supplements. They might interfere with other important trace metals such as copper, and in some people, the long-term use of zinc can cause digestive problems and anemia.

Strong sunlight seems to accelerate macular degeneration. Wearing special sunglasses may decrease the progress of the disease.

TESTS AND ADJUSTMENTS

A comprehensive dilated eye examination is used first to diagnosis AMD. A visual acuity test using an eye chart determines distance vision. After drops are used to dilate the eye, the Optometrist or Ophthalmologist examines the back of the eye looking for signs of AMD and other eye problems. Optical coherence therapy (OCT) is a painless test that uses light waves to achieve high-resolution pictures that help in diagnosis. An effective test to determine if a person has wet macular degeneration is fluorescent angiography. A special dye is injected into a vein in the patient's arm and then flows to the blood vessels in the eye. Photographs are taken of the retina. The dye highlights any problems in the blood vessels and allows the doctor to determine if they can be treated.

Annual eye examinations that include dilation of the pupils are also useful in early detection. Early detection is important because a person destined to develop macular degeneration can sometimes be treated before symptoms appear, which may delay or reduce the severity of the disease. Anyone who notices a change in vision should contact an ophthalmologist immediately.

A number of aids can help people with AMD make the most of their remaining vision. Some low-vision aids include magnifying glasses, special lenses, electronic systems, and large-print books and newspapers. Sound aids include books on audiotape and products equipped with voice synthesizers such as calculators and computers. Using lamps that provide direct lighting for reading or tasks that require close vision, keeping curtains open, and painting walls and ceilings white make it easier for macular degeneration patients to see in the home.

TREATMENT

There is no proven medical treatment for dry macular degeneration. Risk reduction through lifestyle changes such as diet, exercise, stopping smoking and protecting eyes with sunglasses are beneficial. According to the American Academy of Ophthalmology (AAO), people with AMD may benefit from a specific mix of vitamins and minerals. Taking this mix may slow the disease. ARENDS 2 (Age-Related Eye Disease Study 2) analyzed individuals with large amounts of drusen who took certain supplements. The study found that some benefit was obtained from the supplements. The supplements studied were: (1) Vitamin C (500 mg), (2) Vitamin E (400 IU), (3) Lutein (10 mg), (4) Zeaxanthin (2 mg), (5) Zinc (80 mg) and (6) Copper (2 mg). Both over-the-counter formulations and prescription formulations of these supplements are available. The optometrist or ophthalmologist should be consulted before beginning this regimen.

Treatments for wet macular degeneration are available that may slow disease progression and preserve existing vision. These treatments may also recover some lost vision if started early in the disease. Medications are used to stop the growth of new blood vessels and are considered first line treatment for all stages of wet macular degeneration. These drugs include bevacizumab (Avastin), aflibercept (Eylea) and ranibizumab (Lucentis), which are injected directly into the eye every 4 weeks.

Photodynamic therapy involves the injection of verteporfin (Visudyne) intravenously (into a vein, usually in the arm) and then shines a focused laser light into the abnormal blood vessels. Laser photocoagulation is effective in sealing leaking or bleeding vessels. Laser photocoagulation usually does not restore vision but does prevent further loss. The surgery can be performed in a doctor's office or in an eye clinic on an outpatient basis.

—*Billie M. Taylor*
Updated by Patricia Stanfill Edens, RN, PhD, FACHE

See also: Aging process; Cataracts; Disabilities; Health care; Nearsightedness; Reading glasses; Smoking; Vision changes and disorders

For Further Information

"Age-Related Macular Degeneration (AMD)." National Eye Institute, U.S. Department of Health and Human Services, Nov. 2018. nei.nih.gov/health/maculardegen/. Collects facts about macular degeneration, including symptoms, risk factors, and treatment options.

Al-Zamil, Waseem, and Sanaa Yassin. "Recent Developments in Age-Related Macular Degeneration: A Review." *Clinical Interventions in Aging*, vol. 12, 22 Aug. 2017, pp. 1313-30. doi:10.2147/cia.s143508. Reviews the clinical and pathological aspects of age-related macular degeneration (AMD), diagnostic tools, and therapeutic modalities presently available or underway for both atrophic and wet forms of the disease.

Boyd, Kierstan. "Vitamins for AMD." American Academy of Ophthalmology, 21 May 2018. www.aao.org/eye-health/diseases/vitamins-AMD. Explains which vitamins might help slow macular degeneration.

Gheorghe, Andreea, et al. "Age-Related Macular Degeneration." *Rom. J. Ophthalmol.*, vol. 59, no. 2, Apr. 2015, pp. 74-77. doi: 10.1001/jama.288.18.2358. Reviews the current knowledge on Age-Related Macular Degeneration, including pathogenesis, ocular manifestations, diagnosis, and ancillary testing.

Mayo Clinic Staff. "Wet Macular Degeneration." Mayo Clinic, Mayo Foundation for Medical Education and Research, 11 Dec. 2018. www.mayoclinic.org/diseases-conditions/wet-macular-degeneration/symptoms-causes/syc-20351107. A collection of information on wet macular degeneration.

"What Is Macular Degeneration?" American Macular Degeneration Foundation. www.macular.org/what-macular-degeneration. Explains types, stages, causes, risk factors, and so on for macular degeneration.

MALNUTRITION

Relevant Issues: Health and medicine

Significance: Malnutrition refers to both excess and deficient intakes of calories or nutrients; physical, psychological, and social factors all contribute to malnutrition in the aging population.

Key Terms:

anemia: a condition marked by a deficiency of red blood cells or of hemoglobin in the blood, resulting in pallor and weariness; results from a lack of certain vitamins and minerals

antioxidant: a substance that reduces damage due to oxygen, such as that caused by free radicals

calorie: the energy people get from the food and drink they consume, and the energy they use in physical activity

intrinsic factor: a substance secreted by the stomach that enables the body to absorb vitamin B12

obesity: a condition characterized by the excessive accumulation and storage of fat in the body

Malnutrition literally means "bad nutrition"—that is, impaired health caused by an imbalance of specific nutrients or a deficiency or excess of energy (calorie). However, malnutrition is most commonly thought to denote undernutrition or deficient intake, meaning consumption of inadequate amounts of calories and nutrients to promote health.

Malnutrition in the elderly is a complex phenomenon. Contributing factors include poor physical health, functional disability, psychological problems, and socio-environmental factors. The frail elderly, who are typically underweight and may suffer from chronic illnesses, may require higher nutrient and caloric levels just to sustain health. Some of the illnesses associated with such malnutrition are emphysema, cancer, stroke, and end-stage Alzheimer's disease. Without adequate amounts of such nutrients as protein, vitamin B6, iron, and zinc, the immune system is compromised, leaving the elderly susceptible to infections and further deterioration. For example, bedridden elderly are prone to bed sores, which are aggravated by malnutrition.

Undernutrition among the elderly often results from other conditions, such as chronic diseases, poverty, isolation, depression, or poor dental health. The most severe form of undernutrition is called protein energy malnutrition (PEM). In PEM, body fat stores are used up to provide energy, and eventually muscle tissue is broken down for body fuel. This type of wasting away is often associated with diseases such as cancer, end-stage Alzheimer's disease, emphysema, and other chronic degenerative diseases. PEM is sometimes identified among the elderly living in long-term care facilities and among those who are hospitalized. PEM is accompanied by multiple nutrient deficiencies.

MALNUTRITION AND VITAMINS

Classic vitamin deficiency diseases, such as scurvy (vitamin C deficiency) and pellagra (niacin deficiency), are not as common among the elderly as conditions related to long-term inadequate nutrient intakes. Years may pass before the symptoms of long-term nutrient inadequacies surface.

Heart disease is thought to be associated with overnutrition: excess dietary fat, saturated fat, and cholesterol. However, low intakes, and consequently low blood levels, of certain B vitamins also have been linked to heart disease. High levels of an amino acid derivative called homocysteine are associated with heart disease. Vitamins B6, B12, and folate are involved in clearing this from the blood. High levels of homocysteine are not always a result of a poor diet. Many elderly, especially those over sixty, develop a common stomach condition in which damaged stomach cells produce less stomach acid. Stomach acid is needed for the absorption of those B vitamins. Thus, inadequate absorption causes higher homocysteine levels in the blood and places one at risk for heart disease.

Absorption of vitamin B12 requires a special protein called intrinsic factor. Some aging people produce less of this substance. As with other B vitamins, stomach acid is required for vitamin B12 absorption. Without intrinsic factor or stomach acid, a deficiency disease known as pernicious anemia develops. As vitamin B12 is responsible for the maintenance and growth of nerve cells, its absence may lead to paralysis of the nerves and muscles; if not identified and treated with an injection of vitamin B12, this condition may cause permanent damage to the spinal cord.

Researchers continue to investigate the role of antioxidant nutrients in retarding aging. Inadequate intakes of antioxidant nutrients such as beta carotene and vitamins C and E may be related to increased risk of several diseases, such as cardiovascular disease, cancer, cataracts, and even immune dysfunction.

MALNUTRITION AND MINERALS
Osteoporosis is one of the best-known mineral deficiency diseases of aging. During adolescence and into early adulthood, bones become thicker and denser as calcium is deposited. Between ages thirty and forty, bone loss begins to exceed bone formation. If calcium intake has historically been poor, an inadequate amount of calcium has been deposited to compensate for bone loss during aging. Bones become brittle and susceptible to fracture. Osteoporosis is a major cause of disability and death for the elderly and places a heavy financial burden on society.

Research has revealed that osteoporosis is not exclusively a calcium-deficiency disease. Calcium is only one of several known osteoporosis risk factors. Other factors include hormone status, body weight, physical activity, and vitamin D. Vitamin D works more like a hormone in the body and is responsible for enhancing calcium absorption. For several reasons, vitamin D levels in the blood often decline as one ages. The primary source of vitamin D in the diet is milk, but many elderly people tend to decrease the amount of milk in their diets for various reasons. Even though the body can make vitamin D if the skin is exposed to sunlight, the elderly often avoid sun exposure, use sunscreens, or are homebound, making sunlight a less reliable source of vitamin D. In addition, the body must activate functional vitamin D, and activation declines with age.

Aging individuals may suffer from iron-deficiency anemia. The cause may be blood loss rather that dietary inadequacy. The most likely causes of anemia are gastrointestinal blood loss caused by chronic use of drugs such as aspirin, or blood loss from tumors. Low intake of zinc in the aging population can cause problems such as poor immune response and reduced taste perception for salt. One of the best sources of zinc is meat, but because some elderly people may not be able to afford meat or chew it, zinc intake may be inadequate.

OVERNUTRITION
As people grow older, many suffer from diseases caused by overnutrition, such as heart disease, diabetes (type II), osteoarthritis, some cancers, and gout. The prevalence of obesity increases with aging and often contributes to such diseases. The most important risk factor for heart disease is a high intake of saturated fat. Other contributing substances are dietary fat and cholesterol. Although overconsumption of dietary sodium is blamed for high blood pressure (hypertension), obesity is also an important factor. Obesity is also associated with endometrial and breast cancers and osteoarthritis.

Type II diabetes, also known as noninsulin-dependent diabetes mellitus, typically begins in adulthood and is characterized by the inability of body cells to use insulin. Many elderly people with diabetes suffer severe complications such as kidney disease, loss of vision, heart disease, and destruction of sensory function.

MALNUTRITION AND BRAIN FUNCTION
Proper nutrition is important for normal brain function. Dietary inadequacy of vitamins B12 and C have been associated with short-term memory loss; low intakes of riboflavin, folate, vitamin B12, and vitamin C have been associated with poor performance in problem-solving tests; and inadequate intakes of thiamine, niacin, zinc, and iron have been associated with diminished cognition, degeneration of brain tissue, and dementia. Brain communication chemicals called neurotransmitters are synthesized from components of protein. One example is serotonin, which the body makes from an amino acid (protein building block) called tryptophan. Senile dementia is loss of brain function beyond that which is considered normal memory loss due to aging. There is evidence that people with senile dementia of the Alzheimer's type require more calories to maintain weight, perhaps because of the fidgeting and pacing behaviors that accompany the disease. Further complications include an inability to remember to eat or how to use utensils. It is important that these people maintain adequate body weight, so they must be provided with nutritious meals and snacks that are easy to eat.

TREATING MALNUTRITION
The biggest challenge faced by nutritionists is matching the type of nutritional support to the aging individual to best promote health. Special screening initiatives have been promoted to help increase public awareness of

malnutrition in the elderly population so that needy individuals can be identified. Special attention must be given to drug and nutrient interactions. Medications may compromise nutrition by altering absorption or increasing excretion of nutrients. Attention must be given to physiological declines in the senses of smell and taste. Poor dentition and improperly fitting dentures also can affect food consumption. Elderly people who have suffered from strokes may have difficulty swallowing, causing inadequate food intake. Poverty, depression, alcoholism, and social isolation are important contributing factors to malnutrition.

Special attention must be given to frail aging people who are recovering from illness to ensure that they are receiving enough calories as well as adequate amounts of other nutrients. Without both caloric and nutrient adequacy, the frail person may deteriorate rapidly. Therefore, nutritional supplementation in the form of liquid meal replacement or other fortified products may be necessary. For the overnourished and obese individual, nutritional support must provide high-quality, nutritious foods within a reasonable caloric intake to prevent further weight gain. Malnutrition as a result of poverty is exacerbated by lack of nutritional knowledge and poor food choices. Therefore, overall treatment of malnutrition involves addressing numerous psychosocial issues as well as the diet.

—*Wendy L. Stuhldreher*
Updated by Bruce E. Johansen, PhD

See also: Alzheimer's disease; Antioxidants; Caloric restriction; Cancer; Diabetes; Heart disease; Nutrition; Obesity; Osteoporosis; Sensory changes; Vitamins and minerals; Weight loss and gain

For Further Information

Batsis, John A., and Alexandra B. Zagaria. "Addressing Obesity in Aging Patients." *Medical Clinics of North America*, vol. 102, no. 1, Jan. 2018, pp. 65-85. doi:10.1016/j.mcna.2017.08.007. Explores how obesity affects the aging population and outlines both the benefits and detriments of weight loss in older adults. Emphasizes the need for lifetime prevention in a primary care setting.

"Healthy Eating." National Institute on Aging, U.S. Department of Health and Human Services. www.nia.nih.gov/health/healthy-eating. A collection of articles from the National Institute on Aging about nutrition, including advice on how and what to eat.

Leslie, Wilma, and Catherine Hankey. "Aging, Nutritional Status and Health." *Healthcare*, vol. 3, no. 3, Sept. 2015, pp. 648-58. doi:10.3390/healthcare3030648. Explains how malnutrition affects older adults and presents options for challenging malnutrition in older adults.

Longo, Valter. *The Longevity Diet: Discover the New Science behind Stem Cell Activation and Regeneration to Slow Aging, Fight Disease, and Optimize Weight.* Avery, an Imprint of Penguin Random House, 2018. The culmination of 25 years of research on aging, nutrition, and disease across the globe, this unique program lays out a simple solution to living to a healthy old age through nutrition.

Nagaratnam, Nages. "Malnutrition and Malabsorption in the Elderly." *Advanced Age Geriatric Care*, 27 Nov. 2018, pp. 225-33. doi:10.1007/978-3-319-96998-5_25. This review provides an overview of the causes and management of malnutrition and malabsorption in the elderly.

Stauder, Reinhard, et al. "Anemia at Older Age: Etiologies, Clinical Implications, and Management." *Blood*, vol. 131, no. 5, 1 Feb. 2018, pp. 505-14. doi:10.1182/blood-2017-07-746446. Reviews current concepts around anemias at older age, with special emphasis on etiologies, clinical implications, and innovative concepts in the management of these patients.

Trull, Armando. "Malnutrition Is a Threat to Healthy Aging." NCOA, National Council on Aging, 27 Sept. 2016. www.ncoa.org/news/press-releases/malnutrition-threat-healthy-aging/. The National Council on Aging asks older adults and their caregivers to learn the warning signs of malnutrition and ways they can stay healthy during Malnutrition Awareness Week™, typically the last week of September.

MANDATORY RETIREMENT

Relevant Issues: Economics, work

Significance: As baby boomers approach retirement age, mandatory retirement based on age has come under increasing attack.

The issue of whether legislation supporting mandatory retirement should exist has been exacerbated by the growing number of elderly people within Western societies. A study of data from the United States, West Germany, Great Britain, and Australia revealed that attitudes toward retirement differ sharply according to country, with the Americans most strongly opposed to mandatory retirement and the Britons most accepting of it. Measures of political ideology are significant predictors of attitudes toward compulsory retirement; that is, acceptance of government intervention in various areas of the labor market is positively related to the acceptance of government regulation of retirement age.

Several studies on retirement have reported that compared to people not yet retired, recent retirees exhibit lower income, more physical and mental illness, lower self-esteem, and less life satisfaction. These findings, however, have been challenged by longitudinal studies using data from large samples that claim to show that the way individuals adapt and cope following retirement is largely predicted by how they adapted and coped before retirement. The main thing that does change for most people when they retire may well be the amount of discretionary time they have. As the opportunities and responsibilities of work are abandoned with retirement, new opportunities and responsibilities for decision-making appear.

Planning is needed for retirement, particularly for some of the business aspects of retirement, such as career changes and possible job searches, financial management, housing, health management, and legal arrangements. Leisure and volunteer activities may also require systematic information and assessment. As the average life span has increased, retired people have become healthier and more capable of living independent and productive lives. A growing number of people believe that it is economically, socially, politically, and culturally imperative that older people continue to make contributions to society and that retirement should be seen as a transition from one activity to another rather than a withdrawal from useful, productive living.

LABOR PROBLEMS

Many economists, government officials, and industrial leaders, fearing an impending labor shortage, believe that the trends of early retirement should be reversed. Many also believe that the cost to society of supporting huge numbers of people who are no longer working is too great. The fact that fewer younger workers are paying into Social Security, while more older workers are drawing money out, has raised concerns about the health of the Social Security program and has added to the pressure to create incentives to keep people in the workforce.

Despite the increased recognition of the value of older workers, many have faced major adjustments in their career plans. Midlife and older workers have been especially vulnerable in three main areas: losing their jobs unexpectedly, retiring earlier than planned, and staying in positions no longer challenging to them. In the 1980s, people in the over-fifty age group were hard hit by layoffs. It is estimated that 20 percent of workers between fifty-five and fifty-nine years of age who leave the workforce do so unwillingly; of this population, 18 million people have stated that they want to work or to get a better job.

Legislation has made mandatory retirement illegal in most sectors of the American workforce. However, it has been relatively easy for employers to get around these laws, and many have sought to do so because of intense economic pressures. During the 1960s, the retirement age dropped from sixty-five to sixty-two years old. However, the affordability of retirement has changed because of changes in pay, pensions, and saving rates. A Harris Poll found that 76 percent of retirees would like to be working and that 86 percent opposed mandatory retirement. Another Harris Poll found that life satisfaction among sixty-five year olds was significantly higher for those who were employed than for those who chose to retire early and then decided they had made a mistake.

Mature workers who stay in their jobs do not escape from the implications of the trends already discussed. A decrease in the number of middle-management jobs has meant less chance for promotion. Many mature employees who remain in organizations feel that they have reached a plateau, often at a much earlier age than they had planned. For many, this has produced feelings of burnout and anxiety about their future security.

AGE STEREOTYPES

Although it may be officially denied, many older workers have been victims of age stereotypes and age discrimination. This is based on the attitudes toward aging that exist in the United States, as well as on financial realities. Bias toward hiring and retaining younger workers, while squeezing out mature employees, often exists because of a pervasive youth culture and the feeling that young people are more flexible and comfortable with technology. In addition, cutting older workers can be attractive because their salaries tend to be higher than those of younger workers. Health benefit costs are also a consideration.

In October of 1996, the U.S. Congress passed amendments to the Age Discrimination in Employment Act of 1967 (ADEA) that allow cities to force police officers and firefighters to retire at age fifty-five. Many of these older workers have valuable experience and can serve ably for many more years. Such legislation has created renewed interest in redefining retirement criteria in terms of a functional age concept that would give attention to individual variability in the maintenance and development of behavioral competence.

Although inflation has forced many older people to find part-time employment or to continue working past their anticipated retirement age, stereotypes of aging may hinder the acceptance of older people in the workplace. It is particularly important to assess attitudes toward the elderly in the working-class population, which will be the first to feel the impact of increased numbers of older workers in the labor force. As very young workers and retired people who seek employment are both competing for the same low-status jobs, it is also important to assess the attitudes of young people toward the elderly in the labor force. Studies have indicated that there are significant differences in perceptions between male and female subjects and between high school students and adults. In general, students, more than working adults, consider older workers to have poor coordination, to be prone to accidents, and to have problems learning new methods. Students also tend to think that older workers are overpaid, often absent because of illness, and too costly for employers.

The increased life span means that retirement can last for fifteen to twenty years or longer, during which three additional subtransitions may occur: onset of sickness and disability, institutionalization, and widowhood. The growing trend of early retirement causes a further extension of the retirement period through earlier entry into this role by relatively young elderly people, widening the gap between retirement and traditional concepts of old age. Some researchers have found that many people experience conflicting role expectations and strain after early retirement. It has been suggested that three distinct stages emerge during the extended retirement period: preaging (early) retirement, active (engaged) retirement, and passive (stabilized) retirement, each with its own characteristics and needs. These developments require long-range planning, with individuals and society adjusting to specific situations and needs as they arise.

Preparing for retirement can sometimes be problematic as it means that one is aging and moving into another life cycle change. The impact of retirement on older citizens is often neglected in the counseling arena. In the American youth-oriented society, it is hard to get people to discuss the need for providing counseling services for the millions of people who are considering retirement. A preretirement counselor must be trained as a counselor plus understand what a person will face in retirement. Limited counseling is given to retirees by most employers, but it usually only concerns pensions.

—*Jane Cross Norman*

See also: Age discrimination; Age Discrimination in Employment Act of 1967; Early retirement; Employment; Johnson v. Mayor and City Council of Baltimore; Massachusetts Board of Retirement v. Murgia; Retirement; Retirement planning; Social Security; Stereotypes; Vance v. Bradley

For Further Information

Hannon, Kerry. "Is It Time to Abolish Mandatory Retirement?" *Forbes*, 2 Aug. 2015. www.forbes.com/sites/nextavenue/2015/08/02/is-it-time-to-abolish-mandatory-retirement/#3f47843a40db. Hannon argues that since "old age" cannot truly be determined, mandatory retirement is difficult to establish and often ends up as a tool for ageism.

Ilmakunnas, Pekka, and Seija Ilmakunnas. "Health and Retirement Age: Comparison of Expectations and Actual Retirement." *Scandinavian Journal of Public Health*, vol. 46, no. 19, 2018, pp. 18-31. doi:10.1177/1403494817748295. This paper analyzes the role of health in retirement decisions by modeling the relationships between self-assessed health (SAH) status, expected full-time retirement age, and actual full-time retirement age.

Levmore, Saul. "A Provocative Argument for Mandatory Retirement." *Forbes*, 6 Nov. 2017. www.forbes.com/sites/nextavenue/2017/11/06/a-provocative-argument-for-mandatory-retirement/#4397885720db. Levmore argues that setting a mandatory retirement age can increase productivity and make room for newer hires.

Sewdas, Ranu, et al. "Why Older Workers Work beyond the Retirement Age: A Qualitative Study." *BMC Public Health*, vol. 17, no. 1, 22 Aug. 2017, p. 672. doi:10.1186/s12889-017-4675-z. This study offers important new insights into the various preconditions and motives that influence working beyond retirement age.

MARRIAGE

Relevant Issues: Family, psychology
Significance: Longer life expectancies now allow seniors to spend more than one-third of their married years together after their children have left home; for most, these years are characterized by happiness, intimacy, and social support.

Individuals change over time, and so do their relationships. Marriage is no exception. As couples get older, they move into the stage that gerontologists call post-parental marriages, referring to the time of life after the children have grown up and left home. This stage of marriage has been extended significantly as elders live longer and have fewer children. At the beginning of the twentieth century, it was typical for at least one of the parents to die before the last child had left home. By the end of the same century, parents were spending an average of thirteen years, or about one-third of their married life, together after their last child had left the house.

BENEFITS OF MARRIAGE IN LATER LIFE

Many demographic studies of technological societies during the second half of the twentieth century showed that married men and women live longer and enjoy better physical and mental health than unmarried men and women. Although it can be argued that healthier people are more apt to marry than those in poor health, there is a lot of evidence that close relationships contribute to better mental and physical health. Other research shows that happily married people are healthier and better adjusted than either unmarried people or unhappily married people and that suicide rates for men are higher for those who are divorced, separated, or widowed than for those who are married.

Marriage also has economic benefits, especially for women. On average, both divorced and widowed women have lower incomes and fewer assets than all men and married women their age. Each year, a greater proportion of older women fall below the poverty line, a situation called the feminization of poverty. This occurs because of the combined facts that women generally spend fewer years in the workforce, have lower salaries and fewer benefits, take more financial and physical responsibility for their children, have more chronic illnesses and medical expenses in later years, and have longer life expectancies than their spouses.

The benefits of marriage also include social relations. Regardless of the increasing number of divorced and widowed individuals among older adults, the social world is still one of couples. Widows and widowers report being excluded from their long-term social groups and activities once they are one-half of a couple. However, women seem to be able to form new social groups with other women, while men seem to become isolated without a spouse.

Although marriage vows traditionally include "in sickness and in health," young couples do not often consider that their role may include caregiver to an aging spouse. However, as life expectancy gets longer, there is a good chance that one or another spouse may spend the last years of their marriage in this role. A large number of Alzheimer's disease patients are cared for at home by their spouses, and the major caregivers for married people with other lingering illnesses are also usually spouses.

THE QUALITY OF POST-PARENTAL MARRIAGES

Research on long-term marriages shows that older husbands and wives tend to be very much alike. They not only agree with each other when making plans or solving problems, but they also tend to give similar answers when asked individually about goals and favorite activities. Part of this may be because of the tendency for people to marry others who are similar to themselves, but part of this similarity between couples in late life comes from learning from each other and sharing a lifetime of experiences on which they base their opinions.

When discussions between middle-aged and elderly married couples have been compared, researchers have found that the older husbands and wives, regardless of the topic, show more positive and caring communication styles. They are more approving and respectful of each other, and they express less anger and aggression than the middle-aged couples. Several interpretations of these findings have been suggested. One is that age itself brings more tranquility and that couples no longer experience the same levels of intensity in their emotions. Another interpretation is that, as the years ahead become fewer, the motivation to change one's spouse decreases. Still another explanation is that married couples continually become closer and closer and that by late adulthood they approve of and respect each other more than ever before.

In the late 1990s, only about 5 percent of people over sixty-five were divorced, while 33 percent were widowed. The rate of divorce for this age group has skyrocketed in recent years; by 2019 it had tripled. A cause of marital distress in older couples is a shift in dominance patterns, with women who were traditionally subordinate to their husbands becoming more dominant as they age. This happens for a variety of reasons. One is simply the trend of women's progress in many arenas. Older women are now more likely to have worked for a time outside the home. Also, men are usually older than their wives and tend to age more quickly, so it is not unusual for a younger, healthier wife to become the designated driver of the couple or the one who takes care of the family finances or other tasks that the husband once controlled. Evidence that women have always taken on more dominant roles as they age is supported by anthropological studies in a variety of societies. In almost one-half of the societies studied, women become more dominant with age; in none of the societies do older men become more dominant.

One often discussed cause for marriage problems in later life that has not held up well to the light of research is retirement. Popular belief has been that retirement brings about a variety of marital problems that were either not present earlier in the marriage or were present but not apparent. However, research on the quality of life after retirement has shown that couples report the same level of marital happiness that they did before retirement. The only problems that retirement seems to bring are those associated with lowered income.

SEXUALITY IN LATER YEARS

Another popular belief about marriage in older adults is that sexuality loses its importance with age and that older marriages are companionate instead of intimate. Research on sexual activity in older couples has shown that this is not true. Although many older individuals report that they no longer engage in sexual relations, the major reason cited for this is lack of a partner. When older couples are interviewed, about one-half report having sexual relations with their spouse on a regular basis, even up to the age of seventy. When illness, disability, or side effects of medication makes sexual intercourse difficult, many older couples find ways to be sexually intimate throughout their marriages.

The false stereotype of older marriages not being sexual has caused difficulties for many older couples who move into nursing homes. Before passage of the Patients' Rights Act of 1980, it was not uncommon for spouses to be separated at night into male and female wings of the facility and to be denied the private atmosphere conducive to intimate relations. However, some older couples living with their children complain about the lack of privacy and time alone together.

HIS AND HER MARRIAGES IN OLD AGE

According to many sociologists, there are two views of all marriages: his and hers. This seems to be especially true in late adulthood. For most couples in this stage of life, marriage is more central for the husband than it is for the wife. Several reasons for this have been suggested. First is that women have traditionally found other facets of life to attend to while their husbands were absorbed in their careers. If they did not work outside the home, women forged close bonds with their children and with other family members. They developed hobbies and were involved in volunteer work. They formed close relationships with other women. Those who had jobs were more apt to form social relationships with their coworkers than their spouses did. When men retire, they depend heavily on their wives to be spouse, friend, confidante, and social partner. When retired, married men are asked to name their best friend, they typically respond, "my wife." Wives, in contrast, typically name a female friend or relative. Another reason that men are invested so heavily in their marriages in old age is that other men become scarcer and scarcer as the years go by. It is not unusual for a man in his seventies to have outlived all of his friends, coworkers, and brothers, and to find himself in a society of women.

This difference in viewpoint of marriage between partners is especially apparent when a spouse dies. Although men and women react similarly to the death of a spouse, women are surrounded by the social support of their children, their relatives, and their friends. Men, in contrast, have often lost their entire social group by the death of their spouse. It is suggested that this is one of the factors behind the high suicide rate for older men.

HOW TO TALK TO SENIORS ABOUT CARING FOR A PARTNER

How Do They Feel?

Caring for a partner in the senior years of life can bring a rollercoaster of different feelings. Of course, seniors will feel some degree of sadness over the fact that their loved one's health is declining. Some will feel they must devote themselves fully to caregiving, even resisting outside help. Others may worry that they are unprepared to supply the necessary amount of care.

The shift in relationship roles can also bring more complex emotions. There may a profound sense of loss if their partner's physical or mental state means they are no longer able to offer familiar expressions of love and support. Being thrust into the role of primary decision-maker, rather than an equal partner in a relationship, can be distressing and overwhelming. Caregivers can often feel lonely, abandoned, or even depressed as the realities of their situation become clear. When demands are especially challenging, such as in caring for someone with dementia, feelings of resentment, anger, and frustration may surface. These, in turn, can trigger guilt and self-doubt.

Some seniors are able to adopt a pragmatic approach to dealing with these challenges. In these instances, they are able to avoid becoming weighed down by the emotional aspects and cope in various ways. This may involve recognizing the limits of care they are able to supply, as well as carving out time for recreational activities to maintain their own mental and physical well-being.

How Do I Start The Conversation?

Talking to seniors about caring for a partner requires a great deal of sensitivity and an understanding of the emotional environment. The senior with whom you are engaging in conversation needs to know that their concerns are being heard. The optimum setting for beginning the conversation is one in which it's understood that solutions and a framework for care will be mutually determined, not imposed. If the partner requiring care is still in sound mind they should be included in discussions as much as possible. However, it is also important to give the caregiver a chance to voice their feelings privately, even if they don't ask to do so.

One of the key subjects you should raise is the possibility of the caregiver losing sight of his or her own needs while caregiving. There is often a tendency to think that devotion to a partner means placing all their needs at the forefront and abandoning one's own. This generally results in fatigue, burnout, and resentment, which are counterproductive to dispensing practical and loving care. Gently suggest ways the caregiver might maintain their own well-being, but avoid telling them what they should or must do. Conveying examples or stories of how others have successfully handled such situations can introduce the subject in a nonthreatening way and help to spur discussion.

Throughout the conversation, you should avoid lecturing and use a calm, empathetic tone of voice. Don't let your own emotions get out of hand, especially if dealing with your parents. Try to initiate discussion by finding out what the caregiving spouse would find helpful and steer the conversation to setting achievable goals. It may be necessary to recommend additional caregiving help, whether from you, another family member or friend, or a professional. Many seniors will initially resist such a suggestion, whether for reasons of pride or financial concerns. Rather than getting frustrated by their refusal, mutually discuss ways in which small steps can be taken to improve the situation. Even if a caregiver resists relinquishing control now, they may be willing to seek help if circumstances change. Knowing that they have your support when it's needed can be invaluable.

In all instances, let the caregiving partner know how valuable it is to have someone to talk to a therapist, counselor, social worker, or health-care professional. You may suggest support groups as a method of providing an excellent network of friendship and support as they move through the stages of caring for their partner.

—Leah Jacob

CHILDLESS MARRIAGES IN OLD AGE

About 60 percent of married couples are also parents. The remaining 40 percent of couples with no children often experience a more stable relationship over the years. Couples who do not have children start out happy and do not experience the middle-aged dip in marital satisfaction that seems to be caused by the presence of children.

Whether childless couples are happier in old age than those with children has not been firmly established. Elderly parents report that a major cause of concern and anxiety for them is the problems of their adult children; examples include financial problems, divorce, business failures, and health problems. Couples with no children are spared that distress in their later years. However, elderly parents also report that a major source of happiness and pride is the achievements of their adult children, listing such examples as grandchildren, affluence, professional attainment, and concern for parents.

Childless couples tend to have higher incomes in later years, not simply because of the lack of college tuition, weddings, and other direct costs of having children but also because both spouses have been able to work and pursue careers full time without taking time out for parenting responsibilities. Similar to women who never marry, working women who marry and have no children have more education, higher incomes, and better retirement benefits.

In middle adulthood, childless couples are more apt to be caregivers for aging parents than their siblings who have children. However, as they have only one generation to care for, they are not caught in the generational squeeze familiar to those who have both children and aging parents making demands on their time and resources.

One stereotype of childless couples in the later years is that of being lonely and having no one to care for them. Research has shown that this is not an accurate portrayal of this group. Childless couples have levels of social support in old age that are similar to those of couples with children. The difference is that their social support comes from friends and other relatives instead of children and grandchildren. In fact, several studies have shown that happiness, life satisfaction, self-esteem, and satisfaction with social support are all unrelated to the amount of contact older people have with children and grandchildren.

REMARRIAGE IN LATE LIFE

A number of older adults who have been divorced or widowed marry again. More older men remarry than older women, partly because there are a greater number of women in older age groups than there are men and partly because marriage is more central to the lives of men at this age. Remarriage often includes differences in the wife's and the husband's experiences. For remarried men, the relationship with the wife takes precedence to the relationships he might have with his children, other relatives, and friends. For the woman, the opposite is true: The relationship with the new husband becomes a marginal relationship compared to that with her children, other relatives, and friends.

Remarriage in the later years tends to be happier than remarriage in young adulthood or midlife and happier if the participants have been widowed rather than divorced. The biggest problems for remarried couples of any age are stepchildren, and it can be argued that this is especially true in later life. The adult children of both spouses often view the new spouse as an intruder in the family, and they may worry about sharing their inheritance and about having the responsibility of caring for another aging family member.

—*Barbara R. Bjorklund*

See also: Alzheimer's disease; Caregiving; Childlessness; Communication; Divorce; Facility and institutional care; Friendship; Men and aging; Parenthood; Poverty; Remarriage; Retirement; Sexuality; Social ties; Suicide; Widows and widowers; Women and aging

For Further Information

Birditt, Kira S. "Growing Older Together: Couple Relationships and Aging." *The Gerontologist*, vol. 57, no. 2, 2017, pp. 381-82. doi:10.1093/geront/gnx002. The book covers a wide variety of topics, including marital quality, diversity in the couple tie, sexuality, equity, transitions including caregiving, the empty nest, retirement, and chronic illness.

Brown, Susan L, and Matthew R Wright. "Marriage, Cohabitation, and Divorce in Later Life." *Innovation in Aging*, vol. 1, no. 2, 2017. doi:10.1093/geroni/igx015. This article reviews recent scholarship on marriage, cohabitation, and divorce among older adults and identify directions for future research.

Browning, Dan. "Financial Pros and Cons of Getting Married Late in Life." *Next Avenue*, 20 Feb. 2018. www.nextavenue.org/financial-pros-cons-getting-married-late-life/. Using his own experience, Browning describes the potential cons of remarrying in old age.

Cornell University. "Love, Factually: Gerontologist Finds the Formula to a Happy Marriage." *ScienceDaily*, 17 June 2015. www.sciencedaily.com/releases/2015/06/150617134613.htm. A review of a study of a random national survey of nearly 400 Americans age 65 and older, asking how to find a compatible partner and other advice on love and relationships.

Gottman, J. M. *The Seven Principles for Making Marriage Work*. 2nd. ed. Harmony Books, 2015. The author is a research psychologist who studies married couples and is often able to predict problems and intervene. Much of his work is based on studies of long-term successful marriages.

Hsieh, Ning, and Louise Hawkley. "Loneliness in the Older Adult Marriage." *Journal of Social and Personal Relationships*, vol. 35, no. 10, 2017, pp. 1,319-39. doi:10.1177/0265407517712480. The authors used a contextual approach to characterize each partner's ratings of the marriage as supportive (high support, low strain), ambivalent (high support, high strain), indifferent (low support, low strain), or aversive (low support, high strain) and examined how these qualities associate with own and partner's loneliness.

MASSACHUSETTS BOARD OF RETIREMENT V. MURGIA

Date: Decided on June 25, 1976

Relevant Issues: Law, values, work

Significance: In this case, the Supreme Court determined that mandatory retirement of uniformed officers in the Massachusetts State Police does not violate equal protection under the law.

Massachusetts Board of Retirement v. Murgia involved Robert Murgia, a uniformed officer in the Massachusetts State Police who was forced to retire against his wishes at age fifty by the Massachusetts Board of Retirement. Four months before his compulsory retirement, Murgia passed an annual physical and mental test that strongly implied that he was still capable of satisfactorily performing the duties of a uniformed state police officer. Murgia sued the Massachusetts Retirement Board, claiming age discrimination and a denial of equal protection of the laws by virtue of this "arbitrary" retirement age set by Massachusetts law. A district judge dismissed Murgia's complaint, saying no constitutional question was involved. However, the U.S. Court of Appeals upheld Murgia's claim and ruled that compulsory retirement at age fifty by itself does not further any substantial or rational state interest. The U.S. Supreme Court reversed the federal appeals court.

The majority opinion of seven members of the U.S. Supreme Court held that a Massachusetts state law that makes it mandatory for state patrol officers to retire at age fifty does not deny equal protection of the laws. Maintaining a government job is not a fundamental right, and the law in question protects the public by assuring the physical and mental preparedness of its state police. People over the age of fifty are in middle life; thus, the Massachusetts Retirement Board and the state law do not discriminate only against its senior citizens. Furthermore, it is a legislative and not a judicial task to make distinctions about fitness for uniformed police work.

The Massachusetts legislature, said the Court, sought to protect the public's safety and welfare by reminding citizens that the arduous duties of controlling prison and civil disorders, patrolling highways in marked cars, and apprehending criminals are hard work. Clearly, men above middle age are not usually physically able to perform such strenuous duties all the time. The court noted the substantial economic and psychological effects that mandatory, premature retirement can have on people but said that these individuals can continue to contribute to society in some other way.

Justice Thurgood Marshall dissented, saying that the right to work is the very essence of personal freedom and opportunity, and it is the purpose of the Fourteenth Amendment to secure that important right for citizens discriminated against and deprived of governmental employment simply because they reach a certain age. Once terminated, middle-aged and elderly citizens cannot easily find alternate work; and mandatory, arbitrary retirement of physically capable people such as Murgia is economically and emotionally damaging. Retiring state police officers for no other reason than they are fifty years old, said Marshall, is the height of a state's irrationality and thus violates the equal protection of the laws.

—*Steve J. Mazurana*

See also: Age discrimination; Age Discrimination Act of 1975; Age Discrimination in Employment Act of 1967; Employment; *Johnson v. Mayor and City Council of Baltimore*; Mandatory retirement; Retirement; *Vance v. Bradley*

MATLOCK (T.V. SHOW)

Created By: Dean Hargrove
Principal Cast: Andy Griffith
Date: Aired from 1986 to 1995
Relevant Issues: Culture, law, media, work
Significance: This television series depicted an older attorney and amateur sleuth who capably solved mysteries and vindicated clients in the courtroom, appealing demographically to older viewers.

First aired by the National Broadcasting Company (NBC) on September 20, 1986, the *Matlock* television series starred sixty-year-old Andy Griffith as Ben Matlock, an amiable Atlanta attorney who was famous nationwide. Seeking justice, Matlock questioned witnesses, visited crime scenes, and cleverly exposed liars in dramatic courtroom scenes. Characterized as a country lawyer in the big city, Matlock defended underdog protagonists against greedy, corrupt villains in murder cases about stolen inheritances, mistaken identities, spurned lovers, art thefts, and blackmail. Violence was minimized in episodes. The predominantly wealthy suspects often arrogantly underestimated Matlock's intelligence to unravel their ruses, yet Matlock consistently and competently exposed wrongdoing. "Matlock is a good man, but he wants to win. He's very shrewd," Griffith noted. Plots also involved Matlock's daughter, also an attorney, and his interactions with younger colleagues. Don Knotts later joined the cast as Les Calhoun, Matlock's meddling retired neighbor.

Matlock quickly gained fans and was ranked among the top twenty television shows every week. Television movies featuring Matlock won ratings sweeps. Griffith credited viewer interest to the show's humor and Matlock's eccentricities, such as always wearing a gray suit, eating hot dogs, and playing a ukulele. In 1992, NBC canceled *Matlock*, hoping to attract a younger audience to gain more advertising dollars. Although ranked third with adults over fifty, *Matlock* was eighty-third with

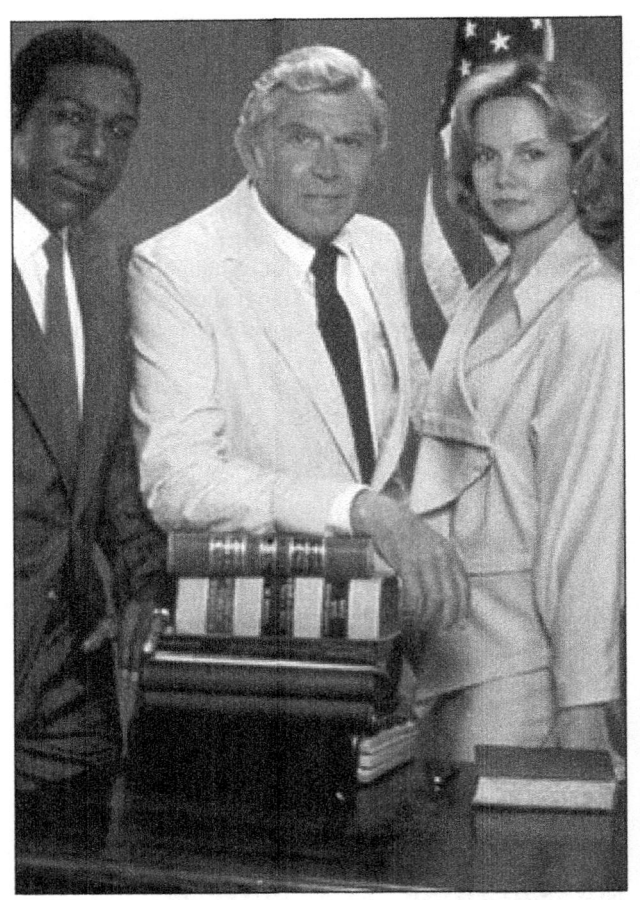

The original cast (from left): Kene Holliday, Andy Griffith, and Linda Purl. Purl left the show after the first season. (via Wikipedia)

viewers under fifty. At that time, 44 percent of NBC viewers were over fifty. The American Broadcasting Company (ABC) added *Matlock* to its schedule, airing shows through 1995. Syndicated *Matlock* reruns were broadcast on cable networks.

—Elizabeth D. Schafer

See also: Communication; *Murder, She Wrote*

MATURITY

Relevant Issues: Psychology, sociology, values
Significance: The achievement of maturity in middle and late life enriches the individual's ability to make decisions and enjoy the rewards of a lifetime.

The mature adult of any age is often defined as one who has made personal choices and has committed to them. Choices relate to life partners, work, religion, friends, interests, and hobbies. Mature adults are balanced in terms of attention to and understanding of self and others. They have a set of inner principles that guide their lives. Although these attributes are basic for all mature adults, there are aspects of maturity that change with age.

There is no single way to achieve maturity in middle and late life. Sociologists and psychologists have not been able to define one pattern of living or one personality type that leads to maturity in aging. They find so-called successful aging among people who are actively involved in life and among those who are disengaged or withdrawn from social life; they find contented, fulfilled older people with many different lifestyles and personality types.

Early psychologist Erik Erikson described the course of life as a group of stages and suggested that there are tasks in every stage that must be accomplished for successful development. In midlife, the task is to be productive, what Erikson termed "generativity." Mature, middle-aged adults use their skills to be productive in areas that represent their commitments. For example, mature, middle-aged people may contribute a great deal to their chosen field of work or may share in satisfying marriages or friendships. One who is active in church may be given a responsible position because of experience, while one who has coached soccer for years may be asked to manage a soccer league. Thus, maturity at midlife often relates to the individual's use of accumulated skills to enhance humankind.

During midlife, most people begin to gain a different perspective on life. With the realization of mortality, individuals begin a process of introspection that continues into late life. Midlifers often think about what they still want to accomplish. This examination of goals sometimes leads to significant changes, such as divorce or career switches. The world generally views these as midlife crises.

In late life, this introspection turns toward finding meaning in one's life. Erikson's task for late life is finding integrity. Young people may be considered egotistical if they focus too much on themselves, but many psychologists claim that older people need to be introspective. To mature in late life is to find the meaning of one's life and to be able to see oneself in the context of all humanity. Family members are sometimes able to help older relatives during the life review process by supporting them with positive memories. Older people working on this process often forgive themselves and others for the inevitable "wrongs" of life and think about positive influences they have had on family, friends, and their work.

The components or personal attributes of maturity remain the same throughout adulthood. However, the tasks of midlife and old age differ in that the focus of the first is on fulfillment of goals, while the focus of the second is on feeling satisfied with the accomplishment of some, if not all, of these goals.

—*Virginia L. Smerglia*

See also: Creativity; Erikson, Erik H.; Middle age; Midlife crisis; Old age; Wisdom

For Further Information

Cox, Tony, and Sandra Aamodt. "Brain Maturity Extends Well Beyond Teen Years." NPR, National Public Radio, 11 Oct. 2011. www.npr.org/templates/story/story.php?storyId=141164708. Cox discusses with Sandra Aamodt, neuroscientist and co-author of the book Welcome to Your Child's Brain, the emerging science about brain development that suggests that most people don't reach full maturity until the age25.

Howard, Jacqueline. "You're an Adult, but Your Brain Might Not Be." CNN, Cable News Network, 21 Dec. 2016. www.cnn.com/2016/12/21/health/adult-brain-development/index.html. This article discusses emerging research on the true process of maturity in the brain.

Osho. *Maturity: the Responsibility of Being Oneself.* Griffin, 2000. Osho outlines the ten major growth cycles in human life, from the self-centered universe of the preschooler to the flowering of wisdom and compassion in old age.

MEASURE OF MY DAYS, THE (BOOK)

Author: Florida Scott-Maxwell

Date: Published in 1968

Relevant Issues: Death, family, health and medicine, religion

Significance: Scott-Maxwell reflects upon love, death, and wonder in her eighties, thus providing a model for the struggle to gain identity and meaning in later life.

Disengaged from careers in fiction writing and Jungian psychology, Florida Scott-Maxwell entered her eighties armed with a newly found passion for reflection on humanity and on her own rich life. Not one to romanticize old age, Scott-Maxwell, in her book *The Measure of My Days*, rages against disappointment, illness, uncertainty, and most of all, the threat of becoming a burden. Yet her awareness that life's crucial task is the achievement of balance leaves her little room for self-pity. She finds that pain gives rise to energy, and energy stimulates vitality and love.

Scott-Maxwell declares that the chief aim of old age is the protection of one's identity, a sacred self that vacillates between differentiation from others, on one hand, and assimilation to the masses, on the other. The temptation to hide from the struggle for identity competes with the need to assume responsibility for one's existence. Responsibility derives from openness to personal experience; even immortality, as experienced here and now, is a real part of one's self.

Scott-Maxwell asserts that in old age, one's soul serves as one's best companion. The soul cries, exults, and remains silent, but, in the main, waits. At times, the elderly are too full of life inside to die; at other times, they feel too full of illness not to die. In neither state of mind does Scott-Maxwell mourn for herself or for her losses; rather, she mourns for the incomprehensibility of life and for what she deems confused and arid times. Scott-Maxwell concludes, though, that all people possess a reservoir of "unlived life" that passes to the next generation.

—*Gregory D. Gross*

See also: Old age

MEDICAID

Relevant Issues: Government program, health insurance, low income, elderly, long-term care

Significance: Medicaid, a low cost health insurance program jointly funded by the federal government and states, offers health resources and support to low income persons of all ages, children, pregnant women, the disabled, and the blind.

Medicaid is a low-cost health insurance program jointly funded by the federal government and states for persons of all ages with low income, pregnant women, children, the blind, and the disabled. The federal government pays the state a percentage or the Federal Medical Assistance Percentage (FMAP). The program is, however, administered by the states. Eligibility and programs offered vary somewhat among states. The individual state requirements can be accessed online at Medicaid.gov by searching for "State Overviews." This article addresses Medicaid as it applies to older adults.

There are 7.2 million low-income seniors who receive health-care coverage through Medicaid and are dually enrolled in Medicare. Combined with the 4.8 million person with disabilities who are covered with Medicaid and Medicare, 12 million people, or 15 percent of all Medicaid enrollees, are dually eligible for these services. For seniors who meet the low income eligibility guidelines, programs are available for care such as nursing home, skilled nursing facility, adult day care, adult health day care, assisted living, home health care, and non-medical home care.

Several programs are available to Medicaid eligible seniors including long-term care options. The senior must meet both financial qualifications and have a medical care need. A medical need might be that the person requires a skilled nursing facility or nursing home level of care or has mental impairment such as dementia.

To qualify for Medicaid insurance, the applicant must have a limited income level that is below the federal poverty level (FPL) as determined by their state or have very high medical bills when income and assets are reviewed for eligibility.

For those enrolled in Medicare, Medicaid can provide what Medicare covers, which includes Part A for hospitalizations; Part B for physician services, X-ray and lab services, outpatient services, and durable medical equipment; Part C, a Medicare managed care plan like a HMO or PPO that is offered by private companies; and Part D, which helps pay for prescription drugs. However, Medicaid covers more services than Medicare coverage such as skilled nursing facility care beyond 100 days paid by Medicare, eyeglasses, hearing aids, and prescription medications. Medicare acts as the primary insurance with Medicaid paying the remainder to the state payment level limit.

Medicaid can cover long-term care in an institutional setting as detailed in the Social Security Act. This can include hospital services, intermediate care facilities, nursing home care, and services in an institution for mental diseases for persons 65 years or older with mental illnesses.

APPLICATION PROCESS FOR SENIORS

Applications for Medicaid health coverage should be made in the state where the person resides as every state has its own requirements. Applications are taken at the state office, in a community office, by phone, or online. The applicant process includes a proof of income, a current tax bill, a social security number, and copies of the home mortgage if the applicant owns their home. Generally the applicant must be 65 or older, have a disability, or be blind and be a U.S. citizen and resident of the state where they apply. If the person has other assets such as a car, bank account, stocks or bonds, these will need to be reviewed in the application process. Approval may take up to 45 days to complete. After approval, the applicant will have an assessment to see if they qualify for long-term care covered options or skilled care. Persons with chronic illnesses or disabilities may qualify.

Applicants for long-term care coverage in a nursing home require a Preadmission Screening and Resident Review (PASRR) to determine the appropriate place to receive the level of care they need and to provide that care.

PACE

Programs of All-Inclusive Care for the Elderly (PACE) provides an option of care for certain frail elderly in the community who are usually eligible for both Medicaid and Medicare. This managed care model of health services offers comprehensive medical and social services coordinated by a team of interdisciplinary professionals such as doctors, nurses, therapists, dietitians, socials workers, and personal care assistants to help beneficiaries live in their communities and out of a nursing home. States can elect to offer the PACE program to Medicaid recipients as a benefit option. Social and medical services are provided in settings such as adult day health centers, inpatient hospitals, and at the person's home. In some cases, PACE may cover services not provided through traditional Medicare. PACE is only available in 31 states and is a program under Medicare.

Eligibility for the PACE program includes the person is age 55 or older, eligible for nursing home, resides in a state and service area for PACE, and able to live safely in their community. Once the person is enrolled in PACE, the program becomes their source of Medicare and Medicaid benefits.

—*Marylane Wade Koch, MSN, RN*

For Further Information

"How Does the Medicare PACE Program Help Older Adults?" eHealthMedicare. www.ehealthmedicare.com/faq/how-does-the-medicare-pace-program-help-older-adults. Defines and provides information on services provided through the PACE program and criteria of eligibility. PACE is not provided in every state.

"Long Term Care Services and Support." Medicaid.gov. www.medicaid.gov/medicaid/ltss/index.html. Explains that long-term care (LTC) is needed by many with chronic illness and disabling diseases and how Medicaid is the primary payer for LTC in this country. LTC includes a continuum of care from community care to institutional care such as nursing homes.

"Medicaid and Long Term Care for the Elderly" Paying for Senior Care. www.payingforseniorcare.com/long termcare/resources/medicaid.html. Lists long-term care options offered through Medicaid and links to details on each.

"Medicaid Application." Medicaid.gov. govtbenefits.org/medicaid-application. Explains how to apply for Medicaid and offers an online process.

"Medicare and Medicaid Programs; Programs of All-Inclusive Care for the Elderly (PACE)" A Proposed Rule by the Centers for Medicare & Medicaid Services, 3 June 2019. www.federalregister.gov/documents/2019/06/03/2019-11087/medicare-and-medicaid-programs-programs-of-all-inclusive-care-for-the-elderly-pace. Provides a summary as well as details of updates to requirements of PACE. The changes are designed to "provide greater operational flexibility, remove redundancies and outdated information, and codify existing practice."

Program of All-Inclusive Care for the Elderly (PACE). Medicaid.gov. www. medicaid.gov/medicaid/ltss/pace/index.html Provides description and eligibility guidelines.

"Seniors & Medicare and Medicaid Enrollees." Medicaid.gov. www.medicaid. gov/medic aid/eligibility/medicaid-enrollees/index.html.

"State Overviews." Medicaid.gov. www.medicaid.gov/state-overviews/index.html. Provides state profiles information with current information about eligibility, enrollment, quality of care, and any documents needed utilized by the specific state.

MEDICARE

Relevant Issues: Economics, health and medicine

Significance: Medicare is a national health insurance program for people aged sixty-five years and older, for people with permanent kidney failure, and for people with specified disabilities.

Medicare is designed primarily as a health insurance supplement for older Americans receiving Social Security. The program consists of two components: Part A, or hospital insurance (HI), helps pay for hospital and related costs, while Part B, or supplementary medical insurance (SMI), helps pay for physician services, medical equipment, and other health-care expenses. Part A is financed by a payroll tax, with the employer and employee each paying 1.45 percent of the employee's total wage. To participate in Part B, beneficiaries are required to pay a monthly premium ($135.50 per month in 2019, or higher depending on income). Medicare, in contrast to Medicaid, is not considered a form of public assistance, and benefits are not dependent upon financial need.

BENEFITS

On the average, Medicare covers less than 60 percent of the health-care costs of its non-institutionalized elderly enrollees. Under Part A, or HI, beneficiaries must pay a deductible for hospital care, which is equivalent to the approximate cost of one day of hospital care ($1,364 in 2019). Medicare then pays the full cost for the first two months in the hospital, 75 percent of the costs for the third month, and 50 percent of the cost of stays beyond three months. Medicare also covers part of the costs of post-hospital care in a nursing home for a maximum period of one hundred days. Although Medicare does not pay for long-term nursing home care, it does pay most of the costs of hospice care for terminally ill patients. Because late-stage care is especially labor-intensive, approximately 25 percent of Medicare funds are spent on patients who are in the last year of life.

As the premiums of Part B, or SMI, are much less expensive than those of private insurance policies, about 98 percent of the elderly participate in the SMI program. In 2019, in addition to premiums, beneficiaries were required to pay a deductible of $185 per year, and they were also responsible for coinsurance payments of 20 percent of allowable physicians' charges. Physicians may bill the government directly, or the patients may pay the physician and obtain reimbursement from Medicare. Medicare generally does not pay for prescription drugs, a source of real hardship for many seniors with chronic health conditions. Some private companies provide managed care options that combine Parts A and B under one contract for all covered services.

Many elderly people purchase private health insurance policies to pay for services not provided in Parts A and B. These so-called Medigap policies are regulated by law. Medicare recipients who are poor may qualify for Medicaid assistance to help pay for coinsurance, medication, and other medical expenses. In addition, when poor people under Medicaid do not qualify for Medicare coverage, the states are able to "buy into" the Medicare program on their behalf.

The most significant limitation on Medicare's coverage is that it does not provide for most of the costs of long-term nursing home care. Because of the great expense (around $80,000 per year or more in 2016), long-term care places a substantial burden on many of the nation's elderly and their families. Of the 52 million adults over 65 in 2019, about 2 percent, or 1.2 million, lived in nursing homes. Although one-half of direct payments for long-term care are paid by public funds, about 80 percent of these funds come from Medicaid, and individuals can participate in Medicaid only after they "spend down" their assets and become indigent. In view of the potential impact on the budget, it is unlikely that Congress will expand Medicare coverage to include long-term care. For a short period in the 1980s, an

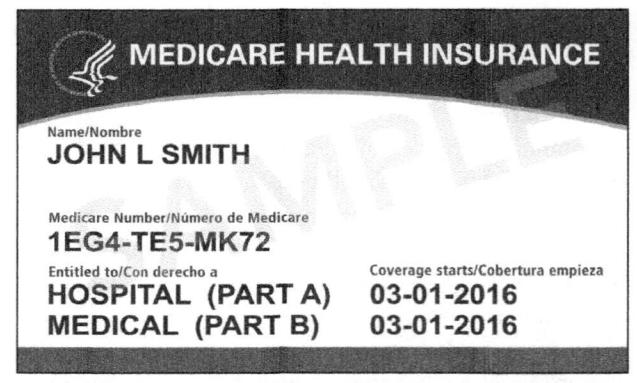

Sample for the new United States Medicare program cards that began rolling out in 2018. (via Wikimedia Commons)

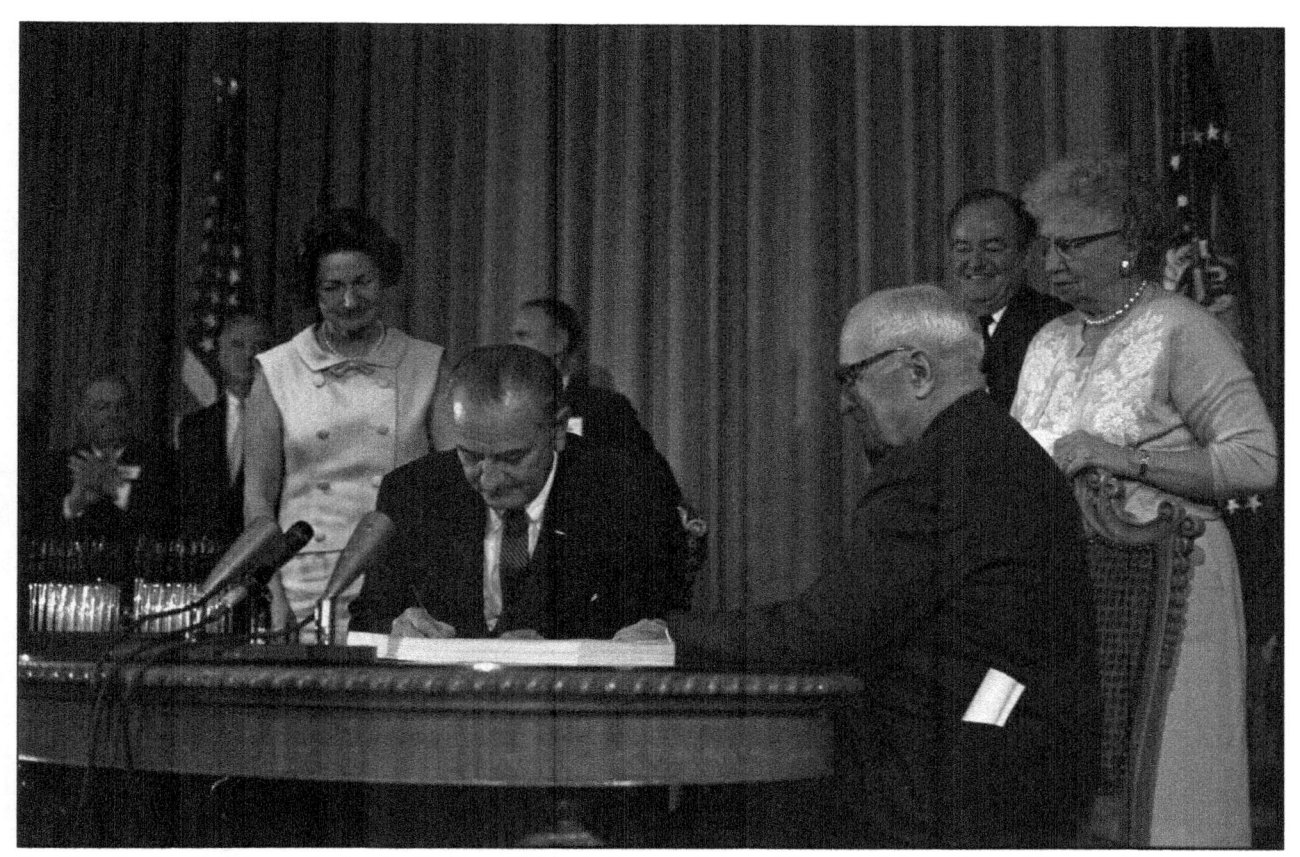

President Lyndon B. Johnson signing the Medicare Bill at the Harry S. Truman Library in Independence, Missouri. Former president Harry S. Truman is seated at the table with President Johnson. (via National Archives and Records Administration)

attempt was made to fund long-term care through Medicare premiums, but the strong protests caused Congress to terminate the program.

BEGINNINGS

The evolution of the 1965 Medicare Act really began during the New Deal period. In 1934, President Franklin Roosevelt's Committee on Economic Security announced that it was considering a national health insurance program; this provoked such a public outcry that the idea was dropped to promote the passage of the Social Security Act. President Harry S Truman resurrected the proposal as part of his Fair Deal, and, in 1949, Congress gave some consideration to the Murray-Wagner-Dingell Bill, which would have provided comprehensive medical services to all citizens. A coalition of Republicans and southern Democrats, however, killed the bill.

In 1951, Wilbur Cohen and other advisers of the Federal Security Agency drafted a more modest proposal that limited coverage to the beneficiaries of the Old Age and Survivors Insurance program. The public was especially sympathetic to the special health needs of the aged, who were widely perceived as more deserving than other groups. Congress, nevertheless, held no hearings on the proposal until 1958, when the Forand Bill was introduced and debated. Labor unions were the strongest supporters of the bill, while the American Medical Association (AMA) led the opposition. In 1960, Congress passed a conservative alternative, the Kerr-Mills Bill, which provided federal grants to the states for assisting those in severe financial need.

President John F. Kennedy's New Frontier platform included a proposal for a compulsory health insurance law for aged Social Security beneficiaries, and he appointed Cohen as head of a task force to draft such a bill. Supported by about 60 percent of the public, the

Medicare bill was finally passed by Congress after the overwhelming Democratic victory in the elections that followed Kennedy's assassination in 1964. President Lyndon B. Johnson's initial proposal, a key element of his Great Society, was limited to hospital insurance, but the House Ways and Means Committee, led by Representative Wilbur Mills, expanded the bill to include both an SMI component and a Medicaid program for the indigent. After Congress passed the bill, President Johnson flew to Missouri, where he signed the legislation in the presence of former president Truman on July 30, 1965.

GROWTH OF THE PROGRAM

When Medicare began, the nation's economy was very strong, and medical technology was much less advanced and must less expensive than it became two decades later. Also, because the large baby-boom generation was just beginning to enter the workforce, the percentage of the population relying on Medicare was relatively small. As a result, the financing of the program was not especially difficult for the first few years. In order to minimize the AMA's opposition to Medicare, the early administration policies were designed to encourage hospitals and physicians to participate in the program, and there were almost no limits to the charges allowed.

In 1972, Congress tried to contain runaway costs by enacting maximum limits on payments, by allowing an option for enrollment in health maintenance organizations (HMOs), and by establishing professional review organizations (PROs) to determine reasonable rates. In 1974, Congress expanded Medicare to include chronic renal disease patients and the disabled. In 1977, the Health Care Financing Agency (HCFA) was established to administer Medicare under the Department of Health and Human Services (HHS). As costs continued to rise more rapidly than inflation, Congress, in 1983, passed Social Security amendments to increase the tax rate. About the same time, President Ronald Reagan convinced Congress to establish the prospective payment system (PPS), which pays hospitals according to fixed scales for about five hundred conditions. As a result, hospitals began to "cost shift" Medicare losses to private patients, and they tended to put pressure on physicians to discharge patients as early as possible.

Growth in Medicare costs has reflected the general increase in health-care expenditures in the United States. While national health expenses were only $247 per person in 1967, by 1994 they had grown to $3,510. The aging of the population was one of the major reasons for the growth of Medicare. In 1967, 19.5 million people were enrolled for Medicare coverage; by 1996, the number had grown to 38.1 million. Medicaid expanded even more rapidly—from 10 million people in 1967 to 37.5 million in 1996. As medical technology became more efficacious, the level of usage increased accordingly. The ratio of aged Medicare users of any type of covered service was 367 per 1,000 enrollees in 1967, while it was 821 per 1,000 enrollees in 1994. Likewise, Medicare enrollees with end-stage renal disease grew from 66,700 recipients in 1980 to more than 250,000 in 1995, an increase of 285 percent.

By the 1990s, there were almost constant political battles about how to finance the ballooning costs of Medicare. The public has strongly supported the Medicare program, and few politicians have been willing to support any decrease in its funding. In 1994, Republicans and President Bill Clinton had a major confrontation about limiting the program's growth. The Republicans proposed reducing the growth of Medicare by $270 billion over seven years, much more than the Clinton administration favored. After heated debates, the two sides eventually agreed on a compromise of $137 billion in reductions. Informed observers generally agreed that the dispute helped boost the popularity of President Clinton and the Democrats.

As part of the Balanced Budget Act of 1997, Congress created the Medical Payment Advisory Commission (MedPAC). The purpose of the sixteen-member nonpartisan commission was to collect data and to make recommendations to Congress about possible ways to solve the long-term financial problems of the program. At the same time, Congress expanded the options for the delivery of services. Seniors were given two more expensive options: government-subsidized private insurance and Medicare medical savings accounts (MMSAs). In 1998, the Clinton administration advocated expanding Medicare to include the cost of prescription drugs and to allow early retirees to purchase coverage in the system. Conservatives replied that the additional costs would be prohibitive.

The Medicare Prescription Drug Improvement and Modernization Act of 2003 (MMA) made the biggest changes to the Medicare program in 38 years. Under the MMA, private health plans approved by Medicare became known as Medicare Advantage Plans. The MMA also expanded Medicare to include an optional prescription drug benefit, Part D, which went into effect in 2006. The Part D monthly premium varies by plan (higher-income consumers may pay more). As of early 2019, more than 45 million Medicare beneficiaries—about three-quarters of the Medicare population—had Medicare Part D coverage (Medicare beneficiaries can also obtain prescription coverage from an employer or retiree program, or from Medicaid if they're eligible for both Medicare and Medicaid).

The 2010 Affordable Care Act (ACA) brought the Health Insurance Marketplace, a single place where consumers can apply for and enroll in private health insurance plans. It also made new ways to design and test how to pay for and deliver health care. Medicare and Medicaid have also been better coordinated to make sure people who have Medicare and Medicaid can get quality services.

In 2015, Congress passed the Medicare and CHIP Reauthorization Act (MACRA), which changed the previous payment system for doctors who treat Medicare patients. It revises the Balanced Budget Act of 1997 and constituted the largest change to the American health-care system since the Affordable Care Act. MACRA implemented a Merit Based Incentive, transitioning from a fee for service system to a pay for performance system. This model will require the provider to give information on the quality of service being given, how valuable it is to the patient, and accountability the provider has to the treatment being performed.

By early 2019, there were 60.6 million people receiving health coverage through Medicare. Medicare spending reached $705.9 billion in 2017, which was about 20 percent of total national health spending.

CONCERNS FOR FUTURE FINANCING

Medicare spending projections fluctuate with time, but as of 2018, Medicare spending was expected to account for 18 percent of total federal spending by 2028, up from 15 percent in 2017. And the Medicare Part A trust fund was expected to be depleted by 2026 (Medicare will continue to exist, but claims will have to be covered by payroll taxes, which won't be enough to fully cover all Part A claims). But Medicare per capita spending has been growing at a much slower pace in recent years, averaging 1.5 percent between 2010 and 2017, as opposed to 7.3 percent between 2000 and 2007. Per capita spending is projected to grow at a faster rate over the coming decade, but not as fast as it did in the first decade of the twenty-first century.

In 2003, legislation was proposed by Democratic Congressman John Conyers (MI) to establish a single-payer health-care system in the United States. Although the bill, called the United States National Health Care Act, or Expanded and Improved Medicare for All Act, originally only had 25 sponsors, as of 2017 there are 120 cosponsors and the highest level of support since first introduced. If the bill is passed, most medical care would be paid for by the federal government for all ages, essentially ending the need for private health insurance and premiums. An initial analysis by the Physi-

---

> **SENIOR TALK:**
>
> **How Do You Feel About Medicare?**
>
> When you qualify for Medicare, you may be pleased to have access to Medicare health insurance. The fact that you will be covered by a comprehensive medical care plan may give you a feeling of comfort and security. You might feel confused or overwhelmed by aspects of the coverage, how and when to enroll, and if you must do so. There are many components to Medicare coverage, and you might worry that you'll misunderstand and get it wrong. To alleviate that fear, you can gather the information by calling one of the government help lines set up to answer questions or seek advice from a trusted health professional. The clarity you gain can help you feel reassured and more empowered to make important medical choices. You'll know what is covered, what is not, and what you have to do to make up the difference with private insurance, if need be. Unless you learn how Medicare works, you may be shocked if you are charged for something you thought was covered.
>
> —*Leah Jacob*

cians for a National Health Program (PNHP) estimated that immediate savings would total $350 billion a year. The Act was not debated when the ACA was implemented, but both Democratic Representatives Bernie Sanders (VT) and Pramila Jayapal (WA) proposed similar bills to establish a single-payer system. It is expected that universal health care will be a major debate topic in the 2020 Congressional and Presidential elections.

—*Thomas T. Lewis*

See also: Baby boomers; Facility and institutional care; Hospice; Hospitalization; Long-term care; Medical insurance; Medications; Terminal illness

For Further Information

Blumenthal, David, et al. "Medicare at 50—Moving Forward." *New England Journal of Medicine*, vol. 372, no. 7, 2015, pp. 671-77. doi:10.1056/nejmhpr1414856. In part two of this Health Policy Report marking the 50th anniversary of Medicare, the authors review several potential strategies for addressing the challenges to the effectiveness and sustainability of the program.

———. "Medicare at 50—Origins and Evolution." *New England Journal of Medicine*, vol. 372, no. 5, 2015, pp. 479-86. doi:10.1056/nejmhpr1411701. In part one of a two-part report marking the 50th anniversary of Medicare, the authors review the history of the program's passage into law and how it has been modified over the past five decades.

Brockett, Patrick L., et al. "Potential 'Savings' of Medicare: The Analysis of Medicare Advantage and Accountable Care Organizations." *North American Actuarial Journal*, vol. 22, no. 3, 2018, pp. 458-72. doi:10.1080/10920277.2018.1436445. This article reviews current literature on Medicare Advantage plans, compares them to Accountable Care Organizations, examines the administrative costs of Medicare Advantage plans and Medicare privatization, and analyzes the profit efficiency of the different lines of business of private insurers including Medicare Advantage plans.

Centers for Medicare & Medicaid Services. Department of Health and Human Services, 27 June 2019. www.cms.gov/. Government-funded office designed to communicate general information and policy changes to both Medicare and Medicaid programs.

Cotton, Paul, et al. "Medicare Advantage: Issues, Insights, and Implications for the Future." *Population Health Management*, vol. 19, no. S3, 2016. doi:10.1089/pop.2016.29013.pc. This supplement offers the perspectives of experts, researchers, and administrators on Medicare Advantage today and the important role it can play in Medicare for years to come.

Dalen, James E., et al. "An Alternative to Medicare for All." *The American Journal of Medicine*, vol. 132, no. 6, 2019, pp. 665-67. doi:10.1016/j.amjmed.2019.01.007. Presents possible solutions to the need for health coverage for all Americans.

Krieg, Gregory, and Ryan Nobles. "The Fight over 'Medicare for All' Is Only Beginning." CNN, Cable News Network, 30 Aug. 2019. www.cnn.com/2019/08/30/politics/medicare-for-all-bernie-sanders-elizabeth-warren-kamala-harris-joe-biden-2020/index.html. Explains universal health-care plans proposed by Bernie Sanders and Kamala Harris within the context of the upcoming 2020 elections.

Marmor, Theodore. *The Politics of Medicare*. 2nd ed. Routledge, 2017. A fascinating historical account that explains how the Medicare Act was passed in 1965.

Medicare, www.medicare.gov/. The official U.S. government site for Medicare.

Moeller, Philip. Get What's Yours for Medicare: Maximize Your Coverage, Minimize Your Costs. Simon & Schuster, 2016. A coauthor of the *New York Times* bestselling guide to Social Security Get What's Yours. Moeller presents an essential companion to explain Medicare, the nation's other major benefit for older Americans.

O'Brien, Sarah. "Here's What You Should Know about Medicare Costs If You're Nearing Age 65." CNBC, 29 Aug. 2019. www.cnbc.com/2019/08/29/heres-what-you-should-know-about-medicare-if-youre-nearing-age-65.html. Reveals some of the costs associated with Medicare that many don't know about.

Starr, Paul. *Remedy and Reaction: The Peculiar American Struggle over Health Care Reform*. Revised ed., Yale U P, 2013. Tracing health-care reform from its beginnings to its current uncertain prospects, Starr argues that the United States ensnared itself in a trap through policies that satisfied enough of the public and so enriched the health-care industry as to make the system difficult to change.

MEDICATIONS

Relevant Issues: Health and medicine

Significance: Older people are the largest users of prescription medications; in fact, 50 percent of all drug consumption is attributed to them.

MISUSE OF DRUGS

Belief by the aged and the population at large that there is a "magic bullet" for every complaint is widespread. Older adults living at home consume between three and seven drugs daily, whereas those living in nursing homes take, on average, four to seven different medications. In addition, when five or more drugs are ingested, the incidence of drug poisoning rises 50 percent; when eight or more are taken together, the incidence rises 100 percent.

Overuse, underuse, and erratic use of medications constitute a major problem among older people. Between 12 and 17 percent of hospital admissions among seniors involve adverse drug reactions. Of these, approximately 80 percent are reactions from commonly prescribed medications. Drugs for mental and nervous system disorders are among the ten most prescribed drugs, yet these disorders account for less than 7 percent of problems in older people. It is estimated that 40 percent of older people living in their own homes experience drug reactions. Overdoses involving barbiturates, sedatives, tranquilizers, and alcohol are common occurrences.

PHYSICAL CHANGES OF AGING

Absorption, distribution, metabolism, and elimination of medications change in older persons compared to younger people. As a person ages, lean body mass, decreased functional tissue, and an increased number of fat deposits create differences in the ability of the body to use standard doses of drugs. Chemical changes in the body also affect how drugs act on the body. The type, the intensity, and the duration of drug action depends on these changes.

The time required for medication to enter the general circulation is termed absorption. In older people, reduced gastric motility influences absorption. Increase or decrease in movement of medications through the digestive tract may enhance or interfere with their purpose. For example, coated tablets may pass through the digestive tract slowly and be delayed too long. Because of the delay, their action may inadvertently begin in the stomach, causing nausea and irritation.

Distribution, or transport, depends on a healthy circulatory system. Some older people have decreased cardiac output or impaired circulation that may delay delivery of medication to the target site, delay the release of a drug from storage tissue, and stall excretion of a drug. A drug like Coumadin (Warfarin), a common blood thinner, attaches to protein in the blood. Some is available for use, and some stays bound to the protein.

Older people have less protein in the blood, so more drug freely circulates, creating a climate of potential toxicity. As a result, the dose of a protein-bound drug like Coumadin may need to be adjusted downward to avoid too much circulating drug. Also, a person in a poor nutritional state would need close monitoring of drug effects or reactions.

Medicines come in various forms, such as capsules, coated beads, layered tablets, or plastic matrix tablets. Drugs are prepared by manufacturers in a certain way to provide the most therapeutic effect—to make certain that an accurate dose reaches the target area. Altering the form in any way may change drug effects or destroy their effectiveness altogether. Medications are prepared with special coatings or substances to avoid destruction by stomach acid. Crushing or manipulating tablets meant for sustained release spills all of a drug in one location and destroys its intended long-acting effect.

In older people, the amount of fatty tissue increases in relation to a decrease in muscle mass. Vitamins such as A, D, E, and K are fat-soluble. Fat-soluble medications are stored and not readily passed, potentially resulting in toxic accumulation. Generally these vitamins must be taken with food to ensure more efficient absorption and distribution in the body. Elders should seek the advice of a physician, pharmacist, or nurse before taking fat-soluble supplements.

Relative body water declines in older people. When there is a decrease in relative body water, drug levels are elevated and sustained. This means that water-soluble drugs are not distributed evenly or adequately. Cimetadine (Tagamet), a drug sold over the counter and often taken by elders for gastric irritation, is water-soluble. Digoxin, an often prescribed heart medication, is also water-soluble and must be closely monitored in older adults. Elders must drink plenty of fluids and remain well hydrated to derive benefit from these drugs.

Each person metabolizes medications in a unique way. Genetic differences and ethnic variations explain why people react to drugs in different ways. Body composition, weight, and gender, as well as nutritional status and disease, determine how drugs are metabolized. Smokers metabolize drugs more rapidly and experience both adverse and toxic drug effects.

The liver is the organ that breaks down, detoxifies, and removes by-products of drugs metabolized by the body. Decreased blood flow through the liver decreases metabolism, which means that ingested drugs will stay in the body longer. Because common drugs such as acetaminophen (Tylenol) and ibuprofen (Advil or Motrin)—two widely used drugs for pain—are detoxified in the liver, they must be taken with caution and only when needed. Routine use of these common over-the-counter (OTC) medications should be discouraged as their excessive use can cause irreversible liver damage.

Many drugs, including antibiotics and some cardiac drugs, are excreted by the kidneys in the urine. Kidney function is very important in older adults, as toxic accumulation of drug by-products, particularly antibiotics, can cause retention of substances that will damage kidneys. Diuretics are drugs that remove water from the body and decrease the amount of fluid circulating in the bloodstream. Many older people take diuretics as treatment for high blood pressure and other heart ailments. When taking these drugs, timing and hydration are two important factors. "Water pills" should be taken in the morning and not in the evening to accommodate less frequent trips to the bathroom and allow for undisturbed sleep.

Because of visual and perceptual changes associated with aging, older people often confuse pill colors or misinterpret shapes. Some elders cannot read the small print on drug labels. Impaired hearing and unclear instructions by health-care providers preclude proper timing of medications. Lapses in memory interfere with routine dosing and aggravate existing symptoms. Stiff hands make opening bottles difficult. Some elders skip meals, especially when alone, and inadvertently skip medications ordinarily taken with meals. Some medications have embarrassing side effects that cause older people to eliminate doses when away from home or when at social gatherings.

POLYPHARMACY

The use of multiple medications is common among older adults. Some older people see many doctors for a variety of ailments. Elders take over-the-counter (OTC) medications as well as prescription drugs and are often unaware of potential toxic effects. Laxatives interfere with the action of blood pressure drugs, and calcium-based antacids and those containing aluminum and magnesium cut the absorption rate of tetracycline antibiotics by 90 percent. Use of OTC medications can also mask signs of serious infection or serious undiagnosed disorders. Some OTC medications, like inhaled sprays used to relieve temporary symptoms of asthma, are dangerous in diabetics and those with high blood pressure. The underlying airway disease remains undiagnosed, and the OTC medications can cause dangerous or potentially fatal reactions.

NECESSARY INFORMATION

For satisfactory treatment it is important to know how often a person sees a physician, what medications are prescribed from all sources, and what OTC medications the older person is taking. Equally important are questions about herbal remedies. Diverse populations of elders follow cultural preferences and do not consider herbs "medicines." Similarly, most older adults do not include vitamin and mineral supplements in the category of medicines. Therefore, it is important to ask older people what medications they take, how often they take them, and what vitamins, minerals, or other supplements they use.

Some clinics that follow an older clientele have so-called brown bag days. Elders are asked to put all medicines they have at home in a brown paper bag and bring them to the clinic for review. Expired drugs, different doses of the same prescribed drugs, herbal remedies, and OTC drugs are commonly found by health-care personnel. Elderly clients are advised to throw away expired medications, keep the most recently prescribed dose of the one-and-the-same drug, and dispose of all other multiple doses. They are also asked questions about their herbs and OTC medications. Because of vision changes and cultural differences, labels should be read and questions asked if information is unclear. Communication problems lead to drug problems.

Medication problems increase with the use of multiple pharmacies and physicians. Some pharmacies have a central repository of information that can locate all medications prescribed for one person. To some degree this controls duplication and provides the margin of safety needed. However, it does not record OTC medications or information on supplements.

HOW TO TALK TO SENIORS ABOUT MEDICATION ORGANIZATION AND MEDICAL INFORMATION

How Do They Feel?

Seniors may feel overwhelmed when trying to remember and manage all their medical information. The effort to stay organized, together with the stress of dealing with health conditions, often causes worry and anxiety. This can be exacerbated by common fears regarding health care, such as negative drug interactions or what will happen in the event of an emergency. Many older adults prefer not to think about their health, finding it scary or an unwelcome reminder of aging. Some seniors may also simply be unaware of the importance of keeping their health information organized or of the best practices for doing so.

Even seniors who are generally organized may struggle to remember what medications to take and when. The hassle of managing multiple prescriptions, each with different and sometimes complex instructions, can be deeply confusing and frustrating. This may lead to incorrect administration of medications or neglecting to take them at all, both of which can be dangerous. Seniors who are made aware of steps for better organization are often greatly relieved and more willing to participate in their own care.

Many seniors are very receptive to methods of organizing their medical information and medications. Even those who may not be naturally organized often understand the safety benefits of having information easily accessible and feel more comfortable knowing things are under control. However, some older adults are resistant to any attempt to change their normal way of doing things. They may see suggestions regarding organization as attacks on their independence or ability to manage their own affairs. This can be especially challenging if personality changes associated with cognitive decline deepen their stubbornness or even cause them to lash out angrily. Open communication is critical to get past such resistance.

How Do I Start The Conversation?

You can play an active role in raising the importance of medical information and medication organization to seniors. When initiating the conversation, do so in a gentle, caring, understanding manner. Be aware that the subject of health and medical care can stir up strong emotions. Try to keep your own emotions in check and be prepared to keep calm no matter how they react. You might begin simply by asking how they feel about the current organization of their medical information. Another strategy is to mention the experience of someone else who benefited from a certain method of organization and let the senior respond. Listen actively and empathically as they share any concerns or opinions. When you are tuned into their needs and feelings, you will be more able to steer the conversation appropriately.

Be particularly careful to avoid using scare tactics or otherwise making the senior panic about the future. Never overload them with too much information at once. The aim is not to arouse anxiety about an urgent need to organize their records and medications. Instead, try to create a sense of calmness, showing that being organized will be manageable and beneficial. You might ask what type of organizational methods work best for them, and try to help them put them into practice. If they're unsure, try presenting a few options and letting them choose one to try. If possible, make it clear that you are only there to help and that they are in control of decisions. For example, if they feel that a folder or binder will be effective for managing their records, let them choose the type and color, and listen to their ideas about placing the information in order. Where your help is required, engage in discussion so that they still feel part of the process.

As seniors become more comfortable with getting organized, you can bring up additional suggestions, but continue to avoid framing them as what they "should" or "must" do. Open-ended questions are often an effective, nonthreatening way of doing this. You might ask where they think they can safely store important information, such as in a drawer or closet. Ask which family members or other trusted individuals will be told this location in the event of emergencies. Similarly, you can ask what their biggest challenges with medications are, and then work with them (and the doctor or pharmacist, if necessary) to fix these issues. At all times, nonjudgmental support and open communication are key.

—Leah Jacob

A close relationship with a local pharmacist is an important resource for older patients. Printed information given to elders at the time of drug dispensing is helpful. At that time, the pharmacist should review side effects of the medication; discuss when and how to take it; alert the older person to prominent adverse effects; and advise the person to seek medical advice if any unusual changes in feeling, behavior, or function occur.

PREVENTING PROBLEMS

Several strategies can be used to decrease adverse interactive effects of medications associated with the normal physical changes of aging and ensure a smooth therapeutic course. If an older person takes multiple medications, a pill box that holds a seven-day supply is a good idea. The box is labeled by day of the week, and the compartments of the box are loaded once a week. Each compartment can be opened only on the day of the week marked and at the preset time the medicine is to be taken. Another method to ensure accuracy is a check-off chart. Medicine bottles are color-coded with colors easily identified by the older person. The chart lists the name of the medication in the same color as the medicine bottle. When the medicine is taken, the chart is checked off.

Elders should be advised to take medications on time. If a dose is missed, it is inadvisable to double up on the medicine. The dose should be taken as soon as remembered and the next dose rescheduled according to the time frame prescribed.

Medicines retain their potency when stored in cool, dry places, unless otherwise directed. The worst place to store medicines is in the bathroom medicine cabinet, where humidity will either decompose the drug or decrease its potency. Dark containers prevent light from entering and thus prevent medicines from decomposing. Elders should not change containers. In this same vain, it is inadvisable to mix old and new medicines. Elders are advised to use all pills contained in one bottle and to safely dispose of expired or unused medications.

The best advice to elders is to be aware of what to do if feeling poorly after ingesting medications. Phone numbers of the pharmacist, physician, or nurse should be readily available for quick reference.

—*Maureen C. Creegan*
Updated by Patrick Richardson, MSN

See also: Fat deposition; Gastrointestinal changes and disorders; Health care; Malnutrition; Nutrition; Overmedication; Vitamins and minerals

For Further Information

Koronkowski, Michael, et al. "An Update on Geriatric Medication Safety and Challenges Specific to the Care of Older Adults." *Official Journal of the American Medical Directors Association*, vol. 24, no. 3, 21 June 2016, pp. 37-40. www.ncbi.nlm.nih.gov/pmc/articles/PMC4915389/. In this review, the authors discuss recent medication safety literature pertaining to the classes of medications commonly prescribed to older adults: anticholinergics, psychiatric medications, and antibiotics.

"Medicines and You: A Guide for Older Adults." FDA, U.S. Food and Drug Administration, 7 Oct. 2015. www.fda.gov/drugs/resources-you/medicines-and-you-guide-older-adults. A guide about medications directed specifically at seniors.

Rochon, Paula A. "Drug Prescribing for Older Adults." UpToDate, 19 Feb. 2019. www.uptodate.com/contents/drug-prescribing-for-older-adults. A stepwise approach to optimized prescribing of drug therapy for older adults is reviewed. Drug treatments for specific conditions in the older population are discussed separately.

Wiese, Bonnie. "Geriatric Depression: The Use of Antidepressants in the Elderly." *BC Medical Journal*, vol. 53, no. 47, Sept. 2011, pp. 341-47. www.bcmj.org/articles/geriatric-depression-use-antidepressants-elderly. Describes how depression presents in older adults and stresses the need of assessment in choosing antidepressants for treating the disorder.

MEMENTO MORI (BOOK)

Author: Muriel Spark
Date: Published in 1959
Relevant Issues: Death, family, religion, values
Significance: This novel presents one of few serious examinations in fiction of attitudes among elderly toward death.

Scottish-born novelist Muriel Spark takes the title of her tragicomic novel *Memento Mori* from jewelry and other tokens sometimes worn in the past to remind humans of the shortness and uncertainty of life; the Latin term memento mori means "remember you must die."

For Spark, a Roman Catholic convert, death is the central fact of life. Only three characters in her novel remember this fact. Most, however, receive anonymous calls, each in a different voice, warning the person that he or she must die. Their reactions range from the Christian to the paranoiac. Jean Taylor, dumped into a public geriatric ward when she is no longer of use as a companion/servant, needs no phone reminder; a Catholic convert, she turns the horrors of the ward into a Christian acceptance of suffering and death. Charmian Colston, a Catholic, is not alarmed; she moves out of her house to avoid her jealous husband and possibly homicidal servant and calmly awaits death. Retired policeman Henry Mortimer, a stoic searcher for truth, alone understands that the telephone voice is that of death itself. For him, death is the end of weariness and suffering.

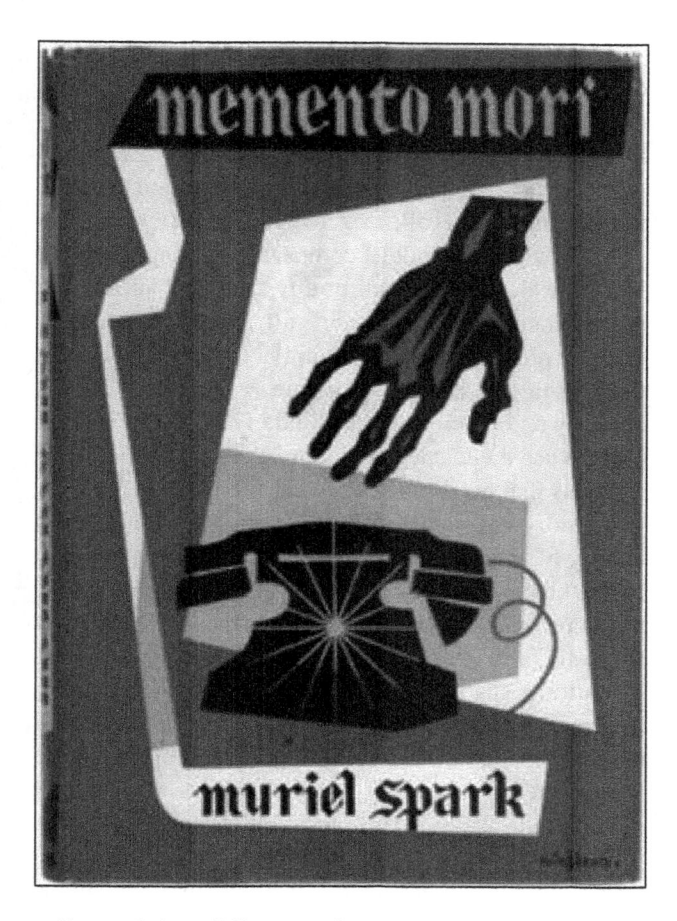

Others cannot face their own mortality. Dame Lettie Colston, noted prison reformer, reveals the shallowness of her reforms when she regrets that harsh punishments, such as flogging, can no longer be used to punish the caller. Increasingly paranoid, she isolates herself and thus inadvertently causes her own violent death. Most characters, such as her brother Godfrey Colston, simply refuse to acknowledge time and change, tragically or comically reliving the emotions, problems, and views of the past. For example, Alec Warner, a former sociologist, can only collect useless statistics; in him, Spark satirizes the approaches of social sciences to this central fact of human life.

—*Betty Richardson*

See also: Death and dying; Death anxiety; Religion

MEMORY LOSS

Relevant Issues: Biology, health and medicine, psychology

Significance: The past contributes to present self-identity and allows people to function on a day-to-day basis in a changing world; without memory, life would be stripped of the ability to live independently.

Key Terms:

cued recall: the retrieval of memory with the help of cues

episodic memory: a type of long-term memory that involves conscious recollection of earlier experiences together with their context in terms of time, place, associated emotions, and so on

free-recall test: participants study a list of items on each trial, and then are prompted to recall the items in any order

procedural memory: a type of long-term memory involving how to perform different actions and skills

recognition memory: the ability to recognize earlier encountered events, objects, or people

source memory: recalling the source of learned information, such as knowledge of when or where something was learned

spatial memory: part of the memory responsible for the recording of information about one's environment and spatial orientation

Many older persons become anxious when they forget things previously learned. When they complain of forgetfulness, older adults are typically referring to a decline in their ability to recall recent events. They complain of difficulty recalling the names of acquaintances, family members, and dates of events that will occur in the near future. They complain that as they get older it takes them longer to remember. Older adults say their most often memory lapse is not being able to recall a word that was on the "tip of the tongue." What is most worrisome to them is forgetting where they had placed an object, not doing something they should have done or forgetting something someone had told them.

There are a number of myths regarding memory loss and aging. One myth concerns a widely held belief that memory decreases across the board as one ages. A faulty underlying assumption that helped promulgate this myth is the belief that memory is a unitary construct. However, cognitive scientists theorize that memory is really a collection of dozens of different memory processes with many of them being driven by different underlying neurobiological mechanisms. As one ages, one finds that some types of memory actually improve. It is true that older adults can experience a number of memory problems, but the deficits are not as global as one might expect. A second myth is the belief that aging, particularly for individuals seventy years or older, can cause profound memory loss that results in the person becoming incapacitated. Aging is not the culprit; rather, the memory loss is typically due to a neurological disease or some other risk factor that is associated with advanced years.

To older adults, significant forgetfulness—whatever the cause—represents a threat to independence and their ability to think clearly. While many people report they forget things, research confirms that significant forgetfulness is not an inevitable consequence of aging. Surveys of older people show that as many as 20 percent of adults over age eighty-five report they have never had significant trouble with their memory.

MEMORY THAT DECLINES WITH AGE

Specific kinds of memory loss begin much earlier than middle age but become more noticeable once one reaches the mid-sixties. Generally, as one gets older, it is not the oldest memories that are forgotten but rather the recent past that is difficult to recall. Episodic memory refers to specific events and experiences in life. Recalling episodes from a family vacation, or a game of basketball that was played, or meeting a well-known actor, are considered episodic memories. These tend to fade as one ages.

Research shows that older adults have more difficulty on a free-recall test than young adults. In a free-recall test, participants are shown a list of words or pictures and are asked to recall as many of the stimuli as possible. If a delay exists between the presentation of the items and their recall, larger memory deficits are revealed for the older adults compared to younger people. Not only does free-recall ability decline, but another type of memory called cued recall begins to weaken as one gets older. Cued recall is similar to free recall except that during the test period a cue is given to help aid memory recollection. In this kind of research it is common to use a cue such as a word that rhymes with the stimulus that needs to be recalled.

Memory theorists state that age brings on deficits in a variety of areas. For example, younger people perform better than older adults at remembering medicine labels, the names and faces of people, songs they have heard on the radio, and television programs they have watched. In addition, spatial memory declines with age as shown by poorer memory for the location of specific buildings on familiar streets, or the layout of museums that have been visited.

Part of the challenge for older adults can be explained by greater difficulty they have in reinstating the circumstances under which they acquire information. This is referred to as source forgetting. If a person is not able to recall as many details that were a part of the original context in which the information was encoded, the probability that the item or event will be recalled is greatly diminished. However, source forgetting does not explain all the memory difficulties brought on by advanced age. It has been found that cognitive processes necessary for efficient memory performance change over time and ultimately reduce the likelihood of retaining information. One such process is the rate of rehearsal. Rehearsal is a specific type of control process that is used to facilitate the transfer of information from short-term storage to a more permanent storage. If a problem develops with the rehearsal mechanism, subsequent memory transfer will be adversely affected. In the case of older adults, evidence suggests that the rate of rehearsal is slowed compared to younger adults.

As people age, they become more susceptible to risk factors that could lead to devastating memory loss. These factors are not directly related to the aging process but arise due to injury or disease impacting the brain. Once the brain is damaged, whether it be due to alcoholism, a closed head injury such as a stroke, or a poorly understood disease, the aged brain is not able to adapt and recover as well as a young brain.

MEMORY THAT STAYS INTACT OR IMPROVES WHILE AGING

Tasks that are least likely to cause memory problems for older adults tend to be meaningful, highly practiced, and well learned. Fortunately, there are a handful of memory processes that are particularly resistant to forgetting. One such process is the memory for motor skills referred to as procedural memory. Memory researchers have compared speeds of different typists of different ages. Although they found that on a simple reaction-time task older subjects were slower than younger ones, no differences were found in typing speeds. Although this was somewhat puzzling at first, it was later discovered that older adults were better at adopting compensatory strategies—such as looking further ahead on the page and anticipating upcoming keystrokes better—than their younger counterparts.

One common test of short-term memory found on intelligence quotient (IQ) tests is the measure of digit span. This involves the test administrator calling out different sequences of numbers and then having the participant immediately repeat back as many of the digits in their correct order as possible. Some of the sequences must be repeated in the same order they were read aloud; in other instances they must be recited in reverse order. Research has shown that the digit span stays relatively stable through the age of seventy years. However, memories that stay intact are not limited to those recently acquired. Recognition memory changes only slightly as one advances in age, even when the items to be recognized were encoded days before they were asked to be recalled. In addition, semantic memory processes—such as memory for words—tend to be robust toward any kind of decline associated with aging. Studies that do show some performance loss of semantic knowledge in aging individuals reveal that the decline is due to a slower speed at which older people can access their knowledge.

Research indicates most people will not develop significant memory impairment as they age. People's ability to remember autobiographical material, for example, does not normally decline with age. Although age-related forgetfulness may cause older adults to take longer to absorb new information, they are just as capable as younger people to retain and recall it. In fact, vocabulary and reasoning skills often improve as a person ages.

WHAT CAUSES FORGETFULNESS?

The oldest and most common explanation for forgetting is decay. The decay theory holds that if unused, memory traces will vanish. In the 1880s, German psychologist Hermann Ebbinghaus developed the "curve of forgetting," which illustrates just how rapidly memory decays. People forget 80 percent of what they have learned after one month of having learned it. According to an alternative theory of forgetting, the interference theory, memories do not so much disappear as lose themselves in the crowd of memories. As people age and their experiences multiply, they tend to become neglectfully absentminded. The interference theory holds that a lack of a precise cue to trigger recall of the memory causes the forgetting. Still another theory holds that age-related memory loss is behavioral, brought on by negative cultural stereotypes rather than by physical deterioration.

People who believe memory inevitably declines with age tend to believe that trying to do something about the problem is futile. Adherents say it is virtually impossible to compensate for age-related memory loss. It is important to remember that age-related memory deficits are accompanied by general cognitive slowing. Thus, age-related memory loss is considered normal.

The degree to which memory is lost can be a function of good health, intellectual stimulation, daily activity, and a positive attitude. Research indicates it is possible to do something about forgetfulness. However, no magic wand exists to make age-related forgetfulness better. Scientists have been searching to find drugs (called "smart drugs") to boost memory. Sugar, for example, enhances memory by fueling the active neurons in the brain, which require high quantities of blood sugar. Little or no strong evidence showed substances such as ginkgo, choline, or lecithin improve memory. Staying physically fit and problem solving mental activity also contribute to managing age-related memory loss.

Older adults use an array of strategies to enhance or improve memory. The more effective tools and techniques for the older adult require the user to pay close attention and be organized. They rely on memory retrieval cues such as an image, a number, a word, a sentence, an acronym, a face, an auditory signal, or a smell. External memory aides include reminders from other people, to-do lists, address books, alarms and timers, strings around the finger, calendars, and appointment books. Another useful memory aid involves repeating a new acquaintance's name several times during a conversation.

Evidence points to the fact that to be successful, forgetful older adults must invest themselves in compensating for age-related memory loss. They must be motivated, have a positive attitude, and be willing to put in the effort it will take to manage their forgetfulness.

Age may make older people more forgetful, but it has little or no effect on the ability to think. Most people remain both alert and able as they age, although it may take them longer to remember things. Older people are less likely to have major memory problems if they believe in themselves and work to improve their recall. Indeed, older people's perception of themselves—their self-confidence—can be improved. Older adults who use their minds are not as likely to lose them, or at least not as fast.

BIOLOGICAL FACTORS

The root causes of age-associated forgetfulness are largely biological—a decline in the efficiency of cortical processing in the brain. Psychological and sociological factors may also lead to a decline in mental energy or attention span. Forgetfulness that is greater than expected in healthy aging can often be treated medically. Age-related forgetfulness is usually not accompanied by other thinking impairments and is not severe enough to grossly interfere with daily living and be linked to a neurological disease.

Many older adults fear that forgetfulness is a sign of a brain disease called dementia. Dementia seriously affects a person's ability to perform daily activities. The symptoms of this disease include severe memory loss, impaired thinking, and altered personality. Other signs of dementia are asking the same question repeatedly, becoming lost in familiar places, being unable to follow directions, being disoriented, losing track of time, and neglecting personal health, hygiene, and safety. Dementing illnesses are usually categorized by their suspected causes, including degenerative, vascular, infectious, toxic, or metabolic. The World Health Organization (WHO) reports that 47.5 million people have dementia with 7.7 million new cases being added each year. Alzheimer's disease accounts for 60 to 70 percent of all dementia diagnoses. In the United States, it is the sixth leading cause of death with an estimated one in three seniors dying of some form of dementia. The National Institute on Aging (NIA) ranks it as the third (behind heart disease and cancer) leading cause of death for older people.

Age-related memory disorders may be due to cardiovascular disease, poor vision and hearing, fatigue, depression, infections, or medication side effects. Other common causes of memory disorders are strokes (which are blockages or bleeding in the blood vessels in the brain), thyroid disease, and vitamin B12 deficiency. Untreated high blood pressure (hypertension) can also cause mild memory impairment and lengthen recall time.

Another contributor to cognitive decline is the fact that the brain gradually begins to shrink as early as age forty—especially in the frontal regions that play a critical role in remembering. Brain mass steadily shrinks as people enter their sixties and seventies, at approximately 5 to 10 percent per decade. Research done by the National Institute on Aging shows that the most dramatic memory decline does not occur until about age seventy. A significant loss of neurons in the regions of the brain responsible for memory—the hippocampus and forebrain—probably contributes to age-related

Performance on Memory Tasks in Late Adulthood

Memory Declines	Memory Remains or Improves
Working memory	Procedural memory
Cued recall	Digit span
Explicit memory	Semantic memory, particularly for vocabulary words
Episodic memory	Implicit memory tasks
Source memory	Reasoning skills
Spatial memory	Long-term autobiographical memory

memory difficulties. The forebrain delivers the critical neurotransmitter acetylcholine to the hippocampus and many regions of the cerebral cortex.

Such psychological factors as stress may even make people forgetful. High concentrations of cortisol, a hormone released by the adrenal glands in response to danger, threat, and aggravation, correlate with higher levels of forgetfulness.

—Bryan C. Auday and Fred Buchstein
Updated by Bryan C. Auday, PhD

See also: Alzheimer's Association; Alzheimer's disease; Brain changes and disorders; Dementia; Psychiatry, geriatric; Reaction time

For Further Information

Baddeley, Alan D., et al. *Memory.* 2nd ed., Psychology P, 2015. This book, co-written by two stalwarts within memory research, is one of the best introductory textbooks on the subject.

Jebelli, Joseph. *In Pursuit of Memory: The Fight against Alzheimer's.* Little, Brown and Company, 2017. Some of the primary symptoms of Alzheimer's disease are related to memory problems. This book is written for the general educated public by a neuroscientist who has spent his career studying Alzheimer's.

Schacter, Daniel L. *The Seven Sins of Memory: How the Mind Forgets and Remembers.* Houghton Mifflin, 2001. Although this book was written a number of years ago, it remains one of the best on the topic of how we can forget.

Schwartz, Bennett L. *Memory: Foundations and Applications.* 3rd ed., Sage, 2018. This book provides a solid introduction into the major areas of memory theory. The author includes mnemonic memory improving tips within most of the chapters.

Surprenant Aimeìe M., and Ian Neath. *Principles of Memory: Essays in Cognitive Psychology.* Psychology P, 2009. Surprenant and Neath summarize the vast literature in memory and propose seven general principles of memory: (1) Cue-Driven, (2) Encoding-Retrieval, (3) Cue Overload, (4) Reconstruction, (5) Impurity, (6) Relative Distinctiveness, and (7) Specificity.

MEN AND AGING

Relevant Issues: Economics, family, health and medicine, recreation

Significance: As life expectancy for men grew from about forty-eight years in 1900 to a projected eighty years by 2010, issues surrounding men and aging has received considerable attention.

The statistics of life expectancy have undergone considerable change over the centuries. In classical Greece and Rome, the average life expectancy was between twenty and thirty years, although this figure is perhaps misleading because factored into it is a high infant mortality rate. Certainly most of the classical writers and thinkers whose work has survived lived into what would today be considered old age. Socrates, for example, was about seventy when he drank the hemlock that ended his life.

By 1900, life expectancy for males in the United States was about twice what it had been in ancient Greece and Rome. Men born in 1900 lived on average just short of forty-eight years, women three years longer. A great demographic change occurred, however, in the next several decades. Life expectancy for men born in 2017 was seventy-six years. It is estimated that by 2030 this figure will have advanced to a life expectancy for men of only seventy-nine years. While this is a general increase over time, the United States has, and is projected to continue having, one of the lowest life expectancy rates for high-income countries.

REASONS FOR INCREASES IN LONGEVITY

The increases in life expectancy for men have been directly related to several factors. As industry has become increasingly automated, fatal accidents in factories have declined substantially. In the United States, government agencies oversee the implementation of safety precautions in the workplace. The Occupational Safety and Health Administration (OSHA) enforces strict regulations to ensure the safety of all workers, particularly in the heavy industries that employ large numbers of men.

As medical science has advanced, the spread of such devastating diseases as polio, diphtheria, influenza, and bubonic plague has been checked by immunization or by effective treatment with sophisticated medications. Preventive medicine is widely practiced throughout the industrialized world, with massive immunization programs offered free of charge or at affordable fees by various health agencies. The United States and Canada have been exemplary in their attempts to eliminate the kinds of air and water pollution that once led to illness and death among large populations. Such disabling and often-fatal illnesses as cholera, amoebic dysentery, typhoid fever, yellow fever, and malaria are well controlled in North America.

Even diseases that remain incurable, such as diabetes and acquired immunodeficiency syndrome (AIDS), have become manageable. Medical science has also made huge advances in the treatment of cancer and cardiovascular disease both by publicizing ways to avoid such diseases and by aggressively spearheading their treatment when they do occur. The media have worked to inform the public about health and longevity.

Most American men understand the relationship between diet and good health, the value of regular exercise, the advisability of limiting alcoholic intake, and the need to avoid tobacco. Antismoking campaigns have succeeded in driving smokers from public places and conveyances and have reduced substantially the numbers of smokers in American society. The use of alcoholic beverages among men past thirty has also been in steady decline.

Perhaps the most important factor resulting in increased longevity for men and women in much of the industrial world is the easy and virtually universal availability of medical treatment. In many countries, socialized medicine has put medical care within the reach of all citizens, regardless of their economic levels. In the United States, insurance programs offered by many employers and the growth of health maintenance organizations (HMOs) have made medical care easily accessible to much of the population. Many of those who are not covered by insurance qualify for Medicaid. For those over sixty-five, Medicare pays a substantial portion of their medical expenses, although it still does not cover prescription drugs, which have become increasingly sophisticated and expensive.

All these factors have contributed to increases in life expectancy for men, although their life expectancy remains considerably lower than that of women. Many factors explain this disparity, although as more women enter the workforce and are subject to the same sorts of stresses as men, some demographers think that the gap between male and female life expectancy will be narrowed.

WHY WOMEN LIVE LONGER THAN MEN

There is no clear answer to the question of why women outlive men. On the surface, it might seem that men are subjected to more stress in the workplace than women are. Certainly more men have jobs that pose physical dangers than women do. With the increase in the numbers of working women, trends will soon be identified to test the hypothesis that stress in the workplace accounts for the shorter life expectancy of males.

Most biologists discount the role that stress plays in causing the disparity in life expectancy between the sexes. They point out that this disparity is not limited to humans but that in nearly all animal species, females outlive males, suggesting that the disparity is genetic or in some way biologically determined rather than environmental.

Some research has implied that women outlive men because of their sex hormones. When premenopausal women are producing estrogen, their incident of heart disease and high blood pressure is substantially less than it is after the menopause, when their production of estrogen diminishes or ceases. Thus, up to age forty-five or fifty, most women seem to have built-in protection against heart disease, although after the menopause the incidence of heart disease among women is comparable to that among men.

THE AGING PROCESS

All organisms undergo the aging process, during which irreversible changes occur that ultimately lead to ill health, disability, and death. In humans, the aging process is usually so gradual as to be barely perceptible on a day-to-day or month-to-month basis, although serious illness, severe emotional stress and shock, and other such factors can accelerate the process so that it becomes noticeable. The hair of some people who have undergone a great emotional shock, for example, will turn white within a month or two.

The changes that take place in men are not only obvious changes such as wrinkling of the skin, increased brittleness of the bones, or increased fat deposits in the abdomen. Some changes are functional, making it difficult or impossible for people to perform tasks that they were once able to perform with ease. Sometimes, the aging process involves stooped posture, a shuffling gait, reduced muscular coordination, or lapses in memory.

The effects of aging are different for everyone; they have little direct relationship to age. Some men are old at sixty, while others continue to be active and functional into their nineties. Any generalizations one makes about aging are filled with exceptions and fraught with inconsistencies.

Aging is partly cultural and partly genetic. Men who have led hard lives, received little medical treatment, and had little mental stimulation tend to age more rapidly than those who have had easier lives, have had easy access to medical treatment, and have been stimulated mentally. In the United States, it has been observed that educational level has a correlation to life expectancy: On the whole, college graduates live three years longer than high school graduates. This disparity may exist because college graduates usually have less physically demanding jobs than high school graduates or because college graduates often have a broad range of interests to keep them alert and involved. Also, educated people probably demand more sophisticated medical assistance than those who are less educated.

The genes one inherits appear to have a direct relation to longevity. Men whose parents and grandparents lived to be eighty years old can expect to live six years longer on average than men whose parents and grandparents died before sixty. Apparently within the genes of all living organisms there is a mechanism that controls life span, that imposes a maximum upon how long the organism can live: three months for the common housefly, about twenty years for dogs, about forty-five years for horses, and about two hundred years for some tortoises. By 2019, the oldest documented human life was 122 years, although undocumented claims have been made of anywhere from 140 to 160 years. Some biologists see no reason that life expectancy among humans should not eventually exceed 100 years and that ages of 150 or more will be attainable by some people.

Research by Michael Rose, an American evolutionary biologist, suggests that maximum life spans can be extended through genetic engineering. Rose extended the lives of his selectively bred, experimental fruit flies by 100 percent, thereby doubling their life spans. Other researchers, by manipulating the gene that sets puberty in motion, were able to extend the average life spans of some platy fish by as much as ten months. Obviously, these experiments have little immediate relevance for humans, but they challenge the long-held belief that there are upper limits to the life spans of all organisms. The Human Genome Project, which is unraveling the intricacies of the human genome, offers the promise that one day the human life span and the years of healthy, productive living among humans will be extended substantially.

DEFINING OLD AGE

Specific designations of old age vary from culture to culture and from person to person. To a ten-year-old, someone who is thirty seems old. In most cultures, men are considered old when they leave the workforce, when they cease to be economically productive. In male-dominated cultures, which still prevail in most parts of the world, women are often categorized in reference to their husbands, so that when a husband is considered old, his wife is also considered old, although she may continue to work strenuously at her household duties.

In contemporary American culture, many people, through early retirement, leave the workforce long before they are technically considered old. Because the Social Security Act of 1935 set sixty-five as the age when benefits began, in the eyes of many sixty-five has been considered the beginning of old age. This is the age at which Chancellor Otto von Bismarck of Germany granted the first old-age pensions in a system established under his direction in the 1880s. At that time, few people lived much beyond sixty-five. Today, men and women receive equal benefits under Social Security, despite discrepancies in life expectancy.

In contemporary culture, one can identify at least four stages through which men normally pass as they make the transition from middle age to old age, from working full time to full-time retirement. In the first stage, many early retirees, who cannot really be viewed as old, continue to work but at less demanding, less remunerative jobs than they held during most of their lives. Often they work only part-time. Many early retirees try to live solely on the income from this work because, if their children are now independent, they can live on less money and permit their savings to compound. This stage of retirement often lasts, for men, anywhere from five to ten years.

Most male retirees eventually begin to pursue one or more kinds of leisure activity, such as golf, tennis, swimming, or travel, gradually reducing their work schedules and devoting more time to such non-work activities. During this stage, many men begin to feel a diminution in their physical strength brought about by the heart's reduced ability to supply blood to the muscles. In a twenty-year-old male, the heart typically pumps 6.5 liters of blood per minute, whereas in his eighty-five-year-old counterpart, only about 3.5 liters per minute are pumped through the circulatory system.

Older men can, however, substantially improve their heart action through moderate exercise. Many begin to pursue exercise programs to strengthen their bones and muscles and to improve their heart action and blood flow. Such programs usually involve light exercise, some weight lifting, and a commitment to devote at least twenty to thirty minutes a day to it. In time, however, many men find athletics and travel too strenuous and revert to less physically taxing activities, such as reading, gardening, or walking. Such people are still healthy and well able to cope with the daily routine of living and looking after themselves.

The final stage that affects those who live into old age is the period when health begins to break down and when the older person cannot easily live independently and look after himself. At this stage, some men need help in getting out of bed or up from chairs. They might not be able to dress and groom themselves. They may need to have someone feed them. Because women live longer than men, they are often available to look after husbands whose health declines to the point that they require some custodial care. Widows are more numerous in most cultures than widowers. Often widows who have attended their husbands through terminal illnesses have no one to look after them as they weaken, so they enter group-living facilities, retirement communities, or nursing homes. The populations of such facilities are disproportionately female.

HOW MEN ADJUST TO OLD AGE

Most men work outside the home longer than women typically do, although various social changes have altered that situation. Before World War II, most wives were stay-at-home mothers, whereas most men went daily to a place of business and were away from home for five or six days a week during most of the daylight hours. If women worked outside the home, they usually had done so before marriage and/or after their children had been raised, so their work for pay was not continuous and their total number of years in the workforce was considerably less than that of the typical man.

When retirement comes to a married man who has been used to leaving the house five or six days a week to go to a job and to mingle with other people, a rude awakening often occurs for both husband and wife. The husband wakens in the morning and sees sprawled before him a long day with little to fill it. The wife, even the working wife, has usually grown used to having time to herself during the day after the husband goes to work or before he comes home. Wives of newly retired men often comment that they married their husbands for better or worse but not for lunch. The adjustment to retirement can be traumatic for both husbands and wives, particularly if the initial withdrawal from the workplace is total. Sociologists note that retirement is generally more difficult for men than for women because married men are less likely to bond with other men than women are with other women. Often, a man's chief social outlet is the workplace. When this outlet is no longer available, many men feel abandoned and despondent.

Some companies and educational institutions have introduced graduated retirement systems under which men reduce their workloads slowly over a period of two or three years, thereby easing into retirement rather than plunging into it. Where it is possible for men to take a graduated retirement, it is usually desirable for them to leave the workforce in this way. Their reduced schedules will enable them to develop new interests, make new friends, and find activities to fill their days when their retirement becomes total. Also, a graduated retirement helps wives adjust to having their husbands around more than they have been accustomed.

One cannot reasonably define old age as the point at which one retires. Most current retirees can look forward to two or more decades of not working full time. As life expectancy increases and early retirement becomes more usual, it is thought that many men retiring after 2020 will spend almost a third of their lives in retirement, which is almost as much as most of them will have spent in the workforce. Perhaps old age is best defined in terms of how well one functions physically and mentally. Active retirements keep men from deteriorating, and the availability of first-rate medical services makes debilitating diseases less of a problem for the elderly than they once were. Although physical deterioration cannot be avoided altogether, it can, in most men, be forestalled by regular exercise, proper diet, and mental stimulation.

THE MALE SEX DRIVE

As men age, the level of testosterone that is secreted in the testes diminishes steadily. The endocrine glands, however, continue to produce sex hormones. Most people think that as testosterone levels in the blood decrease, the male sex drive diminishes, and sexual activity becomes less often as well as less satisfactory. Research into this matter does not support popular opinions about declines in the sex drives of older men.

Actually, almost no correlation has been found between the level of testosterone in the blood and a man's sexual prowess. What seems to determine the sexual activity of older men is their general health and social customs. If they believe that sex is for the young, then they may suffer sexual dysfunction even in middle age. If they have had fulfilling sex lives, then their sexual activity is likely to continue well into old age.

Attitude has a great deal to do with human sexuality at all ages, but particularly in old age. Physical changes and disorders, however, can be a factor. Impotence, permanent or temporary, can result from some kinds of illnesses. Men whose prostate glands have been removed may be unable to perform sexually in the ways to which they have been accustomed. Prostate disorders are common in older men. It has been said that every man, if he lives long enough, will be afflicted by prostate cancer. In men over seventy, a malignancy in the prostate often goes untreated because it is a slow-growing type of cancer. Men in their seventies who have prostate cancer will probably die of something else rather than be killed by their cancers. In younger men who have prostate cancer, radiation and, more drastically, removal of the prostate gland may be indicated.

All men over the age of fifty should have annual prostate screenings, which involve both a digital examination of the prostate and a test that reveals prostate-specific antigen (PSA) levels in the blood. In many cases, the digital examination does not reveal cancer in its earliest, most manageable stages, but if PSA levels are elevated, cancer is usually present.

THE ILLNESSES OF OLD AGE

Among American men over sixty-five, the most common illnesses are arthritis, hypertension, hearing impairment, heart disease, and cataracts. Most of these illnesses are manageable, and treatment of one may cause decreases in others. For example, by controlling hypertension, which is easily done with a broad spectrum of readily available medications, a man's likelihood of developing heart disease is reduced substantially. Visual and hearing problems are easily dealt with in most cases through corrective lenses, laser surgery, or hearing aids. The removal of cataracts from the eyes has become a routine, outpatient procedure.

In old age, responses to stimuli are generally reduced. Many elderly men find it virtually impossible to deal with several stimuli simultaneously, which can make driving or the operation of machinery dangerous for them and for others. Men aware of their reduced response time can adjust by driving more slowly, avoiding crowded highways, and generally exercising considerable care on the road. As long as their vision is adequate, many men can continue driving well into their nineties.

The most common causes of death among elderly men are, in the following order, heart disease, cancer, cerebrovascular diseases (strokes), chronic obstructive pulmonary disease (COPD), and accidents, often drowning or falling. All these causes except for accidents can be managed well if they are detected early and treated aggressively and consistently.

As people age, they lose brain cells at a steady rate, although humans have so many brain cells that losing even a million a day should not quickly result in perceptible changes in the person. As brain cells are lost, the surviving cells in most people increase the number of connections that they make with other cells, thereby eliminating substantial neuronal loss. In some older people, however, the cells are unable to make the connections that in most people are made routinely. Two of the most frustrating illnesses of old age are Alzheimer's disease and Parkinson's disease, both diseases of the nervous system that can have devastating outcomes for their victims, who usually succumb to the disease.

To date, there is no cure and little palliative treatment for either of these two diseases in their advanced stages. Many men who have Parkinson's disease continue to function for many years, although tremors will affect their extremities. Alzheimer's disease in essence robs its victims of their personhood. Their memories are virtually wiped out. They do not recognize members of their families. They are constantly disoriented and cannot focus long enough to read or to follow what is going on in television shows or films. Of all the research on aging that is currently afoot, research on these two diseases is perhaps the most important.

—*R. Baird Shuman*

See also: Aging process; Cancer; Cardiovascular disease; Cultural views of aging; Death and dying; Divorce; Early retirement; Employment; Genetics; Heart attacks; Heart changes and disorders; Home ownership; Hypertension; Impotence; Life expectancy; Longevity research; Marriage; Middle age; Midlife crisis; Old age; Pensions; Prostate cancer; Prostate enlargement; Remarriage; Reproductive changes, disabilities, and dysfunctions; Retirement; Rhinophyma; Sexuality; Smoking; Sports participation; Stress and coping skills; Strokes; Urinary disorders; Widows and widowers; Women and aging

For Further Information

Bribiescas, Richard G. How Men Age: What Evolution Reveals about Male Health and Mortality. Princeton U P, 2016. This book provides new perspectives on the aging process in men and how we became human, and explores future challenges for human evolution?and the important role older men might play in them.

Le Couteur, David G., et al. "Sex and Aging." *The Journals of Gerontology: Series A*, vol. 73, no. 2, 2017, pp. 139-40. doi:10.1093/gerona/glx221. A series of review and research articles that explore the relationship between sex and aging in animals and humans.

Linden, Dana Wechsler. "Why Men Have Such a Hard Time with Aging." *The Wall Street Journal*, Dow Jones & Company, 2 Mar. 2017. www.wsj.com/articles/why-men-have-such-a-hard-time-with-aging-1488164880. Discusses how traditional thinking about masculinity can make it more difficult for men to accept the changes aging may bring.

Oregon State University. "Aging Men: More Uplifts, Fewer Hassles until the Age of 65-70." *ScienceDaily*, 20 Feb. 2014. www.sciencedaily.com/releases/2014/02/140220095001.htm. A new study of how men approach their golden years found that how happy individuals are remains relatively stable for some 80 percent of the population, but perceptions of unhappiness—or dealing with "hassles"—tends to get worse once you are about 65-70 years old.

Stibich, Mark, PhD. "How Is Aging Different for Men and Women?" *Verywell Health: Healthy Aging.* 5 Oct. 2018. www.verywellhealth.com/is-aging-different-for-men-and-women-2224332 Compares aging with men and women and highlights differences.

Thompson, Edward H. *A Man's Guide to Healthy Aging. Stay Smart, Strong, and Active.* The Johns Hopkins U P, 2013. Refuting the ageist stereotype that men spend their later years "winding down." This book will help men reinvent themselves once, twice, or more—by managing their health, creating new careers, and contributing their skills and experiences to their communities.

MENOPAUSE

Relevant Issues: Biology, health and medicine

Significance: The hormonal changes that take place with menopause at midlife have long-term effects on the health and well-being of women.

Key Terms:

endometrium: the innermost lining layer of the uterus, and functions to prevent adhesions between the opposed walls of the myometrium, thereby maintaining the patency of the uterine cavity; during the menstrual cycle, the endometrium grows to a thick, blood vessel-rich, glandular tissue layer

estrone: the major postmenopausal estrogen derived from the conversion of androgens, mainly androstenedione, produced by the ovaries and adrenal glands

Once a secret passage dreaded by women as the final loss of youth, menopause—the cessation of monthly menstruation—is now being encountered by the baby boomers, and they are not going quietly into this next stage of life. Women in their forties and fifties have formed support groups with names such as the Red Hot Mamas and Crone Societies. Social media, television programs, books, and articles in newspapers and magazines offer advice on recognizing and managing the changes that occur with the onset of menopause. Increased numbers of studies on the physiology of menopause, as well as the overall physiology of aging, have accompanied this popular trend.

Until a few hundred years ago, humans typically lived about twenty to forty years. The average life expectancy of an infant born in 1900 was forty-eight years. By the end of the twentieth century, the average female life expectancy in the United States was almost eighty years. It is clear that many more women today live beyond the age of fifty than at any time in human history.

When a woman reaches fifty to fifty-five years of age, her ovaries run out of eggs. The depletion of eggs marks the end of the menstrual cycle (menopause) and is accompanied by dramatic hormonal changes—the most obvious is a significant drop in estrogen production by the ovaries. Changes that ultimately lead to menopause may begin as early as thirty-five years of age, and the period preceding menopause, during which estrogen levels begin to decline, is referred to as perimenopause. Menopause is clinically defined as complete once a woman has gone one year without a menstrual period.

THE MENSTRUAL CYCLE PRIOR TO MENOPAUSE

Each month, in response to hormones secreted by the pituitary gland, which is located in the brain, an ovarian follicle consisting of an oocyte (egg, or ovum) and surrounding cells is readied for ovulation. This process usually takes about two weeks. Although typically only one egg is released, many follicles actually begin to develop. Typically, all but one degenerate before reaching maturity. During the two-week period prior to ovulation, the follicular cells surrounding the egg secrete increasing amounts of estrogen. Peak estrogen secretion is reached just prior to ovulation. Estrogen plays many important roles; one of the most important is to stimulate the inner lining of the uterus, the endometrium, to grow in thickness as it prepares for implantation of the fertilized egg.

At ovulation, the egg is released from the ovary and enters the oviduct or Fallopian tube. The remaining cells of the follicle collapse back into the ovary and form the corpus luteum, a structure that secretes both estrogen and progesterone. Estrogen and progesterone together act on the endometrium to make it a hospitable place in which an embryo may implant itself, should fertilization take place. The corpus luteum secretes these hormones for about ten days. If fertilization does not occur, it ceases to function. Without the hormones secreted by the corpus luteum, the uterine lining is not maintained and is soon sloughed off in menstrual flow. If fertilization occurs, the corpus luteum does not degenerate, but instead persists almost to the end of pregnancy.

As a result of cyclic fluctuations in the levels of a finely orchestrated set of hormones, a woman's menstrual cycle repeatedly supplies eggs for possible fertilization and readies the uterus (womb) for pregnancy. Near the age of fifty, this cycling becomes irregular and eventually stops. Many events lead to this change. Not all are well understood, but it is clear that cycling stops with the end of available ovarian follicles.

THE OVARIES FROM BIRTH TO MENOPAUSE

A female infant is born with all the follicles she will ever produce. Her reproductive potential is determined even before she emerges from the womb of her mother. It is estimated that, at birth, each ovary contains as many as ten million immature follicles. After birth, many of these follicles degenerate, so that at menarche (the onset of menstruation at puberty) there are an estimated 250,000 to 500,000 follicles per ovary. Between menarche and menopause, only about four hundred follicles reach maturity and are ovulated. Because many follicles begin to develop each month and then degenerate, the huge reservoir of follicles with which she began life is depleted as a woman approaches menopause. Without the cyclic maturation of follicles, estrogen production drops significantly. Investigators have learned about the

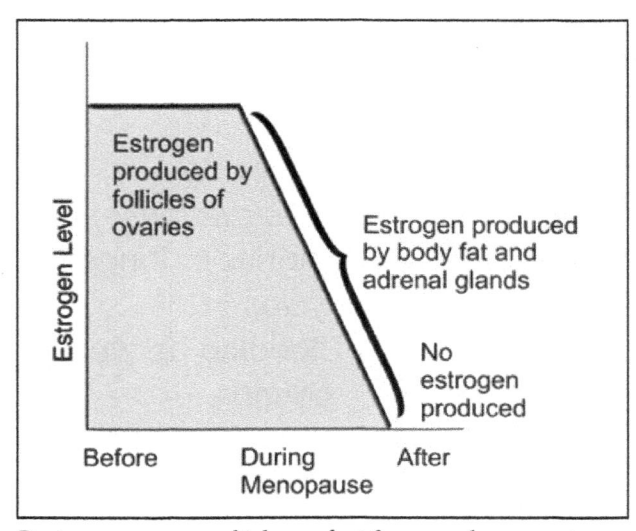

During menopause, which may last for several years, estrogen production diminishes; after the menopause, estrogen is no longer produced by the body. © EBSCO

declining number of follicles that accompanies aging by studying ovaries surgically removed from living women or those taken from cadavers. They have learned about hormone levels by analyzing blood samples taken from women of different ages and varying menstrual stages.

Although the ovaries at menopause no longer produce follicles for ovulation, it is important to point out that the ovarian tissues are not quiet. For several years beyond menopause, the remaining tissues secrete androgens ("male" hormones such as testosterone), which are converted to estrogen by fat cells in the body. The adrenal glands also secrete androgens that are converted to estrogen. "Estrogen" is a generic term that refers to a family of closely related molecules. For example, the estrogen secreted by ovarian follicles is estradiol, while

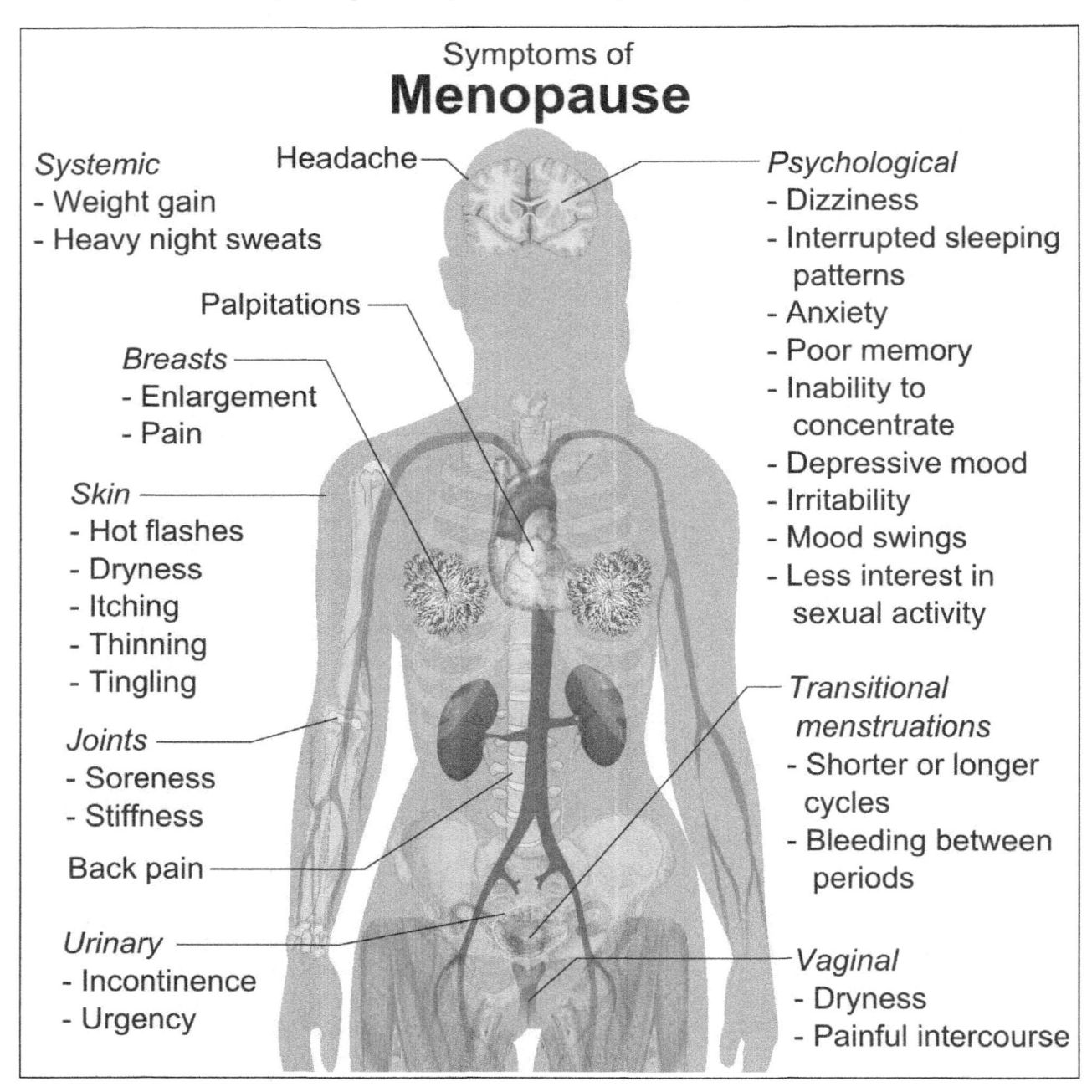

Symptoms of Menopause

Systemic
- Weight gain
- Heavy night sweats

Headache

Palpitations

Breasts
- Enlargement
- Pain

Skin
- Hot flashes
- Dryness
- Itching
- Thinning
- Tingling

Joints
- Soreness
- Stiffness

Back pain

Urinary
- Incontinence
- Urgency

Psychological
- Dizziness
- Interrupted sleeping patterns
- Anxiety
- Poor memory
- Inability to concentrate
- Depressive mood
- Irritability
- Mood swings
- Less interest in sexual activity

Transitional menstruations
- Shorter or longer cycles
- Bleeding between periods

Vaginal
- Dryness
- Painful intercourse

the main estrogen formed in postmenopausal women is estrone.

THE EFFECTS OF ESTROGEN

Estrogen circulates in the blood and interacts at specific sites called receptors in a variety of target tissues, including the endometrium, lining of the vagina, urinary tract, skin, bones, blood vessels, muscles, and brain. A decline in estrogen levels produces wide-ranging effects. The endometrium is not stimulated to increase in thickness, so cyclic menstrual bleeding stops. The vaginal lining tends to become thin and dry, which may lead to itching and discomfort or pain during intercourse. The urinary tract and bladder lose muscle tone, leading to more frequent feelings of the need to urinate and possibly to urinary stress incontinence (leakage of urine with sneezing or coughing). The loss of flexible connective tissue beneath the skin leads to wrinkling. Thinning of the bones (osteoporosis) may result in fractures. Reduced levels of estrogen also appear to be correlated with development of atherosclerotic plaques (hardening of the arteries), which can lead to heart attacks or strokes. Decreased estrogen in many women leads to hot flashes or night sweats, which may cause sleep disturbances and resulting fatigue and irritability. It is believed that hot flashes result from a disruption of signals in the hypothalamus, the part of the brain that regulates body temperature. Finally, emerging studies suggest that estrogen also plays an important role in memory and cognition. The risk of Alzheimer's disease and other forms of dementia appear to increase in women with early menopause or late puberty, and decrease in women who have had three or more pregnancies (where estrogen levels are very high). The effects attributed to pregnancy, however, may actually be the combined effects of estrogen and T cells of the immune system; studies are ongoing.

Adult women of any age who have had a bilateral ovariectomy (both ovaries removed), which sometimes is done with a hysterectomy (removal of the uterus), immediately cease menstruation and often report having hot flashes and vaginal dryness. Estrogen replacement therapy reverses the effects of low estrogen on many of these symptoms.

SYMPTOMS AND CONSEQUENCES OF ESTROGEN REDUCTION

Women who go through a natural (not surgically induced) perimenopause and menopause report a wide variety of symptoms related to fluctuating levels of estrogen and other hormones, such as follicle-stimulating hormone (FSH) secreted by the pituitary gland. As estrogen gradually declines during perimenopause, women in their forties may experience menstrual irregularities, lighter or heavier menstrual flow, premenstrual syndrome (PMS), or menstrual cramps that they had not had before. Although some women passing through this decade experience a gradual increase in the time between menstrual periods and gentle waning of menstrual flow, others have frequent and heavy bleeding with clots. Some women never have hot flashes; others report being incapacitated by frequent and intense hot flashes that interrupt their sleep or disrupt their work. Similarly, women report a spectrum of mild to severe problems with vaginal dryness and urinary tract problems. Decreases in muscle mass and increases in weight have also been reported.

Hot flashes and mood swings generally abate once a woman has her last menstrual period and her hormonal secretions settle into postmenopausal levels. (However, some women report hot flashes well into the postmenopausal years.) Vaginal dryness and urinary symptoms both result from low levels of estrogen and will continue in many women for the rest of their lives. Likewise, low estrogen levels can lead over time to osteoporosis and cardiovascular disease. Over their lifetimes, one in five women will develop osteoporosis. The dowager's hump (kyphosis) and broken hips, common signs of osteoporosis, show up at advanced ages, but they are the result of bone loss over many decades. Men and women alike begin to lose bone around thirty-five years of age, even when estrogen support is still quite high. With the abrupt drop in estrogen levels at menopause, however, women experience accelerated rates of bone loss. Cardiovascular disease is the number one killer of women over the age of fifty. By comparison with men, strokes and heart attacks occur relatively infrequently in women prior to menopause, but with the loss of the protective effects of estrogen, postmenopausal women become increasingly vulnerable to heart and blood vessel disease. Finally, research-

> ### SENIOR TALK:
>
> #### HOW DO YOU FEEL ABOUT HYSTERECTOMY?
>
> Although hysterectomy is among the most common surgical procedures for American women, the prospect of undergoing any major surgery can be daunting. Although having a hysterectomy as an older adult removes some of the considerations that can be particularly distressing for premenopausal women—such the sudden cessation of menstruation, the loss of the ability to become pregnant, and the early onset of menopause brought on by a hysterectomy—needing to have a hysterectomy at any age can be overwhelming.
>
> Common reasons for needing a hysterectomy after menopause include cancers of the endometrium and the cervix, as well as abnormal postmenopausal bleeding and persistent uterine fibroids, which can be indications of gynecological cancer. If your doctor suspects that you have cancer or you have been diagnosed with cancer, you are likely to feel distressed, anxious, and afraid. It can be helpful to speak to your doctor, surgeon, or a therapist about these concerns. Having a hysterectomy due to cancer enables the doctor to see the spread of malignant cells and remove the cancerous tissue, thereby greatly improving your prognosis. Having a hysterectomy can be a relief for many women with gynecological cancer. When gynecological cancers are discovered in their early stages, having a hysterectomy greatly reduces the risk of recurrence. Older women who need to have a hysterectomy due to chronic pelvic pain or uterine prolapse may also be relieved to undergo the surgery, as the procedure can often alleviate most or all of their symptoms.
>
> —Leah Jacob

ers have found evidence suggesting an association between a lack of estrogen and the occurrence of Alzheimer's disease, but there is still much to learn about this link.

TREATMENT OPTIONS

Women who live many years beyond menopause will experience the long-term effects of low levels of estrogen. A vigorous debate is taking place between those who characterize the menopausal years as hormone-deficient and in need of treatment by means of hormone replacement therapy (HRT) and those who characterize those years as a normal part of the female life experience needing only sensible living habits to maintain good health. Proponents of HRT argue that osteoporosis and cardiovascular disease are critical public health issues. Opponents point out that the effects of long-term use of HRT are still unknown and that women who take supplemental hormones are potentially at risk for equally devastating diseases, such as breast and uterine cancers.

As the debate continues, pharmaceutical companies are developing new "designer estrogens." These drugs are also called selective estrogen receptor modulators (SERMs). They act like estrogen but only at certain estrogen receptor sites and therefore have more narrowly defined actions than estrogen itself. For example, raloxifene (Evista) is known to mimic estrogen at estrogen receptors in bone (therefore protecting against osteoporosis) but not at estrogen receptors in the breast and uterus (which means it protects against cancers of the breast and endometrium). Raloxifene may protect against heart disease, but it does not block hot flashes.

Women seeking natural ways to increase their levels of estrogen may include phytoestrogens (estrogens from plants such as soybeans) in their diets or in supplements. To treat vaginal and urinary symptoms, estrogen creams may be applied to the vagina.

Unlike earlier generations, today's women have a growing number of options available to treat the symptoms of perimenopause and menopause. A woman and her health-care provider need to consider her individual health risks, including her history of cancer, estrogen levels, and symptoms to determine the most appropriate course of action to alleviate or prevent the consequences of low levels of estrogen.

Whether hormonal or other treatment is sought, a woman will improve her later years by eating a diet rich in calcium and vitamin D (to combat osteoporosis) and low in fat (to combat cardiovascular disease and weight gain). She is well advised to stop smoking; smoking has been implicated in heart disease, osteoporosis, and earlier onset of menopause, as well as in lung disease. She should exercise aerobically to stimulate the heart and maintain a healthy body weight and do load-bearing exercises (including walking) to facilitate strengthening the bones. She will find that Kegel exercises (squeezing the muscles at the floor of the pelvis) will improve bladder control and sexual pleasure.

THE BIOLOGICAL SIGNIFICANCE OF MENOPAUSE

The overall process of aging involves a variety of physiological declines, but the human female reproductive system is shut down noticeably early. Is there a selective advantage to the human species to have women stop reproducing relatively early and then to live beyond their reproductive years? Two opposing hypotheses have been proposed to explain menopause. One is the grandmother hypothesis based on studies of the Hadza people, contemporary hunter-gatherers in Tanzania. The Hadza grandmothers play an important role in providing adequate food for their grandchildren while their daughters are bearing and nursing new young. The argument is that the postmenopausal grandmothers are assured of their own genes being passed on through their daughters by contributing to the survival of their daughters' children.

The opposing hypothesis of reproductive shut down is based on studies of populations of baboons and Serengeti lions, both similar to humans because they live in social groups that involve female kin relationships. Because all mammals require considerable maternal care following birth, this hypothesis holds that a female becomes infertile early enough to ensure that her last offspring would be able to survive on its own after she died. For early humans, assuming that maternal care was needed until the child reached about ten years of age, females entering menopause between forty-eight to fifty-five would have lived to be fifty-eight to sixty-five years old.

Whatever investigators conclude is the evolutionary significance of menopause, all agree that it is a significant feature of the reproductive life of human females. The future is expected to bring a more detailed understanding of the physiology of perimenopause and menopause. As research continues on hormone replacement therapies as well as alternative non-hormonal options, better-tailored treatments can be devised to assure healthy, productive, and fulfilled lives to women during the decades beyond their reproductive years.

—*Margaret Anderson*
Updated by Kerry Cheesman, PhD
and Maryann Cheesman, RN

See also: Aging process; Biological clock; Change: Women, Aging, and the Menopause, The; Estrogen replacement therapy; Infertility; Middle age; Midlife crisis; Ourselves, Growing Older: A Book for Women over Forty; Reproductive changes, disabilities, and dysfunctions; Sexuality; Women and aging

For Further Information

Dalal, Pronobk, and Manu Agarwal. "Postmenopausal Syndrome." *Indian Journal of Psychiatry*, vol. 57, no. 6, 2015, p. 222. doi:10.4103/0019-5545.161483. This article attempts to understand postmenopausal symptoms, the underlying pathophysiology and the management options available.

Faubion Stephanie S. *The Menopause Solution.* Time Inc. Books, 2016. Drawing on the latest information, leading women's health expert Dr. Faubion covers common questions, lifestyle strategies, and treatment options.

Gittleman, Ann Louise. *Before the Change: Taking Charge of Your Perimenopause.* HarperOne, 2017. Offers a gentle, proven, incremental program for understanding your body's changes and controlling your symptoms during perimenopause to help you feel great through this vital phase of life.

Halloran, Laurel. "Is It Hot in Here? Menopause Symptom Management." *The Journal for Nurse Practitioners*, vol. 10, no. 9, 2014, pp. 759-60. doi:10.1016/j.nurpra.2014.07.002. Reviews the most common complaints of perimenopause and discusses complementary therapies used to treat perimenopausal issues and recent research regarding hormonal treatment of perimenopausal complaints.

"Menopause." Office on Women's Health, U.S. Department of Health and Human Services, 23 May 2019. www.womenshealth.gov/menopause/. A compilation of resources on menopause.

Santoro, Nanette, et al. "Menopausal Symptoms and Their Management." *Endocrinology and Metabolism Clinics of North America*, vol. 44, no. 3, 2015, pp. 497-515. doi:10.1016/j.ecl.2015.05.001. Explains core symptoms of menopause and their management.

MENTORING

Relevant Issues: Economics, psychology, work

Significance: Older individuals can either serve as mentors or be mentored by others, particularly in the workforce; this type of relationship, whether formal or informal, can occur at any point in an individual's career or life stage.

Mentors are people who serve as close, trusted, and experienced counselors or guides. Additionally, mentors function as teachers, tutors, or coaches. Technical, interpersonal, and political skills can be conveyed in a relationship from the mentor to the person being mentored. Not only does the less experienced (often younger) person benefit from this type of relationship, but the more experienced (often older) individual may enjoy the opportunity to share earlier acquired knowledge, skills, and abilities.

OLDER WORKERS AND MENTORING

The concept of mentoring in the work environment has evolved over time from the formal arrangement of apprenticeship to an informal protégé situation involving advice and back to a more formal relationship. Mentoring seems to work well in many employment situations. For example, women with mentors advance in a career more quickly than those without them. Further, it is more likely that a person who has been mentored will, in turn, mentor others. Mentoring is a useful tool that can be used to establish and enhance networks and references.

Older workers may act as mentors for younger colleagues. People anticipating a transition to retirement enjoy the role of mentor and look forward to having an opportunity to share acquired history, culture, and informal dealings in work situations. These workers are often skilled in the oral tradition of passing information from person to person. Older workers hired at a new company or in a new field or returning to work after an absence may also appreciate the guidance offered by having a mentor.

Older workers often face prejudice and discrimination in the workplace. This situation, sometimes called the gray barrier, describes a situation in which an older worker is not hired or does not get promoted as quickly as other workers. When knowledge, skills, and abilities are equal among employees, the gray barrier can be one explanation for the older employee's lack of employment progress. Although little real research exists on this issue, numerous personal narratives and anecdotes confirm that such a barrier exists. Additionally, it is clear that hiring and promotion activities occur to the detriment of older workers. Age discrimination exists in government, profit, and nonprofit fields.

While the situation may be changing in the government sector as a result of the influence of organizations like the American Association of Retired Persons (AARP), mandated employment practices, and numerous labor union activities, the pace of change is relatively slow. Having a mentor can often ameliorate this situation. Successful older workers also report pushing through the gray barrier by using political savvy, establishing credibility, fitting in with the current management style, and understanding the nature of the customer base.

STAGES OF FORMAL MENTORING RELATIONSHIPS

Formal arrangements for mentoring in the workplace can be established through meetings, instruction manuals, and regular appraisal sessions. During the initiation phase, which typically lasts between six months and one year, the mentor's knowledge, skills, and abilities are acknowledged without question. The mentor serves as a source of support and guidance. Mentors begin to recognize the potential of others requesting mentoring. A time period of two to five years typically outlines the cultivation stage. Mentoring relationships gain self-confidence and mutual respect. Differences of values and styles of operation are explored. Mentors begin to allocate challenging work, actively coach individuals, and sponsor individuals in new work situations.

Mentoring relationships should not last indefinitely; a separation phase typically takes six months to a year. Just as it is not advisable to begin mentoring relationships precipitously, neither should they be terminated without care. One reason is the experience of simultaneous freedom in decision-making coupled with anxiety of evolving away from the mentor relationship. Most successful mentoring relationships, however, are measured by the success in moving away from the closeness of this type of work situation. As is true of other work systems, successful mentoring should include ongoing information gathering to redefine and inform the mentoring process. Both the mentor and the person being mentored are excellent resources of information for change during the process.

ENTRY-STAGE ISSUES

Older workers are often presented with unfamiliar work environments and cultures when returning to the world of work. A mentor can exert a strong influence in determining how to adjust to culture differentials. The initial weeks at any job are often the most critical. Mentors can smooth over many of the usual problems in the workplace while at the same time establishing boundaries for untoward circumstances at work. Many times, there appears to be no place to turn when attempting to understand a new workplace. Early stages of work, for both older and younger workers, are the times when aspirations and ideas meet reality. This matching of culture and individual can be as important for the older worker as the skill, knowledge, and ability level brought to the job.

Mentors can ensure the appropriate level of challenge for an older worker to avoid unpleasant situations during the initial period of adjustment. At the same time, when high expectations do not match the nature of the job requirements or settings, a mentor can offer a different perspective for the older worker. Many work situations assign initial job tasks that may be more challenging than usual. This type of increased responsibility for the older worker can be especially perplexing if not mediated by a mentor arrangement.

Early in the career development of an older worker, a clear set of goals and objectives should be mutually agreed on. These goals emphasize vocational or educational work outcomes as well as social outcomes in the workplace. An orientation that discusses roles, responsibilities, and expectations should follow. Frank and open discussion of personal characteristics, skills, and specific objectives of the mentor relationship is important. A period of training for overcoming shortcomings and deficits should follow. Equally important is a trial period or a preparatory time for testing the relationship before any long-term commitments are made by the mentor or the older worker. Following the trial period, an extensive review of expectations and applications should take place.

The concept of group mentoring should be explored as an alternative. Small businesses or self-employed individuals may not be able to take advantage of the formal mentor relationship often found in larger organizations. These group mentoring relationships often take the form of membership in professional organizations and trade associations. In addition to the provision of an effective career development tool, important networking opportunities are established and enhanced.

BENEFITS AND DRAWBACKS

Mentors can bring a broader overview of the work environment and the relationship of functional areas. Communication on work activities maintains a dynamic perspective of work functions. Job description changes, salary modifications, and work assignment evolution are important parts of the communication base. This type of mentor relationship helps alleviate the initial feelings of being overwhelmed and the ongoing feelings of being lost in a large, faceless workplace. In addition to the career or work function mentors often perform, an additional psychosocial function also exists. Aspects of the workplace such as competence, self-esteem, and perception by others can be better observed through the eyes of a mentor.

Mentoring is not a panacea without problems. Older workers often find it difficult to find a mentor willing to work with them. Often, the willingness to work with older workers is undermined by the same prejudice and discrimination originally present in the hiring process. Mentors who are not satisfied with a work situation may use a mentoring opportunity to sabotage the potential successful work situation of someone else. This can be avoided by developing several mentoring relationships, either concurrently or sequentially. The pejorative notion of mentors manipulating workers has gained some acceptance. This stereotype is usually overstated; a cooperative working relationship is more indicative of the mentor's role.

Older workers sometimes resist entering into a mentoring relationship because the formal definition of mentoring is a relatively new workforce concept. Workers who were trained in another era and have not been introduced to the benefits of a mentoring relationship may be reluctant to embrace such a practice. Workers trained without mentors find that they may understand the informal nature of mentoring but do not see the value of formalizing the relationship. Additionally, work attributes of power and achievement are emphasized through formal mentoring relationships. Older workers often have been trained in a more passive work setting.

—*Daniel L. Yazak*

See also: Age discrimination; Ageism; Communication; Employment; Retirement; Wisdom

For Further Information

Dessler, Gary. *Human Resource Management.* 16th ed. Prentice Hall, 2019. This book provides readers with the daily tools and skills they need to function as successful managers—in both human resources and business in general.

Gomez-Mejia, Luis R., David B. Balkin, and Robert L. Cardy. *Managing Human Resources.* 9th ed. Prentice Hall, 2018. This book prepares all future managers with a business understanding of the need for human resource management skills.

Herr, Edwin L., and Stanley H. Cramer. *Career Guidance and Counseling Through the Life Span.* 6th ed. HarperCollins, 2004. The book examines the current changes in the organization and content of work, the implications of the global economy for the practice of career development, best practices in career services, and perspectives on the research findings supporting career counseling and other career interventions.

Mathis, Robert L., and John H. Jackson. *Human Resource Management.* 16th ed. Cengage Learning, 2018. A leading resource in preparing for professional HR certification, this edition ensures you are familiar with all major topics for professional examinations from the Society for Human Resource Management and Human Resource Certification Institute.

MIDDLE AGE

Relevant Issues: Biology, demographics, family, health and medicine, psychology, sociology

Significance: Middle age is a period in life filled with change and requiring major adaptations on the part of the individual and society.

Middle age is broadly defined as the period between young adulthood and senescence. Although there are no precise age limits associated with this period, it is usually defined as the period from forty to sixty-five. During this period, development continues to occur at a steady pace, but changes become more readily apparent than they were in the past. As a result, this is a period that often has many negative stereotypes associated with it. In spite of these stereotypes, most elderly adults report that middle age is the period that they would prefer to return to given the chance.

PHYSICAL CHANGES

Changes in skin integrity, pigmentation, muscle mass, distribution of body fat, vision, and joints do not begin during middle age but rather reach a level where alterations become noticeable. For this reason, middle age is often viewed as a period of physical decline.

Among the changes that commonly become noticeable in middle age are graying of hair, wrinkling of skin, development of "middle-age spread," decrease in metabolic rate leading to more rapid weight gain, and development of some signs of a arthritis in many individuals. Vision changes abound: Farsightedness develops with the ability to accommodate decreasing; the retina becomes less sensitive to low levels of illumination, so that middle-aged adults require brighter illumination to see as well as they had in the past; and the size of the blind spot typically enlarges as a result of decreased blood supply to the eye.

Changes in the functioning of the sex organs and related endocrine changes are most readily apparent in women in the case of the menopause. The cessation of menstruation, and the signs and symptoms associated with it, is the single most common physical change in middle-aged women. While the hormonal and sex-related changes in middle-aged men are less obvious, there is a comparable decline in testosterone level.

A less well known but definitely important physical change in middle age takes place within the nervous system itself. Demyelination (breakdown of the myelin sheath) of the axon of the neurons results in slower transmission of the neural impulse. This is one factor that results in increased reaction time with age. Therefore, as one gets older, it takes a longer time to respond completely to a stimulus.

HEALTH AND SEX

Middle age is a time when many adults begin to complain about their health and health-related issues. The "aches and pains" of arthritis (inflammation of the joints) usually become apparent during middle age. The decrease in metabolic rate makes the middle-aged adult more easily prone to weight gain, increasing concern with proper diet and exercise. Hypertension (high blood pressure) typically appears for the first time in middle age, requiring more diligent health screenings to allow early detection and treatment. Similarly, cancer screenings and cholesterol checks are more routinely done in midlife in an attempt to promote wellness. Despite these concerns, more than 70 percent of middle-aged adults in a nationwide survey indicated that they viewed their health as excellent.

There is little change in the ability of men and women to function sexually in middle age (although women normally do lose their ability to reproduce by their mid-fifties). In spite of this, sexual activity tends to occur less frequently than it did in young adulthood. This decline in sexual activity may occur, in part, because of job-related stress, family matters, changing energy levels, or routine. Research indicates that sexual activity is greatest in twenty-five- to twenty-nine-year-olds and drops off considerably by the time individuals reach middle age. In a national survey, fewer than 25 percent of adults in their forties to fifties reported engaging in sexual intercourse at least twice a week, while 40 percent reported having intercourse only a few times per month. Although participation in sexual activity in middle age shows a decline, most middle-aged adults remain sexually active and report continued enjoyment of intercourse and sex-related behaviors.

FAMILY

Marital satisfaction appears to increase in middle age. Nearly three-fourths of married couples in a nationwide survey by the MacArthur Foundation indicated that they had very good relationships with their spouse. This increase in marital satisfaction may be related to changes within the family (resulting in more time and energy for each other), lessening of stressors and responsibilities as children develop and work roles change, or the fact that dissatisfied couples have separated by middle age, resulting in fewer marriages but more happy marriages.

Middle age is typically viewed as a time of changing family roles. Although (nuclear) family size tends to have stabilized, three major family changes usually occur during the middle years that require relatively major adaptation on the part of the individual. This is a period in which offspring develop independence. Middle-aged adults report having a difficult time adapting to the independent functioning of their children. As a result, many middle-aged parents with adolescents experience a generation gap before the children leave home. Once the grown children have moved out of the house, and on with their lives, the middle-aged parents may experience the empty nest syndrome. If all the offspring leave home (the nest), the parents are faced with adaptation as they return to the original dyad. In some households, these changes are greeted tearfully, while in other households they are viewed very positively. In still other households, the nest does not remain empty as grown children take turns returning to the home and leaving again because of school situations, social and family relationships, or financial and job-related matters. Rather than the empty nest, these middle-aged parents experience the revolving door syndrome.

As these offspring go off on their own, a second major change is likely to occur within the family with the birth of grandchildren. Adapting to grandparenthood is the single most positive change that middle-aged adults report. The majority of grandparents report that the birth of grandchildren gives them a sense of renewal as well as a sense of continuity. They enjoy experiencing developmental milestones that they missed in their own children's lives or that they barely had time to enjoy. Traditional middle-aged grandparents also report enjoying the fact that they can spend time with their grandchildren without having to be fully responsible for them.

The third major change in family roles involves the fact that elderly parents often develop dependence on their middle-aged children. This is the change to which middle-aged adults have the hardest time adapting. Viewing one's parents (who have always been there for one to count on) as suddenly frail or in need of help requires major adjustments in life. If the development of this dependence occurs prior to the complete independence of all offspring, the middle-aged parents enter the sandwich generation. Most members of the sandwich generation report having a difficult time juggling their responsibilities related to their now-dependent parents and still-dependent children. Often, this conflict comes to an end with the death of one's parents. This loss not only requires major adaptation but also leaves individuals with a heightened sense of their own mortality, as they begin to think more about their own death.

PLANNING FOR THE FUTURE

With middle age comes the realization that life is finite, that there is less time ahead than in the past. Along with this notion comes psychologist Erik Erikson's notion of generativity. This concern for the future spurs many middle-aged adults to do what they can to make the world a better place through mentoring, volunteering, charitable contributions, or political involvement. At the same time that they are thinking about the future of the world, they are planning for their own futures. Major concerns usually include planning for retirement and planning for health-related issues and death.

Middle-aged adults have typically begun planning financially for their retirement and begin to think about how and where they would like to spend their time. Studies indicate that better planning leads to a happier future. Access to health care is a major issue for all age levels. Concerns about health insurance (including long-term care and catastrophic coverage) are common. Often of greatest importance is concern with end-of-life issues. All adults have the option of creating an advance directive: a living will or durable power of attorney for health care. By so doing, they can make their medical wishes known for the future, as well as appoint an individual to make sure that these wishes are carried out.

Clearly, the time from forty to sixty-five is a period filled with change. The majority of these changes are dealt with in a positive manner. As a result, middle age is often considered (by the elderly) to be the best years of life.

—*Robin Kamienny Montvilo*

See also: AARP; Aging: Biological, psychological, and sociocultural perspectives; Aging process; Biological clock; Change: Women, Aging, and the Menopause, The; Death of parents; Divorce; Early retirement; Employment; Empty nest syndrome; Erikson, Erik H.; 401(k) plans; Grandparenthood; Individual retirement accounts (IRAs); Marriage; Maturity; Menopause; Midlife crisis; Parenthood; Premature aging; Remarriage; Retirement; Retirement planning; Sandwich generation; Successful aging

For Further Information

Schaie, K. Warner, et al. *Handbook of the Psychology of Aging.* 8th ed., Elsevier/Academic P, 2016. Providing perspectives on the behavioral science of aging for diverse disciplines, the handbook explains how the role of behavior is organized and how it changes over time.

Hayslip, Bert, et al. *Adult Development and Aging.* 5th ed., Krieger Pub. Company, 2011. The text examines the development of adults of all ages from a topical rather than a chronological perspective. Special consideration is given to issues regarding personality and psychopathology, clinical interventions, cognitive processes such as learning, memory, and intelligence, social roles in adulthood, physical changes with age, and death and dying.

Santrock, John. *Life-Span Development.* 16th ed. McGraw-Hill, 2016. Through an integrated, personalized digital learning program, students gain the insight they need to study smarter and improve performance.

MIDLIFE CRISIS

Relevant Issues: Biology, death, family, psychology

Significance: Midlife crisis, once thought to be a common, traumatic reaction to the realization of one's own aging and mortality, was found by the late 1990s to be relatively infrequent and atypical.

Key Terms:

generativity: a concern for establishing and guiding the next generation

stagnation: a refusal to grow, an acquiescence to old methods and perspectives

The concept of midlife crisis, which has been called the most celebrated feature of adult development, originated with psychoanalyst Elliott Jacques, who, in 1965, wrote about the fact that most artists undergo a crisis in their late thirties propelled by their awareness of time left to live rather than time since birth. Jacques believed that everyone experiences midlife crisis in some form, as death ceases to be a general concept and becomes a personal matter. People who reach middle age without becoming successfully established in work and family life, or who neglect emotional issues to engage in frantic levels of activity, may experience pronounced psychological disturbance. Jacques noted that midlife crisis for these individuals can include preoccupation with appearing young, over-concern with health, including sexual promiscuity, a search for solace in religion, and a tendency to stop enjoying life. Many of these symptoms made their way into the stereotype of midlife crisis. Healthier people, Jacques stated in his article "The Midlife Crisis," enter into awareness of their own future death "with the sense of grief appropriate to it"; but even for them, midlife crisis is "a period of purgatory—of anguish and depression."

DEFINITION AND CHARACTERISTICS

When Jacques first wrote about midlife crisis, the idea of developmental stages in adulthood was fairly new. In 1980, Solomon Cytrynbaum defined the phenomenon, in his article "Midlife Development: A Personality and Social Systems Perspective," as a "perceived state of physical and psychological distress that results when internal resources and external social support systems threaten to be overwhelmed by developmental tasks that require new adaptive resources."

Whether people experience a crisis or a transition at midlife, certain characteristics can be observed. The process may take a short time, or it may last five to twenty years. The individual's reaction to the process may be open, adaptive, conscious, and masterful, or it may be passive, defensive, and unconscious. An individual also may vacillate between the two. The process can be seen as a series of tasks that must be mastered: accepting one's mortality, coping with biological changes and health limitations, reassessing career and marriage, and reevaluating sexuality and self-concept. If the tasks are not mastered successfully, subsequent stages of life can be unhappy. The process can bring about personality changes, such as increasingly inward focus and greater attention to earlier neglected parts of the personality (particularly those associated with the opposite gender). Women grow more in touch with their independent, competitive, and aggressive aspects, while men become more willing to be expressive, dependent, and sensuous. Some researchers contend that the characteristics that reemerge after midlife transition are any that were earlier rejected or unrealized, not just those that are gender related.

Several studies report that development occurs in stages during midlife transition. One model refers to the stages as "progress" and "regression." Another proposes the stages of destructuring, reassessment, reintegration or restructuring, and behavioral or role change.

Destructuring, provoked by awareness of mortality, biological changes, or a variety of life events, can cause alternating euphoria and depression. Reassessment, which consists of reactions to these precipitators, might involve mourning the loss of goals, denial, transitional partners, and reassessment of one's primary relationship. Reintegration or restructuring involves testing new ways of relating to the important people in one's life, integrating the earlier neglected personality characteristics, and finding and exploring new aspirations. Behavioral and role changes solidify the new dreams and new ways of relating to others.

CONFLICTING ESTIMATES OF PREVALENCE

In 1977, Paul T. Costa created a "midlife crisis scale" with questions pertaining to the feelings usually mentioned in studies of midlife crisis: inner conflict and confusion, preoccupation with death and decline, a sense of meaninglessness, and unhappiness with family and work. In a study of 350 men aged thirty to sixty, there was no increase in these feelings at the middle of the age range. Only 2 percent of respondents met the scale's definition of midlife crisis. A replication with 300 men found similar results. By 1985, some scholars were writing about the "myths" connected with midlife crisis, partly because of disparities in reports of its frequency. Some studies called midlife crisis a rare occurrence; others said 10 percent of people experience it; still others, 70 to 80 percent. A 1994 review of the literature concluded that most studies disconfirm the statement that the majority of people experience a midlife crisis.

Several researchers have noted that people who meet the definitions of midlife crisis have predictors of this painful transition earlier in life—in poor life choices or in high scores on neuroticism scales. Narcissistic people are also susceptible to traumatic midlife transitions. People with enduring personality characteristics such as these experience crises throughout adulthood.

Undoubtedly, people undergo a change in perspective at midlife—a realization that there is no longer time for everything, so new goals must be established and complex choices made. For most, the experience may not properly be termed a "crisis." Some scholars believe that most people experience a midlife "transition," as described by Daniel Levinson in The Seasons of a

Man's Life (1978)—a deeply affecting, sometimes painful reassessment. People in crisis respond with abrupt action in order to avoid their past choices, current responsibilities, and the future's seemingly limited possibilities. Those in transition respond with careful thought, making changes only after assessing the possible consequences.

Another view of what happens at midlife has been inspired by psychoanalyst and human development theorist Erik Erikson. He believes that in the matured adulthood stage, the primary developmental task is to resolve the tension between "generativity" and "stagnation." Generativity is the process of identifying something that is vitally important and taking action so that it is maintained and cared for. Generativity is a way of moving forward, rather than regressing to past patterns by trying to regain lost youth. Stagnation is a refusal to grow, an acquiescence to old methods and perspectives, perhaps because of the belief that it is too late to accomplish new goals, or perhaps because of a fear of change. For some people, the search for generativity may lead to excess—doing so much for others that one is worn out and family relationships are stressed. Other people may stagnate rather than change and grow because of the structure of their lives prior to midlife. People who experienced premature career, creative, or artistic success (perhaps in their twenties), or who enjoyed a career pinnacle in their early forties, may view the remainder of life as anticlimactic and have trouble imagining what remains to be done. Those who have relied too heavily on their spouse's or children's successes rather than developing their own sense of identity also may struggle with establishing goals for the next life stage. Generativity may find outlets through a new approach to one's existing job, a job change, volunteer work, or political activity.

THE MIDUS SURVEY

In 1999, initial results were released from the Midlife Development in the United States (MIDUS) survey, at that time the most comprehensive examination of midlife ever undertaken. The study was funded by the John D. and Catherine T. MacArthur Foundation's Research Network on Successful Midlife Development. The team of twenty-eight researchers was led by Orville Gilbert Brim. The study encompassed 7,861 people aged twenty-five to seventy-four (to give data for comparisons of other life stages with midlife) but focused on ages forty to sixty. Three thousand of the participants completed thirty-minute telephone interviews as well as a two-part self-administered questionnaire. The remaining 5,000 people were involved in eleven other studies. The study's one 1,000 addressed twenty-seven different areas of life, with the intention of developing a concrete picture of what actually happens to people during midlife. The study looked at factors that spur midlife development—including life events, work, family, illness, and culture—and also examined the strategies people use to cope with these issues.

The majority of respondents found midlife a period of greater control over many areas of life, including work and finances; great satisfaction with marriage and family; extremely busy lives; increased autonomy and environmental mastery (handling of daily responsibilities); excellent health; and optimism about health in the future. Although both women and men improved in personal autonomy during midlife, women gained in greater increments. Brim reported that 95 percent of Americans could define the term "midlife crisis" and knew someone who had experienced it. Among MIDUS survey participants, however, only 23 percent reported having had a midlife crisis. Only one-third of this group linked their crisis to awareness that they were aging. For the rest, midlife crisis was provoked by particular life events, some of which had no connection to aging. The survey's researchers concluded, therefore, that only 10 percent of participants had undergone a "classic" midlife crisis (as originally defined by Jacques). These people were likely to have high scores on neuroticism scales (a finding that was in keeping with earlier studies) and were highly educated. The researchers noted that because many earlier studies of midlife crisis had been based on clinical populations, the frequencies those studies reported may not have paralleled the incidence among the general population. They also surmised that the midlife crisis myth persists because nearly everyone knows someone who seems to have experienced it and retains vivid memories of its tumultuous impact on that person.

The MIDUS survey results also addressed other factors that studies have named as contributors to midlife crisis. Most of the postmenopausal women said they felt "only relief" when their menstrual periods ended, and 50 percent went through the menopause with no hot flashes at all. Rather than being concerned about future health and about biological changes associated with aging, participants surprised and concerned researchers with their optimism about their health. However, 70 percent reported being overweight, while 42 percent of women and 24 percent of men said that hurrying on level or slightly sloping ground made them short of breath. Only 23 percent strongly agreed that they worked hard to stay in good health, and most of the smokers did not believe they had an above-average risk of contracting heart disease or cancer.

In addition, 72 percent of participants rated their marriage excellent or very good, and 90 percent said it was unlikely that their marriage would ever end. Of those surveyed, 21 percent were experiencing anxiety or depression—a lower rate than was found in younger adults. Survey participants in their forties said they were dealing with high numbers of negative life events involving children and other family members, but many were showing great resiliency. Only 5 percent of all respondents had consulted a psychiatrist in the past year; 9 percent had talked to a counselor, 20 percent had consulted a family physician about emotional problems, and 19 percent had attended a self-help group during some period in their lives.

—Glenn Ellen Starr Stilling
Updated by Bruce E. Johansen, PhD

See also: Alcohol use disorder; Death anxiety; Divorce; Empty nest syndrome; Erikson, Erik H.; Marriage; Menopause; Middle age; Personality changes; Sandwich generation; Suicide

For Further Information

Clay, Rebecca. "Researchers Replace Midlife Myths with Facts." *American Psychological Association*, vol. 34, no. 4, Apr. 2003, p. 36. doi:10.1037/e300092003-024. Examines a decade-long study by the MacArthur Foundation Research Network on Successful Midlife Development that uncovers data that challenge stereotypes about midlife crisis, menopausal distress, and the empty-nest syndrome.

Lachman, Margie E. "Mind the Gap in the Middle: A Call to Study Midlife." *Research in Human Development*, vol. 12, no. 3-4, 27 Aug. 2016, pp. 327-34. doi:10.1080/15427609.2015.1068048. Explains why more research into midlife is necessary to promote well-being among the middle-aged.

Schmidt, Susanne. "The Feminist Origins of The Midlife Crisis." *The Historical Journal*, vol. 61, no. 2, June 2018, pp. 503-23. doi:10.1017/s0018246x17000309. Tells the history of the midlife crisis and explores its feminist roots. Contradicts stereotypes of midlife crisis as being mainly a male experience

Setiya, Kieran. *Midlife: a Philosophical Guide*. Princeton U P, 2017. Setiya confronts the inevitable challenges of adulthood and middle age, showing how philosophy can help someone thrive. Combining imaginative ideas, surprising insights, and practical advice, Setiya makes a wry but passionate case for philosophy as a guide to life.

Sheehy, Gail. *Passages: Predictable Crises of Adult Life*. E. P. Dutton, 1976. See part 6, "Deadline Decade," pp. 242-340. These chapters discuss the "sense of deadline" and feelings ranging from vulnerability to upheaval that can accompany the midlife passage.

MOBILITY PROBLEMS

Relevant Issues: Demographics, economics, family, health and medicine

Significance: The aging of the society posits important questions about mobility problems and mobility needs in the elderly, as mobility strongly influences the ability to maintain independence and to access various resources.

Mobility is one of the essentials of human wellbeing. Especially for an older adult, daily activities are impacted and determined by mobility. Thus, an inability to meet the needs of mobility could lead to changes in the physical, social, and psychological health of the elderly. As the population is aging, mobility problems will become more severe in the near future.

The physical measurements of mobility include gait and balance. Gait and balance can be assessed by a simple test called "Get Up and Go." The procedure of the test is to begin sitting in a chair with standard height and straight back, then get up from the chair without use of armrests, stand still momentarily, walk forward 10 feet, turn around and walk back to the chair, turn, and be seated. Mobility problems associated with gait include difficulties in sitting balance, transferring from sitting to standing, walking (pace and stability), and turning (such as staggering). Some self-reported information is also helpful to determine physical mobility. The information could include feeling unsteady when walking or needing help when walking. Mobility is often closely related to a history of falls. People with poor mobility are more likely to have falls and to be institutionalized in a hospital or a nursing home.

CAUSES AND CONSEQUENCES OF DECREASE IN MOBILITY

Any health conditions that result in movement restrictions could decrease an individual's mobility. These medical conditions include stroke, Parkinson's disease, hip fractures, severe arthritis, and other neuromuscular diseases. One of the common causes of decreasing mobility in older people is fear of falling, caused by experiencing a fall. Such fear may lead the elderly to restrict their own activity, especially mobility. Regardless of physical trauma, the response to a fall and decreased mobility consequently determines emotional, psychological, or social changes. Thus, these changes affect older people's quality of life significantly.

PRESERVING MOBILITY IN OLDER PEOPLE

There is a cycle in older people of age-related loss of muscle strength, falls, fear of falling, decrease of mobility, and further loss of muscle strength. To preserve mobility in older people, this negative cycle needs to be broken. Two common ways to prevent or delay this cycle and maintain mobility are exercise and trophic factors.

Exercise, particularly strength training (such as weight lifting), preserves muscular performance and

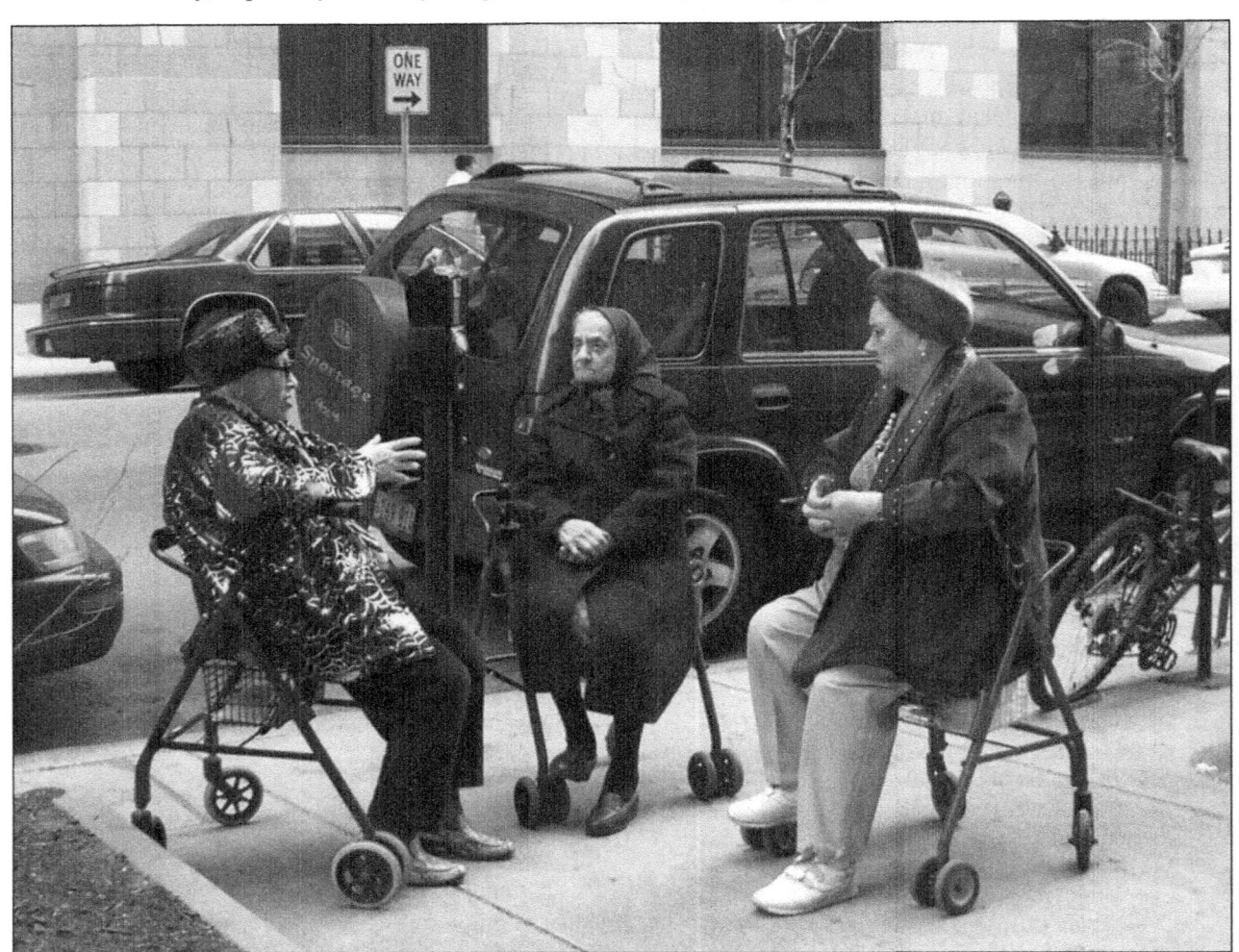

The rollator consists of a frame with three or four large wheels, handlebars and a built-in seat, which allows the user to stop and rest when needed. Rollators are also often equipped with a shopping basket. (via Wikimedia Commons)

mobility. Many research studies have confirmed that higher levels of physical activity are associated with greater muscular performance, better mobility, and a lower risk of falls. Although there is some concern that high levels of physical activity may increase the risk of falls and injuries, physically active older people appear to have less disability even after accounting for the illness due to exercise. In the 1970s, it was questioned whether muscles in older people could even respond to exercise training. However, more recent research shows that strength training increases skeletal muscle strength even in older people, as studies conducted with eighty- and ninety-year-old individuals report increases in strength with resistance training. Strength training affects muscle physiology as well as function in older people. When older and younger individuals are trained in the same program at the same relative intensity, their increments in maximum oxygen consumption are similar. Thus, the fitness response to an endurance training program in earlier sedentary but healthy older people is comparable to that of younger people. Study results are also available to evaluate the effects of strength and endurance training on mobility measured by gait speed and balance. Several randomized clinical trials reported that strength and endurance training improve gait speed by a modest amount, although there are some other trials that have not been successful in finding such an effect. The controversy between findings could be explained partially by the variation in frequency, duration, and intensity of training. Whether or not strength training improves mobility by improving balance in healthy older people is still unclear; however, strength training has been shown to improve balance in weak individuals in nursing homes.

Trophic factors are related to hormones that can enhance muscular performance. The idea of using hormones to improve muscular performance was initiated in the 1980s when it became possible to produce large quantities of hormones with new technologies. The hormones that can enhance muscular performance include growth hormone, estrogen, and testosterone. Growth hormone can increase muscle mass; however, there are side effects from using growth hormones, including glucose intolerance (early stage of diabetes). Also, one study reported that growth hormone supplementation has no effect on mobility and functional limitations. Use of estrogen, also called hormone replacement therapy, is much more common in postmenopausal women. Research evidence indicates estrogen decreases the chance of developing heart disease and osteoporosis in older women. Evidence about the effect of estrogen on muscle strength and mobility is limited and inconsistent. An epidemiologic (population) study reported that estrogen use is correlated with the preservation of muscle strength in postmenopausal women. Testosterone can increase muscle strength in young men, but less information is available on older men, and the effects of testosterone on mobility and functional limitation in older people remains unclear.

In conclusion, regular physical activities, especially strength training, are recommended for older people to preserve their muscular performance and mobility. However, studies show that only 5 to 6 percent of older men and 1 to 3 percent of older women report doing activities like weight lifting to increase muscle strength. A recent U.S. Surgeon General's report affirmed the accumulating evidence favoring the health benefits of strength training in older people. It recommends that cardiorespiratory endurance activity should be supplemented with strength-developing exercises at least twice per week for adults in order to improve musculoskeletal health, maintain independence in performing the activities of daily life, and reduce the risk of falls.

DRIVING AND MOBILITY

Besides the physical factors related to mobility in older people, some other factors also contribute to mobility, particularly outdoor mobility. In the United States, mobility outside the home has mainly relied on the automobile since the time that private vehicles became popular. Changes in housing patterns, such as moving from central urban areas to the suburbs, further the dependence on automobiles. Availability of an automobile and capability of driving an automobile significantly influence one's outdoor mobility.

As the proportion of elderly people rises, the number of older drivers is increasing rapidly. The percentage of persons age 65 and older who are licensed drivers has increased from 61 percent in 1980 to 72 percent in 1990 and 80 percent in 2003. In 2003, about 1 in 7 licensed drivers was 65 or older. By 2029, when the last of the boomers turn 65, the proportion will be close to 1 in 4. Although older people travel less and drive fewer miles than do the rest of the population, they still depend on the car for most trips. National survey data show that for people aged sixty-five years or older, 90 percent of the trips were made by private vehicles. Public transportation accounts for less than 4 percent of trips made by older people. Taxis were rarely used by older people, who considered them either too expensive or not convenient. Walking as a mode of transportation was more often seen in older people than in the younger population. About 10 percent of the trips by older people were done by walking, and the older the individual, the greater was the proportion of walking for transportation. Community-provided transportation services for older people, such as senior citizen's vans, are seen more often.

Older people usually do not depend on automobiles for long trips but use them regularly for short trips, such as going to the doctor's office, grocery shopping, or visiting relatives or friends. Thus, in older people outdoor mobility and independent living are closely associated with the ability to drive an automobile. However, at some point in late life, one has to stop driving due to financial reasons or physical conditions. Some older people give up driving because of limited income and the increased cost of purchasing and maintaining a car, but most older people stop driving because of health problems. The common medical conditions resulting in driving cessation are vision impairment, muscle or joint weakness (or mobility limitations), and mental problems (such as dementia). Currently, the decision of the time to stop driving is mostly made by older people themselves or their family. Medical doctors or other health professionals may provide recommendations to stop driving for older people with certain medical conditions. Police departments may also be responsible for stopping some unsafe older drivers.

Whether it is safe to drive at an advanced age depends on the individual. Some healthy and fit older drivers may drive as safely as younger people, while others may have more difficulties driving in certain situations, such as at night, during rush hours, on snowy days, on highways, or at intersections. As a group, older individuals are relatively safe drivers. Persons age 65 and older have lower rates of crashes and crashes involving injury per licensed driver than younger drivers, the lowest percentage of crashes involving alcohol, and the highest rate of seatbelt use of any age group. However, when adjusting the number of crashes with the total mileage traveled by members of each age group, the older drivers and youngest drivers have the same high-risk levels to be involved in a car crash compared to middle-aged people. Thus, older people drive less and have a lower chance of being involved in a car crash, but for every driven mile, an older driver experiences an increased risk of being involved in a car crash.

To ensure the safety of older drivers and other drivers on the road, some states in the United States have legal restrictions regarding renewal of licensure in older drivers. Several states require vision testing as part of a driver's license renewal. Some states require written or road tests and shorter intervals between renewals for older drivers.

SERVICES AVAILABLE TO MEET MOBILITY NEEDS

Society recognizes the value of older people meeting their own mobility and transportation needs and keeping older drivers on the road as long as possible. Many programs are available to help older drivers retain the skills necessary for safe driving, including the American Association of Retired Persons (AARP), 55 Alive, the Mature Driving Program, and the Safe Driving for Mature Operators by the American Automobile Association (AAA). These courses are offered in many locations around the United States. Some insurance companies provide a reduction in auto insurance premiums for older drivers who have completed such a course. Physical or occupational therapists have developed driver retraining programs to treat individuals whose driving ability has been impaired by disease, injury, or the aging process. These programs can help people adapt to disability and train older drivers with functional limitations to drive. Also, these programs provide the use of special adaptive driving equipment, which compensates for many types of deficits in older drivers.

In general, older individuals who experience outdoor mobility problems are usually those who are unable to own and operate their own vehicles. Lack of such ability produces barriers to travel in older people, limits their independence, restricts their activities, and impairs their ability to take advantage of desirable services. People who have never driven or who stopped driving have sig-

> **SENIOR TALK:**
>
> **How Do You Feel About Mobility Problems?**
> Decreased mobility can be frustrating and even depressing. The thought of losing independence and having to depend on other people for daily tasks or even to move short distances can be hard to face. You may also be worried about falling, which could cause further injury or more serious disability. These fears can cause us to avoid going out or moving around at all, and the resulting social isolation and lack of exercise can further negatively affect physical and mental health.
>
> Mobility aids can help overcome these challenges. However, some seniors look down on such devices, seeing them as a reminder of old age. You may be embarrassed to use a mobility aid. It's important to overcome these stigmas and use mobility aids as needed. In doing so, your quality of life can be greatly improved. You may have tried to use a mobility aid but given up because it was uncomfortable. Finding the right type of device and having it properly fit is key. Talk to your doctor or another health professional for guidance and recommendations. Using mobility aids can help you feel safe and secure from falls. You should be able to do things that would otherwise be challenging or impossible, helping you feel empowered, capable, and independent.
>
> —Leah Jacob

nificantly lower numbers of activities outside the home than those who are current drivers. Where they exist, adequate public transportation systems can help older people overcome their mobility problems.

—Kimberly Y. Z. Forrest

See also: Arthritis; Balance disorders; Bone changes and disorders; Canes and walkers; Driving; Exercise and fitness; Fractures and broken bones; Hip replacement; Home services; Multiple sclerosis; Osteoporosis; Parkinson's disease; Sarcopenia; Strokes; Transportation issues; Vision changes and disorders; Wheelchair use

For Further Information

Brown, Cynthia J., and Kellie L. Flood. "Mobility Limitation in the Older Patient." *JAMA*, vol. 310, no. 11, 2013, p. 1168. doi:10.1001/jama.2013.276566. This study identifies mobility risk factors, screening tools, medical management, need for physical therapy, and efficacy of exercise interventions for older primary care patients with limited mobility.

Giannouli, Eleftheria, et al. "Mobility in Old Age: Capacity Is Not Performance." *BioMed Research International*, vol. 2016, 2016, pp. 1-8. doi:10.1155/2016/3261567. This study examines how well real-life mobility is predicted by standard laboratory measures of mobility or, in other words, how closely capacity and performance are linked.

"Maintaining Mobility in Older Age." *ScienceDaily*, ScienceDaily, 7 Dec. 2010. www.sciencedaily.com/releases/2010/12/101207205230.htm. While maintaining mobility plays a significant part in healthy aging, a new study highlights a high degree of inactivity even among an "elite" sample of fit and healthy older people aged between 72 and 92 years.

"Older Drivers." National Institute on Aging, U.S. Department of Health and Human Services, 12 Dec. 2018. www.nia.nih.gov/health/older-drivers. General information on several conditions that may affect an older adult's driving.

MULTIPLE SCLEROSIS

Relevant Issues: Health and medicine

Significance: Multiple sclerosis (MS) is a debilitating disease affecting the central nervous system; the population of older MS sufferers is growing.

In 2018, it was estimated that nearly 1 million Americans had multiple sclerosis, a disorder of the brain and spinal cord that causes disruption in the smooth flow of electrical messages from brain and nerves to the body. The progress of the disease is slow and may take decades to achieve complete nerve degeneration and paralysis. New, effective medical treatments are available to slow the advance of the disease. Although often considered a disease of youth, MS has the potential to become an increasing problem in aging populations. More cases of late-onset MS are coming to light in individuals over fifty years of age.

WHAT IS MULTIPLE SCLEROSIS?

Multiple sclerosis is caused by degeneration of the nervous system. A fatty substance called myelin surrounds and protects many nerve fibers of the brain and spinal cord, the central nervous system. Myelin is important

Main symptoms of Multiple sclerosis

Central:
- Fatigue
- Cognitive impairment
- Depression
- Anxiety
- Unstable mood

Visual:
- Nystagmus
- Optic neuritis
- Diplopia

Speech:
- Dysarthria

Throat:
- Dysphagia

Musculoskeletal:
- Weakness
- Spasms
- Ataxia

Sensation:
- Pain
- Hypoesthesias
- Paraesthesias

Bowel:
- Incontinence
- Diarrhea or constipation

Urinary:
- Incontinence
- Frequency or retention

The initial symptoms of MS may include tingling, numbness, slurred speech, blurred or double vision, loss of coordination, and muscle weakness. Later manifestations include unusual fatigue, muscle tightness, bowel and bladder control difficulties, sexual dysfunction, and paralysis. The most common cognitive functions influenced are short-term memory, abstract reasoning, verbal fluency, and speed of information processing. All the mental and physical symptoms listed may come or go in any combination. The symptoms may also vary from mild to severe in intensity throughout the course of the disease.

THE DISEASE COURSE

The symptoms of MS not only vary from person to person but also may periodically vary within the same person. This makes the prognosis of the disease difficult to foresee. Although the general course of the disease may be anticipated, the symptoms and their severity seem to be quite unpredictable in most individuals. In the "classic" course of MS, as time progresses, chronic problems gradually accumulate over many years, slowly worsening the sufferer's quality of life. The total level of disability will vary from patient to patient.

The typical pattern of MS is marked by active periods of the disease during which the nerves are being ravaged by the immune system. These periods are called attacks, relapses, or exacerbations. The active periods of the disease are followed by calm periods called remissions. The cycle of attack and remission will differ from sufferer to sufferer. Some people have few attacks, and their MS disabilities slowly accumulate over time; in these sufferers, it takes decades to become truly debilitated. Most people with MS have what is known as the relapsing-remitting form of the disease. They suffer many attacks over time, and these attacks occur unpredictably; the attacks are then followed by complete remission that may last months or years.

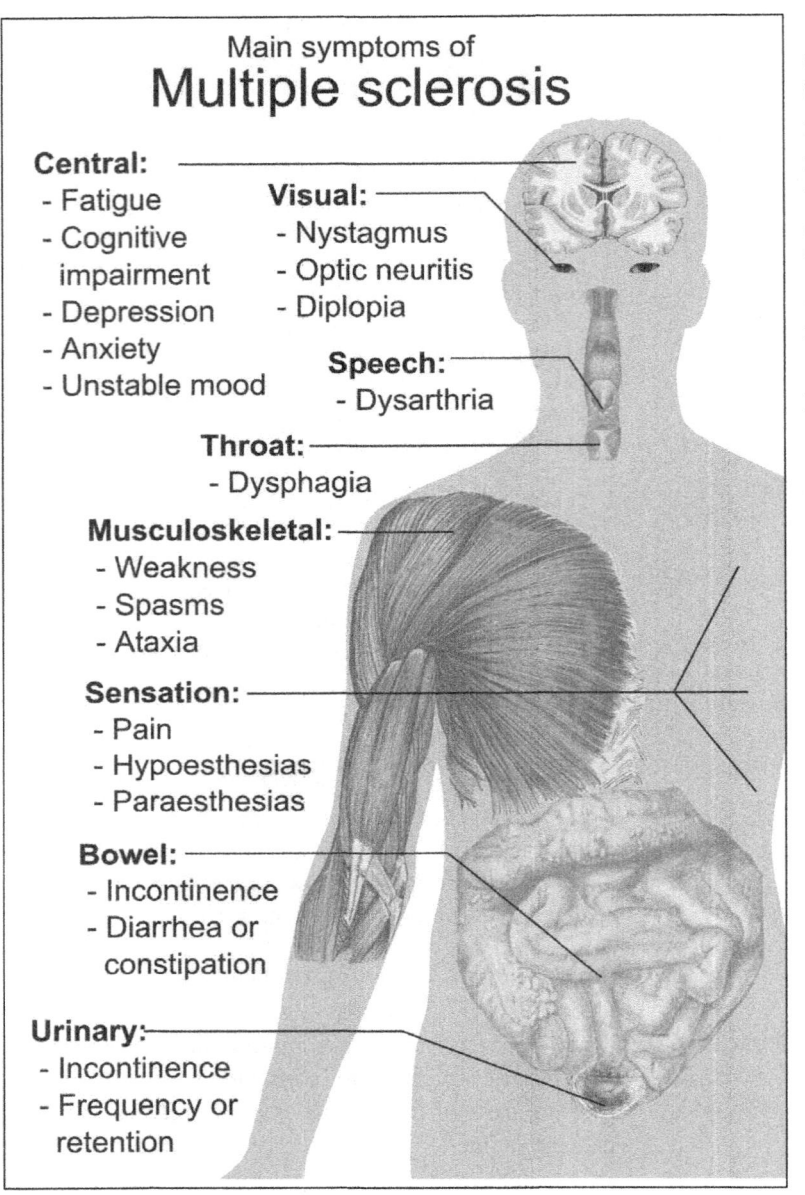

because it speeds up signals that move along the nerve fibers. In MS, the body attacks its own tissues, termed an autoimmune reaction, and a breakdown in the myelin layer occurs along the nerves. When any part of the myelin sheathing is destroyed, nerve impulses to and from the brain are slowed, distorted, or interrupted. The disease is called "multiple" because it affects many areas of the brain. Sclereids are hardened, scarred patches that form over the damaged areas of myelin.

Again, the injuries may take many years to accumulate to complete disability.

The most aggressive form of the disease is primary progressive MS. In this type of MS, the disease follows a rapid course that steadily worsens from its first onset. Although there are still attacks and partial remission, the attacks are quite severe and occur more regularly in time. Full paralysis may develop in primary progressive MS in three to five years. Secondary progressive MS occurs in patients who initially have the relapsing-remitting type and later develop the more aggressive form.

ONSET AND EPIDEMIOLOGY

Both genetic and environmental factors have been implicated in inducing the onset of MS. Viral infection has been suggested as a cause, but no single virus has ever been shown to be associated with MS. Risk may be conferred by exposure to a specific environment during adolescence, but that environment and the genetic risk factors have not yet been characterized.

Researchers Sharon Lynch and John Rose suggested that certain racial and geographic populations are less susceptible than others to the disease. MS is uncommon in Japanese people as well as among American Indians. The disease is more common among Northern European Caucasians as well as among North Americans of higher latitudes. There is an additional sexual dimorphism in the epidemiology of MS; the disease is found more frequently in women, by a ratio of at least 2:1.

The disease usually begins its first manifestations in late adolescence (around age eighteen) to early middle age (around age thirty-five). It is not clear how the interaction between the genetics of the sufferer and the environment may trigger onset. The progressive type of MS is more common over the age of forty, so those with late-onset MS often have the quickest deterioration of motor function. The reason that an older age predisposes someone to primary chronic progressive MS is still not clear.

MEDICAL TREATMENTS

There is no cure for MS, but there are many effective treatments. In most cases, steroidal drugs are used to treat relapses or attacks of the disease. Corticotropin was the first steroidal immunosuppressant to be used widely in MS treatment. The primary effect of the drug is to shorten the duration of an attack, although it does not appear to reduce the severity of the attack. Although it is still used with patients who respond well to it, corticotropin has been supplanted by the use of other drugs. Methylprednisolone is an immunosuppressant and steroid that has replaced corticotropin. It has been shown to control the inflammation that accompanies demyelination. These steroids seem to work by sealing leaking blood vessels in the brain and coating the white blood cells of the immune system so that they cannot attack the myelin easily.

Several federally approved drugs can slow the rate of attacks: Avonex, Betaseron, and Copaxone. Although these drugs do not stop MS entirely, they actually limit the level of myelin destruction, as observed in magnetic resonance imaging (MRI) scans of the brain. Avonex slows down the rate of increased disability, and all three slow down the natural course of MS. University of Western Ontario researcher George Ebers performed experimental treatments on MS patients with interferons. Interferons are proteins produced by the immune system that enter cells and induce them to set up defenses against attack. The myelin sheath is produced by a special nerve cell called a schwann cell; presumably the schwann cells are stimulated to protect themselves by exposure to interferons. Patients treated with human interferons demonstrated a 34 percent reduction in frequency of attack; that reduction was sustained over five years of treatment. More impressive was the 80 percent reduction of MS activity detected in their brains. Steroid treatment was rarely required in these patients.

As additional therapy, patients with MS should participate in a regular exercise program. Exercise is vital to the maintenance of functional ability in MS sufferers. It strengthens muscles, benefits gait, and generally improves coordination. The best type of exercise is aquatic in nature. Sufferers are often heat-intolerant, and participation in a regular aerobic program would be unpleasant. Also, aquatic exercise is a low-impact activity that puts less stress on chronically sore muscles. Exercise programs also encourage socialization of patients and engender peer support.

—James J. Campanella

See also: Disabilities; Illnesses among older adults; Reaction time; Wheelchair use

For Further Information

"Aging with MS." National Multiple Sclerosis Society. www.nationalmssociety.org/Living-Well-With-MS/Diet-Exercise-Healthy-Behaviors/Aging-with-MS. A collection of resources specifically designed for older adults with MS.

Buhse, Marijean. "The Elderly Person with Multiple Sclerosis." *Journal of Neuroscience Nursing*, vol. 47, no. 6, 2015, pp. 333-39. doi:10.1097/jnn.0000000000000172. This article focuses on the current literature in health-related quality of life in older persons with MS.

Jelinek, George. *Overcoming Multiple Sclerosis: an Evidence-Based 7 Step Recovery Program.* Allen & Unwin, 2016. This book explains the nature of MS and outlines an evidence-based 7 step program for recovery. Jelinek devised the program from an exhaustive analysis of medical research when he was first diagnosed with MS in 1999.

Kalb, Rosalind, ed. *Multiple Sclerosis: The Questions You Have, the Answers You Need.* 5th ed. Demos Medical, 2012. A guide for everyone concerned about multiple sclerosis.

Stachowiak, Julie. "Late-Onset Multiple Sclerosis." *Verywell Health*, 17 July 2019. www.verywellhealth.com/late-onset-multiple-sclerosis-3972555. General information on MS in older adults.

MURDER, SHE WROTE (T.V. SHOW)

Created By: Peter S. Fischer, Richard Levinson, William Link

Principal Cast: Angela Lansbury

Date: Aired from 1984 to 1996

Relevant Issues: Culture, media

Significance: Television programs sometimes present characters in stereotypical roles; however, the character of Jessica Fletcher in *Murder, She Wrote* reflected positive aspects of aging.

In 1984, the Columbia Broadcasting System (CBS) introduced what was to become the longest-running mystery drama in the history of television. *Murder, She Wrote*, starring Angela Lansbury as Jessica Fletcher, enjoyed prime-time popularity for twelve years. The series was set in the small coastal town of Cabot Cove, Maine, where the widowed Jessica made her home. A retired English teacher turned mystery writer, she had an uncanny knack for happening upon murders and becoming involved in the investigations. Fortunately, she also had a knack for solving the murders, often outshining the detectives assigned to the case.

The character of Jessica Fletcher was not subject to stereotypes about aging. She traveled regularly, often in connection with her books. She remained active in her retirement, often bicycling around Cabot Cove or taking brisk walks to become acquainted with new surroundings. She was a widow who sometimes reminisced wistfully about her late husband, Frank, but who also entertained occasional flirtations. She had had a successful career as an English teacher but launched a new career as a successful author. She clung to her faithful manual typewriter for years but eventually adapted to writing on a computer. Faithful to long-time friends such as Seth Haslett, the irascible town physician, Jessica also made new friends in her travels. She was sensible without being a fuddy-duddy, adventurous but not foolish, and nurturing but not controlling. She had a sense of humor, and her infectious laugh was often highlighted in the ending shot of the show. Most of all, her keen intellect was reflected in her abilities to use logic, make deductions, remember important details, and, of course, solve murders.

—*Elizabeth Ann Bokelman*

See also: Matlock; Wisdom; Women and aging

NATIONAL ASIAN PACIFIC CENTER ON AGING

Date: Founded in 1979

Relevant Issues: Health and medicine, race and ethnicity, work

Significance: This organization meets the special needs of the rapidly increasing number of older Asian Americans and Pacific Americans, particularly in the areas of health care and employment.

The National Asian Pacific Center on Aging (NAPCA), with its headquarters in Seattle, Washington, is dedicated to serving aging members of the Asian American and Pacific Islander (AAPI) communities across the United States. Their mission is to break down the cultural, racial, and language barriers and help be the voice of APPI adults and their families to increase access to health and social services. These include educating elders about healthy aging, assisting mature workers with employment and training, and preventing elder abuse. According to the United States Census Bureau, this segment of the aging population is growing at a faster rate than any other segment. There are currently 3.2 million Asian American elders and 162,000 Pacific Islander elders across the United States, with the largest population residing in California, Hawaii, and New York. The number of older Americans in this group is expected to increase nearly 145 percent between 2010 and 2030.

Over half the AAPI population in the United States have limited English proficiency (LEP). LEP means that they do not speak English as their primary language and have limited ability to read, write, speak, and understand English. NAPCA serves over 50 different AAPI ethnicities whom speak over 100 different languages. NAPCA created the Helpline to address the issue of LEP for Asian elders' and is a free service available for LEP and non-English speaking Chinese, Korean, and Vietnamese elders. It is a service that helps increase access for elders to health care and health benefit information such as Medicare or Medicaid.

NAPCA is involved in three important national projects dealing with employment of older members (55 years or older) of the Asian and Pacific communities. They are:

1. The Senior Community Service Employment Program. The Senior Community Service Employment Program (SCSEP), is a federally funded program that provides low-income elders with part-time employment and on-the-job training as a not-for-profit community service program or eligible government agency. The goal of this program is to provide the elders with the opportunity to improve their job skills and increase their competitiveness to find full or part-time unsubsidized employment. NAPCA's participation in this program involves more than 1,200 older workers annually across the United States.

2. The Senior Environmental Employment Program. The Senior Environmental Employment Program (SEE), administered by the United States Environmental Protection Agency (EPA), provides part-time and full-time employment for elders ranging from clerical to scientific and field position in EPA offices. NAPCA matches eligible professionals with qualified government agencies from three field offices that include: Washington DC; Chicago, Illinois; and Seattle, Washington.

3. The Agricultural Conservation Experienced Services Program. The Agricultural Conservation Experienced Services Program (ACES), administered by the United States Department of Agriculture Natural Resources Conservation Service, provides part-time and full-time positions for workers to support conservation-related programs.

—*Rose Secrest*
Updated by Shirley Kuan, RN

See also: Advocacy; Asian Americans; Employment

NATIONAL CAUCUS AND CENTER ON BLACK AGED

Date: Founded in 1970
Relevant Issues: Economics, race and ethnicity, work
Significance: The National Caucus and Center on Black Aged is the only national organization whose major focus is improving life for African American and low-income elderly

In 1970, a group of concerned citizens led by Hobart C. Jackson, a nursing home professional, organized the National Caucus and Center on Black Aged (NCBA) to ensure that the 1971 White House Conference on Aging would address the particular needs of the African American elderly. The caucus existed as an advocacy group until 1973, when it received a grant from the Administration on Aging (AoA) to conduct research, train personnel, and serve as a technical resource. In 1978, the NCBA received a major grant from the U.S. Labor Department to operate the Senior Community Service Employment Program (SCSEP) in five states. In 1983, the caucus expanded to include senior housing.

By 2018, the NCBA had become one of the largest minority-focused organizations in the United States, with thirty-two chapters, employment offices in nine states and the District of Columbia, and six owned and managed housing projects. The NCBA was recognized as a national leader in housing, employment, and advocacy on behalf of African American aged. Its website (www.ncba-aging.org/) includes links to a mission and goal statement, a capability statement, membership information, announcements of conferences and meetings, chapter locations with contacts, and historical information about the organization. It celebrated its forty-fifth anniversary in 2015.

NCBA programs include the Senior Employment Program, the Senior Environmental Employment Program, and the Wellness Promotion and Disease Prevention Program.

—*Mary E. Allen*

See also: Advocacy; African Americans; Employment; Housing; White House Conference on Aging

NATIONAL COUNCIL ON AGING

Date: Founded in 1950
Relevant Issues: Culture, law, media, values
Significance: The National Council on the Aging seeks to improve public and private policies affecting older people.

The changing age structure of the United States has thrust the elderly into the center of American politics, both as a political force and as a topic of debate. Since its founding in 1950, the National Council on the Aging (NCOA) has played a vital role in the development of key legislation to improve the life of older people. The primary short-term goal of the NCOA is to promote the dignity, well-being, self-determination, and contributions of aging people, while its long-term goal is to develop a caring, just world where the aging make vital and valued contributions to families, communities, the world, and future generations.

The NCOA is an association of organizations and individuals committed to enhancing the field of aging through leadership, education, advocacy, and service. To accomplish its goals, the NCOA works closely with professionals and volunteers, service providers, consumer and labor groups, businesses, government agencies, religious groups, and voluntary organizations. Members of the NCOA have many opportunities to participate in the development and expression of public policy views through participation in constituent units and through activities of the NCOA Annual Conference, held in even years in Washington, DC.

The advocacy of the NCOA takes the form of testimony before the U.S. Congress and consultation with government agencies and private organizations. The NCOA has also engaged in fact finding to dispel destructive attitudes toward aging and has sought to counter ideas and campaigns that attempt to pit generations against each other. Two major concerns among the elderly are: (1) the maintenance of Social Security benefits and (2) the establishment of a long-term health care program. The NCOA has long advocated national health-care reform based on principles of universal access and comprehensive coverage that includes long-term care for all generations.

The NCOA provides strong lobbying support for the aging and has been instrumental in the development of the Older Americans Act (OAA), the Age Discrimination in Employment Act (ADEA), Medicare, and Medicaid. It also has been active in protecting Social Security benefits for older people and plays a key role in promoting reform of the Social Security system to ensure that the program will be in operation for future generations of the elderly. The NCOA has helped transform the image of the elderly from one of an underprivileged and forgotten segment of society to one of a powerful and effective voting bloc.

The NCOA is a founding member and cochair in the Leadership of Aging Organizations, which meets in Washington, DC. It is also represented among the nongovernmental organizations (NGOs) of the United Nations (UN) and is in touch with developments in aging throughout the world. The NCOA publishes a biennial statement of essential public policy principles, together with specific recommendations in the broad areas of health, economic security, community services, and housing. The organization also releases policy statements that provide access to its positions on Medicare, Medicaid, Social Security, the OOA, and other policy issues that relate to the elderly.

—*Alvin K. Benson*

See also: Advocacy; Age Discrimination in Employment Act of 1967; Health care; Medicaid; Medicare; Older Americans Act of 1965; Politics; Social Security; Voting patterns

NATIONAL HISPANIC COUNCIL ON AGING

Date: Founded in 1980

Relevant Issues: Culture, demographics, family, race and ethnicity

Significance: This advocacy group addresses concerns associated with aging among Latinos, the fastest-growing segment of the national population over age sixty-five.

Founded in 1980, the National Hispanic Council on Aging (NHCOA) is a nonprofit organization whose mission is to promote the health and well-being of Latino elderly people. A membership organization based in Washington, DC, and governed by a board of directors, the NHCOA produces culturally and linguistically appropriate educational materials. The organization publishes a quarterly newsletter called Noticias (available in English or Spanish) and has published several books, including Hispanic Elderly (1988), edited by Marta Sotomayor and Herman Curiel, and Empowering Hispanic Families (1991), edited by Sotomayor.

The NHCOA is also involved in research, policy analysis, demonstration projects, and training. Members, in association with other organizations, address problems commonly encountered by the Latino elderly and their families, including poverty, limited access to health care, lack of affordable housing, and inadequate social services support. Among its accomplishments is Casa Iris, a forty-unit housing project in Washington, DC, built in cooperation with the Department of Housing and Community Development (DHCD). The council also sponsors a program promoting the early detection of cervical and breast cancer. As with other similar groups (such as the National Indian Council on Aging) (NICOA), the NHCOA acts as a network for organizations and community groups interested in their elderly. The council compiles and disseminates research data, sponsors workshops and a semiannual national conference, and maintains a speaker's bureau, thus supplying national leadership in support of the Latino elderly.

In the mid-2000s, Dr. Yanira Cruz became President and CEO of the organization, aiming to become an affiliate-based organization. NHCOA began supporting a network of independent affiliates throughout the country. Annual national conferences allow for professionals in the field to exchange information, analyze current challenges, and seek opportunities to create positive change within the community.

—*Lee Anne Martinez*

See also: Advocacy; Housing; Latinx Americans

NATIONAL INSTITUTE ON AGING

Date: Established in 1974

Relevant Issues: Demographics, health and medicine, psychology, sociology

Significance: The National Institute on Aging, a department of the National Institutes of Health, serves as a catalyst for innovative research, lifestyle-enhancing technologies, and health-care services related to aging.

Funded by public tax dollars, the National Institutes of Health (NIH) is one of eight agencies of the Public Health Service (PHS), which is part of the U.S. Department of Health and Human Services (HHS). The NIH consists of twenty-four separate institutes, centers, and divisions sponsoring biomedical research in the United States. The goal of NIH research is to acquire new knowledge to help prevent, detect, diagnose, and treat disability and disease.

The National Institute on Aging (NIA) was established as one of the National Institutes of Health (NIH) institutes in 1974. It is the main federal agency focusing on aging. The NIA guides and sponsors collaborative activities with other NIH institutes and other research and clinical agencies. This research is conducted on the NIH campus in Bethesda, Maryland, and also at research and training facilities in hospitals, medical centers, and universities.

The NIA's work focuses on diverse and specific areas of science, each in a specialized program emphasizing a different kind of investigation related to aging. The Biology of Aging Program focuses on basic biologic mechanisms involved in aging, the onset of age-related disease, and research and training in biochemistry, endocrinology, genetics, immunology, molecular and cell biology, nutrition, and pathobiology. The Behavioral and Social Research Program (BSR) supports social and behavioral science research on the processes of aging, the place of elders in society, demography and the age composition of the population, and the impact of the aging population on society as a whole. The Neuroscience and Neuropsychology of Aging (NNA) Program supports research on the physiology of the aging nervous system and the behavioral characteristics of the aging brain. It also has a special focus on Alzheimer's disease, concentrating on its epidemiology, causes, diagnosis, treatment, and short- and long-term management. Finally, the Geriatrics Program supports research on the causes, prevention, and treatment of the health problems of elders, covering such topics as physical frailty and osteoporosis, pharmacology, and rehabilitation. The program also provides such services as the physical and mental assessment of elders and specialty training for providers working with geriatric populations.

The NIA also has a public information office committed to fostering public education on aging through press releases, public service announcements, and the dispensation of science-based educational materials on lifestyle practices that affect health and the aging process. The materials produced cover a wide range of topics, including Alzheimer's disease, the menopause, aging and exercise, cardiovascular disease, and effective communication between professionals and older patients. In addition, the office publishes a directory of aging-related resources. The materials are written for use by the general public, patients and family members, health professionals, the media, and volunteer and community organizations. Booklets, brochures, and fact sheets are available via the Internet and in print for little to no cost.

—Nancy A. Piotrowski

See also: Advocacy; Aging: Biological, psychological, and sociocultural perspectives; Aging process; Health care

NATIVE AMERICANS

Relevant Issues: Culture, demographics, economics, health and medicine

Significance: Race, age, ethnicity, and tribal membership define a high-risk population of Native American elders; the heterogeneity of more than six hundred distinct and evolving cultures complicates the picture and challenges assumptions.

Even a superficial understanding of Native American elders requires some background on Native Americans. As the first peoples to inhabit North America and to organize civilizations there, Indians have variably resisted colonization since European invaders "discovered" the Americas in 1492. The complete occupation of the eastern half of the continent can be symbolized by a yearlong event the Cherokee called Nunahi-Duna-Dlo-Hilu-I, commonly translated as the Trail of Tears. In the spring of 1838, the military, led by President (and former Army General) Andrew Jackson, ignored a ruling in favor of the Cherokee by U.S. Supreme Court Chief Justice John Marshall by illegally arresting and interning Southeastern Indians, expelling them from their homelands, and forcing them to march to the Indian Territory (now Oklahoma).

Under armed guard and without preparation, the Cherokees and others were forced on an arduous thousand-mile march through winter snows to territories unknown. Thousands died on the trail in a prelude to apartheid encountered on reservations west of the Mississippi. Subsequently, the reservation system, too, was slowly undermined in an uncoordinated century-long effort to engineer the partial assimilation and near cultural genocide of Native Americans. Nevertheless, according to Robert L. Schneider and Nancy R Kropf, Indian peoples maintained their wide-ranging diversity of languages, religions, lifestyles, cultures, and national governments.

Federal policy toward indigenous North Americans has resulted in the numerical and geographical marginalization of Indians on their own continent. Once the entire population of what is now the United States, Native Americans are often grouped under "other" or "too small to be statistically significant" by contemporary demographic reports. Some individuals have attempted to assuage the effects of the most savage federal policies, but most attempts have been paternalistic lone efforts lacking a critical mass of the electorate to reverse fully the genocidal tide.

The most notable exception was the Indian Self-Determination Act of 1975. Through this single law, tribal governments have increasingly seized control of, and given direction to, federal programs that permeate reservation life. In related developments, the Smithsonian Institution's National Museum of the American Indian (NMAI) is making authentic strides toward the empowerment of Indian communities. They can tell their own stories, start dialogues with one another, and construct their own representations for mainstream America. With NMAI's help, the Internet is linking reservations and bringing Native Americans together in virtual reality. As a consequence, solidarity among indigenous peoples of the Americas is beginning to have real meaning for the first time in history.

DEMOGRAPHICS

Native Americans, including the Aleut and Inuit (Eskimos), are members of 558 distinct sovereign nations that peacefully coexist, by treaty, within the borders of the continental United States. R. John's demographic review in Full Color Aging (1999) asserted that there were 165,842 Indian elders in 1990, defining elders as those with a chronological age of sixty years or more. At the time, this figure represented 8.5 percent of the total Native American population of 1,959,234 individuals, an estimated 52 percent increase among Indian elders from 1980 to 1990. According to a 1998 report by Robert N. Butler, Myrna I. Lewis, and Trey Sunderland, a majority of Indian elders live in five Southwestern states—Oklahoma, California, Arizona, New Mexico, and Texas—while a substantial portion of the remainder reside on widely scattered reservations, trust lands, tribal jurisdictions, and reservation proximal environs near the Canadian border.

U.S. population increased 9.7 percent from 2000 to 2010 (281.4 million to 308.7 million). Native Americans and Akaska Natives increased 26.7 percent (4.1 million to 5.2 million). The total U.S. population in 2017 according to the Census Bureau's estimate was 325,719,178. Native American and Alaska Native population numbered 6,795,785 or 2.09 percent of the total. According to a study published in 2015 led by Kathleen P. Conte, "The number of older Native Americans is expected to increase almost four-fold, with a resulting increase to 918,000 in 2050 from 235,000 in 2010. Moreover, Native Americans aged =85 years are expected to grow nine-fold between 2010 and 2050."

Indian Health Service (IHS) verification of entitlement offers the most reliable count of federally recognized Native Americans. In 1997, IHS reported 1.8 million system users, while researchers estimated 2.2 million people self-identifying as Native Americans. Some allege that recent Native American census counts are 33 percent inflated by a second population that began embracing their distant Indian ancestry after 1970. Much like Irish Americans and Italian Americans, they fall into a category of so-called hyphenated Americans sharing wide-ranging degrees of unverified descent. This second Indian population lacks a legal claim to treaty protections and entitlements. Demographics are further complicated by variations in tribal membership rules and the fact that any given tribe's sovereignty remains vulnerable to the vicissitudes of federal recognition. Though many of the tribes that were previously legislated out of existence have been restored, more than one hundred groups still pursue federal recognition. These anomalies give rise to a third population of individuals who self-identify as "full-blooded Indian" by descent from grandparents with tribal affiliations but who are unable to meet the tests of any single tribe's membership rules.

Putting aside the debate surrounding a Census over count of the gross Indian population, there are strong arguments that the Census specifically undercounts Native American elders. This paradox is understandable considering that younger U.S. citizens are more likely than elders to be influenced by multiculturalism, accepting themselves as hyphenated Americans and self-identifying as "Indian Americans." Simultaneously, elders, who are more rural and more culturally isolated than the Indian population generally, are more susceptible to underrepresentation in the Census count, even as other subpopulations are being inflated.

—*Sherry Cummings and Clifford Cockerham*
Updated by Bruce E. Johansen, PhD

See also: Alcohol use disorder; Cardiovascular disease; Cultural views of aging; Depression; Diabetes; Family relationships; Grandparenthood; Health care; Homelessness; Housing; Hypertension Obesity; Poverty; Religion; Suicide; Wisdom

For Further Information

Braun, Kathryn L. "The Historic and Ongoing Issue of Health Disparities among Native Elders." *Generations*, vol. 38, no. 4, Jan. 2015, pp. 60-69. ResearchGate. www.researchgate.net/publication/292428492_The_historic_and_ongoing_issue_of_health_disparities_among_native_elders. Presents data on demographic and health indicators of native elders, discusses possible reasons for relatively poor health outcomes, and makes recommendations for research and practice.

Butler, Robert N., Myrna I. Lewis, and Trey Sunderland. Aging and Mental Health: Positive Psychosocial and Biomedical Approaches. Allyn & Bacon, 1998. Extremely well respected in social work, geriatric medicine, nursing, and related disciplines for its comprehensive coverage of the aging process and its effects on mental health.

Conte, Kathleen P., Marc B. Schure, and R. Turner Goins. "Correlates of Social Support in Older American Indians: The Native Elder Care Study." *Aging and Mental Health*. 2015, vol. 19, no. 9: 835-43.doi: 10.1080/13607863.2014.967171. This study examined social support and identified demographic and health correlates among American Indians aged 55 years and older.

Coyhis, Don. *Meditations with Native American Elders: The Four Seasons*. Coyhis Pub. & Consulting, Inc., 2007. A day-at-a-time book offering a quotation by a Native Elder at the top of each page in separate entries over an entire year. Each quote is followed by a reflection by Coyhis.

Curyto, K. J., et al. "Prevalence and Prediction of Depression in American Indian Elderly." *Clinical Gerontologist*, vol. 18, no. 3. 1998, pp. 19-37. doi: 10.1300/J018v18n03_04. 309. Great Lakes American Indian elderly from urban, rural, and reservation settings were interviewed and depression prevalence and its correlates were examined.

Goins, R. T., et al. "Adult Caregiving Among American Indians: The Role of Cultural Factors." *The Gerontologist*, vol. 51, no. 3, 9 Dec. 2010, pp. 310-20. doi:10.1093/geront/gnq101. With a sample of American Indian adults, the report estimates the prevalence of adult caregiving, assesses the demographic and cultural profile of caregivers, and examines the association between cultural factors and being a caregiver.

John, R. "Aging Among American Indians: Income Security, Health, and Social Support Networks." In Full Color Aging, edited by T. P. Miles. Gerontological Society of America, 1999.

National Resource Center on Native American Aging. www.nrcnaa.org/. The National Resource Center on Native American Aging (NRCNAA) is committed to identifying Native elder health and social issues.

NEARSIGHTEDNESS

Also Known As: Myopia
Relevant Issues: Biology, health and medicine
Significance: Nearsightedness, a visual defect that impairs the perception of distant objects, is a prevalent problem for elderly people.

Key Terms:

cornea: the transparent layer forming the front of the eye

CAUSES AND SYMPTOMS

Nearsightedness (also termed myopia) represents the most common eye-related abnormality worldwide, affecting approximately one-third of the U.S. population. This condition arises when light from distant objects reaches a focal point in front of the retina, the photoreceptive tissue of the eye. Consequently, vision of distant objects is blurred on the retina, while objects in close proximity to the individual can be clearly visualized. The primary cause of myopia is an eyeball that is too long from front to back. Alternatively, the cornea (the foremost structure of the eye) may exhibit excessive curvature and predispose the individual to myopia. Higher testosterone levels in the womb and genetic predisposition have been advanced as possible causes of this condition. Research has also found that prolonged eyestrain, especially that which often accompanies long periods of reading, can distort the shape of the eye and render it myopic. This is one reason why well-educated individuals typically manifest higher rates of nearsightedness than less-educated individuals.

All children are born nearsighted to some degree; by the age of six months, however, vision begins to improve. Myopia is an uncommon problem in younger school-age children but begins to increase in prevalence as children move into their teenage years. From the twenties until the late sixties, the rate of visual deterioration tends to slow down, concomitant with a decrease in eye growth. By the time people reach their seventies, however, the rate of visual decline accelerates again. Individuals past the age of seventy are fourteen times as likely to experience myopia resulting in legal blindness than those in their twenties.

TREATMENT AND THERAPY

For several centuries, nearsightedness has been corrected primarily through the use of eyeglasses. Concave lenses, in particular, move the focal point of light in myopic eyes closer to the retina. Contact lenses, which employ a similar mechanism, represent another popular method of vision correction. In certain cases of myopia, vision therapy, through the administration of eye-based exercises, may be another conservative treatment option.

As the twentieth century drew to a close, innovative surgical approaches were developed to address myopia in a more long-lasting manner, especially in adults. Most of these procedures change the shape of the cornea to decrease the distance between the focal point of light and the retina. One such procedure is corneal refractive therapy (CRT), which involves the application of custom-designed contact lenses that act, over time, to flatten the cornea. Laser procedures such as photorefractive keratectomy (PRK) and laser in situ keratomileusis LASIK utilize a laser beam to shave off a predetermined amount of corneal tissue, thereby refocusing light onto the retina.

PERSPECTIVES AND PROSPECTS

Recent research indicates that the prevalence of myopia will continue to rise in the future. The impact of myopia on one's quality of life is hard to overstate, especially considering its association with a variety of serious vision-impairing conditions, including glaucoma and early-onset cataract. Despite the numerous treatment modalities available to nearsighted individuals, it remains largely unclear how to slow, if not prevent, the development of myopia. Various methods have been proposed, including participation in outdoor activities/sports, atropine eye drops, and multifocal lenses (designed to provide clear vision across a wider range of distances). Current literature on this topic is relatively limited but shows a modest positive effect with these interventions. Further research is needed to confirm these findings on a larger scale, however.

—Paul J. Chara Jr
Updated by Ariel R. Choi, Sc.B.

See also: Aging process; Cataracts; Glaucoma; Reading glasses; Vision changes and disorders

For Further Information

Higgins, Jeffrey. *Eye Infections, Blindness and Myopia.* Nova Biomed. Books, 2009.

"Myopia (Nearsightedness)." American Optometric Association. www.aoa.org/patients-and-public/eye-and-vision-problems/glossary-of-eye-and-vision-conditions/myopia. General information on myopia.

Russo, Andrea, et al. "Myopia Onset and Progression: Can It Be Prevented?" *International Ophthalmology*, vol. 34, no. 3, 2013, pp. 693-705. doi:10.1007/s10792-013-9844-1. This review assesses the effects of several types of lifestyle and interventions, including outdoor activities, eye drops, under-correction of myopia, multifocal spectacles, contact lenses, and refractive surgery on the onset and progression of nearsightedness.

Saftari, Liana Nafisa, and Oh-Sang Kwon. "Ageing Vision and Falls: A Review." *Journal of Physiological Anthropology*, vol. 37, no. 1, 23 Apr. 2018. doi:10.1186/s40101-018-0170-1. Reviews existing studies regarding visual risk factors for falls and the effect of ageing vision on falls. Then presents a group of phenomena such as vection and sensory reweighting that provide information on how visual motion signals are used to maintain balance.

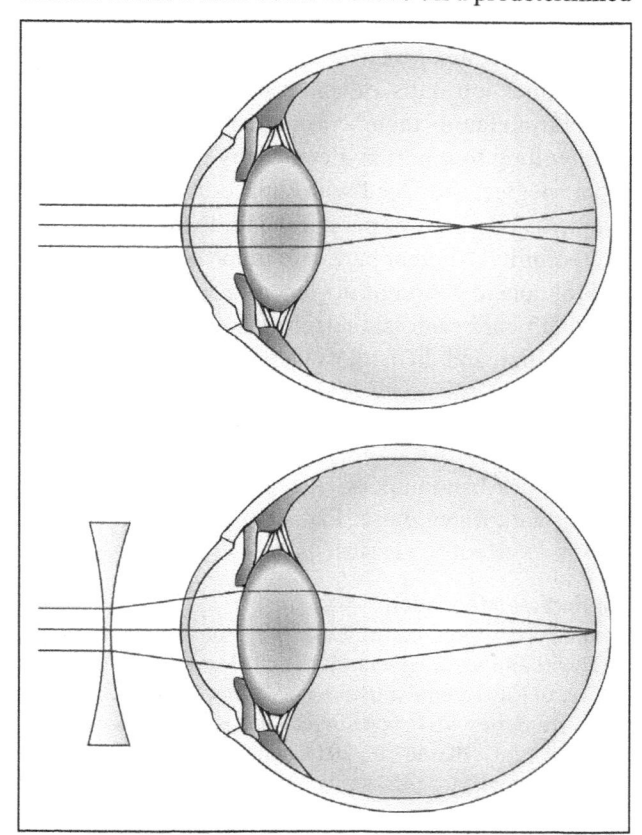

Compensating for myopia using a corrective lens.. (via Wikimedia Commons)

NEGLECT

Relevant Issues: Family, health and medicine, sociology, violence

Significance: Elder mistreatment is a significant problem that can result in both physical and psychological neglect.

Neglect and abuse are underreported, undetected, and affects more than 1 million elderly people each year. Neglect falls within the realm of domestic violence, seen or unseen acts of harm that lead to physical, emotional, or other injury to another person. Indicators of physical neglect include poor hygiene and lack of skin integrity, such as urine burns (skin redness and sores), insect bites, and abrasions; contracture of muscles; dehydration and malnutrition; intestinal blockage with fecal material; and inadequate living environment, such as the presence of physical hazards and insects, as well as insufficient heating and food supplies. Neglect can also be psychological, as elderly patients without social support are at risk for cognitive decline. Possible indicators of psychological neglect include habit disorders, such as sucking, biting, and rocking; conduct disorders, such as antisocial and destructive behaviors; neurotic traits, including sleep and speech disorders; and psychoneurotic reactions, such as hysteria, obsession, compulsion, and phobias.

The typical victim of neglect is a Caucasian woman over the age of seventy-five years, is physically or mentally impaired, and lives with a relative. The person who neglects the elder is most often a family member who serves a caregiver role for the elderly person. The elder is often a source of stress and is dependent on the caregiver.

Several specific stressors may lead caregivers to neglect the elders for whom they are caring. First, family dynamics may have included poor past relationships between caregivers and elders, or may have included a history of marital conflict and family violence. Second, physical and mental impairments among the elderly may cause increased demands on caregivers, which often results in physical, emotional, and financial stress for caregivers. Third, caregivers may be physically or psychologically unequipped to serve as caregivers, resulting in neglect. Fourth, problem behaviors among the elderly, such as combativeness, verbal belligerence, wandering, and bowel or bladder incontinence, may precipitate neglect. A major contributor to elder neglect is caregiver fatigue. Caregivers may feel overwhelmed, unappreciated, isolated, and frustrated and may respond by neglecting elders who are viewed as the cause of isolation and frustration.

Once risk factors for neglect are identified, several steps may be taken to remedy the situation: A community agency may be referred to for monitoring, strategies may be taught to decrease the caregiver's stress, or elders can be placed in another living situation. In cases of documented evidence of neglect, Adult Protective Services (APS) may initiate short- and long-term interventions for both victims and caregivers based on causation. Caregiver support may lead to improved rates of elderly neglect and is an area of active research.

Detection of neglect remains a problem, as it is difficult to complain or report a person who is providing most of one's daily needs. Many victims of neglect fear reprisal or cessation of caring by caregivers or placement in a nursing home. Additionally, elders who suffer from mental impairment with memory loss, who lack communication skills, or who want to hide their predicament from family members or outsiders may be unable or unwilling to report neglect. Many elders who try to report neglect are faced with the stereotype of elderly people as confused or paranoid and, therefore, lacking in credibility. Another barrier to reporting neglect is the lack of consideration of neglect as a specific diagnosis by health-care professionals. Much neglect is subtle in presentation and difficult to identify.

—Linda L. Pierce
Updated by Patrick Richardson, MSN

See also: Abandonment; Adult Protective Services; Caregiving; Elder abuse; Family relationships; Malnutrition; Psychiatry, geriatric

For Further Information

Ayalon, Liat. "Reports of Elder Neglect by Older Adults, Their Family Caregivers, and Their Home Care Workers: A Test of Measurement Invariance." *The Journals of Gerontology Series B: Psychological Sciences and Social Sciences*, vol. 70, no. 3, 2014, pp. 432-42. doi:10.1093/geronb/gbu051. This study evaluates the measurement invariance of a 7-item scale designed to assess elder neglect across three groups of informants: Older adults, family members, and home-care workers.

Day, Mary Rose, et al. *Self-Neglect in Older Adults: A Global, Evidence-Based Resource for Nurses and Other Health Care Providers.* Springer Publishing, 2018. This authoritative resource provides nurses and other health-care professionals with a comprehensive overview and analysis of self-neglect in older adults.

Hoover, Robert M., and Michol Polson. "Detecting Elder Abuse and Neglect: Assessment and Intervention." *American Family Physician*, vol. 89, no. 6, 15 Mar. 2014, pp. 453-60. Endorses a detailed medical evaluation of patients suspected of being abused.

"Preventing Elder Abuse and Neglect in Older Adults." HealthInAging.org, July 2017. www.healthinaging.org/tools-and-tips/preventing-elder-abuse-and-neglect-older-adults. Offers advice on what to do in cases of elder neglect.

NEUGARTEN, BERNICE

Born: February 11, 1916; Norfolk, Nebraska
Relevant Issues: Family, health and medicine, sociology
Significance: Bernice Neugarten conducted groundbreaking research on all aspects of aging, focusing on aging as a normal, rather than a pathological, process.

Bernice Levin Neugarten, who focused on the study of aging people and changes in personality over the life span of adults, began her career with the intention of expanding the field of gerontology. She later came to wonder if there should be a field of gerontology at all. Her daughter, Dail Neugarten, said of her mother, "Given her innate curiosity, Neugarten constantly reinvented the field of adult development and aging, and in so doing, consistently revitalized her students, her colleagues, and herself."

A prolific writer in the field of adult development and aging, Neugarten brought previously unrecognized topics to light during her many years of research. Her research on the menopause, grandparenthood, and parent caring relied on careful and accurate quantitative and qualitative methods. She coined many phrases that are now used in common parlance, including "social clock," "young-old" and "old-old," "age-integrated society," and "age-irrelevance." Important areas of research to which she has contributed include age as a dimension of social organization, the life course, personality and adaptation, and social policy issues.

In 1968, Neugarten edited Middle Age and Aging, a collection of essays that discuss the manner in which society in general divides itself into different age-related roles. Neugarten paid particular attention to "social and psychological processes as individuals move from middle age to old age." She called attention to the question, "What social and psychological adaptations are required as individuals move through the second half of their lives?" Issues regarding health are often omitted in studies of the aging process. Neugarten viewed this as regrettable because, she believed, the issues of physical health must be considered in understanding the social and psychological behaviors in aging.

In 1981, Northwestern University founded the Human Development and Social Policy (HDSP) graduate program under the leadership of Neugarten. HDSP meets the growing need for researchers, decision makers, and professionally trained scholars who can evaluate critical issues that affect daily human life and public policy. Graduates of HDSP have a wide range of career choices that deal with critical issues of midlife and aging populations.

Neugarten's work reflected her belief that an individual's attitude toward health and changing roles through midlife and into old-age are important. Some of these attitudes, according to Neugarten, are changing family roles; work, retirement, and leisure; other dimensions of the immediate social environment such as friendships, neighboring patterns, and living arrangements; differences in cultural setting; and perspectives of time and death. "The aging-society," Neugarten claimed, "brings with it many challenges and opportunities for both aging persons and for the society at large." After her retirement, Neugarten was named professor emerita in the Department of Behavioral Sciences at the University of Chicago.

—*Virginiae Blackmon*

See also: Aging: Biological, psychological, and sociocultural perspectives; Cultural views of aging; Erikson, Erik H.; Kübler-Ross, Elisabeth

NO STONE UNTURNED: THE LIFE AND TIMES OF MAGGIE KUHN (BOOK)

Author: Maggie Kuhn, with Christina Long and Laura Quinn
Date: Published in 1991
Relevant Issues: Law, media, values
Significance: This autobiography by Kuhn, the founder of the Gray Panthers, traces her many accomplishments before and after she became an advocate for older people.

In her autobiography *No Stone Unturned*, Maggie Kuhn writes that she discovered "all injustices, however small or seemingly unrelated, are linked." Throughout her long and extraordinary life, she addressed the intertwined injustices of sexism, ageism, ableism, social elitism, and racism.

Born into an intergenerational home where "men were treated with great deference, but the house was ruled by women," she was the eldest daughter of an older, supportive mother and an adoring, demanding father. Why did she never marry, despite her enjoyment of men and sex? "Sheer luck," she writes.

Kuhn describes how she excelled in academic, social, religious, and career roles, all of which were constricted by society's definition of appropriate female roles. She completed college and studied at Columbia University Teacher's College and Union Theological Seminary. She first pursued a career in the Young Women's Christian Association (YWCA), one of the era's foremost feminist and socialist organizations, advocating full political and economic equality for women. Later, she served as an advocate for hundreds of thousands of women who faced crushing problems in defense production plants during World War II. Kuhn explains how during the 1950s and 1960s, she took progressive stands on civil rights, homosexuality, and Medicare. At a Medicare hearing, President Gerald Ford addressed her as "young lady." She responded, "I am an old woman, Mr. President."

Forced into retirement at age sixty-five, Kuhn organized the Gray Panthers with the vision of a national grassroots organization including young and old activists. She describes her work with consumer advocate Ralph Nader, her challenges to the Gerontological Society of America (GSA) and the American Medical Association (AMA), and her efforts to organize the Older Women's League (OWL), the National Citizens' Coalition for Nursing Home Reform (NCCNHR), and the National Shared Housing Resource Center (NSHRC).

Advocating intergenerational social reform, she writes in *No Stone Unturned*, "We must act as the elders of the tribe, looking out for the best interests of the future and preserving the precious compact between the generations."

—*Anne L. Botsford*

See also: Advocacy; Age discrimination; Ageism; Gerontological Society of America; Gray Panthers; Kuhn, Maggie; Mandatory retirement; Medicare; Women and aging

---

NURSING HOMES. See FACILITY AND INSTITUTIONAL CARE.

NUTRITION

Relevant Issues: Health and medicine
Significance: The requirements for certain nutrients change as people age; in addition, nutrition plays a prominent role in the prevention and treatment of chronic diseases that commonly occur in later years.

Certain functions of the body change as a natural result of the aging process. Many organs are not as efficient as they once were. As these normal physiological changes occur, the requirements for certain nutrients also change. Some changes in the older body are pathological and represent chronic diseases of old age, such as hypertension, diabetes, cardiovascular disease, pulmonary disease, and cancer. Programs designed to prevent or delay the onset of these chronic conditions always include a nutritional component. Even after a disease is established, nutrition maintains a significant role in its treatment.

CHANGING NUTRIENT REQUIREMENTS

Requirements for calories usually decline with age. This decline in caloric need is tied to the common decline in lean body mass and increase in adipose tissue that occurs with aging. This may be because of a decline in energy metabolism. Although some researchers feel that this is associated with an aging body alone, others believe that physical activity also plays a large role in determining what the basal energy metabolism will be. In fact, some experts believe that most of these negative effects can be overcome by a vigorous exercise program.

Changes in protein requirements with age are more controversial because recommendations for both decreased and increased dietary protein intakes have been advocated by different experts. Many believe that dietary protein requirements decrease with age and that this decline is secondary to the decline in lean body mass. Less muscle tissue would require less dietary protein to sustain it. The lower dietary protein recommendation is also congruent with kidney function, which declines somewhat with age as well. The opposing argument claims that higher dietary protein intakes diminish the loss in lean body mass that occurs with aging and that these higher dietary protein intakes are not detrimental to renal function.

Of the vitamins for which there seems to be increased requirements during normal aging, vitamin B12, vitamin D, and vitamin B6 are most prominent. During aging, the amount of hydrochloric acid secreted by the stomach gradually decreases. For many people, this results in achlorhydria (lack of hydrochloric acid in gastric juice) or hypochlorhydria (low levels of hydrochloric acid in gastric juice). The reduction in hydrochloric acid secretion results in less intrinsic factor being secreted. Intrinsic factor is required for efficient absorption of vitamin B12. Therefore, the decrease in intrinsic factor leads to a decrease in the absorption of vitamin B12. This can partially be overcome by ingesting larger amounts of vitamin B12, which will saturate the intrinsic factor carrier system and allow for some free diffusion of vitamin B12. Some of the manifestations of vitamin B12 deficiency are mental changes and dementia. Indeed, many elderly with dementia have subtle vitamin B12 deficiencies.

Although the major dietary source of vitamin D is fortified milk, most vitamin D is synthesized by the skin after exposure to sunshine. The synthesis of vitamin D occurs primarily in the epidermis layer of the skin, where a precursor of vitamin D is metabolized to vitamin D. There is less of this precursor in the epidermis of older people; therefore, less vitamin D is synthesized. Both dietary vitamin D and vitamin D synthesized in the skin must undergo an activation reaction in the kidney. It is also believed that this activation process might be reduced in older people because of the decline in renal function that occurs in aging. Although specific recommendations for older people have not been set concerning vitamin D, additional dietary sources or sunlight exposure are being considered by experts. This is especially important for housebound elders who would benefit by sun exposure on their face and hands for fifteen minutes several times per week.

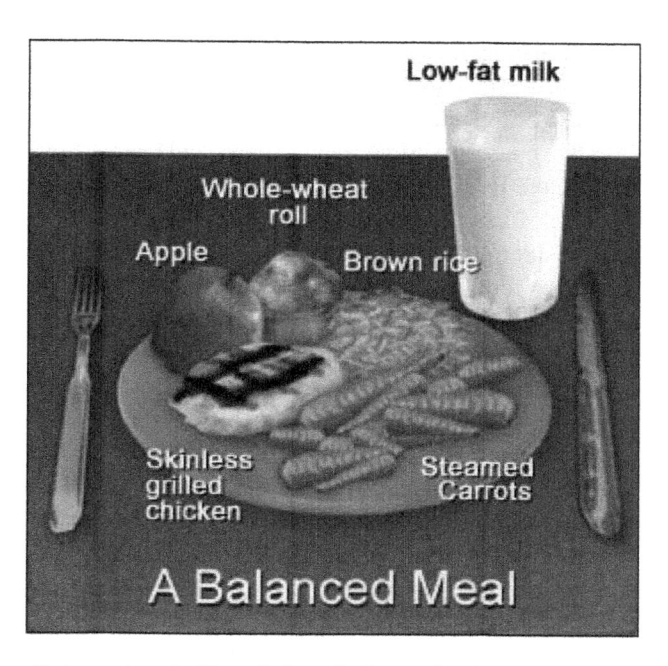

Many elderly have indicators of poor vitamin B6 status, although the cause for this marginal status is not clear. Vitamin B6 requirements are linked to protein intake, so some of the variability may be because of a range of protein intake across many ages and body compositions.

Vitamin A is the only vitamin for which lower requirements have been discussed for the elderly. Preformed vitamin A is found in organ meats, eggs, some fish, and dairy products. Carotenoids found in vegetables and some fruits can be converted to vitamin A. Vitamin A is a fat-soluble vitamin, and excess is stored in the liver. However, vitamin A toxicity can occur when either the liver's capacity to store vitamin A is exceeded or the dose is so large that normal carrying and storage processes are overwhelmed. With a normal, varied diet, sufficient vitamin A will be stored in the liver. The quantity of vitamin A stored will increase as the person ages. Because of the probability of having enough vitamin A stored to cover vitamin A requirements and the possibility that the liver's storage capacity could be exceeded because of long years of vitamin A deposition, experts are considering lowering the recommended intakes of vitamin A for the elderly. However, as carotenoids pose no health risk or threat of toxicity, no recommendation concerning carotenoids has been forthcoming.

Of the minerals, calcium is discussed most often in terms of recommending increased requirements during normal aging. The consensus statement from the National Institutes of Health (NIH) concerning optimal intake of calcium recommends almost twice the current recommended dietary allowance for those over sixty-five years. The reason for the increased calcium intake is based upon a lower intestinal absorption of calcium in the elderly and a decreased conversion of vitamin D to its active form by the older kidney. Vitamin D is necessary for calcium utilization. Higher intakes of calcium are thought to diminish the calcium losses from bone that result in osteoporosis.

Although intestinal absorption of other minerals, such as zinc and iron, may decrease during aging, studies do not suggest a need for an overall increase in dietary intake of these two minerals in general. Furthermore, despite considerable mythology, neither fatigue nor lack of energy seems related to iron status in the elderly. Changes in smell and taste that are common during aging do not seem related to zinc status. However, elderly people with very poor diets, or those who are malnourished, may develop a zinc or iron deficiency that would require dietary modifications.

OSTEOPOROSIS AND CARDIOVASCULAR DISEASE

Most chronic diseases begin to reveal symptoms in middle age. Such symptoms become more severe and impair quality of life in the later years if appropriate therapy is not begun or if such therapy proves ineffective. Chronic diseases for which there is a clear role for nutrition modification in prevention and treatment include osteoporosis, cardiovascular disease, cancer, and diabetes.

Calcium and vitamin D are essential for normal bone matrix to remain viable. Although not the only risk factors in the development of osteoporosis, poor calcium and vitamin D statuses contribute significantly to this risk. Bone health in later years depends upon the peak bone mass determined early in midlife and the rate of bone loss during advancing years. Dietary modification to increase calcium and vitamin D consumption should occur in the young to effect peak bone mass in midlife. However, even increasing calcium and vitamin D consumption in later years can have a favorable impact on the rate of bone loss.

Cardiovascular disease risk includes many factors, such as blood lipid levels, heredity, body weight, exercise level, and smoking history. Diet has been shown to affect blood lipid levels as well as body weight. The blood lipid levels of most concern are the low-density lipoproteins (LDLs), the high-density lipoproteins (HDLs), and the total cholesterol levels. Some discussion has occurred surrounding the cost-effectiveness and ramifications of screening blood lipids in the elderly. Some studies have shown that the risk value of elevated blood lipids is less in the elderly than it is in younger adults. Nevertheless, the consensus seems to be that blood lipid determination in older adults is warranted because the highest incidence of heart disease occurs in people older than age sixty-five.

For those who have high lipid levels, the National Cholesterol Education Program (NCEP) recommends that dietary modification be tried before medication therapy. Such dietary modification includes restriction of dietary fat to no more than 30 percent of total calories, saturated fatty acid intake to 8 to 10 percent, polyunsaturated fatty acid intake to less than 10 percent, monounsaturated fatty acid intake to less than 15 percent, and dietary cholesterol intake to less than 300 milligrams per day. In addition, total caloric intake should be monitored to achieve and maintain desired weight. Studies have shown that therapy that lowers LDL and total cholesterol reduces coronary risk and the total mortality rate. These results include older people. Although some have advocated not restricting the elderly in diet or prescribing medications with possible side-effects, most medical practitioners agree that the high-risk older patient should not be denied the benefits of therapy that can prevent or delay the complications of heart disease.

> **HOW TO TALK TO SENIORS ABOUT DIET ADJUSTMENTS**
>
> **How Do They Feel?**
>
> Seniors may not realize how they would benefit from diet adjustments. Unhealthy eating habits, such as using too much salt or sugar, can be an unconscious response to age-related changes to the senses or appetite. Older adults also may be unaware of healthy eating guidelines, such as reducing red meat consumption. It's common for people to simply follow eating habits they've had throughout their lives. Others may have adopted unhealthy eating habits due to lifestyle changes, such as living alone or living in a senior facility. Some seniors might want to improve their diet but feel unable to do so because of limited finances or lack of access to healthy foods. Limited mobility or low vision can also reduce a senior's ability to prepare meals.
>
> Seniors often face many changes and having to consider dietary changes can be overwhelming or seem unimportant. They might feel frustrated at the suggestion that they should adjust their diet and act resistant. Moreover, trying to sort through diet advice from different sources, including doctors, friends, family members, and advertisements, can be challenging and confusing. This stress can be exacerbated by preexisting anxiety, depression, and other emotional issues.
>
> On the other hand, some seniors view diet adjustments positively. They may be happy to learn of ways to improve and maintain their health. Taking important steps to reduce the risk of chronic conditions such as heart disease or diabetes can feel empowering. Learning about, preparing, and eating healthy foods can also be a fun activity that boosts mental health and slows cognitive decline, especially if done with others.
>
> **How Do I Start The Conversation?**
>
> Diet adjustments can be a sensitive topic for seniors, especially if it means changing long-held habits and giving up favorite foods. When bringing up the subject, you should be aware of their feelings while still communicating the importance of healthy eating. In all circumstances, it is important that your conversations are held in a respectful, empathic manner. The conversation should not be a lecture but a discussion in which the senior is fully engaged. Listening is just as important as relaying information.
>
> You might introduce the topic by sharing an anecdote or story of someone you know who benefitted from a diet adjustment. This can then naturally lead to further discussion. Be sure that the senior has opportunities to express their opinion, and be an active listener. Perhaps ask them to share how they would like to maintain or alter their diet. Questions, asked in a nonthreatening manner, can often be a route to furthering discussions on the subject. Open-ended questions are preferable to avoid a closed yes-or-no response.
>
> Try to avoid saying what a person "should" or "must" do. Effective change is more likely if they feel included in the decision-making process. Avoid becoming overly emotional, and make sure that you do not overreact to their emotional response, including frustration or aggression. Maintain a calm composure, and where relevant gently suggest consulting a qualified professional such as a counselor, doctor, or dietician.
>
> In some situations, an immediate diet adjustment may be required at a doctor's directive. Depending on the senior's physical and cognitive state, you may need to directly oversee the necessary change. In other instances, gradual changes are often more effective. Perhaps start off by replacing an unhealthy item with a healthier alternative a few times a week. Increase the frequency as the senior gets used to the healthier option. Eating meals together also sets a strong example and makes changes seem more normal. For older adults who consistently refuse certain foods, providing options such as smoothies or supplements with needed nutrients may help.
>
> —*Leah Jacob*

CANCER

Diet is known to be a risk factor for several types of cancer common in the older population. Diet is never the sole risk factor, but dietary modification is believed to reduce cancer risk in certain conditions.

There are three phases in the progression of a normal cell into a cancer cell: initiation, promotion, and progression. For cancer to be initiated, the deoxyribonucleic acid (DNA) must be damaged. This damage can occur because of viruses or chemicals. Even after being damaged, cancer will not occur unless the cells are promoted to increase cell division. After promotion, cell division must progress and interfere with normal physiological function. It is at the initiation and promotion stages that most nutrients are thought to have a role in cancer. Some nutrients might help prevent the DNA from becoming damaged, while some might decrease the chance that the damaged cells are promoted. Conversely, some nutrients might increase DNA damage or tumor promotion.

Certain nutrients are believed to increase the risk of cancer. Those include calories, fat, and alcohol. The association between cancer risk and a nutrient appears to be strongest for fat. High fat intake is strongly associated with cancer of the prostate, breast, and colon. There is also an association between cancer and high calorie intake. This might be because diets high in fat are also high in calories. However, it might be that the high caloric intake is really more related to cancer risk than is dietary fat. Nevertheless, high caloric intake is associated with an increased risk of breast and prostate cancer. Alcohol appears to act as a promoter associated with cancer of the esophagus, mouth, and larynx. This is especially true when alcohol is combined with smoking. Alcohol intake has been implicated in the development of breast cancer, although the results are inconclusive.

Certain nutrients seem to reduce the risk for cancer. These include fiber, vitamin C, and carotenoids. The association between fiber and the reduced risk for cancer has been studied for a long time. Fiber may decrease intestinal transit time and thereby decrease the amount of time any potential carcinogen might be in contact with the absorptive surfaces of the gut. Fiber might also trap carcinogens and carry them along to pass through the body unabsorbed. Fiber may also dilute the influence of dietary fat on cancer initiation or promotion. Increasing fiber-rich foods can decrease the proportion of calories coming from fat. However, the reduced risk of cancer associated with high-fiber diets may not be caused by the fiber alone. High-fiber foods such as fruits and vegetables are also high in vitamin C and carotenoids.

Vitamin C, or ascorbic acid, has been associated with a decreased incidence of stomach, larynx, and esophageal cancer. It also appears to decrease the toxicity of nitrosamines, which can be formed when meats are cooked at very high, quick-cooking temperatures and which have been associated with cancer development. Vitamin C, which can act as an antioxidant in certain conditions, can scavenge free radicals, which may have a role in the initiation or promotion stage of cancer development. Carotenoids can also act as antioxidants. Higher intakes of foods that are high in carotenoids, such as fruits and vegetables, are associated with reduced risk of breast, lung, prostate, and cervical cancers.

DIABETES

Another chronic disease that affects millions of older adults is diabetes. In diabetes, the body produces inadequate amounts of insulin, or the insulin produced is not being used effectively. Insulin functions in the body by transporting the sugar from the blood into the cells of the body. The cells then use the sugar (glucose) for energy or store it as fat. If insulin is lacking, the cells are starved for energy, while the sugar in the blood reaches abnormally high levels. Although there are many risk factors for developing diabetes, aging itself is a risk factor. Adult-onset, or type II, diabetes often occurs so gradually that many adults will have had the disease six or more years before it is diagnosed.

Another risk factor for diabetes that is also associated with aging is obesity. More than 75 percent of adults diagnosed with diabetes are obese at the time the diagnosis is made. Indeed, the risk of developing diabetes doubles with every 20 percent of excess weight above desirable weight for gender, age, and height. Therefore, the nutritional prevention of diabetes involves the maintenance of a desirable body weight. Very often this is also the nutritional treatment, although a more rigid dietary structure may also be required.

—*Karen Chapman-Novakofski*

See also: Antioxidants; Bone changes and disorders; Breast cancer; Cancer; Cholesterol; Dementia; Diabetes; Heart disease; Malnutrition; Obesity; Osteoporosis; Prostate cancer; Vitamins and minerals; Weight loss and gain

For Further Information

"Chapter 11. Healthier Older Adults." *A Healthier You*, US Dept. of Health and Human Services. health.gov/dietary guidelines/dga2005/healthieryou/html/chapter11.html.

"Food, Eating and Alzheimer's." Alzheimer's Association. www.alz.org/care/alzheimers-food-eating.asp.
"Lifestyle Changes for Heart Attack Prevention." American Heart Association, July 2015. www.heart.org/HEART ORG/Conditions/HeartAttack/PreventionTreatmentof HeartAttack/ Lifestyle-Changes_UCM_303934_Article. jsp#.
Robinson, Lawrence, and Jeanne Segal. "Eating Well as You Age." HelpGuide.org. Dec. 2016. www.helpguide.org/articles/healthy-eating/eating-well-as-you-age.htm.
Seltzer, Emilee. "6 Vital Nutrition Tips for Seniors." AgingCare.com, 2016. www.agingcare.com/Articles/nutrition-tips-for-elderly-health-and-diets-137053.htm.

OASDI. See SOCIAL SECURITY.

OBESITY

Relevant Issues: Health and medicine
Significance: Obesity is an abnormally high percentage of body fat; it is important to understand the many factors that contribute to obesity in the aging population.
Key Terms:
adiposity: a condition of being severely overweight, or obese
Body Mass Index (BMI): a person's weight in kilograms (kg) divided by his or her height in meters squared

The prevalence of obesity has been increasing in most industrialized nations. The prevalence is higher in certain population groups such as African American women and Latinas. The factors that contribute to obesity are numerous, but the key factor is energy imbalance, which means that more calories are eaten than used by the body. By definition, obesity is an abnormally high percentage of body fat; however, assessing the precise value of this measurement is subject to debate. By 2015, one-third of the population over age 65 were obese; and that percentage has been slowly rising.

MEASUREMENTS OF BODY FAT

Body composition can be measured by several techniques, each with varying degrees of accuracy and cost. One of the best methods is underwater weighing. Using the principle of Archimedes, density is determined from weight of the body both under and out of water. Although this method is relatively easy to perform, people must agree to be submersed and many find the experience unpleasant, especially in the company of medical professionals.

A technique that uses the electrical conductivity of body tissues to estimate fat is based on the premise that lean tissue and fat tissue conduct electromagnetic waves differently. Measuring total body electrical conductivity is expensive. A less expensive technique is bioelectrical impedance, in which electrodes are placed on the arm and leg. Based on level of impedance, one can estimate body fat. This method is accurate provided that the subject is adequately hydrated.

Methods such as computed tomography (CT) scanning and nuclear magnetic resonance imaging (MRI) scanning give an accurate picture of regional fat such as intra-abdominal and extra-abdominal fat. Ultrasonic waves also provide a measure of regional fat. These techniques are impractical for determining total body fat and are expensive. Other accurate total-body composition techniques involve neutron activation, fat-soluble gas, heavy water techniques, and potassium isotopes. All these methods are expensive and impractical for broad scale use.

Simple techniques include height and weight measurement and skinfold thicknesses and circumferences. Skinfolds are a measure of fat under the skin, which perhaps should be more accurately called "fatfolds." The underlying premise is that a certain percentage of the body's fat depot is under the skin. The subject's skinfold measurements can be inserted into standardized prediction equations to estimate body fat. Common sites include the triceps and biceps (arm muscle areas), thighs, and the subscapular (under the shoulder blade) and suprailiac (above the hip bone on the abdomen) regions. Skinfolds are difficult to measure correctly, and practice and skill are required to obtain valid measurements. For the best estimates, multiple skinfold site measures are taken.

If health professionals are interested in assessing obesity on a large scale, the measurement techniques need to be inexpensive and easy to use and to involve little stress on the subject. A more practical technique is measuring height and weight. Measures can be compared to tables of acceptable weights for heights or converted into the body mass index (BMI), also called the Quetelet

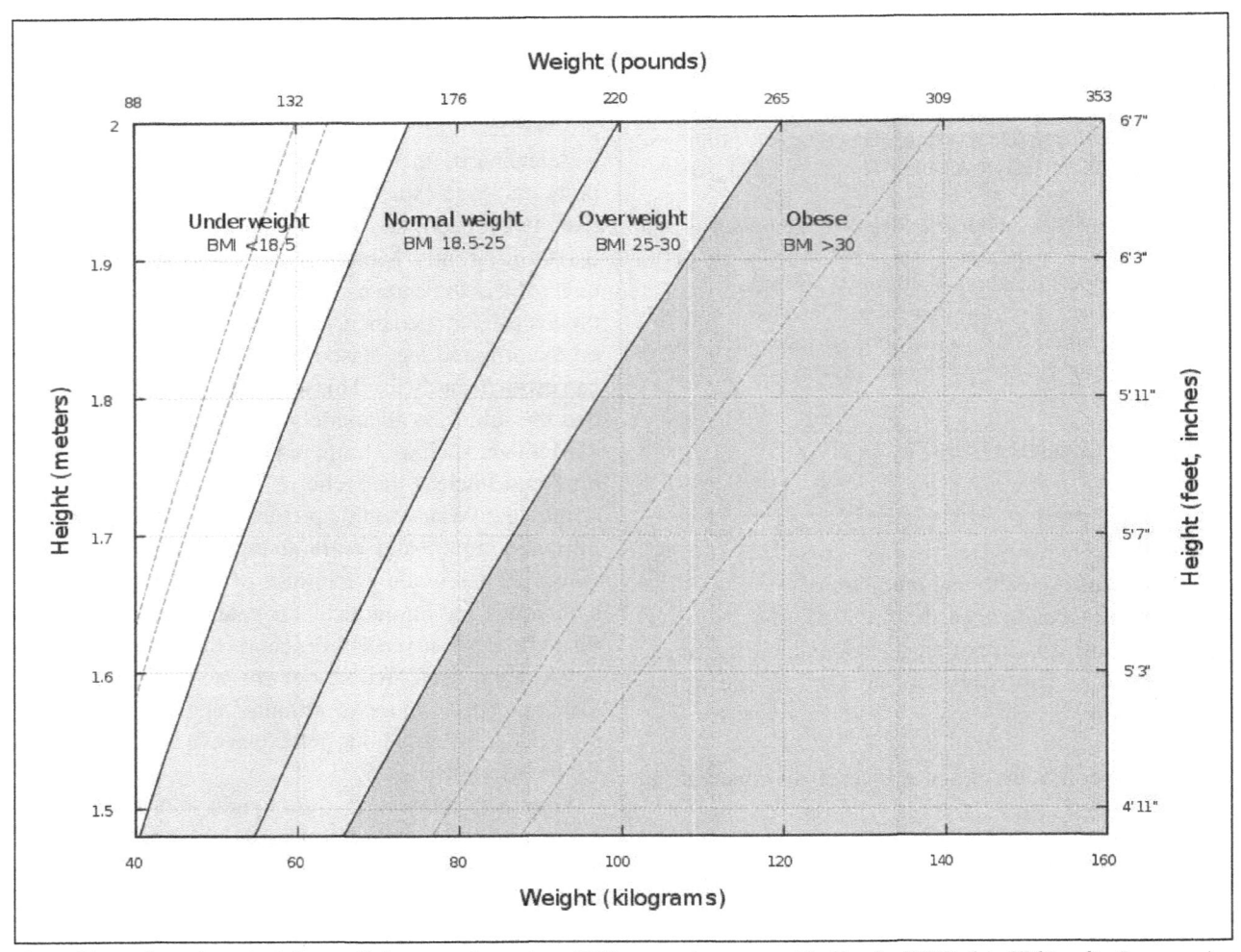

Curved lines show the principle cutoffs between the various BMI categories, as specified by the WHO. (via Wikimedia Commons)

index. BMI gives a measure of weight relative to height. It is calculated as weight in kilograms divided by height in meters squared or as weight in pounds divided by height in inches squared, multiplied by 703. A very simple procedure that provides a close approximation of BMI is height in inches divided by weight in pounds.

In addition to knowing an individual's BMI, it is important to measure where body fat is distributed. Abdominal fat, or central adiposity, is a more potent risk factor for obesity-related diseases than BMI alone. Central adiposity can be measured using a variety of techniques, from sophisticated and expensive techniques such as CT scans to a simple circumference ascertained with a tape measure. Waist circumference provides an estimate of central adiposity that is inexpensive and easy to do. Some experts measure both waist and hip circumference and calculate a waist-hip ratio (WHR). A desirable WHR is under .90 for a man and under .80 for a woman. Waist circumference alone is a useful measure of central adiposity that can be used by health professionals to assess an individual's risk for obesity-related diseases. Thus, two simple parameters, BMI and waist circumference, can be used to define obesity with reasonable accuracy, especially among the older population.

Healthy weight ranges reflect statistically derived values that appear to provide maximal protection against the development of chronic disease. A BMI of 19.0 to 25.0 seems to reflect a healthy weight. Overweight is defined as a BMI between 25.0 and 29.9, and obesity is defined as a BMI of 30.0 or greater. Extreme obesity is defined as a BMI of 40 or greater. For waist circumference, the cutoffs identifying increased disease risk for adults are greater than 40 inches (102 centimeters) for men and greater than 35 inches (88 centimeters) for women. High waist circumference coupled with a high BMI escalates the risk potential for disease.

Body fat composition increases with age. As men age, their fat content almost doubles, while women experience a 50 percent increase as their weight rises only about 10 to 15 percent, reflecting a reduction in lean body mass. When older people become obese, this change of proportion of fat to lean is further exaggerated. Contributing to the problem of obesity in the older population is that energy requirements also decrease with age. For example, basal metabolism, the energy required to rest, declines about 2 percent per decade in adults.

CAUSES OF OBESITY

Although physiological changes in body composition might explain the tendency to gain weight with age, changes in lifestyle can accelerate or retard body composition changes. Numerous labor-saving devices have fostered a reduction in energy output. The physical activity of older people tends to decline as well, further facilitating declines in caloric output.

Many changes in the food supply foster obesity. Numerous snack and convenience foods make it easy to procure and consume excess calories. Eating in restaurants and fast-food establishments provides larger portions of high-calorie, high-fat foods. For elderly persons on fixed incomes, inexpensive food choices are often necessary and are higher in fat and calories. Combining the reduction in energy expended and the increased variety of high-calorie food choices for energy consumed, it is understandable why obesity rates have risen.

HEALTH RISKS OF OBESITY

Obesity is a risk factor for several maladies such as cardiovascular disease, hypertension, diabetes mellitus type II, arthritis, gallbladder disease, gout, and certain cancers. Aging itself is also a risk factor for these diseases. The lowest cardiovascular disease mortality is among those who remain lean throughout life. Obesity increases the risk of high blood cholesterol levels and is estimated to cause 40 to 50 percent of hypertension (high blood pressure). Obese people are five to six times more likely to develop hypertension than lean people. Weight reduction of as little as 10 to 15 pounds in many individuals, however, can reduce the dosage or eliminate the need for drugs to control blood pressure in many individuals.

The rate of type II diabetes rises as BMI increases, with the highest prevalence in those with a BMI higher than 28. This type of diabetes, characterized by the inability of body cells to use insulin, can be corrected with weight reduction. Many elderly with diabetes suffer from related complications, such as kidney disease, blindness, heart disease, and the destruction of sensory function.

Obesity is associated with some cancers. There is a consistent positive relationship between body weight and endometrial cancer, with risk starting at a BMI of 28 to 30 or higher. Postmenopausal women with a BMI of 27 or higher have an increased risk for breast cancer.

Research has estimated that a reduction in BMI of about two units can reduce later onset of knee osteoarthritis and decrease the rate of symptomatic occurrences. Obesity also increases the risk for gall bladder disease, especially among women. Obesity is a risk factor for the development of gout and sleep apnea (episodes of breath cessation during sleep), which is common among those with upper-body obesity.

TREATING OBESITY

People need to reject the notion that increasing weight is a normal phenomenon of aging and begin to make lifestyle changes to prevent weight gain. Dieting alone is not an effective long-term solution because the recidivism rate (and return to obesity) is high. Restrictive dieting can also result in inadequate intake of nutrients.

Drug therapy is not recommended unless the person has a BMI of 30 or higher or a BMI of 27 or higher with concomitant risk factors or diseases. Weight loss surgery is reserved for those with severe obesity or a BMI higher than 35 who also suffer from related disease conditions, but only when all other medical therapies have failed.

Life-long healthy weight maintenance requires a lifestyle that includes regular daily physical activity and consumption of a healthful diet that is calorically matched with energy output. Nothing else has been shown to work as effectively. Weight loss of as little as 10 percent is sufficient to reduce disease risks associated with being overweight. A loss of 5 to 10 pounds helps to lower blood pressure and can improve both blood cholesterol and blood sugar levels. For many elderly, this modest goal is attainable and could provide health benefits. Weight reduction among elderly must be monitored carefully, however, to prevent mistaking disease-related weight loss as the result of voluntary weight loss. With proper guidance, healthful eating patterns coupled with regular physical activity could afford the elderly with marked health benefits that are sustainable and substantial.

—Wendy L. Stuhldreher
Updated by Bruce E. Johansen, PhD

See also: Aging process; Arthritis; Cancer; Diabetes; Exercise and fitness; Gout; Heart disease; Hypertension; Malnutrition; Nutrition; Stones; Weight loss and gain

For Further Information

Fakhouri, Tala H. I., et al. "Prevalence of Obesity Among Older Adults in the United States, 2007-2010." CDC, Centers for Disease Control and Prevention, Sept. 2012. www.cdc.gov/nchs/products/databriefs/db106.htm. This report presents the most recent national estimates of obesity in older adults, by sex, age, race and ethnicity, and educational attainment, and examines changes in the prevalence of obesity between 1999 and 2010.

Nordqvist, Joseph. "Metabolically Healthy Obesity: All You Need to Know." *Medical News Today*, MediLexicon International, 18 Apr. 2017. www.medicalnewstoday.com/articles/265405.php. Discusses the basics of metabolically healthy obesity and calls for the need of more criteria to help define the condition.

Stenholm, Sari, et al. "Patterns of Weight Gain in Middle-Aged and Older US Adults, 1992-2010." *Epidemiology*, vol. 26, no. 2, 2015, pp. 165-68. doi:10.1097/ede.0000000000000228. Examines longitudinal changes in BMI in initially underweight, normal weight, overweight, and obese US men and women using individual-level repeat data from the Health and Retirement Study.

OCCUPATIONS. *See* EMPLOYMENT.

OLD AGE

Relevant Issues: Biology, demographics, family, finances, health and medicine, insurance, psychology, sociology

Significance: Most people born in the United States today will live to be older than previous generations. Life expectancy is about 76 for males and 81 for females.

Although stereotypes tend to present youth as positive and old age as negative, there are benefits to each. Youth has physical benefits, such as strength and speed. Older people have wisdom and resilience. Ageist prejudices are inaccurate. Much of what was believed to be from aging may be from illnesses and injuries. Memory loss is likely to be from Alzheimer's disease and other dementias, not part of normal aging. Furthermore, what has been attributed to aging may be from slower speed. When healthy older people are not rushed, they perform well whether with thinking or exercise. Major roles in public life and politics have increasingly older people. Improved lifestyles and medical advances have made old age productive and enjoyable.

Although old age can be challenging, older people often enjoy life free from previous responsibilities. It can provide opportunities to do things they could not in earlier life.

MIDDLE AGE

Middle age is the stage of life that precedes old age. Often it is regarded as between forty and sixty-five, although not rigidly.

In their book *Aging, the Individual, and Society* (10th ed., 2015), Susan Hillier and Georgia M. Barrow call middle age a transition time. It is a good time for most. People often reach their peak earning power during these years and usually have established careers. They may see their children grown and gone and may experience new freedoms. Married couples may grow closer. In 1950, Erik Erikson called this a stage of "generativity" with, hopefully, a sense of productivity and creativity. Yet, middle age may also bring uncertainties. People tend to think they will always be young, and middle age comes gradually and unannounced.

Middle age is getting more attention as baby boomers are getting older. Some thought that baby boomers, the cohort born between 1946 and 1964, would change middle age as they had changed other aspects of American society. Many baby boomers may try to avoid "middle age" altogether because the stereotypes about the period, in many ways, do not fit them. They may simply give new meaning to "getting older."

For some middle-aged people, simultaneous increased responsibilities of caring for elderly parents and young children can be burdensome. Such situations have become common enough to have the title "sandwich generation."

What was regarded as frightening "midlife crisis" no longer seems as daunting or even inevitable.

WHAT IS "OLD"?

When is old age? It is not abrupt, but a continuum. It is not the same for everyone. There is more diversity among older people because they have lived longer and have more experiences.

Usually, the start of old age is regarded as sixty-five, the retirement age set by the Social Security Act of 1936 and the start of Medicare in 1965. Yet sixty-five may also be considered young. Many researchers divide those over sixty-five into the "young-old," the "middle-old," and the "old-old." Hillier and Barrow believe that seventy-five, eighty, or even eighty-five might describe the beginning of old age.

There are about 48 million Americans over the age of 65, which is about 15 percent of the total population, and an annual increase of more than 1.6 million (census.gov). However, with increased longevity and lower birth rates, the elderly will become a greater portion of the population.

Interestingly, many people may not experience feeling old, because it is gradual and not sudden. Particularly if they are well and maintain their long-term relationships, they may smoothly progress without feeling old. However, there can be major loss of relationships as people die or move away and loss of their own functioning because they are exposed to more illnesses, wear and tear, and injuries. Often, it is loss accompanying aging that makes them feel old.

LIFE SPAN AND LIFE EXPECTANCY

The maximum life span, the age anyone has been known to live is now more than 120 years. Life expectancy (almost 79 years according to the cdc.gov) is the average number of years that one might expect to live. Life expectancy increases the more years people have lived. In other words, those who are older are more likely to live longer than younger people will because they have already survived the earlier years.

LIFE SATISFACTION

The negatives of being old are more stereotypic than universal. Only 1.5 million (1.3 million in 2015 cdc.gov) people are in nursing homes in the United States at any given time.

Many older people are enjoying life, thanks to medical advances and healthy lifestyles. Retirement is a time to play with grandchildren. They golf, swim, and continue with long-term hobbies. They may do new things, such as travel and new hobbies. Some take courses at local colleges. Some give courses or mentor the young.

Not all older people retire, either because they cannot afford retirement or because they enjoy working. Some, who do not need the money, enjoy trying work they could not afford to do years ago or volunteer. Work is not just about money and satisfaction, but also opportunities to socialize.

As reported by Jill Quadagno (Aging and the Life Course, 2017), studies indicate that religion provides comfort, support, and meaning in life to many older people. Churches and synagogues help people in need, offer activities and programs, and provide socialization.

While religion and spirituality add meaning, those with commitment to secular causes and relationships also benefit. It is important to avoid isolation and have reasons to be living. Volunteering, having pets, and learning new things enrich and prolong life.

Mixing generations, such as through visits and programs with children, can enrich all ages. The elderly have much to offer through wisdom, emotional support, and tutoring and mentoring the young.

Meaning in old age can be enhanced. Erik H. Erikson, Joan M. Erikson, and Helen Q. Kivnick, provide stimulating advice in Vital Involvement in Old Age, 1986 (see Further Information Classic Books below).

HEALTH AND INDEPENDENCE

Most older people want to age in place living at home. If affordable and safe, healthy elderly may be able to live at home. They can use resilience and coping mechanisms from mastering previous challenges.

Remaining in private houses may require changes. Stairs are a frequent obstacle, but stair lifts and other adjustments can help. Homes should be reconfigured for safety, such as installation of grab bars in the shower that are secured into house studs (not glued on or with suction cups). Rugs, patterned flooring, thresholds, and other obstacles should be removed. Medic alert pendants to call an ambulance should have automatic fall detectors, be waterproof for shower use, and be tested regularly. Eyeglasses and hearing aids are important to prolong function, safety, and relationships. There should be public pressure for Medicare and other coverage for assistive devices. The elderly should cooperate with using the aforementioned devices and giving up driving when no longer safe.

Family members provide the most assistance, hands-on directly or financially or driving and accompanying elderly to medical appointments. Neighbors, friends, community organizations, churches and synagogues also help. Some employment offers family leave to take care of elderly relatives. There are new programs that may pay relatives to take care of the elderly (if Medicaid and otherwise qualified). Those without family or whose family has moved far away may use "Meals on Wheels," grocery delivery, visiting nurses, maids, and aides. Organizations may help with costs.

Some older people need the intensive care that skilled nursing homes provide and may have coverage from Medicaid and Long-Term Care Insurance. Assisted-living facilities are akin to apartments with communal dining and the option of add-on services as they become needed, such as help with showering, dressing, and other activities of daily living, but they can be costly and not have reimbursement possibilities.

Whatever the venue, it is essential that needs of the elderly are met with dignity and respect. Community and government agencies should prevent elder abuse and report violations to protect everyone.

IMPLICATIONS FOR THE FUTURE

The elderly may be better off financially and educationally than previous generations. However, this can change as the older population increases and younger people paying into programs via employment deductions decrease. Pensions connected with jobs are no longer guaranteed as they were for previous generations.

There are reasons to believe the elderly will thrive. They have better health and education, television and other electronic devices, and wisdom. They can harness and improve community resources to help themselves and their peers.

The outlook is optimistic. As in Robert Browning's poem "Rabbi Ben Ezra": "Grow old along with me! The best is yet to be."

—*Updated by Carol Goldberg, PhD, ABPP*

See also: Aging: Biological, psychological, and sociocultural perspectives; Aging process; views of aging; Death and dying; Driving; Elder abuse; Enjoy Old Age: A Program of Self-Management; Fraud against the elderly; Geriatrics and gerontology; Grandparenthood; Great-grandparenthood; Growing Old in America; Illnesses among older adults; Injuries among older adults; Life expectancy; Life insurance; Longevity research; Men and aging; Middle age; Psychiatry, geriatric; Women and aging

For Further Information

Amen, Daniel G. *Memory Rescue: Supercharge Your Brain, Reverse Memory Loss, and Remember What Matters Most.* Tyndale House Publishers, 2018. Expert physician Dr. Amen reveals how a multipronged strategy—including dietary changes, physical and mental exercises, and spiritual practices—can improve brain health and enhance memory.

Aronson, Louise. *Elderhood: Redefining Aging, Transforming Medicine, Reimagining Life.* Bloomsbury Publishing, 2019. Aronson uses stories from her quarter century of caring for patients, and draws from history, science, literature, popular culture, and her own life to weave a vision of old age that's neither nightmare nor utopian fantasy.

Erikson, Erik H., Joan M. Erikson, and Helen Q. Kivnick. *Vital Involvement in Old Age.* W. W. Norton, 1986. A classic in the field, this book skillfully weaves Erikson's eight stages of psychosocial development into the authors' research with twenty-nine elders in their eighth and ninth decades of life.

Hillier, Susan, and Georgia M. Barrow. *Aging, the Individual, and Society.* 10th ed. Cengage Learning, 2015. This book balances academic research and practical discussions, integrating social and cultural perspectives with the story of the individual aging process. Activities to enhance reader's understanding and skills by providing many opportunities for experiential learning.

Quadagno, Jill. *Aging and the Life Course: An Introduction to Social Gerontology.* 7th ed. McGraw-Hill education, 2017. Quadagno's groundbreaking text examines the relationship between quality of life in old age and its experiential catalysts. Throughout the text an emphasis is placed on the intersectionality of race, class, gender, and culture, and how these classifications affect quality of life.

Schlossberg, Nancy K. *Too Young to Be Old: Love, Learn, Work, and Play as You Age.* American Psychological Association, 2017. Using her own inspirational life as a backdrop, and applying her considerable experience as a psychologist, Schlossberg looks at aging through the lens of Positive Psychology. By taking a broad and comprehensive view on aging issues combined with an approachable discussion on psychological theories, this title will help teach readers the principles of aging well.

Vaillant, George E. *Aging Well: Surprising Guideposts to a Happier Life from the Landmark Harvard Study of Adult Development.* Little, Brown, and Company, 2003. In a unique series of studies, Harvard University followed 824 subjects from their teens to old age. Vaillant uses these to illustrate the surprising factors involved in reaching happy, healthy old age.

OLD MAN AND THE SEA, THE (BOOK)

Author: Ernest Hemingway
Date: Published in 1952
Relevant Issues: Culture, psychology, values, work
Significance: This novel about the struggles of an elderly fisherman highlights issues that accompany aging in physically demanding work.

Ernest Hemingway's novel *The Old Man and the Sea* concerns an elderly and solitary Cuban fisherman, Santiago, who has not caught a fish for eighty-four days. On the eighty-fifth day, Santiago hooks an enormous marlin while in his small boat, but Santiago has gone out to sea too far. He is unable to prevent sharks from devouring his catch as he tows it back to his village after three days of struggle.

Certain experts on this novel note that Santiago has been labeled as useless by his culture because he is elderly and without luck. Despite this label, Santiago continues his fishing. By drawing on his abundant experience and skill, Santiago catches a larger fish than any of the younger, but less experienced, fishermen who have alienated him. Seen in these terms, Santiago's catch is a triumph of the aging individual—possessing the unique

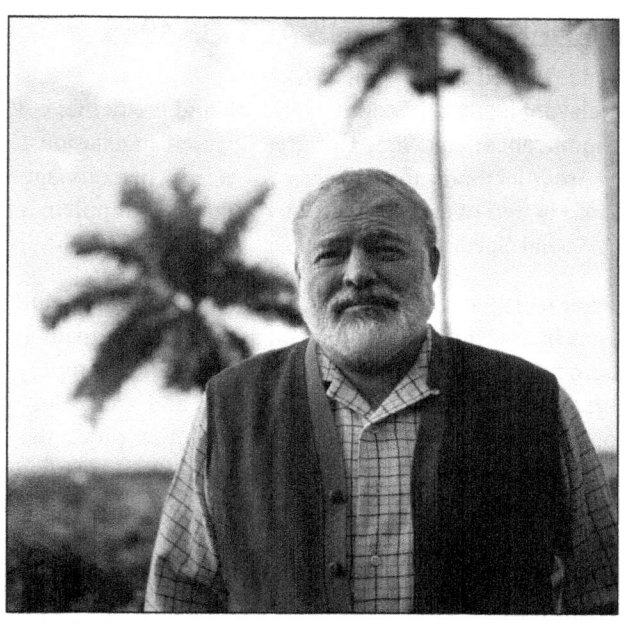

Several of Hemingway's books were influenced by time spent on his boat Pilar, most notably The Old Man and the Sea *and* Islands in the Stream.

abilities acquired only from many years of experience—over a youth-oriented culture trapped by its shortsighted attitudes toward elders. Other commentators, however, have chosen to highlight the fact that Santiago, in an act of desperation, knowingly goes out too far. In doing so, he is making a last attempt to prove to himself, and his critics, that he is still a capable man and member of the community.

Many critics point out that Santiago embodies the values that Hemingway thought one should possess as an elder: determination, humility, hopefulness, wisdom, skill, pride, and courage. Santiago is content with realizing these values in the course of his daily work. This picture of a poor but content elder has been contrasted with Hemingway's depiction of the younger fishermen who, while more successful, are preoccupied by material gain. Seen in this way, Hemingway's Santiago has arrived at a successful approach to life in his later years.

—*Robert Landolfi*

See also: Cultural views of aging; Latinx Americans; Men and aging; Old age; Wisdom

OLDER AMERICANS ACT OF 1965

Date: Passed on July 14, 1965
Relevant Issues: Economics, health and medicine, law
Significance: In 1965, Congress passed legislation to provide funds for services for needy persons aged sixty and over; the law was designed to supplement Social Security benefits.

Prior to 1965, research indicated that many senior citizens in the United States lacked adequate retirement income, health care, affordable housing, gainful employment, and meaningful civil, cultural, and recreational opportunities. In addition, as persons grew older, they were spending increasing percentages of their fixed incomes on medical care. Accordingly, as a part of President Lyndon B. Johnson's Great Society programs, Congress passed the Older Americans Act on July 14, 1965. Several amendments have been made to the act, including the Age Discrimination Act of 1975.

The act created the Administration on Aging (AoA), headed by a commissioner of aging within the Department of Health, Education, and Welfare (HEW). The Advisory Committee on Older Americans, consisting of the commissioner and fifteen people with relevant experience, was also established to provide expertise in designing new programs. In 1978, AoA was transferred to the new Department of Health and Human Services (HHS). Acting on recommendations of the 1992 White House Conference on Aging (WHCoA), Congress in 1993 amended the act by upgrading the commissioner to assistant secretary for aging; in addition, the Advisory Committee on Older Americans became the Federal Council on Aging.

The AoA provides grants to states. To obtain funds, each state must designate a state unit on aging (SUA), which must design a program to utilize the funds. SUAs then identify area agencies throughout each state, which form advisory councils to develop the area plan, hold hearings, represent older people, and review and comment on community programs. SUAs by law must have a full-time ombudsman to handle complaints.

The AoA awards two types of grants: for research and development projects (which make needs assessments, develop new approaches—including clinics to provide legal assistance to poorer senior citizens and multipurpose activity centers—develop new methods to coordinate programs and services, and evaluate the various programs) and for training projects for personnel to run the programs.

Each state receives at least 1 percent of the total funding, and American Samoa, Guam, and the Virgin Islands each receive 0.5 percent. The remaining 49.5 percent is allocated on the basis of the relative size of the state's population. No more than 10 percent of each state's allotment can support SUA administrative expenses. The AoA also provides consultants, technical assistance, training personnel, research, and informational materials to the states. Priority program recipients are those who are homebound because of disability or illness. Meals-on-wheels services provide hot meals directly to their homes, and they are eligible for in-home support services, including home health aides. Low-income minorities are especially targeted.

Programs operating under the act have been criticized largely because, although the quality of services is much better in some states than others, the AoA has neither developed nor enforced minimum standards. Funding for the programs has decreased continuously since 2010, though the number of adults over 60 has increased exponentially. It remains to be seen whether Congress reauthorizes the Act in 2019.

—*Michael Haas*

See also: Advocacy; Age Discrimination Act of 1975; Home services; Home delivered meals programs

OLDER WORKERS BENEFIT PROTECTION ACT

Date: Signed on October 16, 1990
Relevant Issues: Economics, law
Significance: This act ensures that older workers cannot be tricked by employers into losing retirement benefits.

The Age Discrimination in Employment Act (ADEA) of 1967 was designed to deter employers from discriminating against workers over the age of forty. Unscrupulous employers, however, decided to offer early retirement incentives to older workers—often threatening to lay off older workers just before they became eligible for a pension—provided that the workers waived their ADEA rights.

When one of these schemes was challenged, the U.S. Supreme Court ruled, in Ohio v. Betts (1989), that such waivers were perfectly legal. Congress then passed the Older Workers Benefit Protection Act (OWBPA) in 1990 to establish procedural safeguards so that such waivers could not be signed in haste and so employers could not target older workers in staff-cutting programs.

The OWBPA established the following requirements: The waiver must be written in a manner that can be understood by the average employee; the waiver cannot relinquish non-ADEA rights; the waiver cannot refer to rights subsequently established by an amended ADEA; the employee must be advised in writing to consult an attorney before signing a waiver; the employee can take at least three weeks before signing the waiver; and the waiver can be revoked within one week after signing.

The OWBPA provides that the burden of proof about the legality of a waiver falls on the employer. When an employer challenged the OWBPA, the Supreme Court, in Oubre v. Entergy (1998), affirmed that an employee has the right to sue under ADEA if an employer's waiver agreement fails to comply with these six procedural requirements. Moreover, an employee suing for a violation of the OWBPA need not return the severance pay provided in the waiver.

—*Michael Haas*

See also: Age discrimination; Age Discrimination in Employment Act of 1967; Early retirement; Employment; Retirement

ON GOLDEN POND (PLAY)

Author: Ernest Thompson
Date: Play produced in 1978, published in 1979; film released in 1981
Relevant Issues: Death, family, health and medicine, marriage and dating, work
Significance: This play about an elderly couple highlights important issues of aging, including retirement and coping with failing health.

Ernest Thompson's play *On Golden Pond* depicts an elderly couple, Norman and Ethel, on a summer vacation in Maine. They are visited by their daughter, her boyfriend, and his adolescent son. The boy stays the summer while the daughter vacations elsewhere with her boyfriend.

Much of the play concerns difficulties that may occur after retirement. Norman is an always-witty retired professor. In the opening act, however, one sees him searching through "help wanted" advertisements for unskilled jobs. Critics note that Norman is a victim of a youth-oriented culture that often fails to provide a dignified and active role for elders, reducing their self-esteem. Norman no longer believes he has much to offer and is willing to accept any job. In this sense, his relationship with the teenager later in the play represents a triumph. During their summer together, Norman becomes the boy's mentor and is rejuvenated by this relationship.

Health issues that may accompany aging are also central to this play. As Norman nears eighty, he experiences mild senility and heart palpitations. Commentators have noted that the younger and healthier Ethel compensates for her husband's failing health by taking on a parental role in their marriage. Ethel often attempts to structure Norman's time, for example, to help him with his tendencies toward forgetfulness.

Health issues are also a part of the play's treatment of the subject of death. Ethel and Norman have different attitudes toward death. Norman is preoccupied with the subject and Ethel, always the optimist, avoids it. In the final act, Norman has a mild heart attack. Through this experience, Ethel finally faces death. At the end of the play, Norman recovers and the couple appreciates life more than ever as a result of this experience.

A popular film adaptation of *On Golden Pond* was released in 1981. It starred Henry Fonda as Norman, Katharine Hepburn as Ethel, and Jane Fonda as their daughter. The film won Academy Awards for Best Actor for Henry Fonda, Best Actress for Hepburn, and Best Adapted Screenplay for Thompson.

—*Robert Landolfi*

See also: Ageism; Death and dying; Death anxiety; Employment; Family relationships; Heart attacks; Marriage; Memory loss; Successful aging; Vacations and travel

OSTEOPOROSIS

Relevant Issues: Biology, health and medicine

Significance: AS the number of elderly people in the United States grows, an increasing number of women and a smaller, but growing number of men will experience an osteoporotic fracture at some point in their lives.

Osteoporosis is a major public health problem affecting 1 in 4 women and 1 in 8 men over the age of 50. It is estimated that over 200 million women worldwide have osteoporosis. The condition is often silent until a fracture occurs. Bones lose strength over time with bone mass not increasing after the age of 30. One in five older patients who sustain a hip fracture dies within six months of the fracture. One-half of the survivors of hip fracture need some help with their daily living activities, and as many as 25 percent of these patients need care in a nursing home.

Women are five times as likely to suffer from osteoporosis than are men, but men can develop osteoporosis. White and Asian women are most at risk. Risk factors may include family history, ovaries removed before periods stopped, early menopause, insufficient calcium and/or vitamin D throughout life, smoking, insufficient exercise or extended bedrest, certain medications for arthritis and asthma, some cancer drugs and a small body frame.

Bone is a metabolically active, dynamic tissue that is remodeled throughout life. Depending on a number of factors, the process is either in or out of balance. In children, formation exceeds loss, so bone mass increases. In adults, the two are about equal, so bone mass only changes if there is additional or less stress. In old age, bone loss exceeds bone formation, and bone mass is decreased. When bone mass is reduced, the bone becomes mechanically weak and vulnerable to fractures. The gradual loss of bone mineral density, or bone thinning, is a normal part of the aging process; osteoporosis occurs when this process exceeds what are considered normal rates, making bones exceedingly fragile and susceptible to breaks and fractures. There is no known cure for osteoporosis; prevention is the only strategy for combating bone mineral loss and the development of osteoporosis.

The osteoporosis of aging is designated as type I. It has two forms: postmenopausal and senile. Postmenopausal osteoporosis occurs in women between the ages of fifty-one and sixty-five and often results in fractures of the vertebrae and wrist; senile osteoporosis, which occurs in both men and women past the age of seventy, increases the danger fractures of the hip and vertebrae. A side effect of a hip fracture that requires surgery or immobilization is muscle wasting. With less muscle, the person is less stable and more likely to fall and reinjure the hip. Fractures of the hip are a significant medical problem: 12 to 20 percent of such patients die within six months of the fracture, and about one-half lose the ability to live independently.

RISK FACTORS FOR OSTEOPOROSIS

A number of risk factors for osteoporosis have been identified, some of which cannot be changed. For example, the older a person is, the more likely he or she is to develop osteoporosis. Women tend to be more vulnerable than men because, in addition to the accelerated rate

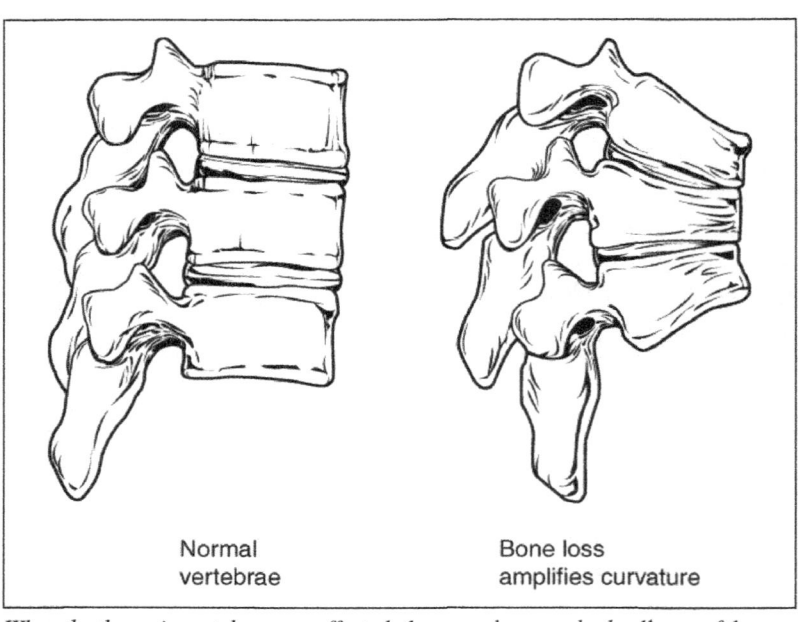

Normal vertebrae

Bone loss amplifies curvature

When the thoracic vertebrae are affected, there can be a gradual collapse of the vertebrae. This results in kyphosis, an excessive curvature of the thoracic region. (via Wikimedia Commons)

of bone loss that occurs at the menopause, women have smaller skeletons than men and, therefore, reach the threshold for bone fragility well before men.

People with large body frames are less likely to develop osteoporosis than those with small body frames, probably because their bone reserve allows them to lose bone for a longer period before reaching the threshold for fracture. Genetic research has also determined that variations in the gene for the vitamin D receptor may contribute to 7 to 10 percent of the difference in bone mass density because of its influence on calcium intake. For those with a family history of osteoporosis, this factor could lead to early identification and intervention.

Several risk factors that can be reversed have also been identified. Even though osteoporosis is a disease of the elderly, identification of risk factors in the young will ensure that preventive measures can be followed. Osteoporosis occurs most often in people with low calcium intake, eating disorders and gastrointestinal surgery to reduce the size of the stomach or to remove part of the intestine leading to poor absorption of nutrients, including calcium. Normal calcium intake throughout life may do the most toward prevention of osteoporosis, even among high-risk populations. About 99 percent of the body's calcium is found in the bones and teeth, and daily intake is meant to keep these stores full. A low dietary calcium intake is associated with a reduced bone mass and an increased fracture rate. Conversely, an elevated calcium intake, particularly in children and adolescents, is associated with an increased mass. Women over 50 need 1,200 mg of calcium daily and men need 1,000 mg from ages 51 to 70 and 1,200 mg of calcium after 70. Vitamin D is necessary for calcium absorption and can be obtained through sun exposure, dietary sources and supplements.

Steroids and other medications can interfere with the bone re-building process. Drugs used for seizures, gastric reflux, cancer and to prevent transplant rejection may also interfere with bone re-building leading to osteoporosis and an increased risk of fracture. Medical conditions such as inflammatory bowel disease, celiac disease, lupus, cancer, and rheumatoid arthritis may increase the risk of osteoporosis.

Physical inactivity is associated with a reduced bone mass. People who are sedentary are more susceptible to osteoporosis than those who are active. During the formative years, exercise helps develop higher bone density. Recommendations include a variety of weight-bearing and vigorous exercises that are done regularly, for thirty to sixty minutes per day, three to five days per week. Variety is essential because no one exercise stresses all bones equally. In the elderly, exercise may have a secondary benefit. Fractures are often precipitated by falls that are caused by a loss of balance or coordination. Maintaining an active lifestyle helps with balance and coordination, as well as confidence, all of which may help in fall prevention. Studies on the elderly have demonstrated that general exercise, such as walking, does not maintain gains in bone density for very long. Many medical experts have, therefore, recommended adding a regular strength-training regimen, performed two or three times per week for twenty minutes, that targets the most common fracture sites.

Other modifiable risk factors include smoking and excess alcohol consumption. Both of these are risk factors for a number of diseases, so they are discouraged in everyone.

TREATMENT AND THERAPY

To prevent osteoporosis, doctors often request baseline information on the bone densities of women before the menopause and of men between the ages of fifty and sixty. The most accurate technique available to measure bone density is dual energy X-ray absorptiometry (DEXA). Although it is an X-ray, exposure to radiation is minimal. The same densitometry machine can do both whole-body and single-site readings.

Osteoporosis therapy includes several options. Estrogen started soon after menopause may help maintain bone density but can cause side effects such as blood clots, endometrial and breast cancer and increase the risk of heart disease. Raloxifene (Evista) mimics some of estrogen's benefits without some of the associated risks. It may reduce some forms of breast cancer. Hot flashes are a common side effect and the risk of blood clots may increase.

Bisphosphonates are the most commonly prescribed medications for osteoporosis. Alendronate (Fosamax), ibandronate (Boniva), risedronate (Actonel, Atelvia), and zoledronic acid (Reclast) are examples. There are side effects, as with any drug. Nausea, heartburn like pain, and abdominal pain are more likely to occur if medications are not taken appropriately. Some people prefer a quarterly or yearly injection, but it may be more expensive. Use of these drugs for longer than 5 years may lead to cracks or fractures of the femur or thigh bone. Osteonecrosis of the jaw bone, or failure of the jawbone to heal after a tooth extraction, may occur. Most dentists will not attempt implants if osteoporosis is present or if therapy is being given. Decisions about therapy with bisphosphonates should take these factors into consideration. Denosumab (Prolia) and teriparatide (Forteo) may be used. Prolia is administered via a shot every 6 months and Forteo is administered by a daily shot for two years and then followed by another osteoporosis drug to maintain bone growth.

PSYCHOSOCIAL FACTORS
Osteoporosis follows the psychological profile of other chronic diseases, causing anxiety, depression, and feelings of hopelessness. Diagnosis often causes a fear of loss of independence, fear of another fall, or fear of financial devastation from long-term health care, all of which lead to further limitation of activities and reduced physical conditioning.

Vertebral fractures, loss of height, protruding abdomen, or compressed lungs can ultimately lead to pneumonia in individuals who contract a viral or bacterial lung infection. Those same patients may experience challenges in tasks of daily living, such as reaching or walking; these limitations may add to feelings of frustration and ineffectiveness. Such people often withdraw from social activities, which are a big part of health and wellness in the elderly.

Pain is probably the primary physical problem associated with osteoporosis. It challenges coping skills and makes it difficult to deal with other aspects of the disease. Pain may be either acute and severe (following a fracture) or chronic (from spinal deformity and associated changes in the body, which often increase over time). Pain management is usually a significant part of the treatment program for people with osteoporotic fractures of the spine.

—*Wendy E. S. Repovich*
Updated by Patricia Stanfill Edens, RN, PhD, FACHE

See also: Back disorders; Bone changes and disorders; Estrogen replacement therapy; Exercise and fitness; Fractures and broken bones; Kyphosis; Malnutrition; Medications; Menopause; Nutrition; Vitamins and minerals; Women and aging

For Further Information
Audesirk G., and T. Audesirk. *Biology: Life on Earth.* 12th ed. Prentice Hall, 2019. This general biology textbook contains several chapters devoted to human and vertebrate animal skeletal systems, development, and nutrition, plus health essays devoted to topics such as osteoporosis.

Compston, Julia, et al. "Bone Histomorphometry." *Vitamin D*, edited by David Feldman et al., 4th ed., vol. 1, Academic P, 2018, pp. 959-73. This volume of Vitamin D presents the latest information from international experts in endocrinology, bone biology and human physiology, taking readers through the basic research of vitamin D. This chapter explains bone histomorphometry, the quantitative assessment of bone remodeling, modeling, and structure.

Demontiero, Oddom, et al. "Aging and Bone Loss: New Insights for the Clinician." *Therapeutic Advances in Musculoskeletal Disease*, vol. 4, no. 2, Apr. 2012, pp. 61-76. doi:10.1177/1759720x11430858. Reviews new evidence on the pathophysiology of age-related bone loss with emphasis upon the mechanism of action of current osteoporosis treatments. New potential treatments are also considered.

Li, Guowei, et al. "An Overview of Osteoporosis and Frailty in the Elderly." *BMC Musculoskeletal Disorders*, vol. 18, no. 46, 26 Jan. 2017. doi:10.1186/s12891-017-1403-x. In this overview, the authors review the relationship between frailty and osteoporosis, describe the approaches to measuring the grades of frailty, and present current studies and future research directions investigating osteoporosis and frailty in the elderly.

Moran, Diana. *Beating Osteoporosis: The Facts, the Treatments, the Exercises.* Green Tree, 2019. Written in association with the National Osteoporosis Society, this practical book is a must-have for anybody affected by osteoporosis. Packed with advice, friendly tips and ideas, and an overview of current research, and what we can all be doing to help ourselves live well.

National Institute on Aging. National Institutes of Health. www.nia.nih.gov. Provides information and resources related to aging including bone changes.

"Osteoporosis." National Institute on Aging. National Institutes of Health. www.nia.nih.gov/health/osteoporosis. General information about osteoporosis.

OURSELVES, GROWING OLDER: A BOOK FOR WOMEN OVER FORTY (BOOK)

Editors: Paula Doress-Worters and Diana Laskin Siegal
Date: Published in 1987, revised in 1994
Relevant Issues: Family, health and medicine, psychology
Significance: *Ourselves, Growing Older* is a guidebook for women over forty in dealing with changes in body, relationships, and health as they and their loved ones age.

Ourselves, Growing Older: A Book for Women over Forty, edited by Paula Doress-Worters and Diana Laskin Siegal, was first published in 1987; it appeared in a revised edition in 1994 as *The New Ourselves, Growing Older: Women Aging with Knowledge and Power*. Doress-Worters and Siegal prepared this volume in cooperation with the Boston Women's Health Book Collective, the authors of *Our Bodies, Ourselves* (1971; revised as *The New Our Bodies, Ourselves* in 1992) and other health-related works. In fact, the idea for this book arose from the challenges associated with writing a single chapter on health concerns for the older woman for *Our Bodies, Ourselves*. It is based on the same principle as *Our Bodies, Ourselves*: that women must know themselves and their bodies to be free from mistaken notions about women and their health and well-being. Written from a feminist perspective, *Ourselves, Growing Older* is a collaborative effort by women in their mid-forties to their eighties aimed at exposing the effects of ageism and sexism on all people, not just on women.

The authors also hope to enable women to stay well as they move into their later years. They examine the ways that culture influences aging in women and argue against the medicalization of the menopause, as earlier women's health activists argued against the medicalization of childbirth. They believe that both of these events should be approached as normal parts of a woman's life, rather than as pathologic conditions. Instead of looking at women's health solely from a biomedical model, the authors also consider the effects of the environment, poverty, and injustice on aging. Their underlying philosophy is that the lives of older women can be rich and fulfilling. They consider this idea to be especially important because the greatest proportion of the older population is female.

Ourselves, Growing Older is divided into three sections. "Aging Well" includes six chapters devoted to dealing with the expected changes of aging and health habits associated with healthier aging. These chapters address diet, exercise, substance use, body image, stress, and other topics. "Living with Ourselves and Others as We Age" includes six chapters on topics ranging from sexuality in the second half of life, birth control and childbearing in midlife, the menopause, relationships, housing arrangements and work, retirement, and economics. The final section, "Understanding, Preventing, and Managing Medical Problems," begins by discussing the needed reforms to the health-care system. Individual chapters cover common health problems of aging: arthritis, osteoporosis, dental problems, incontinence, hysterectomy, heart disease, cancer, diabetes, gallbladder problems, sensory changes, and memory loss. This section concludes with a chapter on death and dying. The final chapter discusses ways to change, both on a societal and on an individual level. Each chapter provides extensive references, and the authors offer more than sixty pages of resources, including other books and articles, agencies, audiovisual materials, and pamphlets.

—*Rebecca Lovell Scott*

See also: Ageism; Arthritis; Cancer; Cultural views of aging; Death and dying; Dental problems; Diabetes; Estrogen replacement therapy; Exercise and fitness; Health care; Heart disease; Housing; Incontinence; Memory loss; Menopause; Osteoporosis; Poverty; Psychiatry, geriatric; Retirement; Sexuality; Stress and coping skills; Successful aging; Women and aging

OVER THE HILL

Relevant Issues: Culture, psychology, values
Significance: This phrase presents a metaphorical image of aging that affords multiple angles for interpretation.

"Over the hill," a popular expression to describe aging, is a metaphoric construct. As simple as it is, the inherent richness of this phrase affords people multiple angles from which to interpret what aging means.

Aging is often seen as a life journey. On the completion of climbing up a hill to the peak, going "over the hill" indicates the beginning of the rest of the journey, and its conclusion.

Aging is coming down the path "over the hill," demonstrating a declining trend in contrast to upward growth. The peak marks the turning point of the developmental course, separating two qualitatively different stages in life: growth and aging.

Aging is a developmental process involving new tasks in a new context. The tasks may be difficult and the path may be rough, as expressed in the Chinese saying, "It is easy to climb up a hill; it is hard to go down a hill." Yet, aging can be exciting: the grass might be greener "over the hill." New growth and achievements are possible in a person's later life.

Aging varies in its internal meaning and motivational structure for individuals. Each person must locate his or her position on the hill of life. Even after going over the "peak" of the "hill," an individual may have some ability to decide the speed and style of descending.

Aging is an indicator of maturity and accomplishment, worthy of celebration. Having gone "over the hill" implies a successful past and opens new prospects for the future, as depicted in an American Indian story in which once over the hill, a person sees another hill ahead yet to conquer.

—*Ling-Yi Zhou*
Updated by Bruce E. Johansen, PhD

See also: Aging: Biological, psychological, and sociocultural perspectives; Ageism; Cultural views of aging; Humor; Maturity; Middle age; Native Americans; Old age; Stereotypes; Wisdom

OVERMEDICATION

Relevant Issues: Health and medicine
Significance: Overmedication of the elderly is a common cause of preventable harm to individuals and results in unnecessary health-care expenditures.

Older Americans are commonly treated for multiple chronic conditions including hypertension, arthritis and diabetes that may require multiple prescription medications for management. The overmedication of older Americans is a serious problem with many dimensions—cultural, economic, political, and medical. Among the contributing factors are a lack of training in aging on the part of some doctors, lack of understanding of bodily changes in the elderly that make prescription drug use by them riskier than for younger people, the absence of drug education programs to teach the elderly and their families safe and appropriate prescription drug use, inadequate research of drug effects on elderly populations, and the inaccessibility of nondrug alternatives for treating chronic diseases of aging.

Approximately 80 percent of Americans over the age of 65 are treated for one chronic condition, and the average older American is treated for two conditions. It is further estimated that up to 40 percent of adults over the age of 65 use five or more medications per day. Unfortunately, some providers may not be aware of all medications that a patient is taking, and with each additional prescription the risk of overmedication increases.

ADVERSE DRUG REACTIONS

Each year, 100,000 Americans die of adverse drug reactions. The elderly are the most vulnerable, especially those who take several drugs daily. They are twice as likely to suffer ill effects from medications as persons in their thirties and forties, and their adverse reactions are more likely to be severe. An estimated nine million older Americans suffer adverse drug reactions each year. Approximately 17 percent of hospital admissions of people over seventy are caused by this problem. Not all adverse reactions are caused by overmedication, but gerontologists (those who study aging) surmise that among the elderly, overmedication is the most common cause. About 40 percent of respondents to a survey by the American Association of Retired Persons (AARP) reported side effects from the medications they were taking.

Because the metabolism of older people slows down and organs tend to function less efficiently, drugs can have a very strong impact on aging bodies. With age, less blood flows into the liver, which becomes smaller and less efficient in metabolizing some drugs. Drug clearance from the body declines with age. For example, reduced kidney function results in drug accumulation. Because the stomach empties more slowly with age, drugs remain there longer. Age-related changes in hormones mean that drugs have a stronger impact on the elderly than on younger people. For example, the elderly are more likely to develop drug-induced hypoglycemia.

With age, the brain becomes more sensitive to the sedative effects of drugs. For example, excess sedation or confusion from too much Valium (diazepam) or Dalmane (flurazepam) may not occur until several weeks after well-tolerated doses were begun.

A well-established resource used by clinicians when prescribing medications to elderly patients is the Beers List, which lists potentially dangerous or inappropriate drugs for use in geriatric patients. According to physician Margaret W. Winker, fat-soluble drugs, including those that affect the brain, are retained longer in the body with age, so that drugs prescribed for problems in the elderly such as anxiety or insomnia must be given in smaller doses and less frequently than they would be given to younger patients. Some narcotic medicines may cause serious side effects in older patients. Winker believes that medications commonly used in the past for insomnia, such as barbiturates, should now be avoided in old persons because they interact with many other drugs, slow respiration, and cause confusion. She also notes that prednisone should not be prescribed for osteoarthritis, the most common form of arthritis, because of its harmful effect on the endocrine system. In addition, the monoamine oxidase (MAO) inhibitors used to treat depression, a common complaint of the elderly, may interact with food to cause high blood pressure. Over-the-counter medicines such as cold remedies and nasal decongestants also interact with MAO inhibitors.

Other common reactions to overmedication include impaired movements, memory loss, anxiety, constipation, palpitations, depression, restlessness, insomnia, blocked thyroid function, mood swings or other emotional imbalances, blurred vision, urine retention, potassium depletion, and lessening capacity to smell and taste. In addition, overuse of drugs can cause nutritional depletion, resulting in such problems as hearing loss, anemia, breathlessness, and weakness. Among nutrients lost are vitamins A and C and beta carotene, all thought likely to help the immune system ward off cancer.

Alcohol and tobacco interact with prescription drugs, increasing risk factors for the elderly who take multiple drugs. Some arthritis medicines, for example, interact with coffee and alcohol to damage the lining of the stomach. When sleeping pills mix with alcohol, breathing can be impaired to a dangerous degree.

Other potential factors related to overmedication include poor doctor-patient communication, and noncompliance on the part of patients. Sometimes an elderly patient will obtain prescriptions from various doctors or pharmacies, so that no one doctor or pharmacist sees the complete picture of the individual's drug consumption. Patients may not tell doctors what over-the-counter medicines they take. They may not understand, for example, that long-term use of laxatives for constipation can damage their intestines. Others may neglect to mention herbal medications that they take, anticipating the doctor's disapproval. Doctors may not have time for a thorough review of drug use history, current symptoms, and potentially harmful side effects. Limited knowledge of English, hearing loss, extreme deference to doctors, and a sense of powerlessness on the part of the patient may also be factors in incomplete drug assessment.

Although overmedication of the elderly affects those who live independently or with families as well as those who are institutionalized, overmedicating is especially serious among nursing home residents. Over one-half of all nursing home residents are prescribed psychotropic drugs (those having an effect on the mind). Geriatricians are concerned that in many cases, no precise diagnosis indicates a need for these powerful drugs. They also believe that nursing home residents are often overdosed with medications marked "as needed." Another problem is that some drugs have very similar names, resulting in mix-ups. Many falls in nursing homes result from over medication.

Sedating is a chemical restraint necessary for unruly or out-of-control patients but often unnecessary for most nursing home residents. Cultural devaluing of the frail and dependent elderly and the convenience of often-underpaid staff may play a larger role in medicating decisions than the health needs of individual residents.

Many hip fractures occur each year among people over sixty-five who use tranquilizers. Both gait and balance are affected by these drugs. Hip fractures are an es-

HOW TO TALK TO SENIORS ABOUT OVERMEDICATION

How Do They Feel?

Some seniors may not be aware that they face a higher risk for overdose. As a result, they may not be particularly concerned that they will be affected. They may not understand the risks of incorrect dosage, taking the wrong medicine, or mixing medications. Other seniors may be very concerned and anxious that something will happen to them. They may vigilantly check every label and carefully track all their medications by writing down the type, dose, and time they took a medication. Their worry may be normal and their caution warranted; however, if they become obsessive or overly anxious, they should consult with their doctor or a therapist or counselor.

Many older adults suffer from depression. Depression may be the result of life-changing events common to many seniors, such as retirement or loss of employment, the death of a spouse or other loved ones, medical conditions and declining health, loss of mobility or independence, or moving. When seniors have the opportunity to discuss their problems and emotions with a qualified counselor or therapist, they will have a greater chance of resolving issues that are causing them emotional pain. If depression is left untreated, they may begin to consider substance use or suicide to cope with these unresolved problems and emotions. Furthermore, depression and other negative emotions can be exacerbated by certain medications. For this reason, it is imperative that seniors have regular consultations with their doctor.

Seniors who have been abusing drugs, either prescription, over-the-counter, or illicit, may have intentionally or unintentionally overdosed. Their substance abuse and possible addiction may cause them shame and embarrassment. These negative feelings can deter them from speaking about their problem and seeking the help that they need. If they have had a near-fatal overdose, they may be more inclined to seek help such as addictions counseling. Others may remain in denial that they have a drug abuse problem.

How Do I Start The Conversation?

It is important to discuss the risks of overdosing with seniors, both as it relates to drug abuse as well as accidental overdoses. How you initiate the conversation will depend on your senior's specific situation. You may choose to call your senior's attention to the high incidence of accidental overdoses among seniors. You might mention the issue while helping your senior organize and track their medication to ensure mistakes are avoided. As you go through the medicines, making clear lists and instructions, you can discuss how accidents are less likely to occur when the label is clear and in large print. Make sure your senior knows to never take medicines in the dark or take anyone else's medicines.

You may also gently raise the topic of the misuse and overuse of over-the-counter drugs or prescription medications, especially those that have a higher risk of causing addiction and overdose. When discussing your concerns about overdosing, always do so in a nonjudgmental and nonthreatening way. Ask your senior about their concerns on the topic and find ways that you can help. Always listen attentively to what they wish to share.

If you suspect that a senior is struggling with cognitive decline or depression, encourage them to seek professional help. If they are reluctant or resistant, try to normalize the concept of therapy by sharing stories of people you both know who were helped by therapeutic intervention. Seniors may be reassured to know that depression and substance abuse problems can be successfully treated by a therapist, psychologist, or psychiatrist.

Drug abuse is a serious issue. If possible, do not hold discussions when the person is intoxicated. It is best to wait until they are sober to raise your concerns, discuss risks, and coordinate the appropriate intervention and treatment.

—*Leah Jacob*

pecially serious problem for women. For either sex, taking more than four prescription drugs is a risk factor for falls.

Although the precise extent of overmedication remains uncertain, pharmacologists who specialize in aging believe that as much as 25 percent of the prescriptions given to the elderly are unnecessary. Other researchers estimate that approximately one-fourth of the elderly are given drugs inappropriate for their complaints. Prescription drugs are most effective for acute, short-term illnesses, but the health problems of the elderly tend to be chronic.

RELATED SOCIAL AND CULTURAL ISSUES

Often when drugs cause elderly patients to become confused or disoriented, these behaviors are attributed to dementia. When reactions to drugs are mistaken for normal signs of aging, elderly persons are unlikely to have their drug use evaluated carefully and adjusted for their individual needs. Relatedly, gerontologists say, when some elderly patients leave a doctor's office without a prescription, he or she feels neglected or believes that a health problem has not been taken seriously.

Given the rising numbers of Americans over sixty-five, the social policy implications of overmedication in the elderly requires further research. Should one consider it acceptable to sedate the old because they are old? How much social control, especially of the frail and dependent old, is appropriate? Do gender and racial differences affect drug prescribing and monitoring? Stanford gerontologist Gwen Yeo suggested, for example, that older Asian Americans may need only one-half of the drug dose prescribed for whites. Will baby boomers resist physical decline more vigorously than their parents and thus demand more careful drug prescribing? The high cost of medications is an increasingly serious problem for low- and middle-income people. Will politically active seniors demand that their expensive drugs be paid for by Medicare or by other government programs? Will resentment of the old increase as their consumption of costly prescription drugs drives up the cost of health care?

In the United States, overmedication of the elderly is both a health and medical problem and a sign of the American tendency to equate aging with illness. Potential dangers of multiple drug use need further study and public discussion. One solution to overmedication is to increase the number of geriatricians trained to meet the needs of an increasingly elderly population. Any senior who takes prescription drugs should heed the advice geriatricians give about medicating the old: "Begin low and go slow." Periodic revaluation of drug use can help prevent over medication.

—*Margaret Cruikshank*
Updated by Patrick Richardson, MSN

See also: Aging process; Alcohol use disorder; Balance disorders; Depression; Facility and institutional care; Gastrointestinal changes and disorders; Health care; Health insurance; Medicare; Medications; Memory loss; Nutrition; Psychiatry, geriatric; Sleep changes and disturbances; Thyroid disorders; Urinary problems; Vision changes and disorders; Vitamins and minerals

For Further Information

"Avoiding Overmedication and Harmful Drug Reactions." HealthInAging.org, Jan. 2019. www.healthinaging.org/tools-and-tips/avoiding-overmedication-and-harmful-drug-reactions. A guide for seniors to help avoid overmedication.

Gorman, Anna. "Has Overmedicating Seniors Become 'America's Other Drug Problem'"? PBS, Public Broadcasting Service, 30 Aug. 2016. www.pbs.org/newshour/health/polypharmacy-americas-drug-problem. Uses expert input and personal stories to illustrate the problem of polypharmacy in geriatric medicine.

Little, Milta O. "The Burden of Overmedication: What Are the Real Issues?" *Journal of the American Medical Directors Association*, vol. 17, no. 2, Feb. 2016, pp. 97-98. doi:10.1016/j.jamda.2015.12.001. Reviews several drug-specific tools and interventions to reduce polypharmacy have been developed and tested across health care settings.

Rochon, Paula A. "Drug Prescribing for Older Adults." UpToDate, 19 Feb. 2019. www.uptodate.com/contents/drug-prescribing-for-older-adults. Provides a step-by-step guide for drug prescribing in older adults and warns against the adverse drug effects of several common medications.

Stockwell, Serena. "Nursing Homes Are Overmedicating People with Dementia." *American Journal of Nursing*, vol. 118, no. 5, May 2018, p. 14. doi:10.1097/01.naj.0000532816.04585.bb. Reviews a Human Rights Watch report that indicates that thousands of patients with dementia in nursing homes are being overmedicated with psychotropic drugs.

PALLIATIVE CARE

Relevant Issues: Long-term, chronic illness, death, family, health and medicine, sociology

Significance: Palliative Care focuses on living with a chronic diagnosis such as heart disease or cancer, and preparing for eventual death from the disease. It is not Hospice care that focuses on late stage disease and death, but rather eases the transition process during a long-term illness with no expectation of cure.

Palliative care (PC) focuses on assisting patients with chronic diagnoses that cannot be cured and their families to have the optimal quality of life and level of comfort while preparing them for the process of dying. Palliative care primarily serves an older population often with neurological, heart or cardiac related diagnoses. Only 14 percent of patient deaths in hospitals are from cancer. Often the aging patient and family struggles to understand the care and long-term effects of the disease. End of life care describes the care given around the time of death, but it should begin much sooner so the patient and family can move through a difficult time, months or even years before death occurs.

Because patients can be overly optimistic at times regarding their chronic diseases and possible outcomes, PC attempts to provide support for the patient and family while being realistic about the process of the disease. Being overly optimistic and not accepting the future of their disease and potential outcome can have a negative effect on quality of life. Providing information about the path the disease will take and the future expectations about the disease allows the patient and family to work through issues in advance of the late stages of the disease and ultimate death. Advanced care planning helps the patient and family to navigate end of life care. Although planning for a peaceful death seems harsh, studies have shown that both patients and families get significant benefits from participating in a palliative care program.

Palliative care is not hospice care. Hospice care focuses on death and dying often shortly before the patient dies from disease. Patients, however, participating in a PC program may transition to hospice care near the end of life. Both PC programs and hospice programs suffer from late referrals, causing unnecessary suffering for patients and families. A referral to the PC team should occur soon after a diagnosis of a chronic disease that has no expectation of cure. The team is trained to approach the patient and family in a positive manner, explaining they are available to help them cope with the disease. PC focuses on patients living with a serious illness with the aim of improving the quality of life for the patient and family far in advance of planning for death.

Because care can be complex depending on the underlying diagnosis, a specially trained team of physicians, nurses and other providers add additional supportive care to the medical plan of care. The growth of palliative care is dramatic over the past 15 years with almost 2,000 hospitals having a PC Team. PC is moving into the community setting as patients do not need ongoing hospitalization in most instances. Companies or organizations including home health agencies and those dedicated to outpatient Hospice and PC as well as physician offices are increasingly moving PC into the community setting. PC is now being seen as a positive addition to health care and moving away from the days when PC programs were compared to "death panels."

Palliative care is designed for patients whose diseases require significant care, often for months or years with no potential for cure. It must be timely and involve all appropriate members of the health-care team beginning with the physician specialists providing medical care. Chronic disease care is often fragmented as patients move through multiple sites of care and health-care providers over an extended period of time. A comprehensive plan of care will provide higher quality of care, deliver optimal outcomes as possible, and save money. The cost of long-term chronic care for patients with diseases such as heart failure, respiratory diseases, cancer and others is significant. Better managing the patient on a day-to-day basis saves money for both the patient and the health-care community. Studies have shown that patients in the late stage of disease who avoided heroic but futile care measures, avoided unnecessary visits to the intensive care unit (ICU), avoided the use of feeding tubes, had appropriately managed pain or did not die in the hospital, described a higher quality end of life. The PC program can assist in managing patients with chronic diseases to a good death while providing the support families need as they care for their loved one long-term up until their death.

PRINCIPLES

Communication about what to expect as the disease progresses; management of emotional needs such as fear, anxiety and depression; managing the patient's physical needs such as pain control, fatigue, breathing difficulties, nausea and loss of appetitive and sleeplessness while coordinating the care of multiple providers across hospital, physician office and home settings; and, referring to death as a natural process are the primary principles of palliative care. Providing a smooth transition through a long-term, life threatening disease from diagnosis to a good death is one of the best gifts a patient and family can receive from their providers.

—*Patricia Stanfill Edens, RN, PhD, LFACHE*

See also: Death and dying; Death of a child; Death of parents; Euthanasia; Family relationships; Funerals; Grief; Health care; Hospice; Hospitalization; Kübler-Ross, Elisabeth; Medicare; Religion; Terminal illness; Widows and widowers

For Further Information

Bodtke, Susan, and Kathy Ligon. *Hospice and Palliative Medicine Handbook: A Clinical Guide.* CreateSpace Independent Publishing Platform, 2016. This comprehensive pocket-size handbook is the essential reference for clinicians and others serving patients with advanced or life-limiting illness. It offers up-to-date, relevant, and highly practical guidance to expertly meet the challenges of serving these patients and their families.

MacLeod, Roderick Duncan, and Lieve Van den Block, editors. *Textbook of Palliative Care.* SpringerLink. link.springer.com/referencework/10.1007/978-3-319-317 38-0. Textbook of Palliative Care is a comprehensive, clinically relevant and state-of-the art book, aimed at advancing palliative care as a science, a clinical practice and as an art. The textbook is available online for free.

"Palliative Care." National Institute on Aging, U.S. Department of Health and Human Services. www.nia.nih.gov/health/topics/palliative-care. Collection of resources about palliative care.

Puri, Sunita. *That Good Night: Life and Medicine in the Eleventh Hour.* Penguin Publishing Group, 2019. Interweaving evocative stories of Puri's family and the patients she cares for. That Good Night is a stunning meditation on impermanence and the role of medicine in helping us to live and die well, arming readers with information that will transform how we communicate with our doctors about what matters most to us.

Schroeder, Karla, and Karl Lorenz. "Nursing and the Future of Palliative Care." *Asia Pacific Journal of Oncology Nursing*, vol. 5, no. 1, Jan.-Mar. 2018, pp. 4-8. doi:10.4103/apjon.apjon_43_17. Discusses the different roles nurses have in palliative care and provides methods for increasing skills in the current nursing workforce.

"Starting a Palliative Care Program." *Palliative Care Program*, Center to Advance Palliative Care. www.capc.org/toolkits/starting-the-program/. The Center to Advance Palliative Care (CAPC) is a national organization dedicated to increasing the availability of quality health care for people living with a serious illness. As the nation's leading resource in its field, CAPC provides health-care professionals and organizations with the training, tools, and technical assistance necessary to effectively meet this need.

PARENTHOOD

Relevant Issues: Family, psychology
Significance: The role of parent continues into late life; for most elders, the positive aspects of this relationship far outweigh the negatives.

Parenthood may not be a universal experience, but more than 80 percent of the adult population has at least one child. With the average life span increasing each decade, this means that most people alive today will spend most of the years of their lives as parents. This is a dramatic contrast to the situation in the early twentieth century, when the average life span was barely long enough to launch children into adulthood.

Today's generation of elders differs also in family composition. Families of the past had few generations but had many members in each generation, giving an older person during his or her lifetime many sons or daughters, a good number of siblings, plus a few grandchildren. Elders are now more apt to have fewer sons or daughters and fewer siblings, but chances are great that they will live to have grandchildren and great-grandchildren. In fact, most people in the United States over sixty-five are members of four-generation families.

Several pervasive, false myths pertain to the parental role in late life. One is that the role of parent ends at some point in the child's life, such as when the son or daughter reaches legal majority or moves out of the family home. This is no longer true of families in Western culture; according to anthropological surveys, it seems not to have been true in the past or in any other cultures. In almost all studies of family structure, contact between parents and their adult children continues after the children have married, even if they have moved to another location and become part of their new spouse's kinship group. In the United States, almost all parents over sixty-five have regular communication of some kind with their adult children. Clearly, the myth of parenthood ending at any point in life is not based on valid evidence.

Another false myth of parenthood in later life is that the family unit now consists of young parents and their children, having shrunk from times past to exclude extended kin, such as grandparents. Census data on family units of the past show that extended families living under one roof were seldom a reality; furthermore, today's families have not excluded their elders, but instead include more generations than ever before. One in five adults between the ages of sixty-five and eighty-nine lives with his or her children and often grandchildren, and the proportion rises to one in two after the age of eighty-nine. Clearly the myth of truncated families is also a false one.

A third myth about parenthood in later life, equally false, is that there is a role reversal at some point in time during which the parents become like children and the adult children take over the parental role. Although this may be true in cases of extreme physical disability or dementia, almost all elders retain their roles as parents. Adult children frequently assist in various tasks of daily living and even bring parents into their homes to live, but in very few instances do parents relinquish their status or do their children stop viewing them in their roles as mother and father.

OLDER PARENTS AND ADULT CHILDREN

In addition to frequency of contact between older parents and their adult children, researchers have studied the types of contact these family members have and also factors that might influence which type of contact older adults have with their adult children. Most communicate via letters, telephone, and e-mail, but 40 percent of parents over the age of sixty-five have face-to-face contact with at least one of their children two or more times a week, and 20 percent see at least one of their children daily.

Among the factors that can affect frequency of contact between older parents and their adult children are gender, with daughters contacting parents more often than sons; race or ethnicity, with African Americans and Latinos contacting parents more often than Caucasians; stage of life, with young and middle-aged adults who have children at home contacting their parents less often than those who have either no children or whose children are already grown; age and health of parents, with adult children having more frequent contact as parents grow older or as their health declines; and socioeconomic group, with working-class families having more contact between parent and adult child than middle-class families.

Although it has been established that the relationship between parent and child is lifelong, the content of the parenting role changes. As children grow up and establish their own families, their childhood needs of parents as providers, protectors, and secure emotional bases change. Part of attaining maturity involves looking to oneself for the fulfillment of needs, perhaps through the process of developing mental representations of one's parents and using them as templates. Other needs formerly fulfilled by parents, such as secure emotional bases, are thought to be fulfilled by spouses. However, more than three-quarters of adults report that their relationships with their parents are emotionally close.

Although older parents do not typically provide financial support to their adult children, they do assist in time of need. This assistance includes lending money to an adult child for specific purposes, such as buying a house or starting a new business, or providing a home once again for an adult child who has serious needs because of illness or financial reversals. Another time older parents are particularly helpful to their adult children is in time of divorce, especially for daughters. Parents not only provide homes and financial assistance for their daughters, but they also may take over some aspects of the parental role if there are grandchildren. Grandfathers, especially, tend to provide the financial support and male influence that was previously the responsibility of their fathers. In some families, especially African American families, mothers play a substantial role in the lives of their adult daughters and often take over the responsibility of raising their grandchildren, even when the daughter is also living in the home. It is estimated that four million American children live in households headed by a grandparent; for one million of those children, the grandparent is the sole caregiver.

Older adults contribute more than tangible assistance to their adult children. Almost one-half of adults report receiving advice and counseling from their parents, particularly concerning health, work, family relationships, and finances. Middle-aged children, in turn, also offer advice to their parents, usually about where to live, how to handle their finances, and how to spend their time. Although more advice comes down from parent to child, older parents are more apt to act on the advice of their children than vice versa. Often the type of advice exchanged is specific to a particular family; that is, some families exchange advice between generations primarily about financial matters, while other families advise each other mainly on strengthening relationships within the family.

BENEFITS OF PARENTHOOD IN LATER YEARS

Becoming a parent is a central goal and ultimate source of meaning for most people. The relationships parents have with their children are thought to shape them as individuals as much as the relationships they had in childhood with their own parents. One of the important psychological tasks of middle adulthood is theorized to be "generativity"—the need to create, to accomplish, to nurture. Although this can be done in many arenas, its most direct expression is found in having children and fostering their development into maturity. According to this theory, individuals who have accomplished this task are able to achieve higher levels of meaning in their lives than those who have not.

Besides individual fulfillment, parenthood also seems to contribute to marital happiness in later years. Older adult couples who are parents often have happier marriages than those who are not parents, although this is not true in the earlier years. Longitudinal research shows that during the years that parents have children living in the home, their assessments of marital happiness is lower than couples who have no children. Once the "nest is emptied," however, marital happiness increases. The difference is not a large one, but it is significant and consistently found in a number of studies. One explanation of these data is that couples who are parents spend more time and effort on effective parenting than on attaining marital happiness. Once the children are launched, they can focus again on each other, pleased that they have accomplished this important task together.

Less esoteric benefits of parenthood for older adults include the contribution adult children make to their welfare and well-being, including financial support and instrumental support. In nontechnical cultures, there is a direct economic benefit to having children, especially sons. Parents provide for children until they are grown, then the children provide for the parents as a fair exchange. This is not the general expectation of parents in the United States. Most parents consider themselves the providers for their children well into adulthood, and it is difficult when situations arise that make them unable to provide, or worse, force them to depend on their children. Although many adult children give to their parents financially and instrumentally, it is difficult when the parents feel they have become a burden. Optimal situations are found when elderly parents feel they are participating in a fair exchange with their children, such as baking a pie for the son who mows their grass each week or clipping grocery coupons for the daughter who drives them to doctors' appointments. Other elderly parents take pride in discussing their life insurance, family jewelry, or other inheritance they will leave for their helpful children.

Perhaps more important that instrumental help, adult children provide social and emotional support for their parents. After physical dependence, loneliness is the greatest fear of older adults. As age increases, the number of friends and acquaintances a person has decreases—some die, some become invalids in nursing homes, and others move away. Older adults who have children rely more and more on them for social and emotional support, especially if they are divorced or widowed. Research has shown that older adults who have close emotional ties to family members have better physical and psychological health than those who are isolated.

NEGATIVE ASPECTS OF PARENTHOOD IN LATER YEARS

If older parents bask in the happiness and success of their adult children, the reverse is also true—having adult children who are troubled and unsuccessful can bring heartache and shame in the later years of life.

Major problems reported by adults over sixty-five include concerns over their adult children's marital problems, financial problems, and physical and psychological health problems. Although these issues are unfortunate at any time, they are especially problematic in later years, when parents have fewer financial or emotional resources to offer.

Other negative aspects of parenthood in later life are intrusive children who often try to make decisions for their elderly parents on matters such as finances, health care, and living arrangements, regardless of the parents' own reasoning abilities. While some adult children no doubt have selfish motives of controlling the family resources, most are acting out of a sense of misplaced responsibility toward their parents or lack of knowledge about the normal aging process. Especially distressing for widowed parents are attempts by children to thwart social encounters with potential for romance. Whether out of loyalty to their deceased parent, motives to protect their future inheritance, or refusal to see one's older parent as having romantic interests, adult children can produce roadblocks when parents show an interest in seeking companionship or romance with a member of the opposite sex.

One surprising aspect of parenthood in old age is that having inattentive children does not pose a significant negative effect. Although adult children can be a major source of social support, older adults who have no children or who have inattentive or disinterested children report similar happiness if they have close relationships with their spouse or with close friends.

The truths of parenthood and aging are that multigenerational families are now common, that almost all older parents have frequent contact with all of their children and most have face-to-face contact with at least one child on a regular basis, and that parent-child role reversals in later years are not typical in physically and mentally healthy families. Parenthood can bring personal fulfillment, social support, and instrumental assistance as one ages. Drawbacks exist, but if one's adult children are reasonably happy and successful, if they allow parents to make their own major decisions as long as they remain capable, and if the parents have some close relationships with other family members or friends, the benefits far outweigh the negatives.

—*Barbara R. Bjorklund*

See also: Childlessness; Children of Aging Parents; Communication; Empty nest syndrome; Family relationships; Full nest; Grandparenthood; Marriage; Maturity; Skipped-generation parenting

For Further Information

Bee, Helen L., and Barbara R. Bjorklund. *The Journey of Adulthood.* 8th ed. Prentice Hall, 2016. This textbook is designed for undergraduate college students majoring in a number of subjects dealing with adulthood and aging. The book is written in a warm and friendly tone but includes research findings from a wide variety of fields that study the aging process. Particularly interesting are two chapters on social roles and relationships in adulthood.

Erikson, Erik H. *Identity and the Life Cycle.* New York: Norton, 1980. Erikson, a leading neo-Freudian, discusses his theory of psychosocial development across the life cycle and the importance of parenthood (or similar generative endeavors) to the well-being of middle-aged and older adults.

Hank, Karsten, and Michael Wagner. "Parenthood, Marital Status, and Well-Being in Later Life: Evidence from SHARE." *Social Indicators Research*, vol. 114, no. 2, 2013, pp. 639-53. doi:10.1007/s11205-012-0166-x. The authors address the question of whether and how parenthood and marital status are associated with various dimensions of elders' well-being, which they define by elements of the individual's economic situation, psychological well-being, and social connectedness.

Pudrovska, Tetyana. "Parenthood, Stress, and Mental Health in Late Midlife and Early Old Age." *The International Journal of Aging and Human Development*, vol. 68, no. 2, 2009, pp. 127-47. doi:10.2190/ag.68.2.b. This study examines the psychological consequences of potentially stressful, non-normative, or "off-time" aspects of the parental role in late midlife and early old age, including co-residence with adult children, stepparenthood, and parental bereavement.

PARKINSON'S DISEASE

Relevant Issues: Health and medicine

Significance: Parkinson's disease arises from a progressive neural degeneration that leads to the death of specific cells deep within the brain; the disease has devastated the lives of millions of people.

Key Terms:

acetylcholine: serves as a transmitter substance of nerve impulses within the central and peripheral nervous systems *anticholinergics*: inhibit the transmission of parasympathetic nerve impulses, thereby reducing spasms of smooth muscles

butyrophenones: any of a class of antipsychotics, as haloperidol, used to relieve symptoms of schizophrenia, acute psychosis, or other severe psychiatric disorders

dopamine: helps regulate movement, attention, learning, and emotional responses

globus pallidus: a structure in the brain involved in the regulation of voluntary movement

phenothiazines: medications used to treat schizophrenia and manifestations of psychotic disorders

striatum: coordinates multiple aspects of cognition, including both motor and action planning, decision-making, motivation, reinforcement, and reward perception

substantia nigra: an important player in brain function, in particular, in eye movement, motor planning, reward-seeking, learning, and addiction

Parkinson's disease (PD) has become a growing problem. In 1999, approximately 500,000 patients were afflicted by this disease in the United States. The Parkinson's Foundation Prevalence Project has estimated that 1 million people in the United States will be living with PD by the year 2020. The number of people affected is higher than all patients of multiple sclerosis (MS), muscular dystrophy, and amyotrophic lateral sclerosis (Lou Gehrig's disease) combined. Most patients are older than forty years of age, although the disease also occasionally affects younger people as well. A rare form of PD also affects teenagers. Statistically, men have a higher incidence of the disease, and Caucasians are more affected than any other race.

SYMPTOMS AND DIAGNOSIS

A human is born with all the brain cells (also known as neurons) he or she will ever have. This means that if, during lifetime, some of those neurons die, they will never be replaced. Extensive research has shown that people with PD have lost most of the neurons that produce dopamine, an important neurotransmitter that delivers messages within the brain. As the available dopamine is decreased, an imbalance of dopamine and acetylcholine occurs in the brain, leading to a lack of movement coordination.

PD is not diagnosed easily because various patients do not show the same symptoms, and there are no proven, specific tests for its identification. Moreover, Parkinson-like symptoms can often arise from head trauma or the use of tranquilizing drugs, such as phenothiazines and butyrophenones. Even carbon monoxide poisoning or Reglan, a common antidote against stomach upset, may provide these symptoms. The general diagnosis involves a neurological examination, which evaluates the symptoms and their severity. If the symptoms are judged as serious, a trial test of anti-Parkinson's drugs (such as primary levodopa) may be administered to establish the existence of the disease. If the patient fails to gain ground, other brain evaluations using such technology as computed tomography (CT) or magnetic resonance imaging (MRI) are used to rule out other diseases rather than certify the presence of PD.

Type A patients display an extensive degree of tremor, often on either the left or right side only, together with muscle rigidity. Type B patients may not exhibit tremors at all but may show a great disturbance in balance and gait, as well as an inability to move easily. A more severe class involves the "Parkinson's plus" patients, whose cases are accompanied by six different types of neurological disorder, such as Shy-Drager syndrome, substantia nigra degeneration (SND), progressive supranuclear palsy (PSP), olivopontocerebellar atrophy (OPCA), or multisystem atrophy.

Despite the scientific breakthroughs in understanding various brain mechanisms, the cause of the disease is still unknown. In some cases, viral infections appear to have triggered the symptoms, such as in the worldwide encephalitis epidemic that took place between 1918 and 1922, in which the mortality rate reached 40 percent. PD has also been found among people whose pyramidal nervous system was damaged by the use of illegal drugs related to the narcotic painkiller meperidine (Demerol).

Comparisons of healthy and PD patients' brains have shown considerable differences in the substantia nigra and the striatum parts. Many of the substantia nigra's pigmented cells are damaged in the patients; instead of the normal black spots, they contain pink staining spheres called Lewy bodies. It is estimated that loss of approximately 80 percent of the substantia nigra's pigmented cells and 80 percent of the striatum's dopamine content results in the appearance of PD symptoms.

HISTORY

Parkinson's disease took its name from nineteenth century British physician James Parkinson, who described the classic symptoms of resting tremor, propulsion, and stooped posture for the first time in a monograph entitled "An Essay on the Shaking Palsy" in 1817. In 1939, neurosurgeon Russell Meyers removed a brain tumor from a patient who also had PD. Further experimental surgery on the same patient involved a lesion in a neurosignal fiber bundle, called the ansa lenticularis, which reduced the patient's PD symptoms to a considerable degree. The same complex surgical procedure was later applied to about one hundred more people, thirty-nine of which showed improvement, while seventeen died.

In the early 1950s, Swedish neurosurgeon Lars Leksell applied a procedure called posterolateral pallidotomy to patients, with mixed results. In this approach, a small-diameter metal probe was inserted into the skull along the front hairline, deep into the globus pallidus part of the brain. However, missing the target by the smallest margin led to blindness or permanent impairment of other functions. Thirty years later, several other Swedish neurosurgeons attempted to implant surgically in the brain parts of the patient's adrenal gland that produces dopamine. Success, however, remained elusive. In 1985, Lauri V. Laitinen proposed a modified procedure of Leksell's original pallidotomy, called PVP pallidotomy. The process involved attaching a calibrated metal halo to the patient's head. The use of CT or MRI pictures with the calibration of the halo allowed the identification of the exact target spot during the surgery.

Transplanting small parts of live tissue from aborted fetuses into the brains of PD patients appeared to gain ground in the war against the disease in the late 1980s. This process, also called fetal tissue transplant, first involved fetal adrenal gland tissue and later fetal brain tissue and served as an attempt to enhance the production of more dopamine in the patient's brain. Pioneering neurosurgeons who used this procedure included Laitinen in Sweden, Z. S. Tang in China, and Robert Iacono in the United States. A fetal bank was established in Huashan Hospital in Shanghai, China, where the fetal brain tissue was held under cryogenic conditions. The actual transplants took place in China, as a long-standing ban on fetal tissue research made this kind of surgery practically impossible in the United States.

TREATMENT

Apart from surgery, type A and B patients can be helped by medication prescription or neurosurgery. The primary medications are classified as anticholinergics, antihistamines, dopaminergics, and dopamine agonists. Unfortunately, all drugs used have side effects that may create a serious impact on the quality of life. Drug therapy attempts to maintain the patient on conservative levels of medication while maintaining mobility. Side effects include dry mouth, constipation, blurred vision, visual hallucinations, lethargy, confusion, and nausea.

Levodopa is the drug of choice for treatment of PD and is marketed as a mixture with carbidopa. Carbidopa is used as a blocker of the breakdown of levodopa in the peripheral organs to allow more levodopa to cross the blood-brain barrier. Through a series of complex enzymatic reactions, levodopa is converted to dopamine. As the disease progresses, however, the patients need much larger quantities of levodopa. During the administration of the medicine, patients appear to have a surge of energy, which quickly wears off as time elapses.

Interestingly, symptoms on the left side of the patient are relieved with an operation on the right part of the brain, and vice versa. Moreover, a brain whose problems arise from the death of some of the neurons can show signs of improvement by deadening some more of those cells in the critically over-stimulated pathways. Thus, the activity that would result if all of the brain's circuits carried action commands appears to be controlled.

During the overall surgical procedure, the patient is awake and only lightly anesthetized, responding to the surgeon's commands to move various parts of the body, such as hands, fingers, eyes, toes, and tongue. With the help of the MRI pictures, the surgeon can pinpoint the cells that are to be neutralized. A probe is slowly entered into the brain, and its tip sends an electric signal back to the control panel, indicating the overall geography of the brain map. Once it reaches the target spot, an electrical shock is applied at the probe tip that kills the overreacting cells. The patient has absolutely no feeling, and the electrical "cauterization" has no effect on the nearby capillaries and the blood flowing in them. The probe is then removed, and the penetrated skin is stitched up. After the surgery, the patient displays much less muscle tightening, as well as dramatic decreases in tremors. In most cases, the patient stays one night in the hospital for observation, and then walks with no help out of the hospital the next day.

Electrical stimulation therapy had developed in widespread use by 2019. Other non-drug therapies also have been tried, such as dancing, which aids in maintenance of balance. New drugs are continually being introduced as well or new uses for older ones. For example, Exenatide, usually used for diabetes, has improved motor function that has been impeded by Parkinson's. Gene implantation in the brain also has been found to reduce severity of motor symptoms. This delicate operation has been used in some Parkinson's patients whose symptoms were no longer controlled by their medications.

—Soraya Ghayourmanesh
Updated by Bruce E. Johansen, PhD

See also: Brain changes and disorders; Illnesses among older adults; Mobility problems

For Further Information

Hammarlund, Catharina Sjödahl, et al. "The Impact of Living with Parkinson's Disease: Balancing within a Web of Needs and Demands." *Parkinson's Disease*, vol. 2018, 29 July 2018, pp. 1-8. doi:10.1155/2018/4598651. This study explores the impact of living with Parkinson's disease (PD) by evaluating nineteen persons diagnosed with PD 3-27 years ago, using semi-structured interviews.

Langston, J. William, et al. "Optimizing Parkinson's Disease Diagnosis: The Role of a Dual Nuclear Imaging Algorithm." *Parkinson's Disease*, vol. 4, no. 1, 23 Feb. 2018. doi:10.1038/s41531-018-0041-9. Highlights how dual neuroimaging strategy can maximize diagnostic accuracy for patient care, clinical trials, pre-symptomatic PD screening, and special cases provided by specific genetic mutations associated with PD.

Marie, Lianna. *Everything You Need to Know about Caregiving for Parkinson's Disease: The Complete Guide for Anyone Caring for Someone with Parkinson's Disease.* CreateSpace, 2016. This comprehensive guide addresses important questions about caring for someone with Parkinson's Disease. Written in easy to understand everyday English, this book is the result of 25 years experience and research in living a life with Parkinson's Disease.

Parashos, Sotirios A., et al. *Navigating Life with Parkinson Disease.* Oxford U P, 2013. A guide for anyone affected by Parkinson's disease: patients, caregivers, family members, and friends. Containing the most up-to-date information, it discusses the available treatments and supplies practical advice on how to manage PD in the long term, emphasizing life-style adjustments.

Rizek, Philippe, et al. "An Update on the Diagnosis and Treatment of Parkinson Disease." *Canadian Medical Association Journal*, vol. 188, no. 16, 1 Nov. 2016, pp. 1,157-65. doi:10.1503/cmaj.151179. A review of the advancements and ongoing research in the management of Parkinson's disease.

PENSIONS

Relevant Issues: Economics, work

Significance: Pension plans enable regular income or annuity payments to a retired former employee who is eligible for pension benefits through advanced age, total earnings, or years of service. Benefits may also be paid following total disability or job termination, with payments made to surviving beneficiaries following the death of the covered worker.

Key Terms:

deferred income: a portion of an employee's compensation that is set aside to be received after the period in which it was earned

group annuity: an employer establishes a group annuity on behalf of its employees by signing a master contract with an insurer; this contract details the agreement between the insurer and employer, such as plan type, contribution requirements and administrative fees

incentives: money that a person, company, or organization offers to encourage certain behaviors or actions, like joining a pension plan

mutual fund: a professionally managed investment fund that pools money from many investors to purchase securities

Americans are becoming increasingly concerned about pension benefits following retirement because they are living longer: In 2016, men in the United States could expect to live approximately eighteen more years after reaching sixty-five years of age, whereas women could expect to live approximately 20.6 more years, according to the Paris-based Organisation for Economic Co-operation and Development, (OECD), Women in Japan could expect to live 24.4 more years, and men 19.6 more years, Many financial and retirement planning professionals recommend that retirees plan for an income of 70 to 80 percent of their final annual work income to maintain a comfortable lifestyle for themselves and their spouses for the duration of the life span.

The U.S. Congress has enacted several laws allowing workers to plan for their retirement that provide strong financial incentives for both employers and employees to set aside additional retirement funds by making them deductible from their current federal income taxes, with deferred income. Monies put into pension plans are allowed to accumulate on a tax-free basis until withdrawn during retirement, thus creating one of the best tax shelters available for persons with middle-class incomes.

A HISTORY OF PENSION PLANS

The Roman Empire was the first government on record to establish pension plans for the provision of housing and board benefits for their disabled and aged soldiers. This practice was followed much later by the governments of France and Britain, as persons holding government offices began passing legislation to make retirement provisions for themselves by the early nineteenth century.

Although various forms of primitive pension plans have been awarded to American war veterans since the founding of the United States, the earliest highly organized American pensions were developed by railroad, banking, and public utility firms beginning in the late 1870s. Metropolitan Life Insurance Company issued the first group annuity contract in 1921, with the Equitable Life Assurance Society following suit and entering the pension business in 1924. In 1940, however, fewer than 20 percent of employees in business and government were covered by private pension plans.

Immediately following World War II, tremendous growth occurred in pension coverage of private citizens. By 1982, approximately 50 percent of all private business workers and 75 percent of all government workers were enrolled in some form of retirement program other than Social Security. As greater taxes began to be imposed on large corporations, particularly those that were highly profitable, financial incentives were established by the federal government to encourage the business sector to create pension plans for its employees.

TYPES OF RETIREMENT BENEFITS

Pension plans offered by private employers are generally identified as being insured or trustee, group or individual, private or public, contributory or noncontributory, fixed or variable benefit, and single employer or multiemployer. Insured plans involve a life insurer as the funding agency, whereas a trust fund plan involves a commercial bank or individual trustee as the funding agency. Both funding methods are employed in a split-funded or combination plan. Insured plans enable the insurance company to invest the contributions and pay retirement benefits using an allocated funding contract or an unallocated funding method.

Allocated funding contracts involve cash-value life insurance or deferred annuities that are immediately purchased for each employee. Individual policies, generally utilized by smaller businesses, are funded through individual insurance such as whole-life or retirement income contracts that deliver payment upon retirement. Group deferred annuity plans involve single-premium annuities that are purchased yearly and then credited to individualized accounts.

Unallocated funding methods make up a vast majority of all insured plans and enable funds to accumulate and be used later to purchase annuities for employees upon retirement. Group deposit administration plans involve the accumulation and investment of employers' deposits to be used later to purchase annuities upon retirement. Immediate participation guarantee plans involve the immediate and full participation of the employer in the plan's investment, with the covered worker being paid directly from the fund following retirement. Guaranteed investment contracts generally involve larger pension funds by which the insurer guarantees somewhat higher rates of interest for a period of several years.

Under a defined contribution arrangement such as a 401(k) plan, profit sharing, or money purchase plan, the employer, employee, or both contribute funds directly into the pension. This money is usually invested into one of several different mutual funds, with many plans leaving the specific allocations up to the individual worker. The money contributed is exempt from current income tax, with the earnings continuing to accumulate tax-free until retirement, when regular withdrawals may begin.

Most pensions will pay benefits either in equal monthly payments or in a lump sum, depending upon the wishes of the retiree. Some plans may require that workers take a lump-sum distribution if they leave their jobs before retirement and the total value of their benefits is a given sum ($3,500 or less, for example). If the value of the benefits is greater than a given sum, workers may be given the choice of an immediate lump-sum payment or monthly payments that begin at retirement as specified in the plan. Choosing to take a lump-sum payment gives workers the choice of investing the money or spending it as they desire. Unless the funds are placed in an individual retirement account (IRA), however, the full amount received is taxable in the year that it was received. The only exception is "forward income averaging," which is available to persons receiving pension funds after 59.5 years of age. If the retiree is under age 59.5, the pension plan administrator is required to withhold 20 percent of pension funds and immediately forward that money to the Internal Revenue Service (IRS).

GOVERNMENT REGULATION OF PENSION PLANS

Because the Social Security system in the United States was never designed to provide, and is not capable of providing, a livable income following retirement, Congress has enacted laws encouraging both employers and employees to set aside additional funds. Some pension plans are designed to integrate the payments that retired workers receive with the amount that Social Security provides.

During the 1930s many U.S. citizens become increasingly more concerned about the need to provide for personal retirement, in addition to that of their spouses and other family members that survived them. This social and increasingly political movement culminated in the late 1940s, when the automobile, coal, and steel unions pushed to make pension plans one of the central issues in their labor negotiations. Pushes by various labor unions for pension benefits were assisted by a National Labor Relations Board (NLRB) ruling in 1948 that employers had a legal obligation to bargain with employees over the specific terms of the pension plans offered. Military pensions are covered by the Servicemen's and Veteran's Survivor Benefits Act of 1957, whereby retired service men and women receive 50 percent of their base pay at time of retirement following twenty years of service, with regular increases as determined by the consumer price index.

The Federal Welfare and Pension Plan Disclosure Act (WPPDA) of 1958—in combination with the Internal Revenue Code of 1921, which qualified taxation issues—provided the initial regulation of pension plans. A pension plan that qualified provided considerable tax advantages to the employer, such as the deduction of employer contributions as a business expense. These contributions are not considered taxable income until after payments begin following retirement. Investment earnings on assets are not taxable, and installment death benefits and lump-sum severance distributions also receive very favorable tax treatment.

The extremely complex Employee Retirement Income Security Act (ERISA) of 1974 allowed comprehensive regulation of pension plans from their inception to termination and greatly strengthened retirement benefits, mainly by reinforcing previous regulations. A major goal of ERISA was to protect the benefit rights of workers regarding pension qualification, participation, funding, vesting, actuarial soundness, plan termination, management of assets, annual reports, and fiduciary responsibility.

This act also established the Pension Benefit Guaranty Corporation, which administers plan termination insurance, thus assuring some level of benefits for pensions that are terminated as a result of inadequate funding. However, this federal insurance would not necessarily replace all benefits in the event that the employer and the related pension plan were not able to remain financially stable. Coverage by the Pension Benefit Guaranty Corporation does not extend to defined contribution plans or to other important benefits such as health or life insurance.

The Retirement Equity Act (REA) of 1984 and the Tax Reform Act of 1986 (TRA) set the minimum standards for pension plans in private industry. Although these and other federal laws made several regulations for pension plans, employers are not legally required to provide any pension benefits whatsoever to workers. Although federal law protects some retired workers in the event that a company attempts to terminate their previously established pension contract, there is presently no similar protection when an employer terminates, for example, the health-care benefits of retirees. An increasing number of workers who retire before age sixty-five and thus are not yet eligible for Medicare find themselves temporarily without health insurance as more companies are legally reducing healthcare benefits for early retirees.

VESTING AND RETIREMENT AGE
The term "vesting" describes the covered worker's right to the monies contributed from the employer to the pension plan in the event that employment is terminated prior to retirement. Cliff vesting involves full vesting not later than following five years of service if the pension is administered by a single employer. Multiemployer pensions involve a collectively bargained plan to which more than one employer makes contributions and within which full vesting must occur no later than following ten years of service. Graded vesting requires that employees be at least 20 percent vested after three years of service and receive an additional 20 percent in each of the next four service years, so that they are fully vested after seven years. Workers have no vesting rights until they complete the appropriate years of service. Contributions made directly by workers to a pension plan, in addition to interest, are always fully vested.

Pension plans generally allow the retirement age categories of normal, early, or late. Normal retirement at age sixty-five corresponds with eligibility for Social Security benefits. Early retirement with an appropriately reduced pension is generally allowable if the employee is at least fifty-five years of age and has paid into the pension plan for at least ten years. Mandatory retirement before age seventy was prohibited in 1978 by an amendment to the Age Discrimination in Employment Act (ADEA). Extremely late retirement (beyond seventy years of age) with increased benefits is then provided, but many pensions now simply pay normal retirement benefits even following late retirement to encourage retirement at age sixty-five.

REGULAR CHECKS ON PENSION PLANS
The Employee Retirement Income Security Act (ERISA) of 1974 requires employers to provide written information regarding pension plans available to their covered employees. Summary plan descriptions, to be received within ninety days by all covered workers after becoming participants, provide information on operation of the pension plan, eligibility of a covered worker or surviving spouse to receive benefits, calculation of the anticipated benefits to be received, and the filing of claims. Federal law also dictates that any changes in the summary plan are to be provided within 210 days of the end of the plan year in which the change took place and that annual reports of the plan be available. Covered workers also have the right to receive an Individual Benefit Statement, which relates vesting status and the accumulated benefits in the plan.

ERISA also established complicated rules that prevent workers from losing pension benefits for a break in service, which depend on the timing of the break in employment and how long the break lasts. Employees can obtain information regarding the financial stability of their pension plan by requesting a copy of the plan's annual federal tax return from the U.S. Department of Labor Disclosure Office.

PENSION RIGHTS FOR SURVIVING SPOUSES
Federal law requires that pension plans provide benefits for surviving spouses. Once an employee becomes fully or partially vested in a pension, survivor benefits are guaranteed upon death of the covered worker. This does not mean, however, that benefits are paid immediately in the event of death of a covered worker before retirement. For example, if the pension allowed early retirement benefits at age fifty-five and the covered worker died at age fifty, the surviving spouse would not receive benefits until the date that the worker would have turned age fifty-five. Additionally, the amount of payment is often only 50 percent of what would have been received if the covered worker had lived until retirement age and then retired.

When a covered worker dies after retirement, joint and survivor benefits require that the surviving spouse receive 50 percent of the previously received benefits, with payments continuing until the death of the survivor. Spouses are able to waive survivor benefits to get a larger monthly pension during the covered worker's retirement, but this is only recommended if the spouse is suffering from a terminal illness.

—Daniel G. Graetzer
Updated by Bruce E. Johansen, PhD

See also: Age discrimination; Age Discrimination in Employment Act of 1967; Early retirement; Employment; Estates and inheritance; 401(k) plans; Income sources; Individual retirement accounts (IRAs); Mandatory retirement; Older Worker Benefit Protection Act; Retirement; Retirement planning; Social Security; Widows and widowers

For Further Information

Ghilarducci, Teresa. How to Retire with Enough Money: and How to Know What Enough Is. Workman Publishing, 2015. How to Retire with Enough Money cuts through the confusion, misinformation, and bad policymaking that keeps us spending or saving poorly. Ghilarducci presents an easy-to-follow program for saving.

———. When I'm Sixty-Four: The Plot against Pensions and the Plan to Save Them. Princeton U P, 2008. Ghilarducci, the nation's leading authority on the economics of retirement, puts forward a sweeping plan to revive the retirement-income system.

Harris, Dan R. The Aging Sourcebook: Basic Information on Issues Affecting Older Americans. Detroit: Omnigraphics, 1998. An often-referenced resource manual that includes information on pensions as related to demographic trends, legal rights, and retirement lifestyle options.

Kotlikoff, Laurence J., et al., eds. *Get What's Yours: The Secrets to Maxing Out Your Social Security.* Revised ed., Simon & Schuster, 2016. Get What's Yours has proven itself to be the definitive book about how to navigate the forbidding maze of Social Security and emerge with the highest possible benefits. It is an engaging manual of tactics and strategies written by well-known financial commentators that is unobtainable elsewhere.

Lowenstein, Roger. *While America Aged: How Pension Debts Ruined General Motors, Stopped the NYC Subways, Bankrupted San Diego, and Loom as the Next Financial Crisis.* Penguin Books, 2009. Lowenstein brilliantly chronicles three fascinating pension cases: the collapse of the over-obligated General Motors, the pension strike that halted New York City's subways and effectively shut down the city, and the scandalous bankrupting of the affluent city of San Diego.

Matthews, J. L. *Social Security, Medicare & Government Pensions: Get the Most out of Your Retirement & Medical Benefits.* 24th ed., Nolo, 2019. Highlights laws and legislation regarding pension trusts and Social Security. The 24th edition is completely updated for 2019.

"Retirement Plans-Benefits & Savings." U.S. Department of Labor. www.dol.gov/general/topic/retirement. An overview of different retirement plans, including pensions.

Pension Benefit Guaranty Corporation. www.pbgc.gov/. PBGC was created by the Employee Retirement Income Security Act of 1974 to encourage the continuation and maintenance of private-sector defined benefit pension plans, provide timely and uninterrupted payment of pension benefits, and keep pension insurance premiums at a minimum.

PERSONALITY CHANGES

Relevant Issues: Biology, psychology, sociology

Significance: One of the fundamental questions regarding human functioning is whether personality changes or remains stable throughout the life course.

Being able to predict what people will be like when they are older is a challenge to both professionals and laypersons. The impact of age upon people entails an investigation into styles of reacting, thinking, and feeling—better known as personality. Trying to unlock and identify the mechanisms underlying personality—as well as determining whether the essential characteristics of people change across the life course—is perplexing. Part of the problem stems from the lack of a comprehensive, universally accepted definition of personality.

This diversity in meaning stems from fundamental differences in how human functioning is viewed and is best conceptualized by clarifying the dimensions upon which personality is described and explained. Those seeking to explain the origin of personality generally concentrate on the roles of inheritance (biology) and experiential (environmental) factors in the development and sustainability of the essential qualities and characteristics of individuals. Another debate exists between the optimistic view that a person's character may change over time and the notion that by the age of thirty the character is stable. Although there are a number of other dimensions used to clarify differences in perspectives regarding personality functioning, the notions of inheritance-experience and change-stability are the primary points of comparison.

STABILITY PERSPECTIVES

Perspectives that emphasize the role of biology in personality development have roots that go back to early Greek philosophy. However, contemporary views can be divided into two camps. The first incorporates theories referred to as psychoanalytic. Austrian psychoanalyst Sigmund Freud's view of human nature personifies this camp. Freud's notions regarding personality development revolve around satisfaction of biological urges and the belief that personality is frozen at adolescence. The second camp incorporates a view of human nature relying upon the biological concept of traits to describe and explain personality. The view that traits are psychological entities subscribes to the assumption that personality is made up of enduring and relatively stable characteristics, and differences among individuals merely reside in how much of each characteristic they possess. These characteristics may incorporate behavioral, mental, emotional, or temperamental traits. However, there appear to be just five dimensions or domains (neuroticism, extraversion, openness to experience, conscientiousness, and agreeableness), along with their associated traits, upon which everyone may be evaluated. Scientific studies originating from this particular camp find that adult personality changes very little and support the notion that by the age of thirty, the character is set. Although some psychological research supports biologically based contributions to the underlying stable nature of personality, there is a great deal of controversy and mixed results regarding whether characteristics or attributes of a more global nature can change well into advanced age.

Perspectives that subscribe to assumptions that people's character may change with age are more numerous and diverse. These views acknowledge the contributions that biology has made in the underlying nature of personality; however, they also emphasize and identify factors external to the person that may be responsible for change later in the life course.

SELF-NOTIONS

There are a number of different positions regarding the role of external factors in personality change. One position has its origins in psychoanalysis. Unlike Freud's view, this view of personality is quite distinct in that growth, development, and change are thought to occur well into advanced age. The defining factor here is the concept of self (who one is). It is thought to evolve over the life course and allow individuals to unite both positive and negative aspects within themselves into an integrated, balanced, and whole notion of who they are. Some individuals never achieve an integrated personality, while others find that age grants them the ability to turn inward (introversion) and explore their inner selves. Whereas in youth, turning toward the outer world (extroversion) is paramount—establishing careers, finding mates—the primary duty of the older person is to turn toward the inner, subjective world—acknowledging eventual mortality and abandoning youthful self-images. Although this position initially focuses on internal biological factors in personality functioning, it also enlists the aid of the external world in its definition and strongly supports the notion of change across the life course as fundamental.

Self, as a defining characteristic of personality, is also used by a number of other positions. Once again, these notions focus upon internal aspects of the individual; however, they are not strictly biological. The notion of self is a psychological construct and is composed of a number of related but separable facets. Similar to the trait concept, it helps explain, describe, and define personality; however, because it is a psychological concept, as opposed to a biological one, aspects of the self are thought to interact with the environment. Many scholars in this area, as well as such related disciplines as sociology, see the developing self as an outgrowth of interactions with others; self and its formation is a social phenomenon. The ways that people view and mentally represent themselves in the past, present, and future are pivotal to understanding whether personality changes or remains stable with age. Research in this area tends to support the potential for personality change, as well as the sustainability of it.

STAGE CONCEPTS

The idea that there is a predictable sequence of age-related changes is another predominant view. Such normative crises models claim that changes in personality emerge as a result of adults progressing through a series of stages (life tasks), which are often marked by age-related role expectations and emotional crises. The notion of the midlife crisis, in which the early to mid-forties is thought to be a stressful period of time in which individuals reevaluate and reappraise their lives and change their personalities and lifestyles, is somewhat of a misnomer; however, the idea epitomizes these crises-model approaches.

Although these views emphasize commonality in personality change, they also leave room for variability in the human experience by focusing on changing personal meanings and values over the life course. This suggests that not everyone reacts in a similar way and that lives may not follow exactly the same course. The defining characteristic of personality advocated by these positions lies within the individual in the guise of age, but it is also impacted by age-related role expectations and life tasks constructed by society that are external to the individual.

LIFE AND HISTORICAL EVENTS

Life experiences and historical events may also play a role in personality changes in later adulthood. Personality psychologists who emphasize life events (marriage, parenthood, retirement) as markers of change define and describe personality according to the various roles that people assume during the life course (spouse, parent, grandparent, worker), as well as to the historical influences (the Great Depression, World War II) embedded within those roles. According to this timing-of-events model, the "social clock" consists of cultural norms and expectations regarding when certain life events should occur. Life events that are anticipated and on time are less stressful than unanticipated, unusual events or events that occur at the "wrong" time. Being forced into an early retirement because of a physical disability would produce stress for many individuals and constitutes a life-altering event that not only is unanticipated but also occurs at the wrong time.

Historical events, such as the Great Depression of the 1930s and World War II, are also pivotal to understanding personality change. Scholars have found that boys whose family incomes were reduced by more than one-third during the Depression were profoundly impacted by the economic hardship. Men and women who had direct contact with war activities during World War II were, as older adults, more assertive and showed greater social competence and self-reliance than their cohorts who had no such experiences.

Overall, these personality models focus primarily upon social cultural constructs, external to the individual, to understand change and stability. Their exploration into both historical and social contexts does not easily support change over stability with respect to the effect of age on personality. However, this line of inquiry does support the importance of including both historical and social contexts in the study of personality development.

—*Rosellen M. Rosich*

See also: Alzheimer's disease; Brain changes and disorders; Creativity; Dementia; Depression; Erikson, Erik H.; Fountain of Age, The; Maturity; Medications; Psychiatry, geriatric; Wisdom

For Further Information

Erikson, Erik H. *Identity and the Life Cycle*. Norton, 1980. Erikson discusses his theory of psychosocial development across the life cycle.

Harris, Mathew A., et al. "Personality Stability from Age 14 to Age 77 Years." *Psychology and Aging*, vol. 31, no. 8, 2016, pp. 862-74. doi:10.1037/pag0000133. The authors study personality stability from childhood to older age.

Lautenschlager, Nicola T, and Hans Förstl. "Personality Change in Old Age." *Current Opinion in Psychiatry*, vol. 20, no. 1, 2007, pp. 62-66. doi:10.1097/yco.0b013e328 0113d09. The short review summarizes some of the most important personality changes in older adults.

Srivastava, Kalpana, and R. C. Das. "Personality Pathways of Successful Ageing." *Industrial Psychiatry Journal*, vol. 22, no. 1, 2013, pp. 1-3. doi:10.4103/0972-6748.123584. Explores how personality traits influence successful aging.

Staudinger, U. M., A. Law, and P. Wink. "Personality Change Predicts Wisdom in Old Age." *Innovation in Aging*, vol. 2, iss._suppl. 1, Nov. 2018,p. 553. doi:10.1093/geroni/igy 023.2044. A longitudinal study on how personality maturation towards adjustment and towards growth might play in the development of wisdom.

PETS

Relevant Issues: Economics, family, health and medicine, recreation

Significance: Elderly people who own or interact with pets often experience psychosocial and health benefits that impact quality of life.

Pet ownership or interaction with companion animals has been found to contribute to psychological, social, and physical health and well-being, all important aspects of quality of life for the elderly. Pet ownership or contact is associated with lower levels of anxiety and depression. The presence of animals appears to increase smiling, touch, and talk. Researchers report that animal interaction also tends to increase happiness and morale, alertness, feelings of affection, and security.

Elderly men and women, particularly those who live alone, may experience loneliness. Pet ownership can reduce loneliness by providing companionship and opportunities for socialization, interaction, play, and affection. Such effects may be direct, as a result of contact with affectionate and playful animals. Pet ownership may also reduce loneliness in indirect ways. For example, elderly dog owners go for walks more frequently than nonowners. During walks, opportunities for socialization with other people often arise. Indeed, there is a growing recognition that pet presence has the potential for giving people an excuse and a topic for conversation and that pets may function as "social lubricants" for their owners.

HEALTH AND ECONOMIC BENEFITS

Pet ownership or contact is associated with better health. Research shows that pet ownership or interaction reduces the risk of cardiovascular disease, heart attack, and stroke. Compared with nonowners, pet owners often have lower cardiovascular risk factors, lower systolic blood pressure, lower serum cholesterol, and lower triglyceride levels. Similarly, of people hospitalized for cardiovascular disease, pet owners have a greater chance of still being alive one year later than do those who do not own pets. Having (and looking at) an aquarium of goldfish has been found to reduce stress and lower blood pressure in people already suffering from high blood pressure. Having a parakeet has been found to increase the health of noninstitutionalized British pensioners. Some aspects of pet ownership encourage

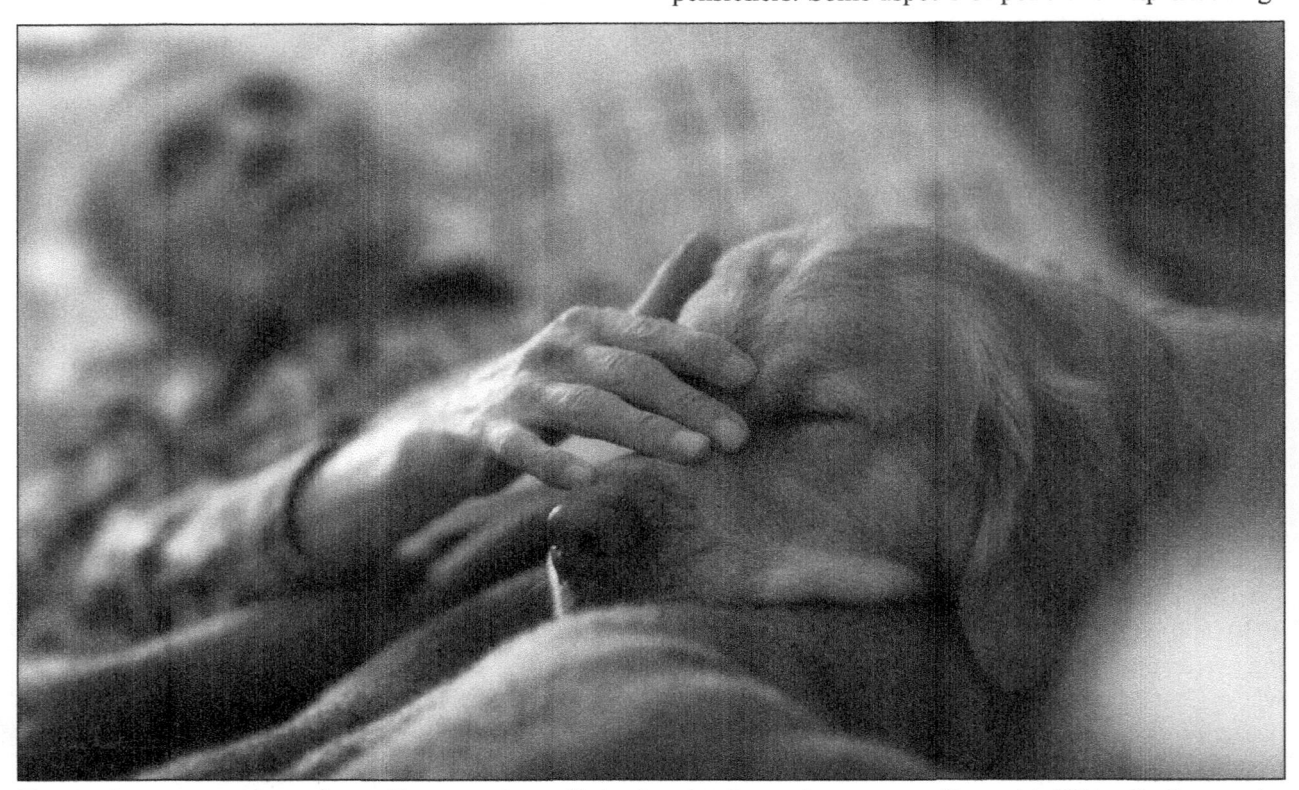

Therapy dogs can provide comfort and love to seniors suffering from loneliness, depression, or illness. (via Wikimedia Commons)

healthy behaviors. Elderly dog owners often get more exercise than people who do not own dogs, probably because they take their dogs for walks.

Pet ownership may also have economic benefits. Senior citizens who own pets visit the doctor less often and live longer than those who do not own pets. A 1990 study of Medicare beneficiaries belonging to a large California health-maintenance organization found that dog ownership was associated with fewer physician contacts.

ANOTHER SIDE

Owning a pet is not for everyone. Animal care can be costly and may be an economic burden that is beyond the means of some. The financial cost of feed, particularly for larger pets, and costs of veterinary care, particularly for older or ailing pets, may be burdensome or unmanageable. Animal care may require energy and strength beyond the abilities of some elderly people, particularly as the person's health declines. Larger, more energetic pets (some dogs, for example) could unintentionally hurt fragile or infirm elderly people by knocking them down. Not all pets are capable of interaction with humans. Goldfish cannot be held and petted. Animals may have been abused or have issues; dogs may bite or cats may scratch. The death of a beloved pet may bring considerable grief and distress.

Concerns about animal care and well-being may keep some from traveling, visiting relatives, and maintaining relationships with family or loved ones. Such concerns may delay or prevent some elderly people from getting the health care they need, as when they postpone surgery that requires hospitalization because they cannot arrange pet care.

Concerns about pet care and well-being keep many elderly people from moving into apartments, nursing homes, or other assisted-living facilities that prohibit pets. For some, giving up a beloved pet to move into an apartment or nursing home may be as emotionally painful as divorce or death. Indeed, many pets that are given up to animal shelters end up being euthanized. As this predicament is recognized, some nursing homes and assisted-care facilities are adopting "pro-pet" policies that allow residents to keep their pets.

PET-ASSISTED THERAPY IN NURSING HOMES

Animal presence or contact has been found to increase social interaction, friendliness, cooperation, and self-care behaviors among elderly residents of nursing homes. Even having a wild bird feeder (and being given responsibility for it) has been found to increase happiness and activity in a nursing home setting. Observations of the positive effects of direct contact and interaction with animals have resulted in a dramatic growth, in recent years, of pet-visitation programs in the United States. In the typical pet-visitation program, volunteers bring their companion animals to interact with nursing-home residents on a regular schedule. Male residents of nursing homes, who tend to be less social and more reclusive than female residents, tend to benefit more and faster than female residents, who may be more adept at getting their needs met by interaction with humans. Research also suggests that the positive effects of contact with animals are not permanent. That is, for the positive effects to be maintained, the visits must be continued on a regular basis. Recognizing this, a growing number of facilities are providing resident companion animals for their patients as part of treatment programming. As nursing-home and other health-care facilities gain experience with pet-assisted therapy, issues have arisen regarding selection, training, and certification of both animals and their owners.

—John W. Engel
Updated by Jackie Dial, PhD

See also: Death and dying; Depression; Facility and institutional care; Grief; Health care; Loneliness; Psychiatry, geriatric; Social ties

For Further Information

Anderson, P. Elizabeth. *The Powerful Bond between People and Pets: Our Boundless Connections to Companion Animals (Practical and Applied Psychology)*. Praeger Publishers, 2008. Explores how some animals initially kept for the work they could do gradually became our companions.

Ballinger, Barbara. "The Healing Power of Pets for Seniors." AgingCare, 20 Aug. 2018. www.agingcare.com/articles/benefits-of-elderly-owning-pets-113294. Reasons for having pets, and advice on finding the right match.

Becker, Karen Shaw. "Conflicted About Getting a Pet Because You Think You're Too Old?" HealthyPets, 04 Jan. 2018. healthypets.mercola.com/sites/healthypets/archive/2018/01/04/pet-ownership-for-seniors. Pets can be good for older owners but caring for ill or older pets brings challenges.

Cusack, Odean, and Elaine Smith. *Pets and the Elderly: The Therapeutic Bond.* Reprint ed., Routledge, 2014. Therapeutic aspects of pet ownership.

Harvey, Jacky Colliss. *The Animal's Companion: People & Their Pets, a 26,000-Year Love Story.* Black Dog & Leventhal Publishers, 2019. The author, a social anthropologist, examines why humans need animal companions of all stripes.

Overall, Christine. *Pets and People: The Ethics of Our Relationships with Companion Animals.* Oxford U P, 2017. A philosophical anthology focusing on ethical issues relating to companion animals, particularly dogs and cats.

Parslow, Ruth A., et al. "Pet Ownership and Health in Older Adults: Findings from a Survey of 2,551 Community-Based Australians Aged 60-64." *Gerontology*, vol. 51, no. 1. Jan.-Feb. 2005, pp. 40-47. doi: 10.1159/000081433. This survey of people aged 60-64 discerned no health benefits and some disadvantages of pet ownership for the age group.

Resnick, Barbara, and Sandra McCune. "Introduction to the Themed Issue on Human-Animal Interaction and Healthy Human Aging." *Anthrozoös*, vol. 32, no. 2, 19 Mar. 2019, pp. 165-68. doi:10.1080/08927936.2019.1569901. Exploring benefits and risks associated with pets and older adults.

PICTURE OF DORIAN GRAY, THE (BOOK)

Author: Oscar Wilde
Date: 1890 (magazine version), 1891 (book)
Relevant Issues: Culture, death, psychology, sociology, values

Though *The Picture of Dorian Gray* was the only novel Oscar Wilde wrote, it is one of his best-known works. It is the story of a young man, Dorian Gray, who lives a life of debauchery but never seems to age or physically show the effects of his hedonistic life. However a portrait of him, painted in the bloom of his youth, is now hidden in the attic, because it has mysteriously begun to show the effects of the life Dorian is living. This story captured the imagination of many other writers through the ages with hundreds of adaptations and retellings in various forms. It raises questions about the avoidance of at least the appearance of aging and the pursuit of youth and beauty at all costs.

SUMMARY

Dorian Gray is a beautiful young man in the prime of his life. He meets an artist, Basil Hayward, who is enthralled with the young man and wants to paint his portrait. During a sitting, Basil introduces Dorian to Lord Henry Wotton, who becomes a damaging influence on Dorian, particularly by giving Dorian a book that practically spells out how to live a life of hedonism. Lord Henry discusses the transient nature of youth and beauty, and Dorian becomes upset, cursing the portrait because in the future it will only remind him of what is past, his youth and beauty. He offers to give his soul if only he can stay young and beautiful forever and the painting can show the ravages of aging and the effects of living a hedonistic life.

Dorian continues his pursuit of pleasure in a pleasure-seeking lifestyle, ruining the lives of many along the way. He sees that the portrait is beginning to change, the face shifting to show the ravages of the life that he is living. He hides the portrait in the attic where it can't be seen by anyone. As Dorian sinks further and further into depredation, he remains young and beautiful while the painting, a representation of his soul, becomes monstrous and hideous. At the end of the novel, Dorian is overcome with the atrocities he has committed throughout his life, but he is unable to find the courage to confess his sins. He decides to destroy the portrait by slashing it with a knife. The servants hear a horrible scream and run to the attic to find the painting beautiful and undamaged, but their master, who they barely recognize, dead with a knife wound to the heart. The portrait and Dorian have returned to their natural state.

ANALYSIS

Wilde's novel was met with immediate controversy. Much of the criticism was directed at Wilde personally as his flamboyant lifestyle was well known. The magazine publisher, who published it first as a series, thought it too scandalous and immoral and deleted about 500 words without Wilde's permission. Critics were appalled at the descriptions of the hedonistic life that Dorian led and upset about the idea that art should exist for art's sake only, an idea that was contradictory to Victorian standards. Wilde published a longer and revised version of the novel, deleting some of the more scandalous parts (including some that were deemed to be homoerotic), with a preface defending his right to free speech and expression and explaining his stance on art. To those who said the novel was morally corrupt, Wilde replied that the novel had a definite moral—you cannot escape past actions.

The novel raises questions about the pursuit of youth and beauty. How far will one go to remain young and beautiful forever? Does the type of life one lives really show on one's face? Is the aging process so terrible that it is worth selling one's soul to avoid it? The points still stand today in a market that consumes an incredible amount of vitamins, supplements, cosmetics, and even surgery to avoid the appearance of aging.

ADAPTATIONS

Wilde's story has definite references to Faust, and Shakespeare allusions abound throughout. Other artists recognized the power of the story immediately, with the first known screen adaptation, a Danish silent film, appearing in 1910. Every few years, another version appears, from various directors and various countries. Possibly the best known version of the movie is a 1945 release with a very young Angela Lansbury in the role of Sibyl Vane, one of Dorian's love interests who he drives to suicide.

There are several made-for-television movies, plays, musicals, and audio productions of the story. It has been updated several times, for example, in a high-school horror novel where the protagonist remains young and beautiful though her reflection in the mirror becomes more and more horrible. Despite the controversy with which it debuted, the story itself remains timeless.

—*Marianne Moss Madsen, MS*

See also: Beauty; Dr. Heidegger's Experiment

PNEUMONIA

Relevant Issues: Death, health and medicine
Significance: Pneumonia, an inflamed state of the lower lung, is a leading cause of sickness and death in those over the age of sixty-five, especially in individuals confined to nursing homes.

Pneumonia has been a common and often lethal disease for centuries. "Captain of the men of death" was a description given to pneumonia by Sir William Osler over one hundred years ago. At the beginning of the nineteenth century, before the advent of antibiotics, pneumonia was responsible for the deaths of about 1 per 1,000 persons each year in the United States. The majority of these cases were caused by streptococcal, also known as "pneumococcal," infections.

In the era of antibiotics, the face of pneumonia has changed. Streptococcal pneumonia is no longer the major threat. In persons under sixty-five years of age and otherwise in good health, atypical organisms, including mycoplasma, are increasingly responsible for new cases of pneumonia acquired outside of the hospital. Pneumonia is generally curable with current antibiotics; this type is sometimes called walking pneumonia. In about 80 percent of cases, it may be treated at home with very good outcomes.

As the body ages, however, its ability to mount a response against dangerous microorganisms through natural defense mechanisms decreases. As a result, both the elderly and those with immune system disorders are susceptible to a wider range of microbiological organisms that can cause pneumonia. Additionally, the presence of concomitant illnesses including diabetes, lung disease, heart disease, and malignant tumors also increases an individual's susceptibility to developing pneumonia.

Sociological factors also play a role. Some individuals who are unable to independently carry out daily activities must enter nursing homes or rehabilitation facilities. Under these circumstances, immobility and exposure to many bacterial and viral illnesses in a closed environment further predispose the body to the development of pneumonia.

SYMPTOMS AND DIAGNOSIS

Pneumonia is an inflamed state of the lower lung, including the lung sacs (alveoli) and the smaller bronchial passages. In the majority of cases, the inflammation is caused by virulent bacteria and viruses that have entered these lower airways in sufficient numbers to overwhelm the lung defenses and cause infection.

Most of the time, the response of the lung defense system is adequate to overcome the infective challenge. The lungs call forth special types of cells, including white blood cells, both locally and from distant sites to help to fight and contain the infection. Some of these cells also promote healing and help decrease inflammation after the invading organism has been dealt with. If the immune system's defenses are sluggish and unable to mount a proper response, or if chronic lung disease limits the ability to eject phlegm and infectious disease through coughing, pneumonia is more likely to develop. In addition, in persons with diabetes and chronic kidney disease the protective white blood cells demonstrate slower entry into the inflamed area to fight off the infection.

Physicians or other health-care workers use many different signs and symptoms to diagnose pneumonia. There is usually a fever of 100 degrees Fahrenheit or higher in younger individuals. In the elderly or immunocompromised, however, this fever may be absent or the body temperature may be lower than normal. A rise in temperature is noted about 80 percent of the time in the diagnosis of pneumonia. In addition, one expects to see coughing that produces phlegm, as well as shortness of breath. The breathing rate, which is normally between ten and sixteen breaths per minute, is usually above twenty breaths. Upon examination, the health-care provider may hear abnormal sounds in the lung, which suggests pneumonia. All these symptoms may be less apparent, however, among elderly over the age of seventy and those with impaired immune systems. The only signs of pneumonia in such cases may be

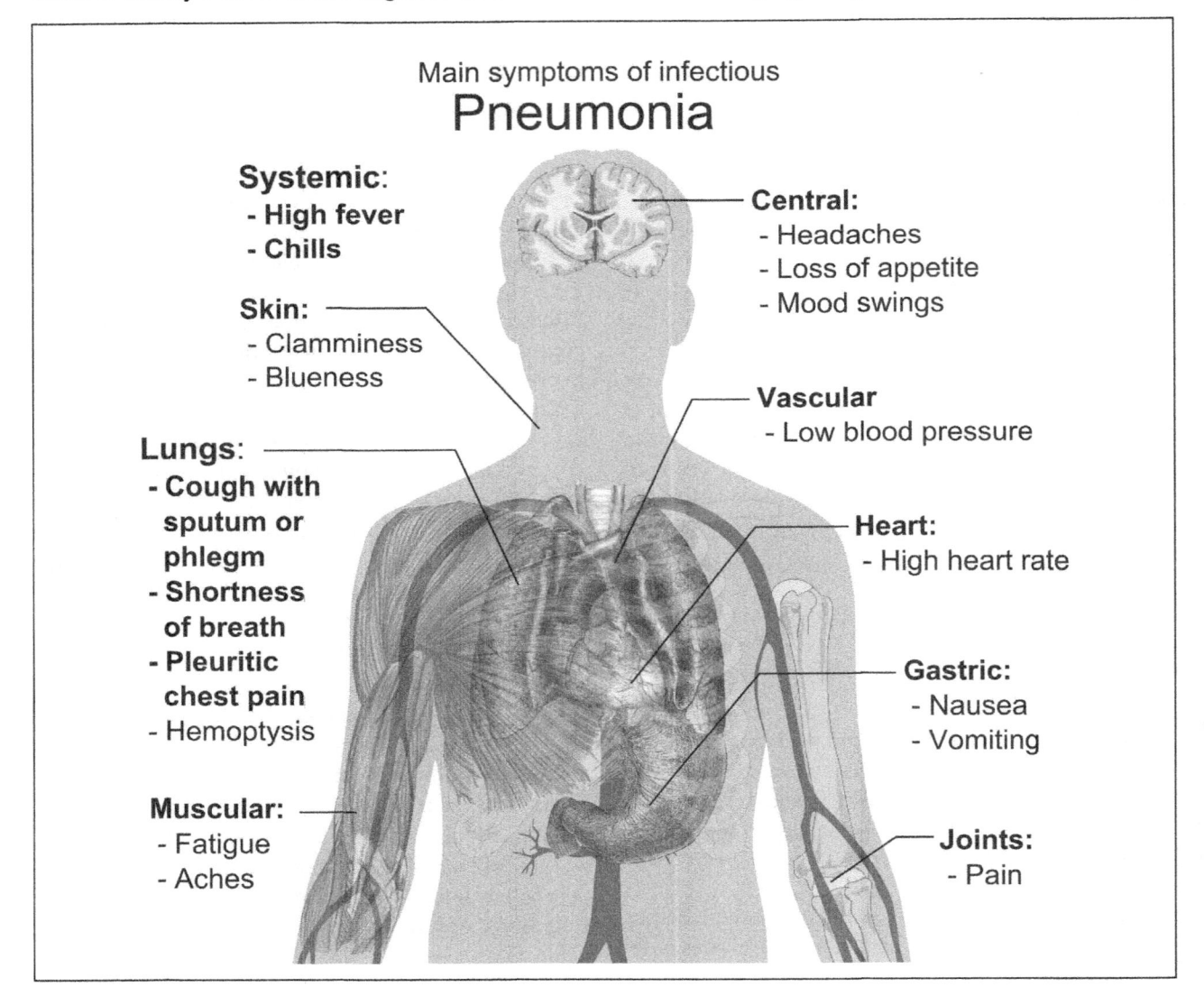

Main symptoms of infectious
Pneumonia

Systemic:
- High fever
- Chills

Skin:
- Clamminess
- Blueness

Lungs:
- Cough with sputum or phlegm
- Shortness of breath
- Pleuritic chest pain
- Hemoptysis

Muscular:
- Fatigue
- Aches

Central:
- Headaches
- Loss of appetite
- Mood swings

Vascular
- Low blood pressure

Heart:
- High heart rate

Gastric:
- Nausea
- Vomiting

Joints:
- Pain

an elevated breathing rate, ranging from thirty to thirty-five breaths per minute, and a change in mental status or confusion.

Strictly speaking, a chest X-ray showing abnormal shadows in the lungs is needed to confirm a suspected diagnosis of pneumonia. This finding may be falsely lacking, however, if the patient is very dehydrated or if the body cannot produce enough protective white cells to create a significant shadow on the X-ray. In practice, many times an X-ray is not taken, because more than 85 percent of the suspected cases of pneumonia acquired in the community will heal with commonly available antibiotics. In patients who display a high fever that does not respond in forty-eight to seventy-two hours and who remain sick with a breathing rate above thirty, low oxygen in the blood, or continued confusion, further imaging may be required. In the most severe cases, a computed tomography (CT) scan of the chest is performed. These severe cases are often encountered among patients who have poor infection-fighting ability, including those receiving chemotherapy for cancer treatment.

Laboratory tests may be required to make a diagnosis of pneumonia and to plan the correct therapy. Testing includes measuring the number of white blood cells and inflammatory markers in the blood, as well as searching for signs of the infective agent in the blood, sputum, and urine. In severe cases of pneumonia, especially those acquired inside the hospital, phlegm may be collected directly from the lower airways using a technique called bronchoscopy to help diagnose the specific type of infection and provide targeted treatment.

Once the diagnosis of pneumonia has been made, the next decision is whether to hospitalize the patient. In general, this assessment cannot be made with absolute certainty, but guidelines for the practitioner are available. When pooled together, these factors suggest and predict which patients would do better in a hospital environment. Factors predicting poorer outcome are age greater than sixty-five, preexisting disease or diseases, cough, mental confusion, fever above 101 degrees Fahrenheit, a breathing rate above thirty-five breaths per minute, and the presence of significant noise in the chest on physical examination.

TREATMENT

Decisions about therapy for pneumonia, especially therapeutic action taken outside the hospital, often need to be made without knowing the infecting organism or organisms. Guidelines for selecting the appropriate antimicrobial therapy in these circumstances often account for factors including patient age, the setting in which the infection was acquired, and local rates of bacterial resistance to antibiotics.

In the elderly, the choice of antibiotic should always include coverage of streptococcal pneumonia. Adequate antibiotic coverage may be achieved using one agent as a monotherapy or through a combination of two or more different antibiotics. In those confined to nursing homes, the antibiotic spectrum needs to be widened to include other potent organisms including methicillin-resistant Staphylococcus aureus (MRSA). For this reason, patient in nursing homes are often initially provided with two antibiotics. These may be given at the nursing home to spare admitting the patient to a hospital. The antibiotics are administered by injection, either intramuscularly or directly into a vein. Once the patient's temperature has normalized, usually after forty-eight to seventy-two hours, antibiotic delivery may be switched to the oral route. In younger individuals who are not confined to an institution, atypical organisms are encountered more often. These organisms respond nicely to macrolide or quinolone antibiotics in an outpatient setting.

Viral infections are also commonly involved in the causation of pneumonia. Antibiotics have no effect on the treatment of viral infections, and their administration is not justified to prevent possible secondary bacterial infections. Prescription of antibiotics in these or similarly inappropriate circumstances contributes to the increasing rates at which antibiotic-resistant bacteria are encountered. Antiviral agents are becoming widely available, however, especially in the treatment of influenza and associated pneumonia. Rapid diagnostic testing for influenza is now available, allowing treatment for this viral illness to be more effective. As with antibiotic selection, health-care providers may use local guidelines to help select the antiviral agent that is most likely to be effective in reducing the severity or duration of illness. One of the most commonly prescribed antivirals for uncomplicated cases of influenza is an

> **SENIOR TALK:**
>
> **How Do You Feel About Pneumonia?**
>
> Pneumonia can be very debilitating. At the onset of symptoms and throughout the course of the illness, you will likely feel weak and fatigued. Some types of pneumonia can even make you feel confused. If you are very ill, you might not be aware of changes to your mental awareness, but your loved ones may notice. You may feel unsure whether your symptoms are a sign of pneumonia. Pneumonia is more likely to be asymptomatic in older adults. Furthermore, older adults may be more likely to ignore or accept symptoms such as shortness of breath or chest pain. The most important thing to do is to contact a doctor without delay if you or a loved one suspect that you are sick.
>
> The feelings of weakness and low energy caused by pneumonia will probably continue for a period of time following the acute stage of the illness. Once treatment begins, most symptoms improve within a few days or weeks. However, feelings of fatigue can last for a month or longer. When we are in a weakened state, it is normal to feel down, frustrated, or depressed. Speaking to a supportive individual or health-care practitioner can be helpful. A prolonged recovery can even cause feelings of anxiety or depression. If this is the case, speaking to a therapist can be highly beneficial. Knowing we will get through the recovery process can help us to feel stronger as we look ahead to good health.
>
> —*Leah Jacob*

oral medication called oseltamivir. However, other antivirals may be indicated depending on case specifics.

PREVENTION

Vaccinations are valuable preventive measures and currently offer protection against influenza and pneumococcal pneumonia. In institutionalized individuals, there is an increased risk of complicated pneumonia caused by streptococcal pneumonia, and these cases, in turn, lead to outbreaks of pneumonia at the institution. The vaccine available in the late 1990s contained antigens (substances that stimulate the immune system) against more than 90 percent of the causative streptococcal organisms.

The Advisory Committee on Immunization Practices (ACIP) recommends that all individuals over sixty-five years of age receive the pneumococcal vaccine. The effectiveness of the vaccine does wane with time, and it is recommended that those who received it before sixty-five have the vaccine administered again after reaching that age. In addition, people under sixty-five years old who have chronic illnesses (such as diabetes, chronic lung disease, liver disease, kidney disease, and heart disease), those without a spleen, and those with impaired immune function due to serious blood diseases should receive the pneumococcal vaccine.

The agents for treating viral infection are not as effective as the antibiotics used for bacterial illnesses. It is, therefore, of paramount importance that these illnesses be prevented. In those over sixty-five years of age and especially those confined to a nursing home, vaccination helps to reduce the severity of the illness in individuals and helps prevent outbreaks of viral disease in institutions. Convincing evidence shows that influenza-related pneumonias are reduced by 40 to 50 percent in those who are vaccinated. In nursing homes, influenza deaths are reduced by 70 to 80 percent in those residents that have received the influenza vaccine. In addition, health-care workers, especially those who work in nursing homes, should be immunized to reduce the chance of transmission to patients under their care.

Pneumococcal and influenza vaccines do work. Their administration is a high priority among health-care providers. Remaining mobile, retaining independence in daily living, and strict handwashing when exposed to a patient with a viral illness are all measures that help to prevent pneumonia.

—*Thomas A. Ramunda, MD*
Updated by Thomas J. Martin, MS II

See also: Death and dying; Facility and institutional care; Hospitalization; Illnesses among older adults; Influenza; Respiratory changes and disorders; Vaccinations

For Further Information

Chalmers, James D. "The Modern Diagnostic Approach to Community-Acquired Pneumonia in Adults." *Seminars in Respiratory and Critical Care Medicine*, vol. 37, no. 6,

Dec. 2016, pp. 876-85. doi: 10.1055/s-0036-1592125. This review article provides up-to-date information on how pneumonia may be diagnosed among adults.

Denys, Gerald A., and Ryan F. Relich. "Antibiotic Resistance in Nosocomial Respiratory Infections." *Clinics in Laboratory Medicine*, vol. 34, no. 2, June 2014, pp. 257-70. doi:10.1016/j.cll.2014.02.004. This review article provides background information on certain strains of antibiotic-resistant bacteria that may cause hospital-acquired pneumonia.

Jain, Seema, et al. "Community-Acquired Pneumonia Requiring Hospitalization among U.S. Adults." *The New England Journal of Medicine*, vol. 373, no. 5, July 2015, pp. 415-27. doi:10.1056/NEJMoa1500245. This article provides population data from a study of community-acquired pneumonia and highlights increased incidence among the elderly.

Kang, Yun Seong, et al. "Antimicrobial Resistance and Clinical Outcomes in Nursing Home-Acquired Pneumonia, Compared to Community-Acquired Pneumonia." *Yonsei Medical Journal*, vol. 58, no. 1, Jan. 2017, pp. 180-86. doi:10.3349/ymj.2017.58.1.180. This article highlights differences in outcomes between cases of pneumonia occurring in the community and those in nursing homes.

Kobayashi, Miwako, et al. "Intervals Between PCV13 and PPSV23 Vaccines: Recommendations of the Advisory Committee on Immunization Practices (ACIP)." *MMWR. Morbidity and Mortality Weekly Report*, vol. 64, no. 34, 2015, pp. 944-47. doi:10.15585/mmwr.mm6434a4. This article reviews current CDC guidelines for intervals between pneumococcal vaccines.

Phua, Jason, et al. "Severe Community-Acquired Pneumonia: Timely Management Measures in the First 24 Hours." *Critical Care/The Society of Critical Care Medicine*, vol. 20, Aug. 2016, p. 237. doi: 10.1186/s13054-016-1414-2. This article provides an evidence-based guide for initial steps in diagnosis and management of severe community-acquired pneumonia.

Postma, Douwe F., et al. "Antibiotic Treatment Strategies for Community-Acquired Pneumonia in Adults." *The New England Journal of Medicine*, vol. 372, no. 14, Apr. 2015, pp. 1,312-23. doi: 10.1056/NEJMoa1406330. This article reviews current recommendations for antibiotic selection for community-acquired pneumonia among adults.

Tomczyk, Sara, et al. "Use of 13-Valent Pneumococcal Conjugate Vaccine and 23-Valent Pneumococcal Polysaccharide Vaccine among Adults Aged =65 Years: Recommendations of the Advisory Committee on Immunization Practices (ACIP)." *MMWR. Morbidity and Mortality Weekly Report*, vol. 63, no. 37, Sept. 2014, pp. 822-25. www.cdc.gov/mmWr/preview/mmwrhtml/mm6337a4.htm. This article reviews current CDC guidelines for pneumococcal vaccination among adults aged greater than 65 years.

POVERTY

Relevant Issues: Economics, race and ethnicity, sociology

Significance: Despite widely held stereotypes depicting older Americans as being secure economically, a significant proportion of the elderly population is impoverished, some elderly subgroups experience extremely high poverty rates, and official guidelines underestimate real levels of elderly economic malaise.

Issues relating to the socioeconomic status of the elderly population are more prominent in public discourse than they have been since the early twentieth century debates that culminated in the passage of the Social Security Act in 1935. During this earlier historical period, there was little question that a huge proportion of the elderly population was destitute and constituted a major social problem in need of public attention.

Contemporary discussions of poverty among the aged, however, are held against a backdrop of decades of marked economic improvement for the elderly. If such debates are to be meaningful, they must be based on detailed social scientific analyses of the economic conditions of the elderly. For example, those considering the myriad proposals for "reforming," or dramatically altering, the structure of publicly funded elderly support programs cannot depend on ideologically driven or "common knowledge" sources, or even objective official guidelines, to provide valid information on, or accurately assess, the needs of the fastest-growing age-based segment of America's population.

ELDERLY STEREOTYPES

In the United States, there have always been popular socially constructed, generalized images of the elderly. Current elderly stereotypes differ dramatically from those of earlier historical eras. From the 1950s through the 1970s, older Americans were commonly viewed as being barely or not able to afford basic necessities, having been relegated to living on small fixed incomes, in poor health and social isolation. It was commonly believed that industrialization and urbanization had weakened nuclear family ties, resulting in the widespread abandonment and neglect of older family members. The perception that the elderly were largely a dependent population led to what some authors call "compassionate ageism," that is, the general acceptance of negative images of the aged, resulting in a willingness to increase public support for their needs. However, the cultural image of the elderly as poor through no fault of their own, and, therefore, deserving of assistance, was to be displaced by the dawn of the 1980s.

The economic progress made by the elderly in absolute terms and relative to other age groups created the current, commonly held image of older Americans as being affluent and greedily seeking even more publicly funded assistance, even though elderly support programs collectively make up a large proportion of the overall federal budget. Macro-level analyses generate findings (for example, the lower rates of impoverishment for the elderly compared to the general population and children, and the relatively large proportion of U.S. collective wealth controlled by those over sixty-five) that lend support to this stereotype. Further support is found in anecdotal evidence involving stories of wealthy older persons receiving Social Security, Medicare, and other benefits that were made possible through withholdings from the paychecks of even the least-affluent Americans in the labor force who are struggling to support their families. This new cultural image depicts the elderly as people who are advantaged and affluent; they retired at relatively young ages with high levels of retirement income because they worked during periods of economic expansion that provided them with generous private and public pensions, and possess political power that has brought them a comprehensive collection of publicly funded programs to provide health care and other services. As a result, many blame the elderly for the economic problems of nonelderly Americans and those of - society.

While it is true that a large proportion of the elderly were poor and needy in the 1950s and 1960s, and that the standard of living for older Americans as a whole has improved substantially, the inherent inaccuracies of all stereotypes apply to these polarized collective images. The move from a sociopolitical atmosphere of "compassionate ageism" to "scapegoat ageism" denotes not only a failure to acknowledge the real socioeconomic diversity within the elderly population during both historical periods, but also a reluctance to recognize the potential consequences of the more recent mind-set. An examination of the social gerontological literature reveals the complexity of ascertaining levels of dependency and need among contemporary older Americans, and points out the inadequacy of the most commonly used standards for determining impoverishment, which underestimate the true extent of the elderly population's economic problems.

POVERTY RATES AND MEASUREMENT ISSUES

One of the greatest success stories of the War on Poverty begun by President Lyndon B. Johnson is the reduction of elderly impoverishment. According to the most commonly used criteria, the poverty rate for Americans over sixty-five in 2017 was 9.2 percent, down drastically from 28.5 percent in 1966. Social Security, Medicare, and other publicly funded elderly support programs are largely responsible for this accomplishment. However, this achievement has generated controversy in the form of resentment expressed by Americans in the labor force over their perception that they are being excessively taxed to provide the annual funding to these programs, that benefits will be severely cut back or eliminated by the time they retire, and that the aged do not really need the assistance. Related ageist slurs have become increasingly commonplace as elderly Americans are collectively referred to by some as "greedy geezers," "woopies" (well-off older persons), or "the generation that hit the lottery."

Objective and critical analyses by social scientists have raised questions regarding the validity of the conventionally used "poverty line" and whether alternative measures of economic jeopardy might more accurately tap into true levels of need among the elderly. Being "poor" in America is defined for all official purposes by applying an income threshold that is determined by a formula established in the 1950s. Persons or households whose incomes fall below it are "poor." Trends in impoverishment for specific groups, for example, the steady reduction in poverty among the elderly and the steady increase among children in recent decades, are almost always expressed in terms of the percentage who fall below the official government poverty threshold. The calculation of the poverty line is based on the cost of the minimal amount of food necessary for survival. Using current food prices, the threshold is established at any point in time by multiplying the cost of this minimally nutritious food plan by three, because a poll conducted in 1955 indicated that food made up about one-third of the average household budget. By this criterion, in 2019, a four-person family with two children would have to receive an income below $25,750 to be poor.

Critics of this measure claim that it has underestimated levels of extreme financial hardship since its adoption. To begin with, the official poverty threshold was never intended to describe a reasonable long-term level of living, but rather the barest requirements for subsistence during periods of emergency. In addition, it has been suggested that, at the very least, the formula should be adjusted to reflect the fact that the costs of basic necessities—housing, clothing, and transportation—are typically much higher than three times the family's food budget. Furthermore, it has been asserted that using the average household budget at any point in time as the basis for this calculation is inappropriate because the least-affluent families in America devote over 85 percent of their budgets to food and shelter alone.

Beyond these general issues relating to the poverty line, the official standards for defining elderly poverty are even more controversial because the income threshold is lower than for those under sixty-five. The underlying assumption is that older people have lower nutritional requirements than their more active younger counterparts, and, because the calculation is based on food costs, the elderly must have less income to be officially poor. In 2019, for example, a household with two adults and an elderly head was poor if its income was below $15,178, compared to a threshold of $16,815 if the head of the household was under sixty-five. For individuals, the poverty threshold was $12,043 for those over sixty-five and $13,064 for the nonelderly. It has been asserted that the assumption of lower nutritional requirements for the elderly is subject to question and that the differential age-based thresholds ignore the dramatic increases in expenditures for many older people for such items as health care and prescriptions, home maintenance, and transportation. One of the architects of the original poverty line formula has stated publicly that if more reasonable food costs were used to calculate the elderly poverty line, the percentage of older impoverished Americans would increase to over 30 percent.

For some time, researchers have responded to the possibility that the poverty line underestimates true levels of economic vulnerability by reporting rates based on both people below the poverty line and the "near poor," that is, those whose incomes are 125, 150, or even 200 percent of the poverty threshold. Although the official definition of impoverishment remains unchanged, some government assistance programs now recognize its inadequacy. For example, people with incomes below 130 percent of the poverty line are eligible for food stamps. However, many assistance programs that serve the needs of the non-affluent aged do not recognize "near impoverishment." In fact, the minimum income guaranteed to the elderly under Supplementary Security Insurance is well below the poverty line. Several authors contend that an accurate measure of financial marginality among the elderly should include the near impoverished, defined as those between 100 and 200 percent of the official income threshold. If this standard is applied, a vastly different picture of levels of need emerges. In 2017, when the elderly poverty rate was 9.2 percent, 30 percent of older Americans had incomes below 200 percent of the poverty line. Those between the line and 200 percent of it, the near poor, may be worse off in real terms than their officially impoverished counterparts, for they are not eligible for need-based assistance programs.

The perspective that conventionally calculated poverty rates underestimate levels of economic malaise among the elderly is not universally shared. There are those who posit that the current poverty line formula creates inflated estimates of elderly impoverishment and that factors currently excluded should be counted as income. "Income," as defined by the poverty threshold formula, includes money received from wages and salaries, private pensions, interest and dividends, Social Security, and public assistance programs. Some contend that a more valid estimate of elderly poverty would result from counting the value of services provided through government programs, tax benefits received by the elderly, and potential income based on the value of home equity in addition to money income. The result would be a significant reduction in the elderly poverty rate.

Critics of proposals to redefine "income" to include factors other than money received believe that such policy changes would place large numbers of older Americans in economically untenable positions. They agree that direct money transfers through government programs should be counted, pointing out that if Social Security assistance money was not counted as income, the elderly poverty rate would have been 39 percent in 2019, which demonstrates the need for and the success of elderly income maintenance programs. Yet, these critics claim that the value of services that the non-affluent elderly could not afford were it not for government programs, such as a temporary stay in a nursing home, does not improve the recipient's ability to cover basic expenses. By the same token, imputed income from home equity does little to assist with increasing home maintenance costs. Charges are common that political motivations underlie suggested policy changes that would reduce levels of elderly eligibility for need-based assistance, in a political atmosphere that features budget reduction and deficit elimination and calls for a more equitable age-based redistribution of publicly funded assistance. The resolution of these debates over whether the current guidelines that officially define poverty should be maintained or amended to include more or fewer of the financially marginal elderly will have a marked effect on the economic well-being of older Americans.

CAUSES OF POVERTY AND DISADVANTAGED SUBGROUPS

Disagreements over the validity of the poverty line notwithstanding, when the conventional poverty threshold is applied, the dominant fact regarding elderly impoverishment in America is its steady and dramatic reduction for several decades. The two most compelling questions that remain are "Why do a significant minority of aged Americans still live in impoverishment?" and "Why does categorical economic diversity within the elderly population produce subgroups with poverty rates much higher than the overall average?" There is a single answer to both questions. Public elderly support programs do not serve the needs of all older Americans equally well. Those who enjoy a decent standard of living fit a profile that includes entering the paid labor force as young adults and contributing to Social Security throughout a long working lifetime, which results in relatively generous Social Security benefits that supplement private pensions, savings, and home equity. By contrast, the elderly poor tend to be people whose labor force participation histories are fragmented or involve the lowest-paying occupations with few or no benefits, and those who suffer from severe physiological or cognitive decline. As a result, the public assistance safety net works well for the healthy middle-class elderly and leaves women, racial and ethnic minorities, and the oldest old overrepresented in the ranks of the elderly impoverished.

Social scientists have sought to analyze the perpetuation of these pockets of severe economic jeopardy within the elderly population. In 2017, for example, when the overall elderly poverty rate was 9.2 percent, the rate was 19.3 for African Americans, 10.9 percent for Asian Americans, and 17 percent for Hispanic Americans. Women experience higher levels of poverty than men in all age and race groups: 10.5 percent of women over 65 lived below the poverty line in 2017, compared to 7.5 percent of men in the same age group "Cumulative advantage" and "cumulative disadvantage" are theoretical concepts developed by economic and social gerontologists to describe processes that perpetuate categorical elderly impoverishment. The former term refers to the fact that those who are advantaged early in life build on those advantages throughout the life cycle, and the latter concept posits that those who historically have had limited access to the structure of opportunities (for example, women and minorities) are affected by those disadvantages throughout their lives, often resulting in impoverishment in old age. Even the higher poverty rate for the oldest old compared to their younger elderly counterparts can be attributed, in part, to these life course processes. Although factors such as failing health, a reduced ability to generate supplementary income, and the higher proportion of elderly women living alone do increase the poverty rate for the oldest Americans, the flow of relatively advantaged cohorts with higher average levels of education and income into the younger elderly age groups also contributes to the perpetuation of age-based economic diversity among the elderly.

Misconceptions and confusion regarding the economic well-being of older Americans are not uncommon because, too often, publicly disseminated information on the topic includes only some of the facts. It is true that, overall, the current cohorts that make up America's elderly population are the most economically secure in its history. It is also true that large numbers of older Americans continue to suffer in impoverishment, and there are only two other industrialized nations in the world with higher current elderly poverty rates than the United States.

—*Jack Carter*

See also: Abandonment; African Americans; Ageism; Homelessness; Latinx Americans; Neglect; Social Security; Stereotypes; Women and aging

For Further Information

Bernstein, Shayna Fae, et al. "Poverty Dynamics, Poverty Thresholds and Mortality: An Age-Stage Markovian Model." *Plos One*, vol. 13, no. 5, 16 May 2018. doi:10.1371/journal.pone.0195734. This paper applies the approach of age-by-stage matrix models to human demography and individual poverty dynamics to extend the literature on individual poverty dynamics across the life course.

Ghilarducci, Teresa. "America's Unusual High Rates of Old-Age Poverty and Old-Age Work." *Forbes*, 2 Mar. 2018. www.forbes.com/sites/ teresaghilarducci/2018/03/02/americas-unusual-high-rates-of-old-age-poverty-and-old-age-work/#1d16804e458a. Exploration on working among the older population in relation to poverty rates and international comparisons.

Hatcher, Daniel L. *The Poverty Industry: The Exploitation of America's Most Vulnerable Citizens.* New York U P, 2016. Hatcher reveals how state governments and their private industry partners are profiting from the social safety net, turning America's most vulnerable populations into sources of revenue.

"Historical Poverty Tables: People and Families—1959 to 2017." United States Census Bureau, 28 Aug. 2018. www.census.gov/data/tables/time-series/demo/income-poverty/historical-poverty-people.html. Tables of historical data on poverty.

Newman, Katherine. "Retirement Should Not Mean Hardship—but Many Older Americans Live in Poverty." *The Guardian*, Guardian News and Media, 24 May 2019. www.theguardian.com/us-news/2019/may/24/elder-poverty-america-hardship-retirement-economics. Discusses the personal experiences of an elderly couple living in Opelousas, Louisiana, the city with the highest rate of elderly living in poverty.

Walls, Barbranda Lumpkins. "Effect of Poverty on Older Adults Revealed in Aging Conference." AARP, American Association of Retired Persons, 24 Mar. 2016. www.aarp.org/politics-society/advocacy/info-2016/effect-of-poverty-on-older-adults.html. Poverty of the elderly and potential solutions were a main topic at the Aging in America conference in Washington.

Wimer, Christopher, and Lucas Manfield. "Elderly Poverty in the United States in the 21st Century: Exploring the Role of Assets in the Supplemental Poverty Measure." *SSRN Electronic Journal, 2015.* doi:10.2139/ssrn.2693201. In this paper the authors consider using an approach adapted from a recent National Academy of Sciences report recommending methods for measuring poverty and medical risk while taking account of assets.

PREMATURE AGING

Relevant Issues: Biology, health and medicine

Significance: People worry about aging prematurely, but with few exceptions, the rate of aging is mainly determined by genes and is beyond individual control.

The best examples of premature aging in humans are the rare genetic diseases Werner's syndrome and Hutchinson-Gilford progeria syndrome (HGPS), the latter also simply called progeria. People with Werner's syndrome age rapidly in their teens and twenties, often suffering from cataracts, heart disease, and diabetes and dying in their thirties. Progeria is even more dramatic. Children with progeria start to show signs of senescence a few months after birth. They age very rapidly, becoming white-haired and bald, developing coronary artery disease, and resembling little wizened octogenarians well before they are ten years old. They typically die of age-related diseases in their early teens. Both Werner's syndrome and progeria remain essentially untreatable. The accelerated rate of aging that characterizes these diseases, once begun, stops only with death.

Fortunately, both diseases occur extremely rarely, as little as once per million or more births. The lesson that these rare diseases teach is that genes control the normal rate of aging. In these families, mutant forms of normal genes lead to aging that is dramatically accelerated. Furthermore, these genes and the proteins that they determine implicate cellular metabolic processes such as deoxyribonucleic acid (DNA) damage and repair in the normal aging that occurs in everyone else.

Considerable evidence from other species such as mice, fruit flies, and higher animals often shows the principal role of genes in determining the rate of aging. In the small roundworm Caenorhabditis elegans, several genes, notably ced-3, control the rate of aging. Phenomena such as programmed cell death in many organisms show that aging is essentially an intrinsic cellular process, under the control of factors in the cell's nucleus, again implicating genes and DNA.

Some well-known risk factors for age-related diseases in humans can be within the control of individuals to affect. Obesity predisposes individuals to heart disease and diabetes. Strong sunlight causes skin cancer and damage to skin cells like that caused by aging. Lack of exercise can cause loss of muscle tone. In these particular regards, a person can prevent premature aging within his or her own genetic makeup.

Most people wish that they could delay aging, or at least avoid the reality or appearance of premature aging. Current fads include diet manipulation with calorie restriction, vitamin supplements, and antioxidants such as flavonoids. Little or no evidence, however, supports the effectiveness of these regimens in humans. Instead, genes appear to take the predominant role in controlling the rate of aging. One cannot determine one's genes, just as one cannot choose one's parents. Nevertheless, a person can try to live a well-balanced and healthy life, get reasonable diet and exercise, avoid too much sun on the skin, and not fret about the rest.

—*R. L. Bernstein*

See also: Aging process; Anti-aging treatments; Antioxidants; Caloric restriction; Cosmetic surgery; Face lifts; Genetics; Gray hair; Hair loss and baldness; Life expectancy; Longevity research; Nutrition; Skin changes and disorders; Wrinkles

For Further Information
Gordon, Leslie B., et al. "Progeria: A Paradigm for Translational Medicine." *Cell*, vol. 156, no. 3, 2014, pp. 400-07. doi:10.1016/j.cell.2013.12.028. This essay summarizes advances made in the understanding of HGPS and discusses the implications of research into rare diseases on basic cell biology, understanding of physiological processes, drug discovery, and clinical trial design.
"Hutchinson-Gilford Progeria Syndrome." U.S. National Library of Medicine, National Institutes of Health, May 2016. ghr.nlm.nih.gov/condition/hutchinson-gilford-progeria-syndrome. General information and resources on Hutchinson-Gilford progeria.
Okines, Hayley, and Alison Stokes. *Young at Heart: The Likes and Life of a Teenager with Progeria.* Accent P, 2015. About to turn 17, Okines reflects on the pains and perks of growing up with progeria: from the heartbreak of being told she will never walk again to the delight of passing her exams and starting college.
Shamanna, Raghavendra A., et al. "Recent Advances in Understanding Werner Syndrome." *F1000 Research*, vol. 6, 2017, p. 1779. doi:10.12688/f1000research.12110.1. Discusses some areas of particular relevance to Werner's syndrome where significant insight has been gathered in recent years.

PRESCRIPTION DRUGS. *See* MEDICATIONS.

PROSTATE CANCER

Relevant Issues: Biology, death, family, health and medicine

Significance: The 1990s showed a sharp rise in the occurrence of prostate cancer; research continues to show a close correlation with aging.

Key Terms:
malignant: tumors can invade and destroy nearby tissue and spread to other parts of the body
prostatectomy: a surgical operation to remove all or part of the prostate gland

The prostate gland is a walnut-sized gland just below the male bladder that encircles the urethra (the tube that carries urine through the penis). Any enlargement or abnormal growth of this gland may cause such symptoms as difficulty or discomfort in urination, excessive frequency of urination (especially at night), or inability to urinate. However, these symptoms by no means indicate cancer in all cases. Cancer is an uncontrolled, excessive reproduction of cells in the gland, which may spread to other parts of the body through the blood stream or the lymph system.

INCIDENCE AND RISK FACTORS
With the exception of skin cancer, prostate cancer is the most often occurring cancer in men; approximately one in nine men will develop prostate cancer. Prostate cancer is seen mostly in older men and in African American men. African American men are twice as likely to die of prostate cancer than white men. Asian Americans and

Hispanic/Latino men have a lower incidence of prostate cancer than white men. It is not clear why these racial and ethnic differences exist. It is rare to see prostate cancer diagnosed before the age of 40; approximately 6 in 10 cases are diagnosed in men aged 65 or older. The average age at which prostate cancer is diagnosed is 66. In American men, prostate cancer is the second leading cause of cancer deaths; lung cancer is the primary cause of cancer deaths. Approximately 1 in 41 American men die of prostate cancer every year. Most men diagnosed with prostate cancer do not die from the disease, and it is estimated that there are 2.9 million men in the United States who are living with prostate cancer today. When a father or brother has the disease, the risk doubles; some studies have shown that when a man has three relatives with prostate cancer, he is more than ten times as likely to get the disease. Inherited genes such as mutations of BRCA1 and BRCA2 may increase the incidence of prostate cancer in a small percentage of men.

DIAGNOSIS AND PREVENTION

Preliminary tools for diagnosing prostate cancer are the digital rectal examination (DRE) and the prostate-specific antigen (PSA) test. The DRE consists of a doctor inserting a gloved and lubricated finger into the rectum and physically feeling for abnormal growths. The PSA test checks the blood for the level of a specific protein produced by the prostate gland; an elevated level does not necessarily indicate cancer but suggests the need for further testing. None of the tests are foolproof.

If any of these tests suggests the possibility of a malignancy, the doctor may combine a transrectal ultrasonography (a procedure in which sound waves are sent out by a probe inserted into the rectum, allowing a computer to create a picture called a sonogram) with a biopsy. If an abnormal area is found by the DRE, tissue will be removed from the abnormal area by insertion of a hollow needle through a tube inserted into the rectum. If an elevated PSA is the indicator, random sections from the entire prostate gland may be taken. The only certain way to detect cancer is to observe the tissue under a microscope.

Perhaps the most important part of the diagnosis is determining the stage of the cancer when a biopsy reveals it to be present. One system is to rank the malignancy from 2 through 10, with the higher numbers being the more advanced stage. The more common system uses a grading of 1 through 4. Stage 1 means the cancer has not spread beyond the prostate gland, is causing no symptoms, and cannot be detected by the DRE. Stage 2 tumors may be felt by the DRE or detected by blood tests but have not spread beyond the prostate. Stage 3 means the cancer has spread to nearby tissues outside the prostate. Stage 4 means cancer cells have spread to lymph nodes or other parts of the body.

Although research is ongoing to find ways of preventing prostate cancer, results have not been notable. High-fat diets have long been recognized as a risk factor; daily consumption of green and yellow vegetables, and especially tomato-based foods, has been shown by some studies to reduce the risk of several types of cancer, including prostate. The validity of such studies has not been universally acknowledged, however, and a strong question has been raised as to whether switching to a low-fat diet after years of ingesting high levels of fat can be effective. Regular amounts of raisins and other dried fruits in the diet have also been suggested as a preventive measure. Exercise is yet another factor. Several studies have suggested that exercise reduces testosterone levels and hence the odds of getting prostate cancer.

TREATMENT

Primary methods of treatment include surgery, hormones, radiation, chemotherapy, and cryosurgery. The

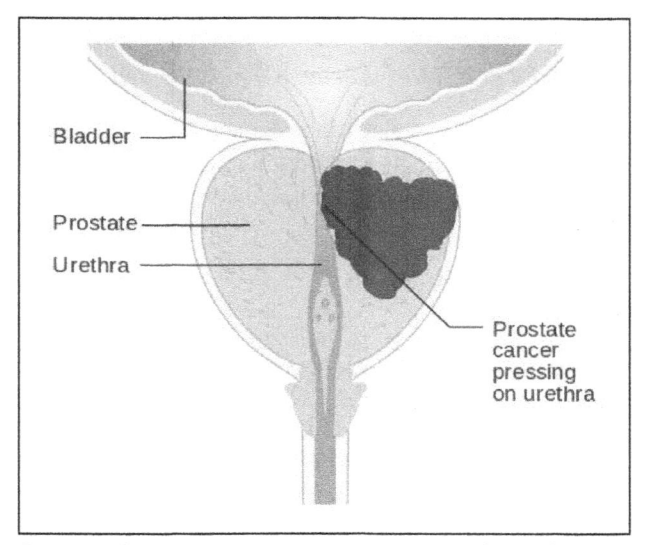

Diagram showing prostate cancer pressing on the urethra. (via Wikimedia Commons)

stage of the malignancy is a primary determinant of treatment methods to be used. For tumors that have not spread outside the prostate, surgery is commonly used to try and cure the cancer. The primary type of surgery used is called radical prostatectomy, which is the removal of the prostate gland and the tissue around it along with the seminal vesicles. There are different ways a surgeon can perform a prostatectomy. There is an open radical prostatectomy approach that can be done through a long single incision that can be approached in two different ways, depending on where the surgeon makes the incision. More common approaches to prostate cancer surgery involve the use of laparoscopic techniques, which involve the use of several smaller incisions and special surgical tools to remove the prostate. The surgeon either holds the tools or uses a control panel that directs the robotic arms that hold the tools in this type of surgery. Laparoscopic radical prostatectomy and robotic-assisted laparoscopic radical prostatectomy involves a shorter hospital stay, less pain and blood loss than open radical prostatectomy. There is also a faster recovery time with laparoscopic surgery. With all types of surgery for prostate cancer, there are often undesirable side effects such as inability to control urine and impotence. Radical orchiectomy (surgical removal of the testicles) may be performed for the purpose of depriving the prostate gland of testosterone that is needed for malignant cells to multiply and grow.

Radiation therapy is often combined with surgery or may be used independently. A machine may be used to direct radiation to the area of the malignancy (external radiation), or radioactive material may be placed directly in or near the infected areas (internal radiation). External radiation is administered on an outpatient basis, whereas internal radiation usually involves a brief stay in the hospital. For stage 3 tumors, radiation is the more common treatment. Like surgery, radiation therapy may have undesirable side effects, such as impotence, diarrhea, or frequent and painful urination.

The preferred treatment for stage 4 cancer is hormone treatment. One form consists of introducing luteinizing hormone-releasing hormone (LHRH) agonists into the body, which prevents the testicles from producing testosterone. An example of a LHRH agonist that is commonly used is leuprolide (Lupron). Antiandrogens may be added to treatment if orchiectomy or an LHRH agonist is no longer working. Antiandrogens block male hormones that stimulate prostate cancer cells to grow.

Chemotherapy is not used in early prostate cancer but is sometimes used if the cancer has spread to other parts of the body. In the elderly man, the risks of chemotherapy and its side effects are considered by the treating physician. Although chemotherapy is not a standard treatment for prostate cancer, there are studies that are exploring its use. The side effects of chemotherapy depend on which drug is used. The effectiveness of cryosurgery—the application of extreme cold directly to the tumor to freeze it and destroy the cancer cells—is not well known.

Sometimes the best treatment for prostate cancer is active surveillance. Prostate cancer cells are notoriously slow growing and are sometimes best left alone. Elderly men with slow growing prostate cancers may never need treatment for their cancer so their health-care provider may recommend active surveillance, which means monitoring the cancer closely. This involves doctor visits about every six months with a PSA and DRE. In addition, prostate biopsies may be done yearly. This allows for close monitoring of any progression in the cancer. If less intense monitoring is desired, then less frequent testing may be done and then this would be referred to as "watchful waiting." Medical experts advise aging males to have a DRE and PSA test annually after age fifty. In the case of high-risk people, these tests should probably begin around age forty.

—Joe E. Lunceford
Updated by Mary E. Dietmann, EdD, APRN, CNS

See also: African Americans; Cancer; Men and aging; Prostate enlargement; Reproductive changes, disabilities, and dysfunctions; Sexual dysfunction; Urinary disorders

For Further Information

Boisen, Samara, et al. "A Cross-Sectional Comparison of Quality of Life Between Physically Active and Underactive Older Men with Prostate Cancer." *Journal of Aging and Physical Activity*, vol. 24, no. 4, Oct. 2016, pp. 642-48. doi: 10.1123/japa.2015-0195. Explores the benefits of physical activity on prostate cancer by comparing patients that are physically active with those who are not.

Espinosa, Geo, and Matthew Solan. *Thrive Don't Only Survive*. Dr. Geo's Guide to Living Your Best Life Before & After Prostate Cancer. CreateSpace Publishing, 2016.

Based on his extensive research and clinical experience on natural medicine for prostate problems, Dr. Geo has created a lifestyle blueprint that men can apply immediately to thrive before or after prostate cancer.

Madsen, Lydia, and Lene Symes. "An Integrative Review of Nursing Research on Active Surveillance in an Older Adult Prostate Cancer Population." *Oncology Nursing Forum*, vol. 40, no. 4, July 2013, pp. 374-82. doi: 10.1188/13.ONF.40-04AP. Summarizes the current state of nursing knowledge regarding the management of older adult men with prostate cancer with active surveillance as the treatment strategy.

Roth, Andrew. *Managing Prostate Cancer: A Guide for Living Better.* Oxford U P, 2015. Roth, a psychiatrist specializing in psychological support for cancer patients, provides the emotional skills and strategies necessary to help patients deal with the challenges a prostate cancer diagnosis brings to everyday life.

Walsh, Patrick C., and Janet Farrar Worthington. *Dr. Patrick Walsh's Guide to Surviving Prostate Cancer.* 4th. Ed., Boston, MA: Little, Brown & Company, 2018. This new edition is updated to maintain its cutting edge as the world's most popular and well-respected resource on prostate cancer.

PROSTATE ENLARGEMENT

Also Known As: Benign Prostatic Hyperplasia
Relevant Issues: Biology, health and medicine
Significance: Problems associated with enlargement of the prostate gland affect more than one-half of all men in their sixties and up to 90 percent of men in their seventies and eighties.

Key Terms:

cystoscopy: procedure in which a lighted optical instrument called a cystoscope is inserted through the urethra to look at the bladder

prostatectomy: a surgical operation to remove all or part of the prostate gland

The prostate gland is a walnut-sized organ of the male reproductive system located just below the bladder. It consists of two halves (lobes) surrounded by an outer layer, or capsule. The prostate gland surrounds the urethra (the tube that carries urine from the bladder out through the penis) just as it leaves the bladder. The primary function of the prostate gland is to produce a milky fluid, which, along with other fluids, makes up semen. Semen carries and nourishes sperm cells and is expelled during ejaculation. There are three main problems that can affect the prostate gland and cause problems for men: benign prostatic hyperplasia, prostatitis, and prostate cancer.

The prostate gland goes through two main periods of growth. During puberty and young adulthood, the prostate grows rapidly, doubling in size. Around age forty to forty-five, the prostate begins to grow again, a condition called benign prostatic hyperplasia (BPH), and continues growing slowly until death. As the name implies, BPH is not cancer and does not turn into cancer. However, it is possible to have BPH and prostate cancer at the same time. Monitoring for prostate cancer is important and may be done in conjunction with examination of the prostate by a blood test that screens for prostate cancer called a prostate-specific antigen or PSA test. The prostate enlarges from within and is kept from expanding by its surrounding capsule. This causes the gland to press against the urethra passing through it, much like a kink in a garden hose. This pressure on the urethra is responsible for the most common symptoms of BPH: difficulty starting or maintaining a stream of urine, the urge to urinate suddenly, the need to urinate more often (especially at night), and leaking or dribbling urine. BPH develops slowly over many years, and the symptoms usually develop slowly as well. This is why symptoms of prostate enlargement caused by BPH are more common among older men. When severe, BPH can cause serious health problems, such as bladder or kidney damage. It is said that all men will have an enlarged prostate if they live long enough.

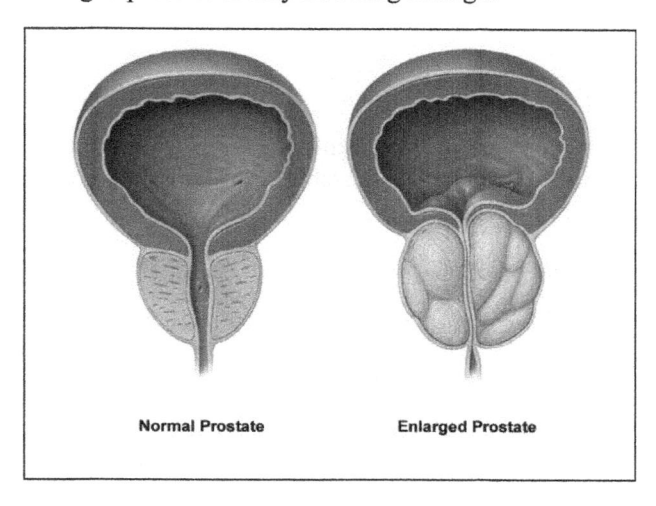

Normal Prostate   Enlarged Prostate

Prostatitis is inflammation of the prostate gland usually caused by a bacterial infection of the urinary tract. Prostatitis occurs in middle-aged men and is associated with BPH in older men. Symptoms of prostatitis may be similar to those of BPH and may also include fever and burning or pain with urination. Prostatitis is generally treated with a course of antibiotics lasting several weeks or several months.

If an enlarged prostate is suspected based on symptoms, a digital rectal examination, and other tests such as urine flow rate, pressure flow studies of the bladder, urinalysis, and cystoscopy may be used. Several treatment options for BPH are available. Surgery may be recommended if there is an inability to pass urine (urinary retention) or inability to control urine flow (incontinence), blood in the urine, inability to completely empty the bladder, bladder stones and decreasing kidney function. Surgery may include a transurethral resection (removing the prostate through a scope, piece by piece), a simple prostatectomy using either an open incision in the abdomen or laparoscopically using a robot (Da Vinci Robotic Surgery) or using heat or a laser to destroy prostate tissue. Other medical treatments involve the use of drugs to shrink the prostate gland or reduce symptoms, though these drugs are not effective in all cases.

Prostate enlargement is extremely common among older men. The symptoms of an enlarged prostate are not a necessary part of getting older, and men need not suffer from such symptoms. Medical experts advise all men over fifty to have an annual examination, including a digital rectal exam to screen for prostate problems.

—*William J. Ryan*
Updated by Patricia Stanfill Edens, RN, PhD, FACHE

See also: Incontinence; Men and aging; Prostate cancer; Reproductive changes, disabilities, and dysfunctions; Urinary disorders

For Further Information

Bazar, Ronald M. *Healthy Prostate: the Extensive Guide to Prevent and Heal Prostate Problems.* CreateSpace, 2011. This book will explain how to cure your prostate problem naturally—without the devastating side effects of conventional medical treatments.

———. *The Prostate Health Diet: What to Eat to Prevent and Heal Prostate Problems Including Prostate Cancer, BPH Enlarged Prostate and Prostatitis.* CreateSpace, 2013. The advice in The Prostate Health Diet will guide readers in customizing your diet for unique constitutions and conditions.

Chughtai, Bilal. *A Comprehensive Guide to the Prostate Eastern and Western Approaches for Management of BPH.* Elsevier Science, 2018. Provides a multidisciplinary approach to BPH and male voiding dysfunction, presenting comprehensive guidance on management.

Foster, Harris E., et al. "Benign Prostatic Hyperplasia: Surgical Management of Benign Prostatic Hyperplasia/Lower Urinary Tract Symptoms." American Urological Association, 2019, www.auanet.org/guidelines/benign-prostatic-hyperplasia-(bph)-guideline. The goal of this revised guideline is to provide a useful reference on the effective evidence-based surgical management of male lower urinary tract symptoms secondary to benign prostatic hyperplasia.

Sobol, Jennifer. "Enlarged Prostate: MedlinePlus Medical Encyclopedia." MedlinePlus, U.S. National Library of Medicine, 26 Aug. 2017. medlineplusgov/ency/article/000381.htm. General information on prostate enlargement.

Gul, Zeynep G., and Steven A. Kaplan. "BPH: Why Do Patients Fail Medical Therapy?" *Current Urology Reports*, vol. 20, no. 7, 6 June 2019, p. 40. doi:10.1007/s11934-019-0899-z. Reviews why patients may fail medical therapy for benign prostatic hyperplasia (BPH) and by doing so, gains a better understanding of the disease process and how to optimize the care of these patients.

PSYCHIATRY, GERIATRIC

Relevant Issues: Family, health and medicine, psychology

Significance: AS people age, mental and emotional problems may result from psychological and social stresses, genetic predispositions, or physical medical conditions; therefore, psychiatric care is a necessary component of geriatric health care.

Psychiatric symptoms can occur at any point in life. Some of these symptoms may result from increased stress in the life of the individual; such stress may be mental, physical, financial, or social. Medical attention, such as visits to a primary care physician or a geriatric psychiatrist, can be beneficial at these times to help the affected person address the stress and decrease or better manage the problematic symptoms. At other times, however, psychiatric symptoms can result from a psychiatric illness that requires specialized medical attention. Although it is possible that such symptoms might go away on their own, it is more likely that, without attention from a health-care professional, the affected individual will suffer more intensely or for a longer period of time than necessary.

As it is difficult to distinguish between these two types of psychiatric symptoms, consultation with a physician is almost always a good idea. Psychiatric symptoms can also be indicative of major physical problems, particularly in older adults; a failure to evaluate and address the symptoms could put the affected individual at risk for major physical health problems or could exacerbate a condition that might already be life-threatening.

SPECIAL NEEDS OF OLDER ADULTS

Advances in medical science are allowing more and more individuals to live longer and more productive lives. Such advances, however, require a keen awareness of the impact of medical procedures and drugs on aging body systems. Simply put, older bodies do not react to drugs, injuries, and medical procedures in the same way that younger bodies do. Slower metabolism of substances, slower healing, and decreased immune system functioning can all play a role in the maintenance of health and mental well-being. In addition, the physical, psychological, social, and financial supports that buffer people from the stresses and strains of daily living may weaken over time, causing older adults to suffer increased vulnerability to psychiatric disorders.

The specialty field of geriatric psychiatry was developed to focus on the treatment and prevention of psychiatric diseases and on the maintenance of mental health in older adults. Because of the nature of social changes that may coincide with aging—including decreases in independence and greater reliance on family or caregivers—geriatric psychiatry often involves collaboration with multidisciplinary medical professionals.

PSYCHIATRIC DISORDERS IN THE ELDERLY

The later years of a person's life can be a great time for enjoying the fruits of lifelong productivity. It is not uncommon, however, for older adults to experience such psychiatric diagnoses as depression, anxiety, substance abuse, and dementia. Even for the most well-adjusted older adults, the challenges of later life can affect mental and emotional well-being. Such difficulties as illness, physical challenges, retirement, geographic relocation, financial and social stresses, and the loss of friends and significant others to death can lead to mild depression and anxiety. For many, these difficulties are eased by support systems such as family and friends. For some individuals, however, these stresses and strains, if not addressed, may result in more serious conditions, such as major depression. Major depression often causes individuals to exhibit decreased levels of activity, decreased levels of pleasure in activities normally enjoyed, and decreased levels of social interaction. Other symptoms may include notable changes in weight (either loss or gain), lack of interest in sex, difficulty sleeping, and suicidal thoughts or extreme feelings of guilt and worthlessness. For some, depression can result in more subtle presentations such as irritability, anger, personality changes, and physical pain.

Changes in physical abilities, such as hearing, vision, mobility, and strength, can also affect mental health; some individuals may become anxious about not being able to take care of themselves or manage daily activities as they once used to do. Certain activities that were once commonly engaged in (such as cooking, bathing, driving, or leaving the home) might be avoided out of fear or anxiety. Often, a critical incident, such as an accident, fall, mishap, or misunderstanding, can lead to avoidance of these activities. Although cessation of the activity is sometimes appropriate (such as when driving ability becomes impaired), the primary issue may simply be fear of reoccurrence of the mishap. In such cases, avoidance often compounds the problem and may lead to the development of phobias and panic, which may impair normal behavior. Older adults also can have problems with alcohol and drugs. For some, this may be a continuation of a lifelong problem, but for others, it can be a new development. Drugs prescribed to take care of pain, insomnia, or even anxiety or depression may create drug dependence and lead to additional physical, mental, and emotional problems. Prescription drugs may also create problems when they are combined with small amounts of alcohol or other prescription or over-the-counter drugs. Symptoms of substance misuse may include falls, accidents, slurred speech, increased sleeping, anxiety, insomnia, irritability, or social withdrawal.

Dementia is characterized by permanent, diffuse, profound, and significant decreases in mental and emotional functioning and abilities. These changes, which can occur gradually (over many years) or abruptly, are usually the result of damage to the brain from a variety of causes. Substance abuse and strokes may lead to localized dementia, while Alzheimer's disease has a global effect on cognition and functioning. The onset of Alzheimer's disease is usually gradual as it progresses through several recognizable, distinct stages. People suffering from dementia at some point usually require the assistance of caregivers and long-term case management.

Some medical conditions common to older adults may first present as psychiatric symptoms. Among the medical conditions that may cause psychiatric symptoms are cancer, diabetes, Alzheimer's disease and other dementias, strokes, hearing loss, vision impairment, and irregular heartbeat or heart palpitations. Symptoms of depression, for instance, can be the first sign of cancer or dementia. Difficulty hearing and understanding oral information can lead to isolation and the misperception of stimuli, fostering opportune conditions for anxiety and paranoia. Memory loss can be one of the first symptoms of dementia. Problems with anger or inappropriate emotional reactions to situations can be an early indicator of strokes and dementia. Confusion can be an indicator of problems with diabetes, hypoglycemia, or dementia.

TREATMENT AND MANAGEMENT

An individual who visits a geriatric psychiatrist for the first time will typically be asked to supply a history, both recent and long-term, of the problems and symptoms. This gives the geriatric psychiatrist a functional picture of the symptoms to help determine causes and the best ways to treat the problem. Sometimes simply describing a problem in detail and receiving some educational information from a professional can help alleviate the concerns an older adult might have. If a problem is determined to be related to stress, the psychiatrist may recommend stress management techniques. Such techniques might involve setting up a daily routine, learning how to identify symptoms of stress, and learning to recognize stressful activities so they can be replaced by healthier, alternative activities.

When the cause or level of symptom severity is more pronounced and more of an ongoing impediment to well-being, regular meetings between a geriatric psychiatrist and the affected individual and his or her family might be suggested. Such meetings, typically called therapy or talk therapy, involve a process in which problems are discussed in greater detail. In the case of depression, for example, individuals might talk about the losses they have experienced and how they feel about them; psychiatrists may then suggest ways of thinking or behaving in response to such feelings that are more adaptive. For cases related to anxiety, discussions may center on specific ways of managing anxious feelings, understanding how certain thinking patterns might be making things worse, and learning new ways of behaving in response to anxiety. If talk therapy alone is not helpful, psychotropic drugs or drugs that affect thinking and feeling might be used to treat some disorders, such as anxiety and depression. In cases of severe depression where psychotropic drugs cannot be tolerated, electroconvulsive therapy may be used.

When psychiatric symptoms result from an underlying medical problem, treatment of the medical problem becomes primary. Typically, geriatric psychiatrists may provide supportive therapy to family members or affected older adults as they go through treatment. In cases where the symptoms might represent a permanent disability, such as with dementia or stroke, supportive therapy may continue for all involved. The affected individual and his or her family or caregivers may be given some educational information regarding what can be expected in the future and how best to design a rehabilitation and adjustment program. This may involve ongoing contact with medical providers or home health assistance.

The geriatric psychiatrist may also recommend behavioral modifications for performing tasks of basic living to allow the affected individual to function as safely and as independently as possible. In these cases, the thoroughness of the initial and ongoing assessments of the individual's functioning and abilities is critical to keep the rehabilitation and adjustment program productive. If a program that was working suddenly becomes less effective or if additional problems develop, further assessment is needed.

—Nancy A. Piotrowski
—Updated by Carolyn Minter, MD
and Miriam E. Schwartz, MD, PhD

See also: Aging: Biological, psychological, and sociocultural perspectives; Alcohol use disorder; Alzheimer's disease; Cancer; Dementia; Depression; Driving; Grief; Hearing loss; Loneliness; Medications; Memory loss; Personality changes; Stress and coping skills; Strokes

For Further Information

Broyles, J. Frank. *Coach Broyles' Playbook for Alzheimer's Caregivers: Bonus Tips and Strategies Booklet.* University of Arkansas, 2006. Coach Broyles was a former college football coach whose wife developed Alzheimer's dementia. He wrote a pragmatic and insightful 'playbook' for caregivers of those with dementia.

Comer, M. *Slow Dancing with a Stranger: Lost and Found in the Age of Alzheimer's.* Harper One, 2015. A poignant memoir written by the wife of a gentleman with early-onset dementia.

Davis, Patti. *The Long Goodbye: Memories of My Father.* A Plume Book, 2004. The author writes an honest reflection about her father, Ronald Reagan, an American president who had to publicly share that he had Alzheimer's Disease. Her message of unconditional love, healing, forgiveness and reconciliation as their extraordinary family lived the journey of her father's disease is an enduring lesson for everyone who has a loved one with dementia.

Hodges, Marian O., and Anne P. Hill. *Help Is Here: When Someone You Love Has Dementia.* Providence Health and Services, 2014. Dr. Hodges provides a useful resource for caregivers, friends, and family members of those with dementia.

Smith, B., and D. Gasby. *Before I Forget: Love, Hope, Help and Acceptance in Our Fight Against Alzheimer's.* Harmony Books, 2016. A touching book by B. Smith and her husband Dan Gasby about their personal experiences in B's diagnosis of early-onset dementia. Offers good strategies and insight into the disease process.

REACTION TIME

Relevant Issues: Biology, health and medicine, psychology

Significance: AS people age, their reaction times to stimuli tend to slow, causing safety concerns about such activities as driving; studies of reaction time have helped researchers learn about the effects of aging on cognitive performance.

Reaction time refers to the amount of time that passes between the occurrence of a stimulus and the execution of a response to that stimulus. Factors that influence reaction time include the need to accurately perceive the stimulus, to decide what action needs to be taken, and to coordinate the actions of the relevant muscular systems involved in the execution of the response. There is little doubt that humans experience a gradual slowing in reaction time as part of the aging process. However, the significance of this finding for performance in everyday life and its relevance to issues such as driving safety is far less clear.

Reaction time remains relatively stable until the age of forty, at which point a gradual pattern of slowing begins. Comparisons between healthy younger and older adults typically show that the responses of older adults take approximately 30 percent longer to execute than those of younger adults. Estimates regarding the rate of slowing indicate that reaction times decrease by approximately 2 percent for every five years of age.

The size of age differences in reaction time varies widely from study to study. Larger age differences are found in studies in which there is greater difficulty in detecting the stimulus, less opportunity to prepare a response in advance, and a change in the rules that indicate the correct response to a given stimulus. In addition, the difficulty of the task has a large influence on the size of age differences in reaction time. More complex or difficult tasks are associated with larger age differences in reaction time. This result is usually thought to reflect a slower speed of information processing in the brains of older adults.

Although older adults almost always display slower responses than younger adults, declines in the speed of cognitive operations may not provide a complete explanation of age differences in cognitive performance. For example, there is evidence that older adults make fewer errors on reaction time tasks than younger adults. This indicates that at least a portion of reaction time slowing in older adults may be explained by a style of performance that places more emphasis on accuracy than on speed. This stylistic difference may manifest itself in everyday life through more cautious driving habits.

Two other lines of research indicate that age differences in reaction time are not as absolute as once thought. First, age differences in reaction time are reduced with extensive practice in a particular task. Second, data suggest that physically fit older adults may not experience slowed reaction times to the same degree as less physically fit older adults.

—*Thomas W. Pierce*

See also: Aging: Biological, psychological, and sociocultural perspectives; Aging process; Brain changes and disorders; Driving

For Further Information
Pedersen, Traci. "As We Age, Loss of Brain Connections Slows Our Reaction Time." *Psych Central*, 17 June 2019. psychcentral.com/news/2018/09/13/as-we-age-loss-of-brain-connections-slows-our-reaction-time/18031.html. Reviews a University of Michigan study that suggests that, as we age, our brain connections break down, slowing up our physical response times.
Shmerling, Robert H. "My Fall Last Fall: Reaction Time and Getting Older." *Harvard Health Publishing*, Harvard Medical School, 14 Mar. 2016. www.health.harvard.edu/blog/my-fall-last-fall-201603149311. Using his own personal experience with taking a fall, Shmerling discusses how it was different because of his age.

READING GLASSES

Relevant Issues: Biology, health and medicine
Significance: With age, the lens of the eye hardens and becomes less able to focus on nearby objects; during middle age, all individuals will require reading glasses for near vision.

The eye gathers visual information and sends that information to the brain, where it is put into a meaningful picture. In order to transmit the information, the lens focuses light on the back of the eye, or retina, where special cells, the rods and cones, process the light information. In order to focus the light precisely onto the retina, the lens must be flexible and able to elongate or shorten. When the lens cannot flex in order to position the light onto the retina, objects in the environment become out of focus or blurred.

The lens gradually loses its elasticity with age. In a very young child, the lens is highly elastic and flexible and has great focusing power. As an individual ages, however, the hardened lens loses its focusing power, and a person begins to notice that close-up objects become blurred. A forty-year-old will notice difficulty reading small print, will have to hold newspapers and books at arm's length, and may have trouble with close tasks such as threading a needle. Once the lens becomes unable to focus on small objects held even an arm's length away, a common complaint is, "My arms are too short."

The inability to focus on near objects as a result of lens hardening with age is called presbyopia and is a completely normal part of aging. Presbyopia is not a disease. Although this condition cannot be prevented, it is correctable with reading glasses. The prescription strength of the glasses will increase gradually as a person advances in age, and the lens of the eye becomes more inflexible. The distance at which the patient works most often should be considered by the eye care professional when determining prescription strength for reading glasses.

—*P. Michele Arduengo*

See also: Aging process; Cataracts; Glaucoma; Nearsightedness; Vision changes and disorders

For Further Information
Mukamal, Reena. "Tips for Choosing the Right Reading Glasses." American Academy of Ophthalmology, 4 Apr. 2018. www.aao.org/eye-health/glasses-contacts/tips-choosing-right-reading-glasses. This article presents the top things to consider before choosing reading glasses.

RELIGION

Relevant Issues: Death, psychology, religion
Significance: Belief in a higher power and being part of a caring community may help maintain a sense of well-being in the face of the almost inevitable losses encountered as a result of aging.

Religion can be a controversial subject. It is commonly described as involvement in an organization of people who share a common theology. Most of the literature on aging and religion seems to assume that being religious includes a belief in an ultimate being, God, and a belief in a relationship with God.

Faith is usually included as part of religion. However, all people have faith in something: in their intellect, in their ability to control their destiny by hard work and determination, in their family and friends and social connections, or just in themselves. Those considered religious have faith in God. Religious faith may be viewed as believing in God, experiencing a relationship with God, and acting on this belief in a way that is thought to be pleasing to God.

Spirituality is sometimes considered synonymous with religion, but one can be religious without being spiritual or spiritual without being religious. Some who equate God with the universe and see themselves as part of God may be quite spiritual but not religious. The other view, and the one that has been most investigated in successful aging, is that God is separate and distinct from the universe: if the universe ceased to exist, God would remain. People holding this belief would probably be considered religious. Some who consider themselves religious and are devout at church attendance and at obeying the strictures of their church may not be spiritual. According to the National Interfaith Coalition on Aging, which became a subcommittee of the Forum on Religion, Spirituality, and Aging as an affiliate with the American Society on Aging (ASA) in 2010, "Spiritual well-being is the affirmation of life in a relationship with a God, self, community, and environment that nurtures and celebrates wholeness." This definition of spiritual well-being seems to include the idea of a connection with God, a caring for self, and an involvement in a corporate body that may minister to the group and to the individual.

Successful aging may have diverse meanings for people. Some would consider successful aging to mean retirement with financial security, having grown children who are doing well on their own, and being in good health. However, success at any point in life often includes overcoming adversity, and successful aging is no exception. If successful aging only included those things mentioned, many people would find successful aging beyond their ability. Dr. Harold Koenig, a noted authority on aging and Director of the Center for Spirituality, Theology, and Health at Duke University, claims that successful aging involves how older people feel, think, and act in whatever circumstances they find themselves. Successful aging, he suggests, is defined by crisis. When crisis comes, religious faith may be the difference between successful aging and facing one's final years with despair.

RELIGION AND AGING

Given this definition of successful aging, the possibility of a special connection between religion and aging is easily understood. When people are young, especially in Western societies, the individual and individual accomplishment are stressed. However, as one ages, it becomes clear that the time left to accomplish goals is shortening. As younger people enter the workplace, elders have a choice: Accept the changing times and find another life-fulfilling goal or fight to maintain their perceived positions. In midlife, focus begins to shift from the outer world and turn toward the inner world by necessity. In fact, retirement may be the occasion that leads some older people to religion. Many people derive their sense of identity from their career so leaving that career behind can create the need to answer one of life's basic theological questions "Who am I?"

When people reach midlife and see the aging process at work in their lives, faith in self and in a sense of control over their destiny may begin to falter. The best efforts cannot always control health or finances. The death of close friends, family members, or a spouse can leave a person feeling at a loss and bring the realization that control over life is, at best, transitory and perhaps only an illusion. People may find themselves looking for something to fill a void in their lives. A resurgence of interest in religion has been noted among the huge cohort of postwar baby boomers that began to reach the fifty-year-old mark around 1996. This could be explained by the fact that many of these people experienced the loss of parents and even the loss of spouses to death by the time they reached their fiftieth birthday.

As people experience the almost inevitable losses that occur with aging, they may feel needs that have not previously been evident. They may sense a loss of connection with the world because of loss of companions. Older people often say that the world they live in has changed since they were young. This may include relatively innocuous changes, such as technological advances, but it often includes such things as loss of homes because of financial reverses and loss of loved ones to death. Religious faith may offer answers in these circumstances by providing a sense of connection with God and with an extended family of believers, helping to soften the blow of losses. Seeing God as an omniscient, omnipresent, omnipotent, and unchanging entity can offer great comfort in the face of changing circumstances.

Other evidence exists for a special connection between religion and aging. Many Eastern religions teach that elders have a clearer vision of divine reality and possess greater wisdom as a result of their age. Hinduism teaches that in contrast to one's earlier years and regardless of what one's vocation was during those earlier years, the final years should be a time of spiritual vocation, of forsaking the world and its vocations and devoting one's self to the soul's salvation. If love of God and others is learned over a lifetime, as suggested by early Christians, spiritual growth should be a natural result of aging.

HEALTH AND RELIGION

According to Andrew Weaver and Koenig, research has consistently shown that nurturing, non-punitive religion is good for mental and physical health. One-fourth to one-third of older adults find religion to be the most important factor in enabling them to cope with chronic illness and other stressors experienced as a result of aging. In one study, 60 percent of elderly people reported that they had become more devout with age, while only 5 percent stated that religion had become less important to them. A 2018 AARP article reported that a study at the University of California found one in five baby boomers is seeking a more spiritual life through organized religion as they age and face health-care concerns.

The connection between mental and physical states is generally accepted by the medical profession. However, there can be reluctance to mention religion as a factor in mental health. Religion's connection to good mental health seems directly related to successful psychological practices, according to Koenig. Psychology and religion overlap in many areas. For instance, psychology speaks of the importance of unconditional, positive regard in the development of self-worth and in the therapeutic relationship between counselor and patient. Religious faith offers the unconditional love of God. Many of the things psychological therapy offers are also offered by religion. Therapy offers a trained listener; most religions offer a God who is always interested and is always listening. Therapy offers to help people gain a sense of self-worth; many religions offer a sense of worth in that each person is loved by God just because he or she exists, not because of having earned that love. Psychology recognizes that suppressed guilt can be problematic; religion offers forgiveness for past mistakes and errors. Anger and hatred toward others is known to be a major factor in maladjustment; religion offers the means to forgive others. Further, involvement in a religious community can offer the social support so important to those experiencing grief over loss, physical problems associated with aging, or the difficulties inherent in caring for a loved one who is ill.

It is generally accepted that many illnesses are stress related. Cardiovascular disease, high blood pressure, ulcers, and autoimmune disease are made worse by stress. Long-term stressful situations may lead to changes in the immune system that can result in illness and infection. Long-term stress has been associated with increases in tumors and loss of brain cells. Stress, by definition, is what one feels when one perceives something as stressful. It might be said that stress exists in the mind of the perceiver. Most religious faith offers the assurance that there is a God in control of life's circumstances. When bad things happen, God is present in that circumstance and will help in some way. This belief can make what would normally be perceived as stressors lose their power to produce anxiety. Holding this kind of belief may be important and comforting to aging people who are experiencing the losses and the changes life may bring.

Other reasons that religious faith may be a significant factor in health maintenance have been suggested. First, a community of caring may be important for maintaining physical and mental health. Second, a belief in a final destination may offer great comfort. If life is seen as a dead end, it may lose its purpose. However, if life is seen as a faith journey with a final destination that offers joy, peace, and a new beginning, it may be easier to face death without anxiety. Third, most religions stress growth throughout life. If one stops being mentally active or focuses on physical problems or on the past, life can quickly lose meaning. Evidence suggests that continued mental activity may be important in helping to prevent dementia. Religious faith usually encourages continued spiritual growth, and this usually entails continued involvement with other people. Fourth, attitude is important. The Christian religion stresses peace, joy, love, and patience as fruits of a growing relationship with God. Few would dispute that these attitudes promote physical health.

PSYCHOLOGICAL THEORIES OF DEVELOPMENT

Psychological development continues throughout life. One theorist who addressed the psychosocial development of adulthood and aging was Erik Erikson. He focused on interpersonal relationships and described eight stages of development throughout the life span, each of which was characterized by a central life task that needed to be completed for successful psychosocial development to take place. The stage of adulthood, from age forty to age sixty-five, is characterized by what Erikson termed "generativity versus stagnation." During this stage, adults must feel that they are accomplishing something important to them in their life. Otherwise, they may feel that life has been without purpose. The final stage, called maturity and termed "integrity versus despair," corresponds to the last years of life. According to Erikson, integrity reflects an emotional integration, a belief that the life one has lived was acceptable and necessary and includes a sense of life's order and meaning.

Erikson believed that failure to successfully negotiate any of these stages would compromise later stages. His theory, while making intuitive sense in many ways, proposes that the only way to achieve generativity or integrity is to complete each previous stage successfully. Misfortunes early in life, non-caring parents, accidents, and illness can all interfere with successful completion of earlier tasks.

However, religious faith may offer an alternative. For those who have faith, past errors can be forgiven, and a new life can be attained. One can achieve intimacy (one of the earlier life tasks, according to Erikson) with God, if no one else. The most basic of skills, learning to trust, is also a basic component of most religious faiths, as trusting God is the first step in faith in God. Religion is the belief that there is an order and a purpose to life, and that life has meaning in spite of circumstances. It offers a sense of continuity between this life and the next.

According to Koenig, the physical illness, disability, and decreasing social, financial, and cognitive resources that often accompany aging can heighten the struggle between integrity and despair. Ill health can adversely affect integrity by interfering with a person's ability to experience hope, meaning, and purpose in life, and can make it difficult to feel loved. These feelings can lead to despair and depression. Studies show that nearly 40 percent of hospitalized patients age seventy or over evidence some form of depressive illness. Religious faith may offer the only sense of meaning and hope that people in these situations can experience. A strong faith in God, an assurance of God's presence in the pain, and a belief in life after death can generate a sense of integrity or peace that might otherwise be impossible.

THEORIES OF FAITH DEVELOPMENT

American psychologist James Fowler developed a theory of faith development that attempts to describe how faith matures across the life span, independent of the content of that faith. Fowler has integrated the developmental theories of Erikson and Jean Piaget, as well as Lawrence Kohlberg's theory of moral development, into his theory of how faith develops across the life span. Fowler defines faith as involving "people's shaping or testing their lives' defining directions and relationships with others in accordance with coordinates of value and power recognized as ultimate." These coordinates of power may refer to God, self, money, job position, family, sex, power, or anything of ultimate concern to the individual. This definition of faith and the stages he describes are meant to be applicable to all religious and nonreligious faiths in all cultures. Fowler carefully differentiates structure from content in his theory.

As is the case with Kohlberg's theory of moral development, Fowler suggests that the faith stages he describes increase in maturity as one ages and that each one is in some way "superior" to the one that came before. Stage 0, undifferentiated faith, occurs from birth until age two, a strictly preliminary stage. Stage 1, intuitive-projective faith, occurs from age two to seven. During this stage, the child begins to form pictures of God, heaven, and hell. Similar to Piaget's early stages and Kohlberg's preconventional stage of moral development, the child is egocentric, incapable of seeing things from another's point of view, and unable to differentiate God's point of view from his or her own.

Fowler calls Stage 2 the mythic-literal faith stage, ages seven to twelve. Cognitively, the child is in Piaget's concrete operational stage, meaning that he or she can begin to use logic and understand what is real and what make-believe is but still interprets things in a very literal or concrete fashion. For the person at this stage of moral development, the world operates, according to Kohlberg, on the rule of reciprocity. At this point, the child's image of God corresponds to that of his or her culture and family. God is seen as operating in a strictly reciprocal manner, giving bad things to bad people and good things to good people. It might be suggested that some people never progress beyond this stage.

Stage 3, synthetic-conventional faith begins during adolescence. The opinions of peers begin to be of major importance to the individual. The young person becomes capable of seeing things from other viewpoints. However, because authority is located outside the self, the characteristic of this faith stage is the tendency to accept faith without critical examination (synthetic) and adhere to group norms (conventional). There is no view of faith independent of the community or family. Fowler suggests that much of church life in the United States works best when members remain at this stage. He claims that perhaps only 50 percent of people in adulthood advance beyond it.

Stage 4, which coincides with the post conventional moral development stage of Kohlberg, is called the individuate-reflective faith stage, beginning in the early to mid-twenties or later. During this time, people are completing Erikson's tasks concerning intimacy versus isolation and are moving toward the generativity versus stagnation conflict. Fowler suggests that it may take a crisis, such as a divorce, health problems, or other loss, to move a person beyond stage 3 into stage 4. At this point, the person moves away from relying on external authority and a need for approval of the group. Faith is questioned, and the individual decides what will form the "faith coordinates" by which he or she will live. This stage of moral development includes the definition of moral values and principles apart from the authority figures that have been the defining force in the past. The individual turns inward, away from the external world, for answers to questions of belief.

The final stage, conjunctive faith, occurs at midlife and beyond. It is said to coincide with the crisis of generativity over stagnation postulated by Erikson and includes a recognition that an overdependence on logic and rational understanding may not make sense in the light of the limits of human reason. Some of the decisions made in stage 4 may be rejected. During this stage, a person must integrate past experience and childhood faith into a new vision of truth. This individual growth is accompanied by a new commitment to justice for everyone, regardless of perceived differences.

Koenig suggests that, although Fowler's stages of faith are intuitively reasonable, scientifically based, and socially conscious, there may be some difficulties with his theory, particularly when one tries to apply it to the aging population. Although the effort to focus on a structure of faith that is totally separate from content is commendable, it may make the theory difficult to apply to individuals. Implying that higher faith stages are more valuable and contain more truth than lower stages may be problematical for two reasons. First, by implying that simple, childlike faith is somehow less mature, contains less truth, and is less valuable than the later stages, Fowler has added content to his theory. Many religious faiths, including Christianity, specifically require the believer to have "faith as a little child." Fowler's theory may be seen as devaluing this simple faith. Second, because Fowler links his theory to cognitive development, people who are not capable of progressing to these intellectual levels may be denied mature faith. In spite of attempting to remove content from his theory, his insistence on looking inside of one's self for truth may be seen as contrary to some religious faiths, including some aspects of Christianity. When considering the elderly, whose reasoning ability may be impaired by illness or advancing age, individuals who maintain simple, devout obedience to their faith are considered to be stuck at a lower stage.

Koenig suggests that the opportunity to advance in faith should be available to all, including an elderly person with a stroke or a slowly advancing organic disease, such as Alzheimer's disease. In his book Aging and God (1994), Koenig offers a complete critique of Fowler's theory and presents a theory of his own, which includes content. Koenig hypothesizes that the most important aspect of Judeo-Christian religion that impacts on mental health is the specific content of the tradition itself. The content of the belief is what determines attitude and behavior, which influence the emotional state. His theory includes a description of mature faith as involving a complete and wholehearted trust in God, regardless of circumstances: believing that God is in control, knows best, and is always present.

Not all people turn to religious faith as they age. Some people never seem to need any religious faith, and some place their faith elsewhere. There is no guarantee that age brings spiritual maturity or even a desire to seek comfort in spirituality. If mature faith is defined as devotion that carries a person through difficult times and does not fluctuate in sorrow or happiness, some faith never matures. In addition, temptations do not automatically lose their appeal at age sixty-five. For some people, the last years of life may bring a more acute awareness of spiritual impoverishment than of spiritual fulfillment. However, a Gallup poll revealed that 69 percent of people fifty to sixty years of age felt that religion was important in their lives, while 70 percent of those sixty-five and up felt the same way. Only 8 percent felt that religion was not important to them during their older years.

—Gayle Brosnan-Watters
Updated by Marylane Wade Koch. MSN, RN

See also: Aging: Biological, psychological, and sociocultural perspectives; Cultural views of aging; Death and dying; Depression; Funerals; Grief; Jewish services for the elderly; Last rites

For Further Information

Koenig, Harold G. *Aging and God: Spiritual Pathways to Mental Health in Midlife and Later Years.* Binghamton, N.Y.: Haworth Pastoral P, 1994. Classic publication with complete treatment of the subject of aging and God covers psychiatry, mental health, theoretical issues, research on aging and religion, clinical applications, nursing homes, Alzheimer's disease, family, and bereavement.

Allen, Kent. "Boomers Becoming More Religious: Long-term Aging Study Finds About 1 in 5 Report Increased Spiritual Activity in Recent Years." AARP. American Association of Retired Persons, 12 Apr. 2018. www.aarp.org/home-family/friends-family/info-2018/boomers-religion-study.html. Research shows one in five boomers are embracing religion as they have extra time on their hands plus feeling of aging and more health issues.

Briggs, David "Investing in Faith: Religion May Help Retirees Stay Mentally Fit." *Huffpost,* 3 Oct. 2012. www.huffpost.com/entry/religion-may-help-retirees-stay-mentally-fit_b_1935797?guccounter=1. Discusses research that links religion and better health outcomes in older adults.

Jackson, Steven. "Why Are Old People So Religious?" *Psychology Today,* 16 Feb. 2016. www.psychologytoday.com/us/blog/culture-conscious/201602/why-are-old-people-so-religious. Provides diverse insights into research that supports that the older one becomes, the more religious one also becomes.

Martin, Emily. "Religious, Spiritual Support Benefits Men and Women Facing Chronic Illness, MU Study Finds." *News Bureau University of Missouri,* 26 Oct. 2011. munews.missouri.edu/news-releases/2011/1026-religious-spiritual-support-benefits-men-and-women-facing-chronic-illness-mu-study-finds/. Discusses how religion and spirituality can help persons cope with chronic illness and experience better health outcomes.

Pew Research Center Religion and Public Life: US Religious Landscape Study 2014. www.pewforum.org/religious-landscape-study/. Information on the religious makeup, practices, and beliefs of Americans.

Pew Research Center Religion and Public Life Demographic Study: "The Age Gap in Religion Around the World." 13 June 2018. www.pewforum.org/2018/06/13/the-age-gap-in-religion-around-the-world/. Includes findings that support young adults are less religious than their elders globally.

RELOCATION

Relevant Issues: Demographics, economics, family, recreation

Significance: Choice and personal freedom remain important as people age. One of those matters of choice is where to live and whether to relocate to a warmer climate or to housing for the elderly.

By the end of the twentieth century, the United States was aging faster than ever. In 2017, the fifty million Americans aged sixty-five and older comprised 15 percent of the population. Projections put the number of persons sixty-five and older at almost seventy million by 2030. While the Caucasian population of the aged was expected to nearly double, even larger increases were projected for African Americans, Latinos, American Indians, Inuits (Eskimos), Aleuts, Asian Americans, and Pacific Islanders.

Relocation upon retirement to Florida or Arizona is a stereotype for the elderly in the United States. Is it accurate? Where do senior citizens actually live? Do they flee ice and snow? Of the top ten states for the sixty-five and older population in 2017, only California, Florida, Texas, and North Carolina would be considered southern. Nine states had sixty-five and older populations make up 18 percent or more of their total population: Florida, Maine, West Virginia, Vermont, Pennsylvania, Hawaii, New Hampshire, Montana, and Delaware. Only two of these states with high elderly populations are considered warm in climate: Florida and Hawaii.

Thus, it seems that retirees do not relocate to warmer climates in droves. Some retirees who do move to Florida become discouraged and migrate a second time north to the Carolinas or Virginia. Other retirees relocate abroad. Others choose to move closer to adult chil-

Population 65+ by State, 2017

State	# Adults over 65	% of All Ages	State	# Adults over 65	% of All Ages
California	5,505,358	14%	Louisiana	697,383	15%
Florida	4,214,635	20%	Oklahoma	602,823	15%
Texas	3,472,712	12%	Connecticut	602,410	17%
New York	3,162,193	16%	Iowa	526,057	17%
Pennsylvania	2,279,687	17%	Arkansas	499,144	17%
Illinois	1,945,398	15%	Mississippi	461,519	16%
Ohio	1,943,136	17%	Nevada	459,059	15%
Michigan	1,667,196	17%	Kansas	449,563	15%
North Carolina	1,630,445	16%	New Mexico	352,601	17%
New Jersey	1,418,603	16%	West Virginia	351,599	19%
Georgia	1,407,810	14%	Utah	335,572	11%
Virginia	1,271,428	15%	Nebraska	295,373	15%
Arizona	1,201,746	17%	Maine	266,214	20%
Washington	1,115,042	15%	Idaho	264,901	15%
Massachusetts	1,108,609	16%	Hawaii	253,560	18%
Tennessee	1,076,602	16%	New Hampshire	236,157	18%
Indiana	1,024,890	15%	Montana	190,523	18%
Missouri	1,007,033	17%	Rhode Island	177,955	17%
Wisconsin	954,557	17%	Delaware	174,128	18%
Maryland	904,671	15%	South Dakota	141,624	16%
South Carolina	864,577	17%	Vermont	116,869	19%
Minnesota	860,209	15%	North Dakota	113,208	15%
Alabama	803,771	17%	Wyoming	91,607	16%
Colorado	772,042	14%	District of Columbia	83,734	12%
Kentucky	711,349	16%	Alaska	82,580	11%
Oregon	708,817	17%			

Source: The Administration for Community Living, which includes the Administration on Aging, 2018 Profile of Older Americans

dren, grandchildren, or siblings or even to share housing with them. Most elderly, however, remain in their own communities.

LIVING ARRANGEMENTS

In the late 2010s, most aging people lived with a spouse or partner (59 percent). About 28 percent of adults over 65 lived alone. Some elderly people congregate informally in neighborhoods; these pods of older persons have been dubbed NORCs, for "naturally occurring retirement communities." In the late 2010s, about 1.2 million adults over 65 lived in facility care. The percentage of those living in nursing homes increases with age, ranging from 1 percent for persons aged 65-74 to 9 percent for persons over 85.

Other levels of housing facilities include apartments or condominiums for those needing no assistance but using a common dining room, assisted-living arrangements within individual apartment or condominium units, nursing care for the bedridden, and special facilities for Alzheimer's patients. Assisted living means help with meals, shopping, money management, telephone use, housework, and medications. These institutions can be expensive. Some facilities may require the resident to buy a condominium, which may trap the individual in that location or generate problems for the estate regarding resale. Others permit a resident to rent a room or apartment.

The wide variety of other care options includes senior centers, hospitals, adult day care, home health care, and hospice. Hospitals have a high representation of the elderly, who account for nearly 50 percent of the days of hospital care. Elders contemplating relocation must also consider the availability of medical facilities such as hospitals, especially if they have special needs.

OTHER IMPORTANT CONSIDERATIONS

Economics may dictate options for relocation. The poverty rate for those sixty-five and older is surprisingly a little less than for younger people, but it still includes 4.7 million elderly, with higher poverty rates among women, African Americans, and Latinx Americans. Investment strategies are a big concern for retirees who are better off financially. Those who wish to relocate and who can afford to do so might choose a place where they always wanted to live. They may move to Mexico for the climate and economy. Estate tax laws and other taxes vary from state to state.

Planning any change is important for the elderly. Planning includes not only the possibility of relocation and financial investment but also the drawing up of a will, the assignment of durable power of attorney, and perhaps the creation of a living will regarding medical care.

Transportation is a concern in choosing living arrangements. First is personal transportation, as stairs become more difficult to ascend. Walking distances and the presence and location of elevators become important. Second, elders may lose the ability to drive a car, so that the availability of alternative transportation (buses, taxis) must be considered. Safety may be a concern, as the elderly may be victims of crime or scams. The elder may no longer be able to or wish to cook. In addition to restaurants, senior citizen centers that serve meals and services that deliver food to homes should be available.

The opportunity for a social life may be a consideration in relocating. Approximately 32 percent of older women lost their spouses by their senior years, three times higher than the rate of men who lost a spouse. Employment opportunities may also be a consideration in relocating, as many seniors want to work, and volunteering is almost expected of active elders. Education is an attractive option for the aging; some colleges and universities are identifying and beginning to appeal to their housing needs and learning wishes.

—Sue Binkley

See also: Adult education; Caregiving; Driving; Early retirement; Facility and institutional care; Home-delivered meals programs; Home ownership; Home services; Homelessness; Housing; Leisure activities; Mobility problems; Poverty; Retirement; Retirement communities; Retirement planning; Safety issues; Senior citizen centers; Social ties; Temperature regulation and sensitivity; Transportation issues; Vacations and travel; Volunteering

For Further Information

"2018 Profile of Older Americans." Administration for Community Living. ACL. U.S. Department of Health and Human Services. 2018 acl.gov/aging-and-disability-in-america/data-and-research/profile-older-americans.

Granbom, Marianne, et al. "Household Accessibility and Residential Relocation in Older Adults." *The Journals of*

HOW TO TALK TO SENIORS ABOUT MOVING

How Do They Feel?

Any lifestyle change for seniors can be very demanding and challenging. Moving, which can be difficult for anyone, can be especially traumatic for older adults who have become used to a familiar environment. The idea of moving, particularly if it entails leaving a family home, can cause deep feelings of loss, along with other complex emotions. Some seniors will resist moving even if it's a medical necessity. In fact, those who must move due to a chronic illness, cognitive decline, or the death of a partner may be especially negatively affected by the change. They may want to be left alone or fear being a burden on others. Many seniors fear losing any independence by transitioning to a different type of living environment. While some level of stress and apprehension regarding a move is normal, be alert for signs of depression.

In some cases seniors are excited to move or pragmatic about the opportunity. They may understand the potential benefits, such as improved safety and amenities at an independent living facility. They may look forward to a new beginning or the opportunity to interact with peers. Of course, positive and negative feelings often come together for major life changes like moving.

Even seniors who move willingly or at least accept the necessity of a move often face negative physical and psychological reactions after relocating. This condition is known as transfer trauma or relocation stress syndrome (RSS). It can manifest as anxiety, depression, and anger. Seniors' sleep patterns may be disturbed, which can, in turn, negatively affect their ability to function in the day. They may exhibit signs of confusion and disorientation.

How Do I Start The Conversation?

Starting a conversation with seniors about moving requires sensitivity. It will be helpful for you to fully consider the issue yourself (or with other family members or caregivers) prior to bringing it up. This way you can have information readily available, such as the types of accommodation that may be suitable. If possible, raise the subject before a move is necessary, so a plan can be made together for the future. This will help the conversation remain low-stress and nonconfrontational. You might bring up the topic in a general manner or by relating a story about another family member or friend who has moved. If the senior mentions moving, you can ask questions or otherwise steer the conversation toward their own living situation.

It's crucial that seniors feel that they are involved in the decision to move. The more they feel they are participating in the decision-making process, the easier they will be able to transition to a new home environment. Ensure that they will have as much a say as possible in selecting and decorating their new place. Planning together to keep things like favorite furniture items, artwork, trinkets, or photographs whenever space allows will help maintain feelings of home and independence. Where possible, make every effort to have your senior visit a new home or community before moving so it can feel familiar upon arrival.

When speaking to a senior about an impending move, engage in the conversation in a gentle way. Listen empathically to what your senior is saying, without judging or informing them what they "should" be doing. Understand that moving can be traumatic and that to them it may represent significant loss of independence and things that have been familiar and dear to them for a large part of their lives. Let them know their concerns are being heard and demonstrate respect and understanding about how they're feeling. Assure them of your support through the transition.

It may be appropriate to raise the topic of keeping in contact with family and friends. Help seniors consider ways of communicating through e-mail, video calling, and other platforms as possible. If they are moving into some form of senior housing, help them explore and make use of any services and amenities that are available. If you know how an individual senior tends to cope with change, you can suggest other support mechanisms that will be helpful.

—Leah Jacob

Gerontology: Series B, 2018. doi:10.1093/geronb/gby131. Examines whether indoor accessibility, entrance accessibility, bathroom safety features, housing type, and housing condition were associated with relocations either within the community or to residential care facilities.

Miller, Jim T. "Specialized Services That Help Seniors Relocate." *HuffPost*, 7 Dec. 2017. www.huffpost.com/entry/specialized-services-that_b_8207446. Describes different options for seniors and their caregivers looking into relocation, including specific institutions.

Nemovitz, Bruce. *Guiding Our Parents in the Right Direction: Practical Advice about Seniors Moving from the Home They Love*. Book Publishers Network, 2013. Nemovitz provides a step-by-step guide through the moving process for older adults.

Roy, Noémie, et al. "Choosing between Staying at Home or Moving: A Systematic Review of Factors Influencing Housing Decisions among Frail Older Adults." *Plos One*, vol. 13, no. 1, 2018. doi:10.1371/journal.pone.0189266. A systematic literature review to identify the sets of factors influencing the housing decision-making of older adults.

REMARRIAGE

Relevant Issues: Culture, family, sociology

Significance: After a marriage ends through death or divorce, demographics make it difficult for older Americans to find another partner.

As the divorce rate rises in the United States, the spouses set adrift for one reason or another must seek out personally and socially acceptable ways of adjusting to their newfound "free" state. The search is exacerbated when the marriage is dissolved by the death of one or the other partner. Typically, women outlive men. Thus, widows find themselves, if they desire remarriage, in direct competition with many other single women—widowed, divorced, or never married—for a relatively smaller population of eligible and suitable men. In the United States, there are six million widows and one million widowers past sixty-five. Social gerontologists, health-care professionals, sociologists, and (to some extent) clergy are involved in helping older unmarried persons find a solution to their unwed status in a manner that is beneficial to both society and to the individuals.

The reasons that people marry vary greatly and have changed over time. Traditionally, a man may be seeking someone to "keep the hearth fire burning"—to help gather food, cook food, bear children, offer companionship, and provide sexual access. A woman may be interested primarily in a protector, a provider of food and shelter, a father for children, a sexual partner, and a companion. Marriage changes the social roles of the man and woman: before marriage, they are two individuals; after marriage, they are a couple, a sort of corporate entity.

All these relationships change with time. Although the married pair still exist as a couple, their roles as homemakers and providers may be switched. Except for childbearing, either person may assume the activities of the other. The end of a marriage, by divorce or other legal means or with finality in the death of one partner, changes the legal and often religious contractual arrangement. Some individuals are content to allow the end of marriage to be just that, with no thought of remarrying. Others, however, seek out another partner.

WHY PEOPLE REMARRY

The reasons that people remarry are in many ways similar to the reasons that they married the first time, but with some exceptions and changes in priorities. For many, the prime reason is companionship. The fires of passion may merely be glowing or be only a fond memory, but the knowledge that another person who cares is close by, especially in the still of the night, is comforting. Childbearing is no longer important in the remarriage of older persons, but social and economic security are very important. One or both partners in the union may provide assets that, when joined, provide a level of living not available to either one living singly. (Conversely, some persons who are living on Social Security income find that their economic status is enhanced by not marrying but simply living together, or cohabitating.)

The loss of a marriage partner, especially through death, may impose heretofore unexperienced burdens on the surviving spouse. For example, a husband may find it more difficult to cope with the death of his wife, not only dealing with the emotional loss but also facing the household tasks of cleaning and cooking. Moreover, although many women are capable, simple household or automobile repairs may prove to be formidable tasks.

In remarriage, older couples find that they often have more time together, further enhancing the companionship aspect. The wives no longer have to share their time with young children, and the husbands, no longer busy carving out a career, do not have to work late or be away from home on business trips.

Not everyone who loses a spouse through death or divorce will remarry. A common reason for not remarrying is the opposition of grown children. The offspring may suggest that their parent is too old for love. The potential marriage partner may be seen as an interloper, usurping the place of the deceased parent. Expected inheritances also play a role in efforts to sabotage a late marriage. Antagonism by the children toward the surviving parent's new romantic interest may quickly put an end to the relationship. In addition, many men and women, after the death of a spouse, simply do not want to remarry. Some have grown accustomed to single life and prefer not having to answer to someone. Others fear the death of a subsequent spouse, with the added burden of the entire grief process again.

MARRIAGE AS A HUMAN INSTITUTION

The formality of marriage is relatively new for the human species. It grew out of a sense of cooperation—basic to human nature—and one of the many kinds of associations formed by humans to help solve the different sorts of problems with which people must cope. Basic problems include the need for food, protection from the elements, and protection from other individuals and from predators. These problems could be solved through group behavior (bands or tribes), but they also could be solved by a pairing of males and females, with the added benefit of easy access for sexual activities and the resulting procreation.

Hearth and home—the household—established the basic unit of human society. Typically, the household consists of some form of family, a grouping of relatives that rises, at its simplest, from the parent-child bond plus the interdependence of men and women. With the inevitable relationship between sexual activity and the production of offspring who must be nurtured, family and marriage arose as a human state.

Over the millennia of human existence, family structures have varied. They have included polyandry (one wife with several husbands), polygyny (one husband with several wives), monogamy (one wife and one husband), and, more recently, serial monogamy (one man or woman married to a series of spouses in succession). Although monogamy is most common on a global basis, serial monogamy prevails in American society, where 41 percent of first marriages end in divorce.

The form or survival rate of marriage notwithstanding, the basic building block of human society, the household, gives identity and support to its members and provides a place for the organization of economic production, consumption of goods and services, inheritance, child rearing, and shelter.

As human culture evolved, the act of marriage took on a life of its own. It became a ceremony or sometimes a series of ceremonies, legal (that is, civil) and also religious, including combinations of the two. Often payment of monies or goods takes place, from the bride's family to the groom (a dowry) or from the groom's side to the bride's family (a bride price). The legal portion of a ceremony is to establish the legitimacy of children of the union and recognition of their place in the family or other kinship group.

Marriage also changes the social status of the couple. Prior to the ceremony, the man and woman exist in society as individuals. After marriage, they are considered to be a familial, inseparable unit, or corporate entity. The history of marriage is complex and encompasses the legal and economic dependence of women upon men. It includes the not-so-ancient concept of the inability of women to legally own or deal with property—real, fiscal, or personal.

In marriage, children are looked upon as the key to an ideal, happy family life. Children demonstrate to society the fruit of the union and the place of that family in the future life. Indeed, many sociologists consider the upbringing of children as the sole and primary function of the family. It is in the family that the children receive their primary socialization—the basic activities of language, correct behavior including eating and proper manners, and toilet training and personal cleanliness. Later, as the children grow, their world is expanded with secondary socialization such as education and the skills needed to live and interact with other individuals.

Ultimately, when the children leave home, they assume adult roles, marry, and establish families of their own. The aging parents of these grown children undergo a metamorphosis, and the parent-child relationship may be reversed. The children may provide financial support for now-retired parents, or the surviving parent if one has died. The children may provide shelter as well. Above all, the children may serve as guides and advisers to the parents, regardless of whether the parents are capable of caring for themselves adequately and making their own decisions.

What if the aging parent, now single as the result of divorce or the spouse's death, decides to remarry? Sociological research has shown that the family dynamics are basically different from those of the first marriage, even if that first marriage was a successful one. In fact, the likelihood that a couple will divorce increases with subsequent marriages. Second marriages have a 60 percent divorce rate and third marriages have a 73 percent divorce rate. The ingredients that made for a successful first marriage do not necessarily guarantee a successful second or third marriage.

PROBLEMS IN REMARRIAGE

About one-third of all Americans will remarry at least once in their lives. The ratio is reduced as the individuals age. Most of the problems in remarriage stem largely from the "baggage" that each partner brings into the new relationship. The marital stresses occur largely in several areas: families, including children (grown or young), relatives, and possibly a divorced spouse; finances; and houses, furniture, and other belongings.

Young children, up to and including older teenagers, often resent the interloper who is now intruding in the cozy relationship they had with the parent, usually the mother. This is especially the case in a "May-December" remarriage in which one spouse, usually the woman, is much younger than the man. Occasionally, she may be young enough to be his daughter's age. Grown children with families of their own see the new spouse as a competitor for their parent's affections or as a freebooter come to take away the inheritance that rightfully belongs (in the minds of the children) to them. Relatives who had formed a close relationship with the couple, on the death of one member of the pair, may feel that they exist in a state of limbo. Are they in-laws, former in-laws, or simply friends? What is their status?

Any finances that the couple brings into the remarriage raise other issues. Do they consider the monies "his and hers" or "theirs"? To clarify the fiscal arrangements and establish ground rules, many couples prepare a prenuptial agreement. Executed with the help of a lawyer, this agreement spells out how the monies are to be handled. This is especially valuable in situations where one spouse has greater financial assets than the other. Occasionally, couples who, as unmarried individuals, relied on Social Security benefits for their income choose to live together as husband and wife without benefit of marriage rather than accept the reduced benefits they would receive as a married couple.

Where to live after the ceremony is a question frequently facing an older couple contemplating remarriage. One or both may have a home with all that goes with it—furniture, neighborhood, nearby friends. There is no simple answer to resolve this situation, and many a potential remarriage has foundered even before it began because of the property, real and personal, owned by the individuals.

One matter that may be important to older, remarried couples is how to spend their day. Perhaps one or both had a full-time job and is now retired. Conflicts can arise with owl/lark personality habits. One partner prefers to stay up catching the late news, then a late talk show, then a late movie, followed by a morning sleep-in. The other prefers to hurry off to bed, not even watching the late news, but instead rising with the sun to work on a favorite hobby or to engage in some early morning exercise. In too many couples, these differences in spending the day can result in a real problem unless there is some serious compromise. Unfortunately, the habits of a lifetime are hard to bend, let alone break, and frequently the late-in-life remarriage becomes seriously damaged.

AGING AMERICA AND THE FUTURE OF REMARRIAGE

Demographic studies clearly demonstrate the differences in the survival rate of women versus men. Data show that almost half of all women more than sixty-five years old are widows and that in the sixty-five- to sixty-nine-year-old age group, there are only eighty-one men for each one hundred women. The ratio becomes even more lopsided as the population ages, so that for persons over eighty-five, there are only thirty-nine men for each one hundred women. Some of the single men over the age of sixty-five will undoubtedly choose not to remarry. The women must choose what to do with the rest of their lives.

Prior to World War I, many older widows and widowers moved in with their married children to fit in as best they could. Unfortunately, modern homes and households do not readily expand to include extended families. Unless the suddenly single older person finds that "special someone" or is able to fit in smoothly as a single, he or she effectively retires from society.

—*Albert C. Jensen*

See also: Cohabitation; Death and dying; Divorce; Family relationships; Marriage; Parenthood; Sexuality; Widows and widowers

For Further Information

"Divorce Statistics: Over 115 Studies, Facts and Rates For 2018." Wilkinson & Finkbeiner, LLP, 2018. www.wf-lawyers.com/divorce-statistics-and-facts/. A collection of statistics on marriage and divorce.

Field, Anne. "Money and Second Marriages, Remarriage and Finances." AARP, American Association of Retired Persons, 30 Aug. 2017. www.aarp.org/money/budgeting-saving/info-2017/second-marriage-money.html. Four couples provide their personal experiences with successfully managing their combined incomes.

Osmani, Nasrin, et al. "Barriers to Remarriage Among Older People: Viewpoints of Widows and Widowers." *Journal of Divorce & Remarriage*, vol. 59, no. 1, 2017, pp. 51-68. doi:10.1080/10502556.2017.1375331. Results of this study showed that older people are more concerned about public opinions and social norms surrounding remarriage.

Shah, Neil. "Remarriage on the Rise, Driven by Older Adults." *The Wall Street Journal*, Dow Jones & Company, 15 Mar. 2015. www.wsj.com/articles/remarriage-on-the-rise-driven- by-older-adults-1426459921.

Wu, Zheng, and Margaret J. Penning. "Marital and Cohabiting Union Dissolution in Middle and Later Life." *Research on Aging*, vol. 40, no. 4, 20 Mar. 2017, pp. 340-64. doi:10.1177/0164027517698024. This study examined the timing and risk factors for subsequent union disruption among individuals who were in a marital or cohabiting union at age 45, focusing particularly on the role of prior union history and children.

REPRODUCTIVE CHANGES, DISABILITIES, AND DYSFUNCTIONS

Relevant Issues: Biology, health and medicine, marriage and dating

Significance: Reproductive changes and disabilities, and the sexual dysfunctions that may arise from them, can greatly affect an elder's quality of life.

Reproductive changes, or changes in a female's or a male's ability to conceive children, begin sometime between the ages of forty and fifty. For most people, these changes are gradual and result in little alteration in ability to maintain sexual relationships. For individuals who value their reproductive ability, including sexual performance and enjoyment, these changes can cause concern. An understanding of the normal changes in female and male reproductive systems can help individuals deal with these changes and adapt their sexual behaviors to accommodate them and increase their quality of life.

The incidence of illness and disability increases as a person ages. Sometimes illness, disability, or changes in the reproductive system can result in sexual dysfunctions or impairment in sexual arousal or orgasm. Sexual dysfunction is not a normal accompaniment to old age and can be treated in a variety of ways. For most people, reproductive aging, illness, or disability might challenge them to be patient, understanding, and creative in their sexual relationships, but it is not cause for ending a sexual relationship that was once enjoyable.

FEMALE REPRODUCTIVE CHANGES

Female reproductive changes are greatly influenced by menopause. Upon arrival of menopause, a woman's ovaries will no longer produce estrogen and progesterone and ripen and release an egg each month; thus, she will no longer have the capability of becoming pregnant. In addition to the cessation of fertility, the severe decrease of estrogen and progesterone will cause several modifications in a woman's sexual anatomy and sexual arousal. A postmenopausal woman may experience changes in the appearance of her genitals. The folds of skin that cover the genital region shrink and become thinner, exposing more of the clitoris. Increased clitoral exposure may reduce sensitivity or cause an unpleasant tingling or tickling sensation when touched. The opening to the vagina may become narrower, especially if a woman is not participating in regular vaginal intercourse. In addition, the natural swelling and lubrication of the vagina occurs more slowly during arousal because the vaginal walls have become thinner and drier. These changes may affect a woman's sexual arousal and response.

Because of decreased vaginal lubrication, more time might need to be spent on foreplay or a water-based lubricant may need to be used. Compared to younger women, an older woman's orgasm will often be shorter and less intense, and it will take less time for her body to move from the height of orgasmic stimulation to a resting state. However, the capacity to achieve orgasm, even multiple orgasms, does not change with age. For many women, engaging in intercourse at least twice a week will cause these sexual arousal and response changes to be reduced or absent.

Although the physical changes related to menopause may cause an alteration in the way some women view sexual relations, in general, if a woman enjoys sexual relations when she is young, she will probably still enjoy those relations after menopause. Sexual desire is largely determined by emotional and social factors, but hormones such as estrogen, progesterone, and testosterone do play a role. Menopause causes a cessation of estrogen production in the ovaries, but testosterone is still produced in the adrenal glands. Thus, for the most part, testosterone levels are unaffected by menopause. Sexual desire is affected mainly by testosterone rather than estrogen, so after menopause most women still produce enough testosterone to maintain their interest in sex.

MALE REPRODUCTIVE CHANGES

Beginning at about the age of forty, men will experience a gradual change in their sexual functioning. These changes parallel those seen in postmenopausal women. Male changes are marked by a gradual, partial decline in the amount of available testosterone in the blood. Less testosterone is produced by the testes, and a growing portion of it is inactivated by bonding with blood proteins.

The gradual decline in a man's testosterone level will affect his sexual response in several ways. As a man ages, it will take longer to achieve an erection. A young man can achieve an erection just by watching someone whom he finds attractive, whereas an older man will probably require more direct stimulation of the penis in addition to visual stimulation or fantasies. Once an erection is achieved, it will not be as firm. Yet a man with good blood circulation to the penis can attain erections

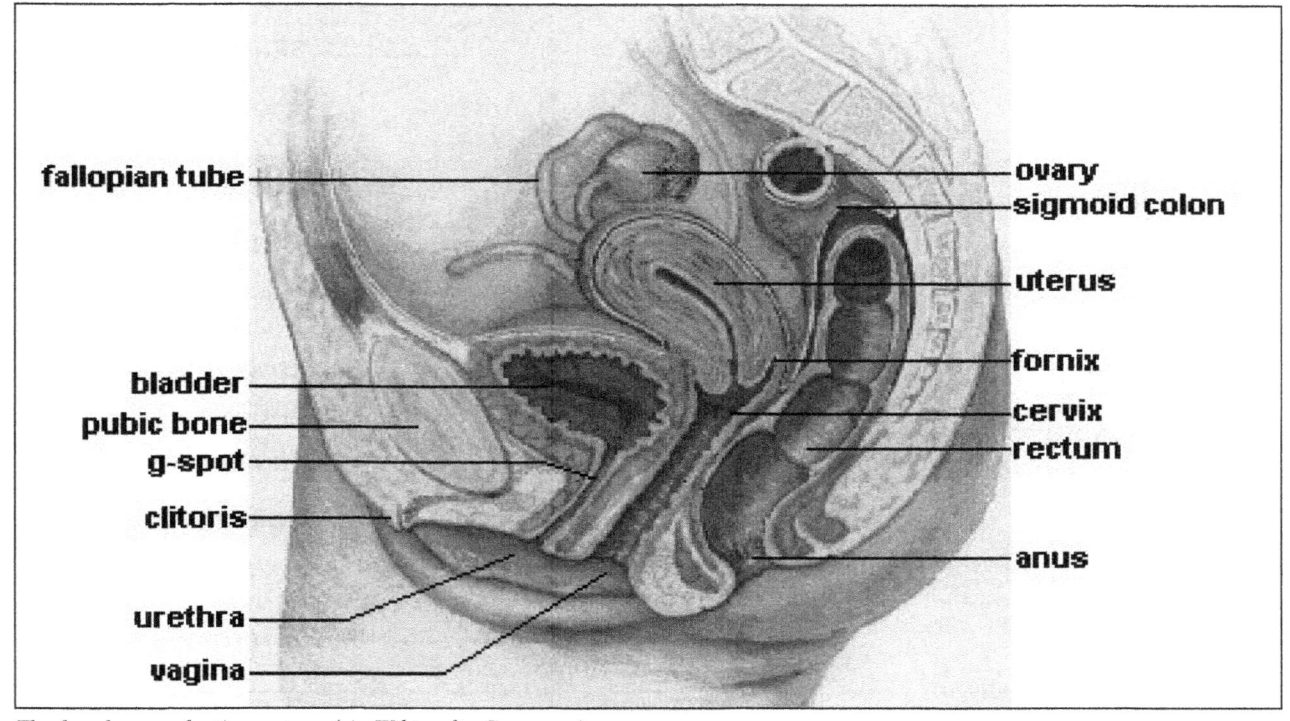

The female reproductive system. (via Wikimedia Commons)

adequate for intercourse until death. As a man ages, he will have more ejaculatory control, enabling longer intercourse and greater partner satisfaction. Although older men find orgasms intensely pleasurable, the actual force of ejaculation and amount of ejaculate become diminished as a man ages. Sperm production declines somewhat during midlife and levels off at about the age of sixty. Despite the reduction in sperm count, most men still produce adequate sperm to father children. After ejaculation, the erection subsides more rapidly, and a longer time is needed between ejaculations. Older men require several hours or a day or two between ejaculations.

Despite these changes, most older men remain interested in sex and enjoy an active sex life. Sexual desire originates in the brain and is influenced by emotional and social factors, but a minimum of testosterone is needed for the desire to actually materialize. Although men do experience a gradual decrease in testosterone levels, the great majority of men produce well above the minimum amount needed to maintain interest in sex into advanced age.

THE EFFECT OF ILLNESS OR DISABILITY

The overall incidence of illness and disability increases with age. The presence of certain illnesses or disabilities may require a modification in sexual activity, but rarely do they warrant stopping sexual activity altogether. Experiencing a heart attack leads many people to stop sexual activity for fear of causing another. Generally, if a person was sexually active before the heart attack, she or he can probably be sexually active again. If one can climb two flights of stairs without symptoms such as chest pain, palpitations, or shortness of breath, then sexual activity can usually be safely resumed. People who have had a heart attack are usually able to have sex two to four weeks afterward, while bypass patients may reach this point in one to three weeks after they leave the hospital. For many people, an active sex life may decrease the risk of a future heart attack.

Atherosclerosis, or hardening of the arteries, can damage small blood vessels and restrict blood flow to the genitals. In men, this can interfere with erection. About half of all impotence in men past age fifty is caused by atherosclerosis. In women, this can interfere

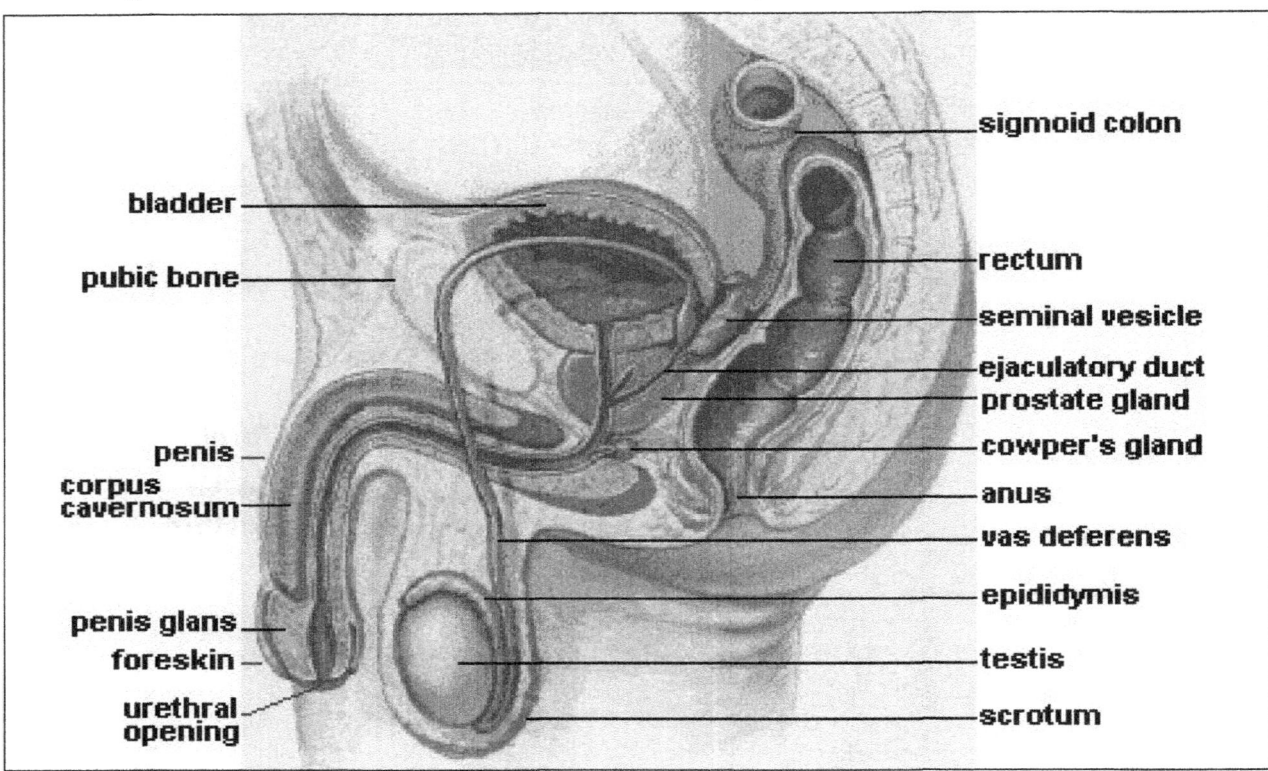

The male reproductive system. (via Wikimedia Commons)

with the swelling of the vaginal tissues. Diabetes can also affect male and female sexual functioning. Diabetes can increase the plaque or fatty deposits in blood vessels. These deposits restrict the flow of blood to the penis, causing about half of men with diabetes to become impotent. The risk of impotence increases with age. Women with diabetes may experience vaginal dryness, painful intercourse, and a decreased frequency of orgasm. Females also may have more frequent vaginal and urinary tract infections.

Although arthritis does not directly affect sexual organs, the pain and stiffness caused by osteoarthritis or rheumatoid arthritis can make sexual relations difficult to enjoy. Certain surgeries and drugs can relieve these problems, but in some cases, the medication actually decreases sexual desire. Exercise, rest, warm baths or showers, changes in positions, and avoiding sexual activity in the evening and early morning hours, when pain tends to be the greatest, can be helpful. Communication is important. Generally, as long as partners communicate openly regarding their desires and capabilities, a satisfying sexual relationship can be maintained.

Prostate surgery for a noncancerous condition such as an enlarged prostate rarely causes impotence. After surgery there will be a decrease in the amount of seminal fluid, but sexual ability and enjoyment should remain unaffected. Prostate surgery for cancer causes impotence 50 to 60 percent of the time; however, this type of impotence can be treated with penile implants. Alternatives to prostate surgery, such as radioactive seed implants, have a lower probability of causing impotence.

Hysterectomy is the removal of the uterus and cervix and in some cases the Fallopian tubes, ovaries, and lymph nodes. This surgery does not interfere with a woman's physical ability to have intercourse or experience orgasm. If the ovaries have been removed, then the woman instantly experiences menopause. Hormone replacement therapy (HRT) can help replace the estrogen and progesterone that the woman's body is no longer producing and reduce the physical and sexual changes that a woman experiences. However, HRT contains certain risks and should be evaluated carefully with a health-care provider.

SEXUAL DYSFUNCTIONS

Sometimes people's bodies do not respond the way they would like them to. A sexual dysfunction is a physiological or anatomical impairment in sexual response that prevents sexual arousal or orgasm. Although not a normal part of aging, sexual dysfunctions are more common among the elderly because of their higher prevalence of chronic illness and the side effects of some prescription medications. Impairment may be due to physiological, anatomic, or psychological factors of which most can be treated.

Changes that a woman's body goes through during menopause, along with medications and alcohol use, can affect a woman's sexual functioning. Reduced vaginal lubrication caused by menopause; use of blood pressure medication, over-the-counter antihistamines and decongestants, alcohol, nicotine, or illegal drugs such as methamphetamines, cocaine, heroin, and marijuana; and reduced vaginal elasticity, a vaginal infection, or poor hygiene can cause persistent or recurrent pain during sexual intercourse (dyspareunia). Dyspareunia is one of the most common sexual dysfunctions. Among older women, dyspareunia may also occur during orgasm because of spastic uterine contractions.

A second type of pain disorder is called vaginismus. Vaginismus is characterized by involuntary contractions of the muscles surrounding the outer one-third of the vagina, thus preventing penile penetration or rendering penetration painful. Vaginismus may be associated with dyspareunia among older women. A psychological fear of penetration causes vaginismus, and that fear might have been brought about by experiencing dyspareunia in the past. Vaginismus may be the result of the woman involuntarily trying to protect herself from painful stimulation associated with intercourse.

Orgasmic dysfunctions are when a woman persistently or recurrently has difficulty reaching orgasm. The use of high blood pressure medications, barbiturates, antidepressants, or alcohol commonly causes loss of pleasure in sexual activity and difficulty in attaining orgasm. Some women have been anorgasmic (never have reached orgasm), and others have reached orgasm but not consistently enough to satisfy themselves or their partner (situational orgasmic dysfunction). Situational orgasmic dysfunction (SOD) can be caused by feelings of guilt or performance anxiety.

Male sexual dysfunctions tend to be related to attaining and maintaining an erection and to ejaculation. Erectile dysfunction (ED), or persistent difficulty achieving or maintaining an erection sufficient to allow the man to engage in or complete sexual intercourse, is the most common male sexual dysfunction. These erectile dysfunctions can be partial (an erection is achieved but cannot be maintained), or they can be complete (an erection is never achieved). It is believed to affect one in every three men over the age of sixty. Four factors are needed for a man to reach and maintain an erection: complete male sexual organs, normal hormone levels, an adequate nerve and blood supply to the penis, and good emotional health. If one or more of these factors are missing, a partial or complete erectile dysfunction may exist. Certain medications and drugs can interfere with nerve or blood vessel function or affect sex hormone levels. Medications used to treat high blood pressure, diabetes, depression, and psychosis commonly cause decreased sexual interest and erectile difficulties. Alcohol, smoking, and illegal drugs such as methamphetamines, cocaine, heroin, and marijuana have also been found to cause erectile difficulties among men.

Ejaculation difficulties are a second sexual dysfunction that can affect older men. These difficulties result in impaired ejaculation (unable to ejaculate) or premature ejaculation (ejaculate sooner than desired). Premature ejaculation is generally considered to be more psychological in origin, while impaired ejaculation can be a side effect of certain medications including antihypertensives, antidepressants, and antipsychotics.

DIAGNOSIS AND TREATMENT

Ultimately adults should be able to discuss sexual changes and difficulties with their partner and physician, but studies have found elders to be reluctant to volunteer information regarding sexual behavior to a physician. Older adults may believe their problems are due to the normal aging process, minimize the importance of their sexual needs and desires, or be embarrassed to discuss sex. Whatever the reasons are, studies have found that when physicians do ask patients if a sexual problem exists, many will volunteer significant concerns.

Before a sexual dysfunction can be diagnosed and treated, a physical examination and medical history are necessary. Blood will be drawn, and laboratory tests will be run to measure blood levels of testosterone and other hormones so hormonal problems can be ruled out. A medical history will include family disease history, alcohol and prescription drug intake, history of smoking, and a sexual history. A sexual history will include a history of present relationship with partner; level of communication with partner about sexual matters; social situation, including other life stressors; how illness affects sexuality; number and gender of sexual partners; desired level of sexual activity; satisfaction with frequency and variety of sexual activity; presence of pain during sexual activity; quality of orgasm; and, for men, the frequency, duration, and firmness of erections and the quality of erection and ejaculation.

The cause of a dysfunction is either psychological or physical or a combination of the two. Psychological causes of dysfunction include emotional stress, tragic sexual events such as rape, partner dissatisfaction, negative body image, and guilt. Physical causes can include heavy alcohol use, certain medical conditions, prescription medications, and over-the-counter medications. Limiting alcohol consumption, treating medical conditions, and altering prescription and over-the-counter medications will oftentimes remedy the problem. If this is not the case, there are specific treatments available for each type of sexual problem. It is important to note that while many women do experience sexual dysfunctions, there has been very little research on the diagnosis, treatment, and causes of dysfunctions in women.

The origin of the dysfunction will determine how it is treated. If the problem is caused by drug therapy, an alternate drug or lower dose of the drug can be prescribed. When dysfunctions are psychological in origin, both the person experiencing the dysfunction and his or her partner (if there is one) are referred to a sex therapist. Also available are hormone therapies and penile injections and implants.

—*Catherine Schuster*
Updated by Kerry Cheesman, PhD
and Maryann Cheesman, RN

See also: Alcohol use disorder; Communication; Estrogen replacement therapy; Hypertension; Infertility;

Marriage; Medications; Men and aging; Menopause; Prostate cancer; Prostate enlargement; Psychiatry, geriatric; Sexual dysfunction; Sexuality; Stress and coping skills; Urinary disorders; Women and aging

For Further Information

"Attitudes about Sexuality and Aging." *Harvard Health*, Harvard Medical School, Mar. 2017. www.health.harvard.edu/staying-healthy/attitudes-about-sexuality-and-aging. Debunks several myths about sexuality and aging.

Buttaro, Terry Mahan, et al. "Sexuality and Quality of Life in Aging: Implications for Practice." *The Journal for Nurse Practitioners*, vol. 10, no. 7, 2014, pp. 480-85. doi:10.1016/j.nurpra.2014.04.008. Discusses prescriptive and herbal therapies that older patients may be using to augment sexual health, as well as potential barriers to conversations about sexuality in aging.

Gunes, Sezgin, et al. "Effects of Aging on the Male Reproductive System." *Journal of Assisted Reproduction and Genetics*, vol. 33, no. 4, 11 Feb. 2016. pp. 441-54. doi:10.1007/s10815-016-0663-y. Discusses the structural and functional changes in the male reproductive system during aging.

Heidari, Shirin. "Sexuality and Older People: A Neglected Issue." *Reproductive Health Matters*, vol. 24, no. 48, 9 Dec. 2016, pp. 1-5. doi:10.1016/j.rhm.2016.11.011. Reviews present studies and ideas about aging sexuality and calls for more research on the topic.

"Sexuality in Later Life." National Institute on Aging, U.S. Department of Health and Human Services, 30 Nov. 2017. www.nia.nih.gov/health/sexuality-later-life. General information for older adults about sexuality and the changes they may experience.

Shirasuna, Koumei, and Hisataka Iwata. "Effect of Aging on the Female Reproductive Function." *Contraception and Reproductive Medicine*, vol. 2, no. 1, 3 Oct. 2017, p. 23. doi:10.1186/s40834-017-0050-9. This review discusses how cellular deterioration and inflammation accelerate reproductive failure in women.

Sousa, Avinash De, et al. "Sexuality in Older Adults: Clinical and Psychosocial Dilemmas." *Journal of Geriatric Mental Health*, vol. 3, no. 2, 2016, p. 131-39. doi:10.4103/2348-9995.195629. Sheds light on the various aspects of sexuality in older adults and the challenges faced by medical professionals working in this area by reviewing several papers and studies on the subject.

RESPIRATORY CHANGES AND DISORDERS

Relevant Issues: Biology, health and medicine

Significance: Respiratory changes during aging are of fundamental importance because they can affect quality of life and exercise tolerance; they are also associated with overall mortality.

Key Terms:

alveolar sac: tiny air-filled chambers within the lungs that allow oxygen and carbon dioxide to move between the lungs and bloodstream

intrapleural pressure: the pressure within the pleural cavity, a narrow, fluid-filled space covering the lungs and lining the chest cavity

oxygenation: the process of adding oxygen to the body system

ventilation: the act or process of inhaling and exhaling

As time passes, we may notice a gradual decrease in the amount of air we are able to exhale after drawing a deep breath. This happens because as we age bones thin and cartilage loses flexibility, reducing the expansion of our rib cages. Other age-related changes affect us as well; muscles of the diaphragm may weaken, alveolar sacs lose flexibility, and general lung health may decline, which raises the specter of pneumonia. These problems may be intensified by obesity, smoking, and waning of heart function. These changes can serve as reminders to pace ourselves; they should not be incapacitating.

The respiratory system transports oxygen into cells and carbon dioxide out of cells. This is accomplished as air moves in and out of the lungs (ventilation), air within the lungs is distributed to areas perfused by blood (ventilation/perfusion), gas mixtures are exchanged between the alveoli and blood (gas transfer), and gases in the blood are transported to tissues. The respiratory system thus includes components of the musculoskeletal system, the circulatory system, and the nervous system.

VENTILATION

Ventilation is primarily enabled through the diaphragm; auxiliary muscles include the intercostal muscles, located between the ribs, and the abdominal muscles. As the diaphragm contracts, the thoracic cavity enlarges, the lungs expand, intrapleural pressure decreases, and air flows into the lungs. When the diaphragm and intercostal muscles relax, the tissues recoil, and air is expired. The amount of air entering or leaving the lungs during a single normal breath is the tidal volume. The total amount of air that is exhaled following a maximal inhalation is called the vital capacity. The amount of air remaining at the end of a maximal exhalation is the residual volume. Together, vital capacity and residual volume equal total lung capacity.

Most increases in lung volume occur during a person's late teenage years or early twenties. Residual volume increases with age. Air remains trapped in the peripheral airways because of a loss of elastic fiber attachments. These elastic fiber attachments usually keep small conducting airways open and patent. As they age, these fibers tend to lose some of their function. Because total lung capacity remains constant with age and residual volume increases, vital capacity decreases with age. That is, the amount of air that can be maximally exhaled decreases with age. Pulmonary-function tests that indi-

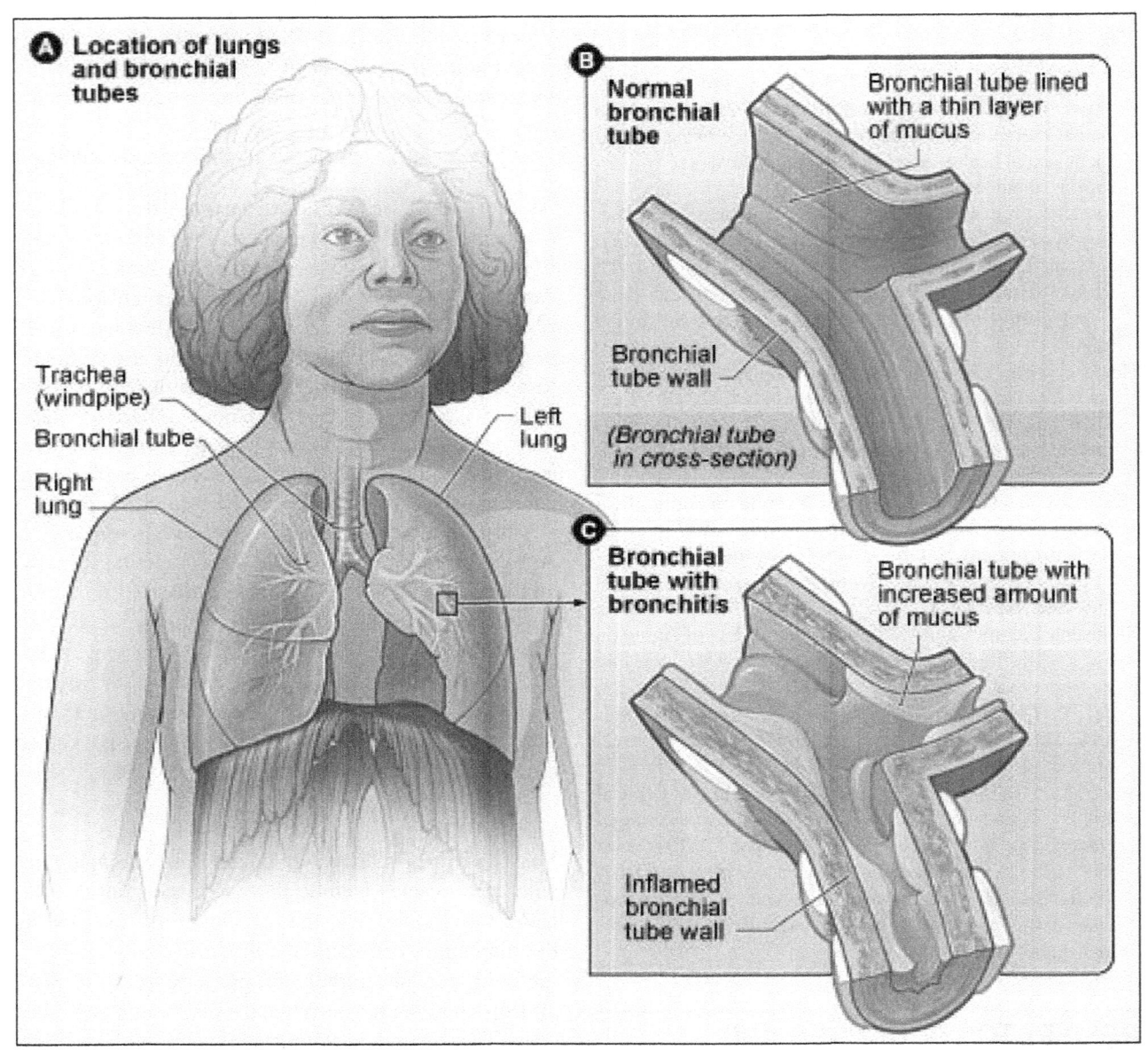

Figure A shows the location of the lungs and bronchial tubes in the body. Figure B is an enlarged, detailed view of a normal bronchial tube. Figure C is an enlarged, detailed view of a bronchial tube with bronchitis. The tube is inflamed and contains more mucus than usual. (via National Heart Lung and Blood Institute)

cate expiration capacity, such as the forced expiratory volume in one second (FEV1), also decrease with age.

During expiration, the small airways at the base of the lung may close, preventing air at the base of the lung from being expired. The lung volume at which this closure occurs is called the closing capacity. The closing volume equals the closing capacity minus the residual volume. Closing volume has been shown to increase as people age. Therefore, older people exhale less air than younger people, and air expired comes more from the upper parts of the lung than from the lower parts. When combined with other conditions, such as smoking or lung infection, ventilation can be significantly impaired, causing blood oxygen to become low.

Every minute approximately four liters of air enter the alveoli of the lung and approximately five liters of blood pass through the lungs. How completely the air and blood mix make up the ventilation/perfusion ratio. Some researchers have shown ventilation/perfusion ratios to be less in the elderly than those found in younger adults. This means that the gases are not mixing as well with the blood, so that less oxygen or carbon dioxide can be exchanged. The lowered ratio, if it occurs, may not be noticed by the average healthy older person. In fact, some scientists have reported a decrease in arterial oxygen content with age, but others have failed to demonstrate this association. Normally, the lungs will increase respiration, or the heart will increase output to overcome the lower ventilation/perfusion ratio. However, when heart disease or chronic pulmonary disease is also present, the decreased ventilation/perfusion ratio may worsen, and the combination of lower blood oxygen and higher carbon dioxide can be more noticeable.

GAS TRANSFER AND BREATH CONTROL

The diffusion of gas from the end branches of the lung (the alveoli) into the blood depends on the total surface area of the alveoli, the thickness of the membrane across which the gas diffuses, and the capacity of the blood to absorb gas. Age-related decreases in gas transfer are usually the result of a loss of alveolar surface area, less perfusion of the lung by blood, or decreases in blood flow, all of which impact the ventilation/perfusion ratio.

The striated muscles of the respiratory system are under voluntary and autonomic control. Autonomic input to the muscles comes from both peripheral chemoreceptors and stretch receptors, which regulate the frequency and depth of breathing. The chemoreceptors are sensitive to the amount of carbon dioxide and, to a lesser extent, oxygen in the blood. The stretch receptors are sensitive to the contraction and relaxation of respiratory muscles. Although a fall in the oxygen content of the arteries can stimulate the chemoreceptors to increase breathing, arterial oxygen content is not normally an important part of the drive to breathe. Chemoreceptors are usually much more responsive to carbon-dioxide concentrations. Researchers have shown that responsiveness to both oxygen and carbon dioxide decreases with aging.

Age-related respiratory changes do not appear to have a substantial impact on the normal, healthy older person. However, these changes do make the aging lung more susceptible to respiratory diseases, and the consequences of cardiac and infectious diseases may be more severe. Certainly, pneumonia and upper-respiratory infections become more serious for the older person who may have decreased ventilation and perfusion, as well as increased closing volume. In addition, chronic respiratory diseases are very common in the elderly.

CHRONIC RESPIRATORY DISEASES

Chronic obstructive pulmonary disease (COPD), the fourth leading cause of death in the United States, usually manifests itself after the fifth decade of life. The term COPD is often used to include both bronchitis and emphysema because these two conditions often coexist. However, some scientists and physicians prefer to differentiate between the two based on the person's symptoms, history, and test results.

Bronchitis is closely associated with smoking and is typified by a productive cough for at least three months during the year for at least two consecutive years. The cough develops because of increased production of mucus and obstruction of the lower airways. The person with bronchitis cannot expire efficiently and so may retain carbon dioxide in the blood. Blood oxygenation may also decrease because of poor gas exchange in the alveoli. The person with bronchitis is often of normal weight or heavier. Although common to both conditions, shortness of breath in a person with emphysema may be more apparent than in someone with bronchitis.

With emphysema gas exchange in the lungs worsens because of alveolar-wall destruction, which decreases alveolar surface area. Measures of expiration decline, and arterial carbon dioxide is often elevated, although less so than is common in bronchitis. The person with emphysema is usually thin and becomes short of breath with little exertion.

Chronic respiratory diseases impair quality of life. When respiratory disease progresses in the elderly, activities may become curtailed. Exertion necessary to perform household tasks or leisure activities may cause such people to become alarmingly short of breath. Combining medication with lifestyle changes and exercise can often be very helpful. Surgical techniques that modify lung capacity also show great promise. In the absence of chronic respiratory disease, changes experienced with aging should not affect a person's quality of life or significantly impact activities. People who maintained an active lifestyle and developed their respiratory and cardiovascular systems generally exhibit less decline than those who have been inactive for a lifetime.

—Karen Chapman-Novakofski
Updated by Jackie Dial, PhD

See also: Aging: Biological, psychological, and sociocultural perspectives; Aging process; Emphysema; Exercise and fitness; Illnesses among older adults; Pneumonia; Smoking; Sports participation

For Further Information

"Common Breathing Problems in Older Adults & What You Can Do About Them." *Kendal at Home*, 27 June 2017. www.kendalathome.org/blog/breathing-problems-in-older-adults. This blog contains a variety of articles concerning older adults.

Guyton, Arthur, and John Hall. *Textbook of Medical Physiology*. 13th ed. Elsevier, 2016. This clear and comprehensive guide has a consistent, single-author voice and focuses on the content most relevant to clinical and pre-clinical students. The detailed but lucid text is complemented by didactic illustrations that summarize key concepts in physiology and pathophysiology.

Jones, Thomas B., ed. *The Merck Manual of Health & Aging* (paperback). Ballantine Books, 2004. Guide to the medical challenges of aging for older adults and those who care for and about them.

Kovacs, Elizabeth, et al. "The Aging Lung." *Clinical Interventions in Aging*, vol. 8, 6 Nov. 2013, p. 1489. doi:10.2147/cia.s51152. This review focuses on the nonpathologic aging process in the lung, including structural changes, changes in muscle function, and pulmonary immunologic function, with special consideration of obstructive lung disease in the elderly.

"Lung Capacity and Aging." American Lung Association, 20 Mar. 2018. www.lung.org/lung-health-and-diseases/how-lungs-work/lung-capacity-and-aging.html. Explanation of age-related lung changes.

Sharma, Gulshan, and James Goodwin. "Effect of Aging on Respiratory System Physiology and Immunology." *Clinical Interventions in Aging*, vol. 1, no. 3, Sept. 2006, pp. 253-60. doi:10.2147/ciia.2006.1.3.253. Explains the functions of the lungs and respiratory system and describes the changes that occur to each as we age.

REST HOMES. *See* FACILITY AND INSTITUTIONAL CARE.

RETIRED AND SENIOR VOLUNTEER PROGRAM (RSVP)

Date: Founded in 1966
Relevant Issues: Demographics, recreation, work
Significance: The Retired and Senior Volunteer Program is a national network of Americans, age fifty-five and over, who volunteer in their communities in an effort to improve the overall quality of life in the United States.

The Retired and Senior Volunteer Program (RSVP) was founded by the Community Service Society of New York in 1966 as a pilot project designed to afford retirees the opportunity to volunteer in ways that utilize their work and life experience. RSVP is one of three National Senior Service Corps programs administered by the Corporation for National Service, established in 1993 to promote community-based service programs. All three Senior Corp programs—the Foster Grandparent Program, the Retired and Senior Volunteer Program, and Senior Companion Program—provide volunteer opportunities for older citizens. More than 450,000 Americans volunteer their skills as part of RSVP annually.

RSVP members are not required to possess any minimum educational background or work experience, only the desire to volunteer on a regular basis. In 2018, RSVP volunteers actively served the needs of communities with more than 500,000 older-adult volunteers. At the local level, RSVP is typically affiliated with service providers, educational facilities, cultural organizations, and government agencies. Opportunities to volunteer vary widely, depending on the needs of the community. Skills or experience with adult day care, childcare, classroom teaching, counseling, public speaking, and tutoring are utilized in most communities. Interested individuals are screened by RSVP staff and matched with the requirements of agencies prior to placement in the community at a volunteer site.

—*Donald C. Simmons, Jr.*

See also: Mentoring; Retirement; Volunteering

RETIREMENT

Relevant Issues: Demographics, economics, law, race and ethnicity, work

Significance: Formal retirement from work is a process that began in the late nineteenth century in Western societies because the industrial system needed to remove older workers in a socially acceptable manner.

Beginning in the nineteenth century, formal retirement with pension payments provided a socially acceptable means for industries to reduce the size of their workforce. The welfare state in Western industrial countries worked with industries to achieve the goal of providing retired workers with a steady source of income. The retirement policies of the welfare state have helped determine the age at which individuals can retire from work. For example, the ability of individuals to receive lower Social Security payments at sixty-two years of age in the United States has been instrumental in lowering the age of retirement for many individuals in the population.

Women and racial minorities have different retirement patterns than Caucasian males because of their different work experiences. The increased size of the baby-boom population may lead to generational conflict in the United States if there are insufficient economic resources to support the current group of workers.

RETIREMENT PRIOR TO THE INDUSTRIAL REVOLUTION

There was no formal universal retirement system in the world prior to the Industrial Revolution. Some occupations, such as the military, did provide care for their incapacitated members in good standing and provided shelter and food for them and their immediate family members. There were also benevolent work societies that cared for their indigent members. However, no universal system existed to provide a steady income for those no longer capable of working. Individuals continued working until their death, or they ceased working and were supported by either their accumulated wealth or their family members. In colonial America, the landed elites, such as George Washington and Thomas Jefferson, used their personal wealth and the services of their slaves to support themselves in retirement.

The economic system did consider the diminished capacity of individuals to work by developing age-graded tasks. The system of slavery illustrated this process, with the younger slaves being engaged in field work and the older slaves doing lighter agricultural tasks or working in the plantation home. Slaves who could not work at all were either supported by the plantation owners or set free and left to the care of the state. In extreme cases, the incapacitated slave would be abandoned and left to die, as illustrated by Frederick Douglass's grandmother, who was left by her owners in a little hut to die after having given a lifetime of service to them.

The family was required to bear the costs of maintaining those elderly who were no longer capable of working. This obligation was a heavy burden on most families, as, in some instances, they had to provide long-term care to their elderly relatives. Proportionally few individuals survived to old age prior to the Industrial Revolution, which limited this burden for most families. In eighteenth and nineteenth century America, many individuals were mobile, as illustrated by the case of Abraham Lincoln, who was born in Kentucky, lived as a child in Indiana, and eventually settled in the frontier town of Springfield, Illinois. These mobile individuals had limited contact with their relatives and were unable to offer them much aid. Propertied and elite elderly individuals, such as Benjamin Franklin in Philadelphia, were venerated by the larger community and received social support from this community, leading a comfortable existence in their older years. Ordinary el-

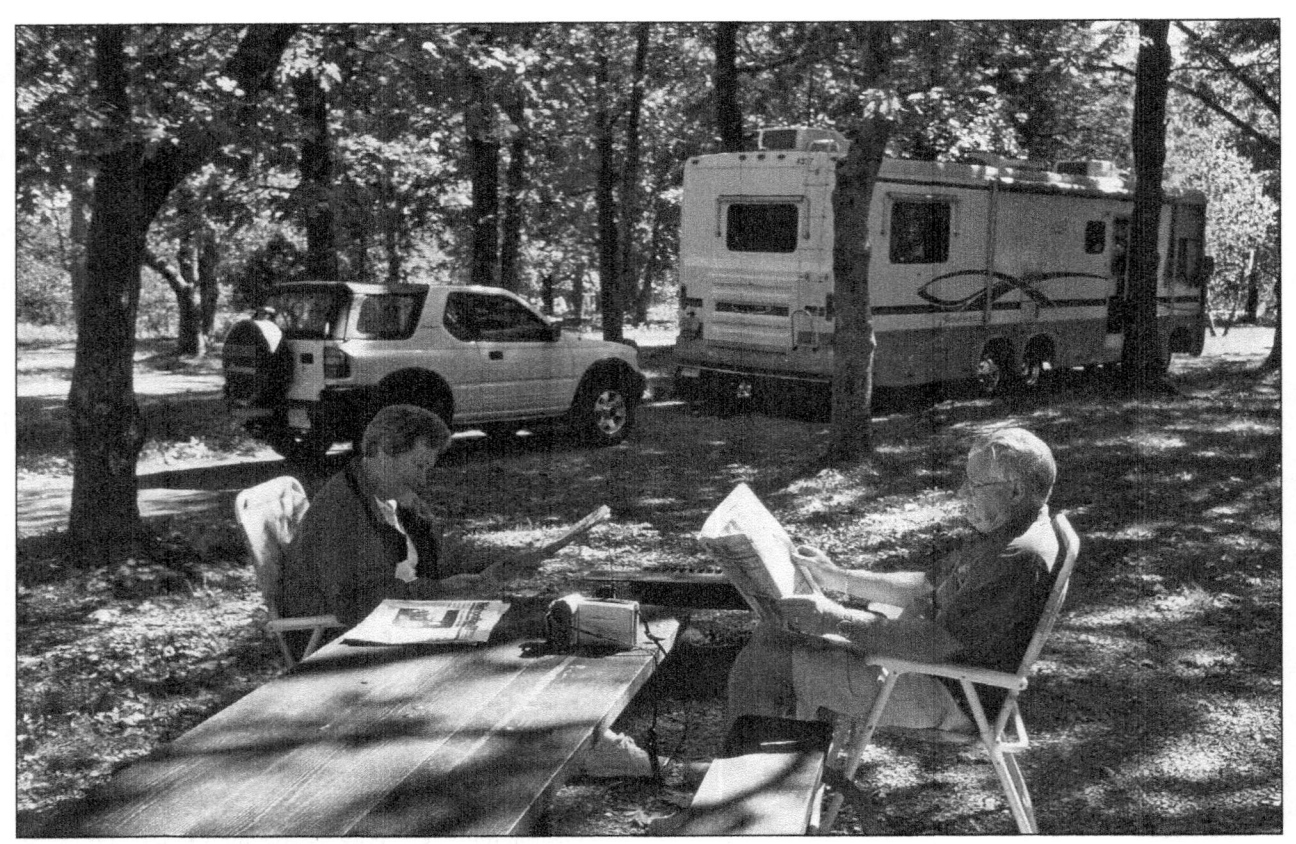

Retirement can mean more time spent on leisure activities, like camping. (Wikimedia Commons)

derly people with limited wealth were dependent on family members for support; without this support, they often endured extreme poverty.

THE INDUSTRIAL REVOLUTION

In the nineteenth century, the evolution of the factory system changed the nature of work. Large numbers of individuals labored in this setting, producing mass goods efficiently and at a low cost. The factory system needed to replace older workers with younger ones, because the physical difficulty of the work made the elderly inefficient workers. There were age-graded tasks in these industries, but not enough for all elderly laborers. As the older workers had no steady source of income if they ceased working, they resisted being removed from the workforce. In the early stages of industrialization, the owners of factories proceeded arbitrarily to dismiss their older workers and replace them with younger ones, sentencing these dismissed workers to a life of poverty. Such a policy created resentment among the workers, as well as discontent in the larger community. Violent labor disputes in the late nineteenth century, such as the Pullman Strike and the steel strike in Homestead, Pennsylvania, demonstrated that management needed a better means of managing their workforce. Part of this management involved the retirement of older workers without creating mass discontent.

One mechanism that industry found to accomplish this goal was to offer retired workers a pension as a reward for their lifetime of service to the organization. The railroad industry in the latter part of the nineteenth century began to offer a pension to its retired workers, easing the economic pain of their being removed from the workplace. However, most industries found that they could not afford to offer such a pension, and such economic incentives were used sparingly until the New Deal era in the 1930s. Companies were engaged in competition with other industries, and they found it unprofitable to offer their workers a pension and not have their competition provide a similar pension for their workers. In the southern United States, the workers were poorly organized and were split along racial lines, so the business community had less to fear from these workers. If a national retirement system was to be developed, a uniform national means of providing a retirement income for the older workers was required.

THE WELFARE STATE

The welfare state was developed in Western industrialized societies to provide an income, as well as health benefits, for the older population. This welfare state, which provided state pensions for all workers in society, was instituted in Germany in the 1870s by Prime Minister Otto von Bismarck. Bismarck, a staunch conservative, was engaged in a political struggle with the democratic socialist parties and needed some way to counter their appeal to the workers. He devised a uniform state pension system as a means of reducing the political radicalism of the workers while tying them to the state. In the twentieth century, many of the other nations in Europe, including Sweden and Denmark, began to adopt such a pension system. Great Britain and France lagged behind other European nations in this development, but after World War II, they and other industrialized Western nations adopted similar retirement systems.

Left-wing and socialist worker parties were instrumental in the development of these retirement systems in Western democratic societies. These parties saw this type of pension system as being beneficial to their constituents. In political campaigns, the adoption of such a system became a major platform of these parties. In many instances, this type of campaign led to political victory and the national adoption of pension support for the elderly, as occurred in Great Britain in 1945 with the victory of the Labour Party.

The United States instituted retirement welfare later than other industrially developed nations. An early attempt at a welfare retirement system in the nation involved the federal government's payments, after 1890, to the 1.8 million individuals who served in the Union Army during the Civil War. This national welfare system was limited in scope, as it naturally excluded Confederate veterans, as well as the elderly immigrants who arrived in the United States after the war. Prior to the 1930s, some states developed pension systems, but their scope was limited, and the dollar amount of their pensions was small.

The Great Depression, which began in 1929 and lasted until World War II, provided the impetus for the creation of a national, although restricted, pension system. The Depression dramatically increased the level of poverty among the elderly and called forth social movements designed to reduce this poverty. In California, the Townsend movement, which advocated a fixed pension for all elderly citizens of the state, formed many clubs throughout the state. In 1934, the movement was instrumental in nominating writer and activist Upton Sinclair as the democratic candidate for governor. Franklin Delano Roosevelt was elected president in 1932 and started the New Deal program designed to help end the Depression. The New Deal came to see the development of a national pension system as an important goal, because such a system would offer aid to the poverty-stricken elderly population while stopping them from supporting more radical relief measures. In 1935, the Social Security Act was proposed by the Roosevelt administration and was passed by Congress. It was modest in scope, offering limited monthly pensions for workers in certain industries. In the South, African American sharecroppers were excluded from the system. After 1935, however, the scope of the program was expanded by successive Congresses, and the system became more inclusive. In 1965, the Lyndon B. Johnson administration passed the Medicare Act, providing medical care and services for those sixty-five years of age and older.

The total number of pension systems available to the American population significantly expanded after 1935. Most individual states offer extensive pension systems for state workers, with the state of California having the largest one in the nation. Many industries, including the automobile industry (which offers high pensions and medical benefits to workers who have thirty years of service), have expanded their pension offerings. By the 1970s and 1980s, individual pension systems, financed by tax subsidies, were instituted. Individual retirement accounts (IRAs) allowed individuals to invest up to $2,000 in most investment plans and claim it as a tax deduction, while supplemental savings accounts (SRAs) allowed workers to invest a larger amount in specified investment accounts and deduct the amount from their gross earnings. These government-subsidized accounts allowed individuals to make investments and defer their taxes on these investments until after they retired, when they would be in a lower tax bracket. These government-subsidized investment plans favored middle- and upper-income individuals, because lower-income individuals did not possess the extra income needed for investment. Although large numbers of Americans have limited pension protection, being dependent on Social Security and Supplemental Social Security for their retirement income, many Americans have been allowed to expand their pension coverage.

THE AGE OF RETIREMENT

When the Social Security Act of 1935 was passed, it specified sixty-five years as the age when individuals or their spouse might receive a retirement pension. This age became accepted as that at which an individual should retire, and a vast majority of Americans prior to the 1960s retired at this age. However, after the Social Security Administration in the 1960s allowed individuals to retire with reduced benefits at the age of sixty-two, there was a decline in the age of retirement, with many Americans retiring before sixty-five. The growth of state pensions, which allow retirement either after thirty years of service or at age sixty, has further increased the number of individuals who retire prior to sixty-five. Many industries, such as the automobile and steel industries, grant retirement and medical benefits to workers after thirty years of service, and this policy has also increased the number of individuals who retire prior to the age of sixty-five.

Many individuals who retire relatively young, such as police officers or military personnel (who can retire after twenty years of service), start a second career. Although some individuals follow a path of full work and then totally retire, others hold "bridge jobs" that provide lower levels of employment before they fully retire from work. This gradual reduction of work allows individuals to ease themselves into the retirement role, which requires some adjustment in their lifestyle. By the age of seventy, most individuals have removed themselves from the workforce or have involuntarily been removed because of illness or disability. Higher status professionals and managers are more likely to continue working beyond sixty-five, as their work activity is less strenuous and as they are in greater demand because of their skills. Many of these individuals can continue to work part-time by consulting with firms and organizations with which they had contact during their career.

In a study that examines the evolution of retirement between 1880 and 1990, Dora L. Costa provides a coherent explanation for the falling age of retirement in the United States. The increased retirement income available to the elderly is a necessary condition for explaining this process, but it does not totally explain it. Another factor is the improved health of the elderly population, which makes it possible for them to be active in their later years. There has been a steady rise in the life expectancy of all Americans, with the current overall life expectancy being seventy-eight years of age, although it is higher for women and lower for African Americans. The education level of Americans has also increased appreciably. In 1945, at the end of World War II, the median formal education of all Americans was approximately eight years of schooling, whereas at present it is more than thirteen years of schooling.

The growth of an elderly population that is healthier and better educated, and possesses more discretionary income, has triggered the growth of a leisure and recreational industry that can serve this market at a competitive low cost. The expansion of cable television and rental films has provided the entire population with inexpensive entertainment in their homes. The development of the Internet, which can be accessed by all individuals with inexpensive computers, has given the elderly access to many sources of information and entertainment. The travel and tourist industry has expanded the services available to the elderly and has given them travel opportunities not available to earlier generations. Prior to World War II, travel to Europe and outside the country was only available for the wealthy or the elite elderly. In the nineteenth and twentieth centuries, wealthy Americans, such as John D. Rockefeller and Andrew Carnegie, or elite Americans, such as Ulysses S. Grant and Theodore Roosevelt, traveled and toured abroad, but such travel was not feasible for the average American. However, the development of low-cost air travel and the packaging of relatively inexpensive foreign tour packages reduced the cost of international travel and allowed lower income individuals the opportunity to travel abroad. Market changes related to leisure and recreation have made retirement more attractive for elderly Americans, who have readily availed themselves of these opportunities when they possess the economic resources.

The increased number of elderly citizens as a result of the aging of the baby-boom population, as well as the falling age of retirement for senior citizens, has prompted policymakers to attempt to reduce the number of retirees by raising the age at which individuals can receive their Social Security benefits. Those individuals born in 1960 and later must be sixty-seven years of age before they can receive full benefits, although there has been no change in the policy of giving reduced benefits for those who retire at sixty-two. This policy change may have some impact on the age of retirement, but because more elderly citizens have other sources of income beyond Social Security, its impact will be minimal. Because there will probably be fewer younger workers to support older workers in the future, it may be necessary to increase the age of retirement.

A larger concern with the increased number of retirees in Western industrialized nations is the impact of this change on economic growth. If the elderly dependent population becomes too large, this increase may reduce the capital available in the society for economic growth. In the 1950s and 1960s, a similar concern arose with the high number of young dependent people (fourteen years of age and younger) in underdeveloped nations. Some demographers supported birth control policies in these nations as a means of reducing their young dependent population, which would make more capital available in these countries and stimulate economic growth.

THE GREAT RECESSION

The financial crisis that started in late 2007 and ended in 2009 is widely regarded as the worst economic catastrophe since World War II. This recession affected most of the world as stocks plummeted, unemployment rates were at record highs, and the real estate industry suffered. The cause of The Great Recession was multifactorial but a direct result of irresponsible lending by the housing and banking industries. Individuals older than sixty-five at the time were minimally affected as they were more likely to already be retired and, therefore, have the cushion of social security benefits. Those who were not yet retired were more likely to want to continue working to offset the effects of an unforgiving recession. However, this was oftentimes not possible as older workers were still vulnerable to the massive layoffs that ensued, leading many to claim their retirement benefits early and subsequently have less funds for retirement.

GENERATIONAL CONFLICT AND RETIREMENT

The increased number of elderly individuals who live a long life because of improved health, while at the same time receiving improved government benefits, has raised the fear of greater intergenerational conflict in American society. It is true that the baby-boom generation born between 1945 and 1964 has placed a strain on the Social Security and Medicare systems. It is estimated that these government transfer programs will pay out more than they take in during the early decades of the twenty-first century. The only means of correcting this situation is to either increase taxes or reduce benefits, neither choice being politically popular. The increased cost of caring for the elderly population led to the establishment of Americans for Generational Equity (AGE), a pressure group that criticizes the redistribution of social transfer payments in favor of the elderly. There are legitimate financial concerns about the increased economic cost of the elderly population for the remainder of society, but a part of this concern involves an ideological battle by conservative groups to end, or at least curtail, all government programs.

Demographer Samuel Preston has statistically demonstrated that, since the 1960s, proportionally more government transfer payments and funding are going to support the elderly and proportionally less are going to the younger population. The Clinton administration's welfare reform package of 1996 is an illustration of this process, with the federal and state governments' transfer payments being cut for children and unwed mothers, as well as illegal immigrants. No such similar reform has been instituted for Social Security and Medicare, and no legislation has been proposed to reduce tax credits for IRA and SRA accounts. The elderly are a well-organized political group, and they can be mobilized to protect their vested interests.

Those who attack high government transfer payments for the elderly usually have no political desire to expand the scope of the welfare state and provide more government aid to children and those in poverty. Rather, they wish to cut or eliminate all government programs that aid the former groups, while also reducing government aid to the elderly. The support by business groups to privatize Social Security or to have a proportion of Social Security taxes go toward private investment is a step in the elimination of the program. Stock investments might aid some middle- and upper-income elderly, but they will be risky for lower-income individuals, as well as for those individuals who have a limited knowledge of personal investment.

Critics of the Social Security system often fail to see the insurance nature of the program and its ability, with full citizen participation, to provide aid to elderly and other individuals who need government support. Partially or totally privatizing the system would reduce funds for the Social Security trust fund required to pay its insurance claims, such as disability claims and Supplemental Social Security claims for the poverty-stricken elderly. The Social Security system is both a retirement system and an insurance system, with no payments for those who fail to survive long enough to collect payments. If an individual and his or her spouse die before retirement, the money they have paid into the system reverts back to the federal government. However, throughout their lives, they have been insured by the system.

In discussing the elderly and their cost for the younger working population, one should differentiate among three categories of elderly. The young-old, between sixty and seventy-five years of age, are relatively healthy and active. The middle-old, seventy-six to eighty-five years of age, experience more health problems and require a higher level of social support. The old-old, those over eighty-five years of age, are a fast-growing segment of the elderly population who experience high levels of health-related problems and require more social services, including long-term care in nursing homes or in their residence. This group places a significant burden on social and medical facilities.

Those individuals who stress the intergenerational conflict approach fail to consider the benefits that the elderly population transfers to the younger population. As a result of the growth of the American economy, the elderly population has accumulated vast amounts of wealth in property, stocks, bonds, and other forms of investments. In the first several decades of the twenty-first century, trillions of dollars of this wealth will be transferred to the younger generation through family inheritance. In evaluating the burden that the elderly population imposes on the younger generation, one should also consider these asset transfers between the generations.

AFRICAN AMERICANS AND WOMEN

Elderly African American workers are often marginalized and have often experienced racial discrimination throughout their work careers. They are more likely to have worked in low-status jobs characterized by sporadic work patterns and low income. This job pattern means that they are less likely than Caucasians to have a pension beyond Social Security or Supplemental Social Security. Some of them work beyond sixty-five years of age because of economic necessity, but, as a group, they are likely to retire earlier than Caucasians, at fifty-five to sixty-four years of age. Their relatively poor health and more sporadic employment are the major reasons for this early retirement. African Americans who have similar work careers as Caucasians have similar types of retirement patterns. The lower life expectancy of African Americans implies that they receive less total retirement income from the system than Caucasians. However, they pay less than Caucasians into the Social Security system, and they are more likely to receive Supplemental Social Security benefits, balancing out inequities in payments from the system.

Women have become more active in the labor force since World War II. They often balance work and family needs. Women are more numerous in lower-paying occupations, such as teaching and social work, and suffer economic discrimination even when they perform the same tasks as men. As a result of these two factors, they have lower wages and a shorter job tenure than men. They also receive lower levels of Social Security benefits than men and are less likely to receive private pensions. The Social Security system discriminates against women when computing their benefits in that it fails to count their child rearing and family work when deter-

> **SENIOR TALK:**
>
> **How Do You Feel About Life After Retirement?**
> Reaching retirement age is often a time of mixed emotions. On the one hand, you might feel relieved to leave behind the stresses of your career. On the other hand, you might feel as if you are facing a void without the daily structure of work life. You may feel overwhelmed as you consider what you will do with your time when you are no longer working. You may even feel like you lack a sense of direction or purpose and feel downhearted and demotivated as a result. Many retirees go through a period of struggling to redefine their identity and sense of self in the absence of their career. It is common to feel nervous about future.
>
> On the other hand, you may have been anticipating your retirement with excitement. The release from work duties may feel gratifying. As you prepare for all the things you would like to do, achieve, and enjoy in your retirement, you may feel buoyed by the energy of possibilities. Looking forward to your retirement does not mean you will not feel some feelings of loss or sadness, rather you may be prepared to move forward to the next stage in your life.
>
> —*Leah Jacob*

mining their benefits. Social Security benefits are determined on the basis of years worked and maximum salary during this work career, which is assumed to be thirty years. If a woman works fewer than thirty years, often because of family obligations, she receives fewer benefits. Women who are married and share in their husbands' benefits usually receive adequate retirement benefits, but divorced, widowed, and single women are likely to suffer economic deprivation.

—Ira M. Wasserman
Updated by Rachel Alison L. Chan

See also: African Americans; Early retirement; Employment; 401K plans; Individual retirement accounts (IRAs); Leisure activities; Life expectancy; Mandatory retirement; Medicare; Men and aging; Old age; Pensions; Poverty; Retired Senior Volunteer Program (RSVP); Retirement communities; Retirement planning; Social Security; Townsend movement; Vacations and travel; Volunteering; Women and aging

For Further Information

Atchley, Robert C. *Social Forces and Aging: An Introduction to Social Gerontology.* 10th ed. Wadsworth, 2004. This standard social aging text discusses retirement, as well as economic and political issues related to aging.

Costa, Dora L. *The Evolution of Retirement: An American Economic History, 1880-1990.* U of Chicago P, 1998. A brilliant study of the economic history of retirement in the United States and the role of the marketplace in shaping retirement decisions.

Hooyman, Nancy R., and H. Asuman Kiyak. *Social Gerontology: A Multidisciplinary Perspective.* 9th ed. Allyn & Bacon, 2010. A discussion of retirement and other issues related to social gerontology.

McDonald, Gail M., and Marilyn L. Bushey. *Retirement Your Way: The No Stress Roadmap for Designing Your Next Chapter and Loving Your Future.* Choices Next, 2019. Packed with practical guidance, useful research, and inspiring stories, this book will motivate you to let go of your stories, add your dreams, and keep exploring.

Quadagno, Jill. *Aging and the Life Course: An Introduction to Social Gerontology.* 7th ed. McGraw-Hill, 2018. This study of the social aging process provides a historic and policy perspective for studying retirement and other aspects of aging.

Ryan, Robin. *Retirement Reinvention: Make Your Next Act Your Best Act.* Penguin Books, 2018. Full of practical advice, this thought-provoking guide offers readers a path for reinventing their own retirements.

RETIREMENT COMMUNITIES

Relevant Issues: Demographics, economics, family, recreation

Significance: Retirement communities are a relatively new alternative for older citizens, who now can live in an age-segregated environment while receiving a varying range of services.

Some people have described retirement communities as halfway stations between preretirement residences and nursing homes, but formal definitions of these communities are as varied as the services they provide. Retirement communities differ greatly in terms of their physical characteristics, organization, amenities and recreation opportunities, fee structure, and other aspects.

VARIETY

The breakdown of retirement communities into categories often includes retirement towns and villages, retirement subdivisions, retirement residences, and continuing care retirement communities (CCRCs). The type of ownership also can be used as a basis for classification. Some are owned by residents and others rented by residents. In one hybrid form, residents buy their dwellings, but ownership reverts back to the corporate owner upon their death.

Many of these settlements have developed an autonomous community life, but others depend to varying degrees on the services of the outside community. A retirement community may take the form of a service-oriented mobile home park, a series of detached residences, or a high-rise public housing project, or even extend to an entire leisure community or a full-service continuing care retirement community.

Services provided may include housing, housekeeping services, recreation, therapy, sit-down meals (including those for special diets), social services, transportation, storage, parking, and, most important, medical care if necessary. In the more modest communities, the services may be limited to housing and one or two meals a day served cafeteria-style. Fees would be correspondingly lower. In CCRCs, there is often an entrance fee, part of which may be refundable upon the resident's relocation or demise (payable to the estate), in addition to the customary, usually high, monthly fee. Some of the newer CCRCs are based on the concept of owner equity, somewhat like a cooperative or condominium. In short, the variety is impressive.

The numbers are impressive as well. In 2018 there were around 2,000 CCRCs in the United States. Unlike nursing home patients, members of retirement communities are expected to be in fairly good health and sufficiently active to participate in community events. Communities offer a variety of programming for residents. A typical week's activities at one community that emphasizes an active social life for residents include such organized events as church services, exercise classes, bingo, cinema, barbecues, ice cream socials, piano instruction, sing-alongs, crafts classes, baking instruction, lunch out, social night, and shopping and banking expeditions. Clubs might be organized around activities, such as a walking club to combine socialization with exercise.

ORIGINS

Although California had a statute as early as 1939, most of the other states that regulate retirement communities at all enacted their legislation between 1975 and 1986. Existing statutes vary widely in purpose, coverage, certification or registration requirements, disclosure provisions, contract content, and enforcement agencies (if any).

Retirement communities started as real estate developments planned somewhat offhandedly by public and private sponsors for an elderly clientele. Sponsors have included government agencies, fraternal lodges, labor unions, religious groups, voluntary associations, and real estate developers. In some way or another, the above were responding to the expressed desire of some older people to live with others of similar age and stage of life, often in warmer climates such as those of Florida and California. The mobility of older citizens in the automobile age, their willingness to relocate, and their desire to live in a special age-segregated environment also help to explain the acceptance and spectacular growth of these communities.

Subsequently, retirement communities were established in northern states—for example, New Jersey and Pennsylvania—as well as in Canada (where they are usually smaller than in the United States but otherwise do not differ in any systematic way). Retirement communities arose in these locations because some older adults preferred to remain in familiar surroundings.

PROS AND CONS

Criticisms of retirement communities, where they occur, are principally focused on the fact that the relatively homogeneous age groups—and often racial, social, religious, and income groups—create an artificial environment. Anthropologist Margaret Mead characterized retirement communities as "golden ghettos" untypical of the natural world. Other critics have stressed the stultifying atmosphere that a group of bored or listless senior citizens leading a hedonistic life in pursuit of happiness can generate. Most observers, however, view a retirement community as a unique opportunity to remain physically and socially active and to be relieved of many household responsibilities.

Other reasons for the success and growth of these communities are the increasing pool of elderly in both the United States and Canada, their longer life expectancy, and their better financial standing, which makes retirement facilities more affordable. The latter is a result of increased government Social Security and Medicare payments, as well as the increasing prevalence and benefits of pension plans and personal retirement savings options. The elderly of the late twentieth century will be among the last Americans to be able to rely to any significant degree on pensions for their retirement, but the elderly of the future have been warned, and many are saving to pay for a comfortable retirement.

RELATIONSHIPS

The tradition of elderly parents moving in with their children or even grandchildren upon retirement or when they become unable to care for themselves is no longer as strong. There may be other "push" factors encouraging the growth of retirement communities, such as the deterioration of older adults' earlier residential neighborhoods, the loss of their friends through relocation or death, or even an excessive number of children in their vicinity. Finally, developers have found the establishment of such communities—especially at the upper end of the scale—very lucrative.

Various polls and anecdotal reports suggest that retirement community residents tend to be satisfied with them, especially because of the socializing possibilities such congregate living affords. Malcontents tend to compare the services of staff unfavorably with the personalized touch of family members. In addition, sometimes the type of retirement community selected may not be tailored to meet the needs and desires of particular residents.

Staff often fulfill a surrogate family role, as do other residents and peers, through socializing and support. Family assistance, support, or merely presence often is unavailable because of estranged relations, lack of sustained contact with family over many years, distance, or simply personal preference. With loners excepted, those who are thus unattached must rely on on-site support systems. Even when the younger family members live nearby, the prevalence of working couples makes it difficult for the younger set to care for older relatives.

A CASE STUDY

Pine Woods Villa is an adult home community in central Florida covering some three hundred acres of land. The site was purchased by an insurance company in 1972 because of its mild climate, rolling hills, woodlands, waterways, and isolation from congested areas. The community was deliberately planned to be relatively small to maximize a friendly village atmosphere.

A sixteen-hundred-seat auditorium in the clubhouse is the hub of social and recreational life. The facility has covered shuffleboard courts, a swimming pool, saunas, whirlpools, and a marina with access to a lake for boating and fishing. Other activities take place in smaller meeting rooms. The retirement community has a closed-circuit television system, cable television, paved and lighted streets, an around-the-clock security system and security gate, and a call-button system linking residents to security for emergencies.

A residents' cooperative association board of directors is responsible for overall policy and financial arrangements. A general manager has day-to-day responsibility for the community and for the paid staff, including a recreation director. In the course of its life cycle, new and younger residents move in as some older settlers move out or die, thus helping to energize the facility and take over voluntary leadership roles. Other types of retirement communities with older clienteles would tend to focus more on health services rather than recreation, or at least on those activities that require less physical exertion.

—*Peter B. Heller*

See also: Facility and institutional care; Friendship; Home ownership; Housing; Laguna Woods, California; Leisure activities; Relocation; Retirement; Retirement planning; Senior citizen centers; Social ties

For Further Information
Alvarez, Ruth. *Find the Right CCRC for Yourself or a Loved One*. 3rd ed. CreateSpace, 2013. Learn how to get family members to move into a CCRC, what to look for when you tour assisted living and nursing facilities, and what accreditations and certifications are important and which aren't.

Breeding, Brad C. *What's the Deal with Retirement Communities?* 2nd ed. People Tested Publications, 2017. Based specifically on popular questions that Breeding has received from older Americans and their adult children, this newly updated and enhanced edition is designed to be the first step in the research process, providing answers in a simple and concise fashion.

"How to Find a Retirement Community: Choosing the Best Community." SeniorLiving.org, 16 Aug. 2018. www.seniorliving.org/retirement/best/. Advice on how to choose the right retirement community for you.

Reisenwitz, Timothy H. "Exploring Senior Living Alternatives to Institutional Care: Differences between Residents and Non-Residents." *Global Business Review*, vol. 18, 2017. doi:10.1177/0972150917693153. This study focused on a particular CCRC and examined the differences between two groups: CCRC residents and non-residents, that is, those who considered CCRC residency but decided against it.

Weinstock, J, and L. Bond. "High Quality of Life in Continuing Care Retirement Communities: A Balancing Act." *Innovation in Aging*, vol. 2, iss. Suppl._1, Nov. 2018, p. 474. doi:10.1093/geroni/igy023.1770. An in-depth qualitative case study of a 321-resident nonprofit life care CCRC to determine how residents themselves define components of quality of life, practices to improve quality of life, and challenges of promoting quality of life in congregated housing.

RETIREMENT PLANNING

Relevant Issues: Economics, psychology, work

Significance: Retirement planning is essential to people throughout life if they are to enjoy their retirement years.

Retirement is a time requiring many significant changes in the life of the individual. At retirement, the individual suddenly has more time on his or her hands, fewer commitments, more time for other people, and a change in level of income. One who plans ahead for retirement generally will have an easier time accomplishing these transitions successfully. Preretirement planning is considered one of the major developmental tasks of middle age according to Robert J. Havighurst's theory of development. In reality, to be prepared adequately for retirement, one needs to begin planning by young adulthood.

FINANCIAL PLANNING

An individual facing retirement must first make a decision about when to retire. This decision has been heavily influenced by changing life expectancies. With life expectancies reaching nearly seventy-seven years and increasing, people realize that they will probably be alive for many years after retirement and need money to live on for quite some time. The age at which one will be able to collect Social Security is also a factor influencing retirement. People born prior to 1938 can collect full benefits at sixty-five, while those born after 1960 must wait until sixty-seven. The existence of private pension plans (if any) will also influence the timing of retirement and the socioeconomic status afterward.

It has been estimated that to be financially secure at retirement, an individual must have at least two-thirds of his or her preretirement income (with three-quarters of prior income giving one a more comfortable margin). To decide precisely what people will need, they should estimate the number of years that they will probably be retired, the style of living that they would like during those retirement years, and the rate of inflation likely between now and retirement. The earlier one starts saving, the more time money has to grow. A twenty-two-year-old who sets aside $50 per month will have approximately $319,000 at the age of sixty-two (with a 10 percent annual return). By waiting ten years until he or she is thirty-two, that individual will have to invest approximately $140 per month to reach that same goal.

Clearly, one needs to begin saving early in life. In planning for retirement, one needs to take into account Social Security and employer pension plans, as well as individual savings for retirement. Annual deposits into traditional or Roth individual retirement accounts (IRAs) or 401K plans are highly beneficial to the individual. Many families today are creating "kindergarten capitalists," investing for their children to better secure their futures.

MEDICAL AND LEGAL PLANNING

No matter how well one plans financially for retirement, there are certain expenditures that one cannot foresee. Most typically, these are medical expenses. While most retired elderly have Medicare health coverage, this does not include coverage for eyeglasses, hearing aids, dental work, or prescriptions. These expenses pose a large financial burden for the retired person, but may still be manageable. When one is hit with a long-term or catastrophic situation, medical expenses mount dramatically, often wiping out retirement savings and any legacy for one's survivors. To avoid this situation, in preretirement planning one might acquire long-term care insurance to cover catastrophic medical expenses. Approximately 70 percent of couples over the age of sixty-five can expect one spouse to require long-term care.

Aside from financial concerns associated with medical conditions, people should have very real concerns about how they will be treated medically in the future if they are unable to make decisions for themselves. The existence of advanced directives should allow people to make their desires known, as well as appoint an agent to make these decisions if so desired. By creating a living will or durable power of attorney for health care, all adults can ensure that their medical treatment will be consistent with their wishes. This is one very important part of planning (like financial planning) that is best dealt with initially by early adulthood.

PLANNING A NEW LIFE

Planning for retirement includes planning ways to make life pleasant and productive. As such, this includes planning where one wants to live both in terms of locale and type of housing. In recent years, large numbers of retirement living options have come to exist. Prior to deciding on the type of housing desired, one needs to decide to which area he or she would like to retire. This decision should be based on a familiarity with the area (including actual time spent there), as well as research into such areas as the cost of living, opportunities available including part-time jobs, volunteering, and leisure activities, and the existence of programs designed specifically for the elderly. By engaging in appropriate research, in the years prior to retirement, the individual or couple can make decisions confidently about which options best suit their desired lifestyle. Much of this research can be conducted on the Internet; information is available on a large number of housing options.

People can plan to remain in their own homes, move to smaller houses that are easier to care for and provide them with additional financial resources, or move to condominiums, retirement communities, senior high rises, or assisted-living situations. Consideration of many different housing alternatives while planning for retirement should leave one ready to initiate changes upon retirement. When an individual or couple has decided on a type of housing and an area for retirement, they would do well to actually "try it out" rather than moving permanently. This trial move can be accomplished at the very beginning of retirement (since most people do not have the flexibility to do this while still working).

People would begin by subletting their house (rather than selling it), renting an apartment or house (rather than buying one) in their new desired location, and getting involved in the types of activities that they hope to engage in throughout retirement. By spending the first year of their retirement in this manner, they are engaging in a trial run (and still continuing to plan for a long and happy future). Too many retired individuals burn all their bridges behind them as soon as they retire, only to find out that living in an area and vacationing there are two different things entirely. After a year of living in the new "desired" situation, the individual or couple is ready to make this commitment permanent or go back to their previous way of life (which they can easily do since they have not made any permanent changes). In so doing, they are able to determine that they do have enough money to live on, a liking of the area in which they have settled, satisfaction with their housing situation, enjoyment of the leisure, volunteer, and work opportunities available, and adequate social support systems available to them.

Middle-aged adults should consider the social lifestyle changes that they will face in retirement. Typically, one will spend a lot more time with one's spouse or significant other than while working. This relationship is likely to be more pleasant if the middle-aged couple deliberately plans to spend time alone together (to "date"), concentrating on one another (talking, holding hands, reminiscing) and continually planning their future together.

The other consideration that requires planning is adaptation to a relatively unstructured day. The individual is no longer faced with a routine. One must think about and plan for activities to fill the gap left by loss of career at retirement. By planning in young adulthood or middle age, individuals can uncover and develop hobbies or hidden talents into which they can channel time and energy in retirement.

CONCLUSION

Retirement is a period involving many major adaptations to a changing lifestyle. These adaptations and transitions occur most smoothly when they have been planned for ahead of time. Planning should include all the following areas: financial, legal, medical, social, housing, and activities. A person who plans accordingly can then look forward to the "golden years" of retirement.

—*Robin Kamienny Montvilo*

See also: Durable power of attorney; Early retirement; Employment; Estates and inheritance; 401(k) plans; Health insurance; Home ownership; Housing; Individual retirement accounts (IRAs); Leisure activities; Life insurance; Living wills; Long-term care; Mandatory retirement; Relocation; Retirement; Retirement communities; Social Security; Social ties; Trusts; Wills and bequests

For Further Information

Hinden, Stan. *How to Retire Happy: The 12 Most Important Decisions You Must Make before You Retire.* 4th ed. McGraw-Hill, 2013. This book delivers all the expert advice needed to ensure a happy, healthy retirement in an easy-to-understand step-by-step style.

Merton, Robert C. "The Crisis in Retirement Planning." *Harvard Business Review*, 19 May 2015. hbr.org/2014/07/the-crisis-in-retirement-planning. In this article, Merton explains a liability-driven investment strategy whose aim is to improve the probability of achieving a desired retirement income rather than to maximize the capital value of the savings.

Quinn, Jane Bryant. *How to Make Your Money Last: The Indispensable Retirement Guide.* Simon & Schuster Paperbacks, 2017. With this book, financial expert Quinn explains how to turn retirement funds into a paycheck that will last for life.

Topa, Gabriela, et al. "Financial Planning for Retirement: A Psychosocial Perspective." *Frontiers in Psychology*, vol. 8, 2018. doi:10.3389/fpsyg.2017.02338.

RHINOPHYMA

Relevant Issues: Biology, health and medicine

Significance: Rhinophyma, a complication of rosacea, is a benign skin disorder characterized by thickening of the skin associated with increased volume and bulbous nose.

Rosacea is a common skin condition that causes redness of the face associated with visible blood vessels, papules and small pustules. It affects more than 16 million Americans and is more common in middle-aged women, but is more severe in men. This condition is commonly misdiagnosed as acne vulgaris, seborrheic dermatitis, perioral dermatitis and lupus.

In the fourteenth century rosacea was attributed to excessive consumption of alcoholic drinks. Although alcohol may exacerbate the condition, rosacea can develop in individuals who have never consumed alcohol. Whereas the actual cause is unknown, rosacea is more common in fair-skinned people who flush easily. The most common triggers are alcohol, hot foods or drinks, caffeine, spicy foods, stress, vigorous exercise, sunlight, and extreme heat or cold. There is no cure for rosacea, but it can be treated with oral and topical antibiotics and avoidance of triggers.

Untreated, rosacea may get worse and lead to permanent damage. It may progress to slight facial swelling, pimples, pustules, and prominent facial pores on the nose, forehead, cheeks and chin. Approximately 50 percent of the people affected by rosacea may also develop eye problems like pain, swelling, redness and abnormal vision.

Rosacea can lead to rhinophyma, a slowly progressive skin condition and rare complication from long-standing untreated rosacea that particularly occurs in men. As the oil glands enlarge it may cause a bulbous, enlarged red nose, along with puffy and occasionally thick bumps on the lower half of the nose and nearby cheeks.

Rhinophyma can be extremely disfiguring, and its mistaken association with alcoholism can cause embarrassment and affect self-esteem. However, alcohol can increase flushing in individuals with the condition. Like rosacea, the exact cause of rhinophyma is unknown and the condition cannot be cured, but the symptoms can be lessened or even eliminated. Diagnosis is clinical but it can be confirmed trough a skin biopsy. Rhinophyma is usually treated with surgery, laser or medications.

Isotretinoin, topical and oral antibiotics along with azelaic acid may be used to decrease inflammation. The excess tissue that has developed can be removed by sharp excision with a scalpel, cryosurgery, electrosurgery, dermabrasion and carbon dioxide laser therapy.

—Lisa M. Sardinia
Updated by Ecler Jaqua, MD and
Miriam E. Schwartz, MD, PhD

See also: Beauty; Skin changes and disorders

For Further Information

Fink, Caitlin, et al. "Rhinophyma: A Treatment Review." *Dermatologic Surgery*, vol. 44, no. 2, 2018, pp. 275-82. doi:10.1097/dss.0000000000001406. Describes treatment options for rhinophyma and their respective risks and benefits.

Krausz, Aimee E., et al. "Procedural Management of Rhinophyma: A Comprehensive Review." *Journal of Cosmetic Dermatology*, vol. 17, no. 6, 2018, pp. 960-67. doi:10.1111/jocd.12770. Reviews the spectrum of procedural techniques for treatment of rhinophyma with a focus on the advantages and disadvantages of each modality.

Zuuren, Esther J. Van. "Rosacea." *New England Journal of Medicine*, vol. 377, no. 18, 2017, pp. 1754-64. doi:10.1056/nejmcp1506630. General information on rosacea, including signs and symptoms and treatment options.

González, L.F., et al. "Electrosurgery for the Treatment of Moderate or Severe 4. Rhinophyma." *ActasDermo-Sifiliográficas* (English Edition), vol. 109, no. 4, 2018. doi:10.1016/j.adengl.2018.03.002. Describes a series of cases of moderate or severe rhinophyma treated with high-frequency electrosurgery in the dermatology department of Hospital Simón Bolivar and in private clinics in Bogota, Colombia, between 2012 and 2016.

Hassanein, Aladdin H., et al. "Management of Rhinophyma." *Journal of Craniofacial Surgery*, vol. 28, no. 3, 2017. doi:10.1097/scs.0000000000003467. Reviews medical records of patients with rhinophyma treated with the subunit method between 2013 and 2016.

ROBIN AND MARIAN (FILM)

Director: Richard Lester
Cast: Sean Connery, Audrey Hepburn, Robert Shaw, Ian Holm, Nicol Williamson, Richard Harris
Date: Released in 1976
Relevant Issues: Culture, media, psychology, values

Significance: This film explores the response of the aging hero and heroine whose powers fade, making it impossible for them to repeat the famous feats of their youth.

Upon the death of King Richard (Richard Harris), Robin Hood (Sean Connery) returns, having served in the Crusades and other wars for twenty years. He goes to Sherwood Forest, where he lived as an outlaw during the struggle against King John (Ian Holm) and the sheriff of Nottingham (Robert Shaw, in a marvelous, humane performance). Many of his band have died or given up the outlaw life. Marian (Audrey Hepburn), with whom he is still in love, has become the abbess of a nunnery.

Marian does not wish to leave the religious life, but Robin's love combines with the new king's machinations against the Church to bring them together again. They live in Sherwood as lovers and as leaders of the fight against royal power. Robin is now in his forties, however; he is battle-scarred and stiff. The adventures that follow show that he no longer has the endurance and strength of his youth. Despite his age, he defeats the sheriff of Nottingham in single combat, though he is wounded. Marian and Robin's friend Little John (Nicol Williamson) help him to the nunnery. Robin has not observed that the royal troops, violating Nottingham's order to withdraw should Nottingham be defeated, have destroyed the uprising.

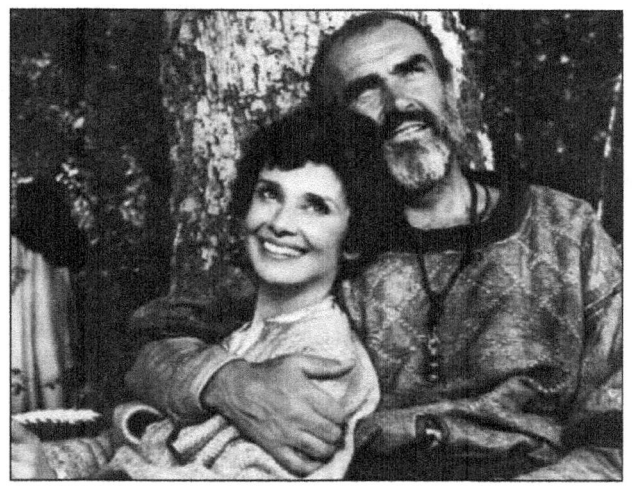

Audrey Hepburn and Sean Connery as Marian and Robin, respectively. (via Wikimedia Commons)

Marian prepares "medicine" that she and Robin both take. She has poisoned them both to protect them from the ravages of age and the destruction of the bright legend that was Robin Hood. When Robin realizes what she has done he says, "I'd never have a day like this again, would I? It's better this way." He asks Little John to bury them both where his last arrow falls in the forest.

Robin and Marian is a subtle and moving examination of the response to the failing of one's powers with age.

—*Robert Jacobs*

See also: Middle age; Suicide

"ROMAN FEVER" (SHORT STORY)

Author: Edith Wharton
Date: Published in 1936
Relevant Issues: Family, marriage and dating
Significance: This short story explores bitterness over sexual rivalry that lasts decades, continuing even after the loved one's death.

Edith Wharton's "Roman Fever" tells the story of two lifelong acquaintances who loved the same man, now deceased. He became the husband of one and, as revealed in a surprise ending, the father of the child of the other. Mrs. Delphin (Alida) Slade and Mrs. Horace (Grace) Ansley, "two American ladies of ripe but well-cared-for middle age," meet in Rome while each is traveling with her daughter. The daughters, like their mothers a generation ago, are seeking romance and marriage.

As the two older women while away the afternoon sitting on a terrace overlooking the Palatine and the Forum, the reader learns that Alida Slade harbors a resentment against Grace Ansley, who had been her girlhood acquaintance and then her New York neighbor for many years. Mrs. Slade is proud of her status as the widow of a brilliant lawyer, but holds a grudge against the other woman for having been a competitor for her husband's hand in those far-off years. Her sense of unease is aggravated by the fact that Mrs. Ansley's daughter is more brilliant than her own.

Mrs. Slade gradually reveals that before her engagement to Delphin, she had used the ruse of writing a letter to Grace inviting her, in the name of her lover, to meet him at the Coliseum, hoping that Grace would catch a chill (the "Roman fever" of the title) and be out of commission for some weeks so that Alida could cement her relationship with Delphin. Grace reveals that she kept the rendezvous—and that Delphin had met her, she having answered the letter. Alida's sense of superiority is dashed, and her wish to hurt the other woman is turned back on herself when Grace reveals that the rendezvous produced a child, the brilliant young woman with whom Alida's own daughter compares unfavorably.

—*Charlotte Templin*

See also: Marriage; Middle age; Widows and widowers; Women and aging

SANDWICH GENERATION

Relevant Issues: Demographics, family
Significance: As longevity has increased in late twentieth century North America, adults have been increasingly obliged to care for two generations, their parents and children, contributing to the growth of the sandwich generation.

People are living longer and having fewer children. This has changed the age composition of the North American population. The "graying" of the population is a major factor contributing to the growing number of sandwich generation families. The expanding proportion of older persons is bringing with it dramatic changes in family structure. People are giving more thought to the nature and extent of services necessary to support older persons and to their views on the respective roles of family and society in providing for these needs.

CARING FOR TWO GENERATIONS

As persons live longer, the aged have a greater need for assistance from their families. The term "sandwich generation," coined in 1981 by Dorothy Miller, MSW, refers to adults who provide financial or task assistance to their parents while also caring for their own dependent children. Adults may assist their parents by providing them with emotional support, financial assistance, transportation, shopping and cleaning, meal preparation, and personal hygiene. At the same time, they may assist their children financially and emotionally and even care for grandchildren. Members of the sandwich generation serve as a support system for both their aging parents and their dependent children. They are "sandwiched" between the needs of two generations, balancing the needs of their children, the needs of their parents, and their own needs, obligations, and ambitions in the home and workplace.

With longer life spans and later childbearing, more middle-aged persons find themselves sandwiched between providing child and elder care. Estimates of the percentage of sandwiched persons vary widely. In 1986, the huge corporation IBM reported that 6.3 percent of its employees were responsible for both their children and parents. By 1991, this figure had risen to 11 percent. In 2013 Pew Research reported that 47 percent of adults in their 40s and 50s have at least one parent over 65 years old while rearing a child under 18 years or financially supporting a grown child. Regardless of the actual percentage, experts agree that the twenty-first century will see even greater numbers of sandwiched persons.

FINANCIAL RESPONSIBILITIES OF SANDWICHED FAMILIES

The financial choices facing sandwiched families are challenging. Even if parents are healthy, sandwiched persons still have to juggle between parents' eventual needs and their responsibilities to their children. Compromises are inevitable. The parents of sandwiched persons may require more financial support than the children of sandwiched persons. Sandwiched families that do not have the financial resources to help parents may bring their parents into their communities or households or offer them nonmonetary assistance.

With limited national financial resources available to older adults in the United States the U.S. government is quick to stress the financial responsibility of families for the health care and other needs of aged family members. Proposed reforms may include increased community-based supportive services and mandated assistance from families. Regardless of the outcome, the growing message has been that families must bear responsibility for aged parents and children. In the United States, this may result in nursing homes for the very rich or the totally destitute, leaving most elderly people in the care of their families.

HELPING CHILDREN

One trend contributing to the financial burden on the sandwich generation is the prolonged financial dependence of children. In 1990, 23 percent of the U.S. population between the ages of twenty-five and thirty-four lived with their parents—an increase of 45 percent since 1970. A combination of attitudes, economics, and demographics underlies this phenomenon. Adult children have begun to marry and establish their careers later in life. In a 1990 Newsweek special issue on "Families in the Twenty-first Century," one article stated that American youth, in a sharp reversal of historical trends, were taking longer to mature. Although more young people were enrolled in college than previously, fewer graduated and many took longer to get their degrees.

Some researchers have blamed the economy for the prolonged dependency of young adults on their parents. In the 1990s, the younger half of the baby-boom generation—that is, adults in their mid-twenties to mid-thirties—seemed to have taken the brunt of economic downturns. Many young adults joined the labor force at a time of stagnant wage growth and have been trapped in a rental market that has seen apartment rents increase at double the inflation rate since 1970. Higher rents have meant that the adults in this age group have been less able than older age cohorts to save for down payments on homes. Unable or unwilling to establish their own households, many young adults have lived longer with their parents. Another stress on young adults is student debt which could explain part of the return to parents' homes. The phenomenon of adult children leaving home and returning several times for brief periods because of economic difficulties or changes in marital status has been called the boomerang effect. Even in 2014, after the job market eased up, nearly 15 percent of 25 to 34 year old young adults still lived with their parents.

HELPING PARENTS

It is believed that one out of six parents or spouses aged sixty-five or older will require some form of assistance—either from their children or other sources. Daughters and daughters-in-law provide care more often than sons. In the United States, the average sandwiched caregiver in the late 1990s was a woman in her forties with a family income of less than $40,000. Parents most frequently required assistance with shopping, transportation, and household chores, such as meal preparation, housecleaning, and laundry. More daughters (69 percent) than sons (59 percent) assisted their parents with personal functions such as eating, toileting, and dressing. Often daughters have helped their parents to use the telephone, make visits, and perform household tasks.

Overall, caregiving daughters have spent an average of 4.0 hours per day and sons 3.5 hours per day on caregiving tasks. Yet, sons have been more likely than daughters to help parents financially in writing checks, paying bills, and assisting in the preparation of income tax returns. Sons have also helped more often than daughters with home maintenance. As aging persons have fewer adult children and perhaps no daughters, sons may be required to provide help with a wider variety of tasks than has previously been the case.

Today's sandwich generation caregivers are ages 40-59 years old although 19 percent are under 40 and 10 percent are over 60. Daughters typically give 12.3 hours of care per month while sons provide 5.6. One-third of all women above the age of eighteen will care for both children and parents during their lifetimes. Many will spend more years helping a parent than in raising their own children. Women's roles as caregivers remain entrenched in the expectations of society and individual families. Caregiving tasks are often viewed as the responsibility of females. Women are the most likely to have little intergenerational support during their middle years. This phenomenon is called the "generational squeeze," because women in the middle generation give significantly more support than they receive.

THE EFFECTS ON WORK

The 1982 Informal Caregivers Survey revealed that 44 percent of caregiving daughters and 55 percent of caregiving sons were in the workforce. Within these two groups, about 25 percent of working daughters and sons reported conflicts between work and caregiving responsibilities. For many, the conflict forced them to cut back on work hours, change their work schedules, or take time off from work without pay. The strains on women have shown up at the workplace. Of caregivers to the elderly, most of whom are women, some 33 percent decreased work hours, 22 percent switched from full-time to part-time jobs, 29 percent have passed up promotions or opportunities for advancement another 28 percent considered quitting their jobs, and 13 percent left the workforce because of caregiving responsibilities.

LOOKING TO THE FUTURE

Longer life spans will continue to put more middle-aged and older family members in the position of providing care to elderly relatives. The chances are increasing that a retired person will also have a living parent who needs care. As a result, care for the disabled elderly may increasingly fall on those who are old themselves.

What the future holds in store for sandwiched persons is an open question. Intergenerational support and cooperation will be more critical. Older persons may help younger relatives with child care when they are able, and as they age, the persons whom they help may provide reciprocal care for them. Parents will probably rely more on friends and volunteers because fewer family members will be able to provide assistance. Communities may need to provide more services to support the independence of older persons when families cannot provide support. With families, friends, and communities working together to balance their needs, older persons will be able to live with dignity, and their younger relatives will be able to meet the demands of their own busy lives.

—*Virginia W. Junk*
Updated by Marylane Wade Koch, MSN, RN

See also: Baby boomers; Caregiver absenteeism; Caregiving; Children of Aging Parents; Death of parents; Employment; Family relationships; Filial responsibility; Full nest; Grandparenthood; Greatgrandparenthood; Middle age; Midlife crisis; Parenthood; Women and aging

For Further Information

Caregiver Statistics: Demographics, Family Caregiver Alliance, National Center on Caregiving. www.caregiver.org/caregiver-statistics-demographics Extensive demographic information on caregivers from the Family Caregiver Alliance (FCA), whose mission is to improve the quality of life for family caregivers and the people who receive their care.

Drake, Bruce. "The Sandwich Generation: Burdens on Middle Aged Americas on the Rise." Pew Research FactTank. 15 May 2013. www.pewresearch.org/fact-tank/2013/05/15/the-sandwich-generation-burdens-on-middle-aged-americans-on-the-rise/. Provides statistics from the 2012 Pew Research survey and highlights the increase in financial and other responsibilities for aging parents and children.

Goyer, Amy. "Five Tips for Sandwiched Caregivers: Ways to Find Balance in a Life with Competing Demands," AARP, 18 July 2016. www.aarp.org/caregiving/life-balance/info-2017/sandwich-generation-tips-ag.html. Offers tips to caregivers of the sandwich generation to manage their stress.

Lemonick, Michael D. "Women Give Way More Elder Care to Aging Parents Than Men" Time.com, 22 Aug. 2014. time.com/3153490/women-aging-parents-better-than-men/. Research study presented at American Sociological Association reveals the gender gap in giving elder care.

Parker, Kim, and Eileen Patten. "The Sandwich Generation: Rising Financial Burdens for Middle-Aged Americans." *Pew Research: Social and Demographic Trends*, 30 Jan. 2013. www.pewsocialtrends.org/2013/01/30/the-sandwich-generation/ Provides insights and statistics into the changing lifestyle and financial burden for middle-aged Americans with care responsibilities for both aging parents and children.

Seagull, Elizabeth A. "Coping with Adult Children Returning Home: A Value Driven Framework" *Michigan Family Review*, vol. 04, iss. 1, Summer 1999, pp. 27-36. quod.lib.umich.edu/m/mfr/4919087.0004.104?view=text;rgn=main. Suggests that when adult children move back parents and children should establish values such as honesty, respect, and courtesy when sharing space and resources.

Tarantine, Dorothy. "The Sandwich Generation: Who's Caring for You?" *HuffPost*, 7 Sept. 2014. www.huffpost.com/entry/baby-boomers-caregivers_b_5733782. Sheds new light on the challenges of the sandwich generation caregivers of today and questions who is caring for these caregivers.

SARCOPENIA

Relevant Issues: Biology, health and medicine

Significance: Reduction in muscle mass with aging that is associated with weakness, decreased physiological functioning, and decreased physical activity, which can result in functional impairment, disability, loss of independence, and increased risk of fall-related fractures.

Key Terms:

Dual Energy X-ray Absorptiometry (DEXA scan): is used to measure skeletal mass and bone density.

Bioelectrical Impedance Analysis (BIA): estimates total body muscle and water composition by measuring resistance to electrical flow.

anthropometry: is the study of human body measurements. Measures the body weight, height, subscapular skinfold, triceps skinfold, mid arm muscle circumference, elbow breadth, abdominal circumference and calf circumference.

handgrip strength: measures the muscular strength in the hands and forearm.

Short Physical Performance Battery (SPPB): evaluates lower extremity function in older adults.

usual gait speed: measures the walking speed on normal pace for a determined distance (usually 10-8 feet).

get-up-and-go test: measures the time a person takes to rise from a chair, walk 10 feet, turn around, walk back to the chair, and sit down.

In 1989, Irwin Rosenberg suggested the term sarcopenia (Greek sarx "flesh"; penia "loss") to describe an age-related loss of muscle mass (also known as lean body mass or fat-free mass). This is differentiated from the general terms "wasting," which refers to the unintentional loss of weight attributable to a loss of both fat and muscle mass from insufficient caloric intake, and "cachexia," which refers to the loss of muscle mass without weight loss as a result of an overactive metabolism. Therefore, the term "sarcopenia" is often used to describe muscle wasting in old age.

PREVALENCE

The extent of sarcopenia in the aged population suggests that about 5-13 percent of persons between 60 to 70 years old are afflicted with this syndrome, whereas 50 percent of those aged 80 years old or more are likely to be affected. Usually after 50 years of age, muscle mass may decline at a rate of 1-2 percent annually. Muscle strength also can decrease by 1.5 percent in adults between 50 to 60 years of age and by 3 percent after 60 years old.

Beginning in the seventh decade of life, approximately 25 percent of people report difficulty in walking and carrying heavy packages. Those older than 70 years of age report decreased ability to carry out common daily activities such as going down stairs or performing housework, and some even have difficulty using the toilet without assistance. These self-reported difficulties in functional ability occur regardless of gender, ethnicity, income, or other health behaviors.

The combination of inadequate dietary intake combined with decreased strength from declining muscle mass results in a progressive decline in physical activity and accelerates muscle atrophy, or shrinkage, as a result of disuse. This condition adversely affects functional mobility, as evidenced by slower walking speeds, shorter walking strides, and a decrease in the amount of work a muscle can tolerate.

ETIOLOGY

The skeletal muscle is fundamental to generate movements and maintain stability. It also stores great quantities of protein for the body. Therefore, when the muscle protein is reduced, this may result in decline of muscle mass. The protein content is determined by assessing the balance between protein synthesis and protein breakdown. With aging, protein synthesis slows, thereby resulting in decreased muscle synthesis. This can be aggravated by poor nutritional status, low caloric and low protein intake.

Nutritional surveys have reported that individuals over age 65 consume an average of 1,400 Calories (kilocalories) a day, or less than 25 Calories per kilogram of body weight (1 kilogram = 2.2 pounds; 1 pound = 3,500 Calories). This average daily caloric intake of 1,400 Calories is approximately 500 Calories less from what is recommended for optimal health for sedentary individuals over 50 years of age. Usually women need fewer calories than men (1,600 versus 2,000 Calories per day respectively) and this number increases when both men and women are more active (2,200 versus 1,800 Calories respectively). Thus, based upon the average energy allowance recommendations, older adults should be consuming 5 Calories more for every kilogram of their body weight if they are to meet or exceed the current U.S. recommended daily allowances (RDAs) for caloric intake and optimal health. Lower caloric intakes imply lower nutritional status: less fat, carbohydrate, and/or protein consumption, potentially leading to nutritional deficiencies in important vitamins and minerals.

The current nutritional guidelines also suggest that adults in the United States only need 0.8 grams of protein per kilogram of body weight daily or 0.36 grams per pound; however, some researchers contend that this value is based primarily on the needs of young adults, not older adults. Based on data that showed that many adults over the age of 60 consume less than 0.8 grams per body weight daily, researchers from several studies suggested that healthy older adults should consume between 1.0 and 1.2 grams of high-quality protein per kilogram of body weight daily. It is also suggested that older adults with acute or chronic illnesses should consume 1.2 to 1.5 grams of protein per kilogram of body weight daily; however it depends on the medical illness, the severity and other factors. This would potentially help to prevent the compensatory loss in muscle mass resulting from long-term deficits in dietary protein intake.

The negative age-related changes in body composition are reflected in decreased muscle, bone density, and water content of the body, with a corresponding increase in body fat. Muscle tissue plays an important role in the regulation of metabolic rate (the burning of calories). It is generally agreed that muscle mass is maintained up to about age 40 and by 80 years of age, regardless of gender, the cumulative muscle mass loss is estimated to average 30 percent with a corresponding decline in muscle strength. Beginning in the third decade of life, metabolic rate, or the rate at which calories are burned by the body, decreases 2 percent to 3 percent per decade. Taken together, the loss in muscle tissue and the decrease in metabolic rate results in a gradual percent body fat increase from the second through the eighth decades of life, resulting in a net percent body fat gain of 20 percent for men and 10 percent for women. Hence, as muscle tissue atrophies, the unused "leftover" space is replaced by fat tissue, which is not used to perform muscular work.

Cross-sectional studies comparing athletes to sedentary controls, as well as studies with non-athletes, suggest that large muscle mass is predictive of higher bone mass. Thus, age-related sarcopenia and osteopenia (loss of bone) may be related. Research suggests that age-related changes in the dynamics of muscular contractions might contribute to bone remodeling imbalances, resulting in bone loss. The loss of motor units, activation, and synchronization of these units not only impairs bone integrity but also contributes to the loss of strength that accompanies muscle mass loss. Muscle strength is the ability to generate a maximal force by a muscle group. This strength is determined not only by total muscle mass but also by the individual muscle fibers. When muscle mass atrophies with aging, there is a decrease in fiber size, fiber number, and selective shrinking of type II, or fast-twitch, muscle fibers. Fast-twitch fibers are responsible for anaerobic, power-type strength activities. In addition, the loss of muscle mass may contribute to the reduction in aerobic capacity as the total amount of mitochondria, the powerhouses of cells, is reduced when muscle mass is lost.

DIAGNOSIS

The diagnosis of sarcopenia is clinical, depending on the signs and symptoms patient reports. In several cases doctors may suggest further work up with specific diagnostic testing. See Table 1.

Table 1. Available diagnostic testing for sarcopenia in clinical practice

Measurement	Diagnostic tests
Muscle mass	DEXA scan BIA Anthropometry
Muscle strength	Handgrip strength
Physical performance	SPPB Usual gait speed Get-up-and-go test

PREVENTION AND TREATMENT

Research is inconclusive as to whether age-related skeletal muscle wasting is preventable.

It appears to be an inevitable part of aging. However, the rate of skeletal muscle loss may be slowed down with progressive resistance (strength) training. This type of exercise has been shown to increase muscle size and strength even in the oldest of old. If strength training is to be used as a potential preventive measure, research suggests that high-intensity training (50 to 70 percent of one's maximal strength) with low repetitions should be implemented no later than 50 years of age; after age 60, strength training is considered to be therapeutic, compensating for the age-related muscle mass wasting.

This is not to say, however, that after the age of 60 strength training should not been done. This situation is quite the contrary. Although sarcopenia may not be preventable after age 50, it has been proven that the frail elderly as well as community-dwelling healthy elderly can increase muscle mass by as much as 17 percent and maximal strength by as much as 110 percent with an aggressive strength training program. Contrary to the "moderate" exercise guidelines used for improving aerobic fitness, low-level resistance training only yields modest increases in strength and muscle mass.

Currently the basic treatment for sarcopenia consists of resistance exercises, protein supplementation, and vitamin D supplement. Unfortunately, there are no medications approved by the U.S. Food and Drug Administration (FDA). However, there are several ongoing studies about the use of potential future medications like Urocortin II, angiotensin converting enzyme inhibitors, beta antagonists, activin IIR antagonists, myostatin antibodies and fast skeletal muscle troponin activators. The use of hormone replacement therapy (e.g., estrogen, testosterone, growth hormone) may also assist in maintaining muscle protein synthesis, but is also under investigation, and should never replace resistance exercises.

—*Bonita L. Marks*
—*Updated by Ecler Jaqua, MD and Miriam E. Schwartz, MD, PhD*

See also: Aging process; Balance problems; Estrogen replacement therapy; Exercise and fitness; Fat deposition; Malnutrition; Mobility problems; Nutrition; Older adults; Weight loss and gain

For Further Information

Dhillon, Robinder J. S., and Sarfaraz, Hasni. "Pathogenesis and Management of Sarcopenia." *Clinics in Geriatric Medicine*, vol. 33, no. 1, Feb. 2017, pp. 17-26. doi:10.1016/j.cger.2016.08.002.

Juby, Angela G., and Diana R. Mager. "A Review of Nutrition Screening Tools Used to Assess the Malnutrition-Sarcopenia Syndrome (MSS) in the Older Adult." *Clinical Nutrition ESPEN*, vol. 32, 2019, pp. 8-15. doi:10.1016/j.clnesp.2019.04.003. This paper evaluates the published literature reporting data on both nutrition and sarcopenia evaluation simultaneously in the population studied, and creates a diagnostic algorithm.

Landi, Francesco, et al. "Sarcopenia: An Overview on Current Definitions, Diagnosis and Treatment." *Current Protein & Peptide Science*, vol. 19, no. 7, 2018, pp. 633-38. doi:10.2174/1389203718666170607113459.

Marty, Eric, et al. "A Review of Sarcopenia: Enhancing Awareness of an Increasingly Prevalent Disease." *Bone*, vol. 105, 2017, pp. 276-86. doi:10.1016/j.bone.2017.09.008.

Tsekoura, Maria, et al. "Sarcopenia and Its Impact on Quality of Life" In: Vlamos P. (eds) GeNeDis 2016. *Advances in Experimental Medicine and Biology, 2017*, vol. 987, pp. 213-18. Springer Cham. doi:10.1007/978-3-319-57379-3_19. Reviews sarcopenia and its impact on quality of life.

SARTON, MAY

Born: BORN: May 3, 1912; Wondelgem, Belgium
Died: July 16, 1995; York, Maine
Relevant Issues: Family, sociology, work
Significance: Sarton gained critical notice and public recognition late in life as a feminist writer and poet; she is best known for her personal journals dealing with change, creativity, and aging.

Eleanor Marie "May" Sarton was born into a cultured and artistic family. Her father, George Sarton, taught at Harvard University. May Sarton nurtured her European roots. Her mother bequeathed to her an intellectual curiosity, a love of art, and a love of nature, all of which became core aspects of Sarton's personality. The beauty of nature and the power of words are themes repeatedly reflected in her writings. Her later poetry and journals clearly mirror the insights gained over time, as she seeks solace in memories and gains wisdom through a renewed understanding of the value of change. Sarton's work is at once her legacy and her reflection upon that legacy as it unfolds.

Sarton's personal history provided both turmoil and inspiration. Her life is recorded in her poetry and prose. Read chronologically, Sarton's works reveal the fire of a young artist-writer tempered over time. The middle-aged Sarton struggles with love, acknowledges her lesbianism, and overtly struggles with inner conflicts concerning her relationships to others and to her writing. As she gains the public attention she craves, she recoils from the demands of fame and seeks solitude. Her work resounds with tension between her contemplative side and her need for attention. Sarton's novels, poetry, and journals reflect the changes brought by time and age and capture with poignant clarity her burdens and joys, the daily struggles of the artistic soul growing older in the modern world. In *Journal of a Solitude* (1973), she notes, "I have written novels to find out what I thought about something and poems to find out what I felt about something."

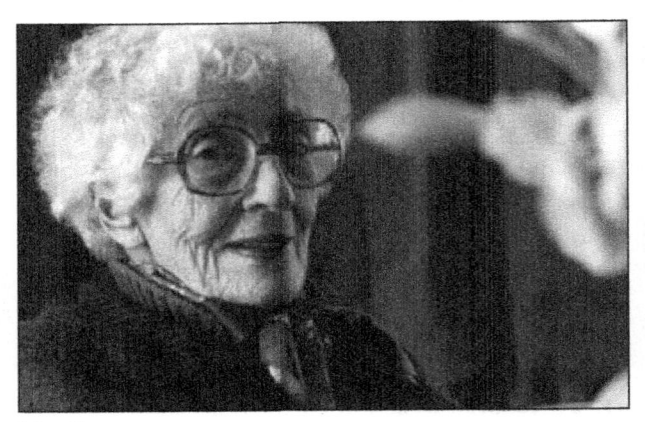

May Sarton

Sarton's novels generally reflect issues faced by independent-minded women or artistic souls in search of a muse. The protagonists of *Joanna and Ulysses* (1963) and *The Poet and the Donkey* (1969) each struggle with the artistic elements of their being in order to bring the muse to fruition, and each has the help of a donkey. Each of these books reappeared in the 1980s as Sarton's audience broadened.

Sarton's body of poetry shows the tenacity of her muse as well. *A Grain of Mustard Seed* (1981) is reflective of her lyricism, but with an edge, as Sarton, the mature poet, puts to pen the political and religious turmoil of the volatile 1960s. In *Coming into Eighty* (1994), Sarton clearly accepts the limitations of age and embraces the poetry that is the fruit of her experience. She states in the preface to the poems, "These poems are minimal because my life is reduced to essences." She notes, "I am a foreigner in the land of old age and have tried to learn its language." Sarton never lost her muse. Through her final years, she continued to write about the limitations and the freedoms that come with age. Her final work, *At Eighty-two: A Journal* (1996), was published posthumously. Sarton's work is a testament to the resilience of the creative human spirit.

—*Kathleen Schongar*

See also: Women and aging

For Further Information

Gussow, Mel. "May Sarton, Poet, Novelist and Individualist, Dies at 83." *The New York Times*, 18 July 1995. www.nytimes.com/1995/07/18/obituaries/may-sarton-poet-novelist-and-individualist-dies-at-83.html. Sarton's obituary in the *New York Times* which gives a detailed account of her life and works.

Sarton, May, and Stefan Martin. *The Poet and the Donkey.* W. W. Norton & Company, 1996. A charming and quick little book about a poet who has lost his muse and is no longer able to write, and the donkey he borrows from his neighbors, who, in time, becomes his missing muse.

Sarton, May. A Grain of Mustard Seed: New Poems. W. W. Norton & Company, 1975. A compilation of intense, spirited verse that explores the realms of religion, politics, nature, violence, and old age.

———. At Eighty-Two: A Journal. W. W. Norton & Company, 1997. Sarton's eagerly awaited journals have recorded her life as a single, woman writer and, in later years, as a woman confronting old age. She completed this pilgrimage through her eighty-second year a few months before she died in 1995.

———. Coming into Eighty: New Poems. W. W. Norton & Company, 1994. Sarton's observations and reflections, many of which came to her as if by magic during the small hours of the morning. Along with the daily events of writing a letter, appreciating her flowers, taking care of her cat Pierrot, these poems wrestle with the larger questions of life and death, the difficulties and rewards of living alone.

———. *Joanna and Ulysses: A Tale.* Revised ed., W. W. Norton & Company, 1987. Joanna, a 30-year old painter, decides to take a holiday in Santorini, Greece, to cope with her mother's death and her general dissatisfaction with life. To get around the steep streets of Santorini, Joanna buys a small, mistreated donkey named Ulysses. The two travel around the town and Joanna comes to terms with her past while searching for the perfect landscape to paint. This is a charming and heartwarming story, with a lot more emotional depth to it than first meets the eye.

———. *Journal of a Solitude.* W. W. Norton & Company, 1992. Sarton records and reflects on her interior life in the course of one year, her sixtieth, with remarkable candor and courage.

———. "'I See Myself as a Builder of Bridges.'" Interview by Neila C. Seshachari. *Weber Studies*, vol. 9, no. 2, 1992. weberstudies.weber.edu/archive/archive%20A%20%20Vol.%201-10.3/Vol.%209.2/9.2SartonInterview.htm A candid interview about Sarton's works, focusing on her portrayal of women and the homosexual themes in many. Sarton's own sexuality is discussed frankly.

SENILITY. *See* ALZHEIMER'S DISEASE; DEMENTIA.

SENIOR CITIZEN CENTERS

Relevant Issues: Demographics, psychology, sociology, recreation

Significance: AS increasing life expectancy has created a larger elderly population and changing family structures have minimized extended families, many elderly people have their social and service needs met through alternate sources.

In 1965, the groundwork was laid for the provision of a variety of social services for the elderly in the United States with the passage of the Older Americans Act (OAA). This legislation provided funding for many programs, including senior citizen centers, which tended to take the form of social clubs for the aged. These centers were needed, to some extent, because of an increase in the population of older persons.

THE AGING OF NORTH AMERICA

In 2017, persons sixty-five years of age or older constituted nearly 16 percent of the U.S. population. By 2030, when most of the baby-boom generation will have retired, it is expected that 1 in every 5 residents of the United States will be retirement-age or older.

In ageist societies, retirees often are excluded from much social participation with those other than age peers. Social isolation, although detrimental to persons of all ages, has been shown to be especially problematic to those in late life. Thus, a place for older people to gather had become important. There were approximately 450 of these seniors' clubs in the United States in 1965.

In slightly more than a decade, however, it became clear that more than just a club-type setting was required. In 1978, amendments to the reauthorization of the OAA called for the creation and support of multipurpose senior centers. This change was the result of recognition that many older persons had a variety of needs that were not being met adequately under other circumstances.

For various reasons, older persons are less likely to live with extended family members than in the past, and even if they do, they may not have someone with them in the home as much as they want or need. Many older persons, therefore, might have to rely on outsiders to meet some of these needs. Multipurpose senior centers developed as community focal points where elderly people could come together for services and activities to help support their independence.

ADULT DAY CARE

Many multipurpose centers offer what is sometimes referred to as respite care or adult day care (ADC). This service is designed to provide the primary caregivers—usually family members—time off so that they do not suffer unduly from the burden of caregiving, which can become a twenty-four-hour-a-day job. Provided on a more long-term basis, it may also enable the primary caregiver—often an adult daughter or daughter-in-law of the elderly person—to return to the work for pay she may have left so that she could provide this care.

ADC centers are often attached to long-term care (LTC) facilities, even though ADC is designed to delay the older person's entry into LTC. In Canada, eligibility for ADC is established along the same lines as for LTC, and it is almost invariably provided by nonprofit organizations. In the United States, ADC is available in some senior residential facilities, some hospitals (nonprofit or otherwise), and some churches.

Wherever ADC services are provided, they enable elders to continue living at home while getting the supervision, assistance, and interaction they need during the day. ADC services may include physical rehabilitation, nursing, and transportation. This latter service may include home pickup and return.

THE NEED FOR ADVANCED SERVICES

The U.S. National Center for Health Statistics indicates that rates of impairment of one sort or another vary by region. This variance leads to a differential incidence of need for ADC services. These different levels of physical need are one factor in the level of demand relative to capacity. Other factors in demand include marital dissolution rates, which are considerably higher in the South than in the Midwest. Spouses are a significant source of care, and lack of a spouse may increase the need for outside caregiving.

ADC centers date back to 1947 in the United States, with one begun at the Menninger Clinic in Kansas. Their growth had been curtailed until recently by the introduction of Medicare and Medicaid legislation, which provided only for payment of medical services rendered by physicians, hospitals, and LTC facilities. With increased efforts at containing costs and finding options that provide for more independence and dignity for elders, health service providers have looked more closely at ADC as an option.

Some organizations have begun to explore novel ways of combining child and adult day care services, which may allow young children and their grandparents or great-grandparents to spend more time together, being cared for in proximate or even interrelated facilities. This could be a great boon to the parents of these children, members of the so-called sandwich generation that have the responsibility of caring for both their children and their parents.

—Scott Magnuson-Martinson

See also: Exercise and fitness; Facility and institutional care; Friendship; Home-delivered meals programs; Home services; Housing; Leisure activities; Long-term care; Older Americans Act of 1965; Retirement; Retirement communities; Social ties; Transportation issues

For Further Information

Malonebeach, Eileen E., and Karen L. Langeland. "Boomers' Prospective Needs for Senior Centers and Related Services: A Survey of Persons 50-59." *Journal of Gerontological Social Work*, vol. 54, no. 1, 2011, pp. 116-30. doi:10.1080/01634372.2010.524283. A survey addressing work/retirement, family, civic engagement, health, caregiving, leisure, and perceptions of senior services.

Pramitasari, Diananta, and Ahmad Sarwadi. "A Study on Elderly's Going Out Activities and Environment Facilities." *Procedia Environmental Sciences*, vol. 28, 2015, pp. 315-23. doi:10.1016/j.proenv.2015.07.040. This study aims to identify the going out activities conducted by senior residents during their daily lives and how the built environment especially in the high densely settlement of the city center support these activities.

"What Is a Senior Citizen Center? Facts & Benefits." NCOA, National Council on Aging, 9 Nov. 2017. www.ncoa.org/news/resources-for-reporters/get-the-facts/senior-center-facts/. General information on senior citizen centers.

SEXUAL DYSFUNCTION

Relevant Issues: Biology, health and medicine, psychology

Significance: Contrary to some myths about aging, sexuality remains a vital aspect of older adults lives. Increasing awareness of sexuality and the aging process, along with understanding, identifying, and treating sexual dysfunction promotes health and wellness on older adults.

Healthy and satisfying sexual function is an important issue for all people, including those in older age groups. Beyond providing physical pleasure, sexual behavior can impact self-esteem and emotional gratification and stability; as well as produce transient happiness, and promote interpersonal closeness, and intimacy. Although normal aging is associated with a general decline in sexual responsiveness and sexual activity, contrary to some beliefs, many older people desire to, and do, continue expressing their sexuality until the end of their life. Lack of public and professional (e.g., medical) awareness of and comfort with addressing the topic can result in missed opportunities in reassuring older adults about normal changes in sexuality, in addition to decreasing the likelihood of diagnosing sexual dysfunction and potential access to effective treatment options.

SEXUAL FUNCTIONING ACROSS THE LIFE SPAN

Five stages of normal sexual functioning, involving physiological and psychological factors have been identified in sexually mature men and women across the life span: desire, excitement or arousal, plateau, orgasm, and resolution. Desire (also known as libido) refers to psychological thoughts, fantasies, and yearnings. Arousal is triggered by physiological and psychological stimuli and involves increasing levels of muscle tension (mytonia) and blood flow and consequent swelling (vasocongestion) in the vulva, clitoris, and breast tissue in women and the penis in men. For both sexes, the arousal stage produces greater mental focus on and drive for sexual behavior, as well as increased respiration, heart rate, and muscle tone. The plateau stage involves a heightened sense of sexual excitement and awareness of imminent orgasm. Orgasm is the climax of the sexual response, involving extreme physical and emotional pleasure, and resulting in several physiological responses, including ejaculation in men and involuntary contractions of the vagina and labia minora in women. Following orgasm, the resolution stage is characterized psychologically by a sense of satisfaction and relaxation and physically by decreasing vasocongestion in both sexes, loss of erection (detumescence) in men, and a refractory period involving temporary inhibition of further arousal and orgasm (especially in men).

Importantly, the sequence and delineation of the stages can vary and overlap among individuals. Also, a range of factors such as individual psychosexual developmental and maturity, family of origin views of sexuality, and sexual history have significant influence on the subjective experience of sex. Additional contributing factors include sexual partner characteristics and associated relationship variables, religious and moral beliefs, sexual orientation, cultural milieu, physical health, body image, and location in the life span. The normal process of aging influences sexual functioning, and age-related factors can contribute to sexual dysfunction and associated treatments.

SEXUALITY IN OLDER ADULTS

Although there is marked variability among individuals, the typical process of aging is associated with mental, psychological, and physical changes in sexual functioning. For both sexes, sexual activity tends to decline in older adulthood. Nevertheless, research suggests that the majority of men and women (60-80 percent) aged 60 and above engage in sexual activity on a regular basis (intercourse at least once per month) and describe themselves as sexually satisfied. Factors that influence the likelihood of active and satisfying sexual functioning in later life include the presence of a healthy and interested sexual partner, level of sexual activity prior to older adulthood, physical and psychological health status, and the type of medications taken for any health conditions.

Factors associated with aging that predict decreased positive sexual functioning in older adulthood include poor health, absence of an interested and willing partner, lack of privacy (e.g., in long-term care facilities), loss of interest, negative body image, and the presence of a sexual disorder. Fears of health risks associated with sexual behavior may unnecessarily contribute to avoiding sexual activity in older adulthood. Although an individual's health status relating to sexual activity should be evaluated and determined by medical professionals, research indicates that, other than acquiring a sexually transmitted infection, there is very low risk of precipitating or worsening a health condition as a result of engaging in sex. For example, the risk of recurrent heart attack resulting from sexual activity among men and women who had previously suffered a heart attack was only 2 in 1 million. Nevertheless, some sexual dysfunctions can be caused by a health condition (e.g., erectile dysfunction and diabetes).

Differences in emotional maturity, openness to change, and adaptation skills may influence sexual functioning in older adulthood. For example, some individuals may view sexual changes associated with aging with a sense of dread and perceive them as signals of impending decline or death. Consequently, sexual activity may be viewed negatively and passively or actively avoided. Conversely, enhanced communication skills accruing from long-term relationships may lead to deeper levels of intimacy and more satisfying sexuality for couples. Also, changes in the family life cycle for older adults may result in more privacy for couples, increased opportunities for sexual activity, and greater freedom for open sexual expression.

In women, the normal process of menopause (the cessation of menses resulting from decreasing ovarian functioning) produces physiological changes such as reduced vaginal lubrication, diminished sensitivity in clitoral, vulvar, and nipple tissue, and lessened clitoral vasocongestion and engorgement during sexual activity. Additionally, menopause is associated with reduced genital tissue leading to diminished vaginal size and elasticity.

Psychological factors associated with menopause may include decreased sexual interest and frequency of sexual activity, reduced sexual responsiveness (including orgasms), greater likelihood of discomfort or pain experienced during intercourse (known as dyspareunia), and decreased sexual confidence related to physical attractiveness and desirability. However, for some women menopause may result in greater sexual interest and activity consequent to eliminating fears of pregnancy or any previous preoccupation or anxiety relating to contraception.

In older adulthood, men typically experience fewer firm erections, reduced intensity of orgasms, and a longer refractory period following orgasm. They may take longer and require more stimulation to achieve an erection. Older men are less likely to report reduced interest and preoccupation in sexual activity compared to same age women.

SEXUAL DYSFUNCTION IN OLDER ADULTS

Sexual dysfunctions can occur across the life span including during older adulthood. Broadly defined, a sexual dysfunction involves a disturbance in the ability to respond sexually or experience sexual pleasure. A number of factors are considered in identifying a specific type of sexual dysfunction including the characteristics of the dysfunction (e.g., specific symptoms and associated consequences), the onset of the condition (present from initial sexual experiences or acquired after a period of normal sexual functioning), and the pervasiveness of the symptoms (situational or generalized), Other considerations aiding in understanding, diagnosing, and treating sexual dysfunction include sexual partner factors (e.g., availability, health) and relationship factors (e.g., concordance in sexual interest, preferences, and communication styles), psychosocial history and vulnerability (e.g., education and perspective of sexuality experienced in the family of origin, body image, exposure to abuse or partner violence), cultural and religious views of sexuality (e.g., regarding appropriate and prohibited expression of sexuality), psychiatric health, and medical factors that influence sexual activity and expression.

The Diagnostic and Statistical Manual, 5th Edition (DSM-5), a guide commonly used by health professional to identify psychiatric conditions, details descriptions of sexual disorders and identifies specific criteria for diagnosing them. Some sexual dysfunctions are experienced by both sexes, while others are specific to women or men. Those conditions specific to women are Female Orgasmic Disorder, Female Interest/Arousal Disorder, and Genito-Pelvic Pain/Penetration Disorder (also known as dyspareunia). Sexual dysfunctions specific to men are Delayed Ejaculation, Erectile Disorder (previously termed impotence), Male Hypoactive Sexual Desire Disorder, and Premature (Early) Ejaculation. Disorders seen in both women and men include Substance/Medication Induced Sexual Dysfunction and the broad categories of Other Specified or Unspecified Sexual Dysfunction. The latter two are employed when full criteria for a condition are not met or there is insufficient information to make a definitive diagnosis. Purely medical illnesses underlying sexual dysfunction are not considered psychiatric disorders so are not included in the DSM-5.

MEDICAL ILLNESS AND DISEASES

Sexual interest and activity typically diminish in individuals confronted with serious medical illness. Some diseases commonly influence sexuality in later adulthood due to their increased incidence and physiologic characteristics. The list of medical illnesses that can potentially impact sexual functioning is long and includes heart disease, stroke, Parkinson's disease, and especially any condition that affects blood supply to genital tissue (e.g., diabetes, atherosclerosis). Some conditions are considered primary causes of sexual disorders because they cause physiological changes that directly inhibit sexual functioning, such as erectile dysfunction caused by reduced blood flow and diminished sensitivity in diabetes. Other illnesses are viewed as secondary causes of sexual dysfunction because impairment results indirectly from a symptom of a disease, such as pain with osteoarthritis, fatigue with multiple sclerosis, or dizziness with Meniere's disease. Sexual functioning may be negatively impacted by surgical intervention such as prostate surgery which is a known cause of erectile dysfunction, or due to such factors as pain or restricted range of motion caused by scarring or inhibition and embarrassment consequent to altered body image. Psychiatric illness may cause sexual dysfunction by hindering sexual performance (e.g., due to depression or panic attacks) or intimacy in relationships (e.g., due to social anxiety).

SEXUAL DYSFUNCTION ASSOCIATED WITH MEDICATIONS AND OTHER SUBSTANCES

A number of medications have been identified as potential contributors to sexual dysfunction in all age groups. Older adults are at heightened risk of medication related sexual dysfunction as a result of decreasing capacity of the liver and kidneys to clear drugs from the system. Older adults are also more likely to take multiple medications, thereby increasing the risk of experiencing side effects, harmful interactions, and toxicity. Drug classes and medications commonly prescribed in older patients that can cause sexual dysfunction include psychiatric drugs (antidepressants, antipsychotics), cardiovascular drugs, antihypertensive drugs, diuretics, and antiulcer medications. Non-prescription, over-the-counter medications, such as antihistamines, and decongestants also can contribute to sexual dysfunction. The possibility of non-prescribed or illicit drug use and abuse causing sexual dysfunction in the elderly should not be overlooked. Alcohol, opioids, sedatives, and anti-anxiety drugs can be associated with sexual dysfunction and procured in virtually all communities and settings by every age group including the elderly.

SEXUAL DYSFUNCTION IN WOMEN

Female Sexual Interest/Arousal Disorder is a condition characterized by reduced or absent interest in sexual activity, erotic thoughts and fantasies, and sexual excitement and pleasure. Sexual encounters are avoided or engaged in for reasons other than seeking sexual pleasure (e.g., as a sense of obligation or to please a spouse). When they do occur, they are experienced with limited physical response (e.g., vasocongestion, orgasm) or emotional and psychological satisfaction. The level of distress associated with the condition varies among individuals; however, older women tend to report less associated distress than younger women. Decreased sexual desire in older women may coincide with changes in body image and sexual confidence stemming from perceived loss of physical attractiveness or illness. Changes in life circumstances associated with aging, such as the loss of a spouse or long-term sexual partner may also lead to decreased libido. Although there are no reliable estimates of the prevalence of this disorder, sexual interest appears to decrease in women as they age.

Female Orgasmic Disorder involves the absence of orgasms, difficulty experiencing orgasm, or significantly reduced intensity of orgasm when they do occur. Wide variability in the subjective experience of orgasm reported by females complicates the understanding, diagnosis, and treatment of the disorder. High rates of women report periodic difficulties achieving orgasm (up to 42 percent) and approximately 10 percent of women report never experiencing orgasms in their lifetime. Distress and preoccupation associated with achieving orgasm is a necessary aspect of the condition; however, older women tend to report less distress than younger women. Menopause has not been identified as causing greater difficulty in achieving orgasm. Individuals with the condition may also meet diagnostic criteria for Female Sexual Interest/Arousal Disorder.

Genito-Pelvic Pain/Penetration Disorder is associated with the following symptoms: difficulty engaging in satisfactory sexual intercourse, vulvo-vaginal, or pelvic pain during intercourse, anxiety and fear of pain associated with intercourse, and significant muscle tension during intercourse or attempts at intercourse. The condition is more common in older women and can be associated with age-related physical changes such as vaginal dryness and loss of tissue. In addition to physical factors, anxiety and fear are significant components of the condition. Approximately 15 percent of all women report pain during intercourse, however accurate estimates of the disorder, including among older women are lacking.

SEXUAL DYSFUNCTION IN MEN
Delayed Ejaculation is a disorder involving marked delay or inability to ejaculate despite seemingly adequate stimulation, opportunity, and desire. The definition of what constitutes a significant delay is usually subjective and largely determined by the perception of the individual with the condition. For the diagnosis to be made, associated symptoms must be experienced in at least 75 percent of sexual encounters for six months. Significant distress accompanies the condition and relationship difficulties may result from sexual partners attributing symptoms to their lack of desirability. Age-related changes in physiology, including decreased testosterone production and nerve sensitivity contributes to increasing incidence in older men, especially after age 50. Precise prevalence data, however, are lacking.

Erectile Disorder is characterized by impairment in the arousal phase of sexual response and is defined as the consistent or recurrent inability to attain and/or maintain penile erection sufficient for sexual performance and satisfaction. Transitory or periodic difficulties with erections occur with many men across the course of their sexual life span. However, in order to make the diagnosis of Erectile Disorder, symptoms must be experienced at a minimum of 75 percent of sexual encounters for six months. Many men evidence shame, decreased feelings of masculinity, lowered self-esteem, and depression resulting from erectile difficulties, which in turn can maintain or worsen symptoms. There is a strong age-related increase in erectile difficulties, especially after age 50. Both physiological and psychosocial factors influence increased erectile dysfunction in older men. These include greater likelihood of illness and need for medications and adaptation to life changes such as retirement, change in social status, and death of a spouse. Approximately 40-50 percent of men aged 60 to 70 experience erectile problems. A considerably lower percentage of this age-group meets full criteria for diagnosing Erectile Disorder.

Male Hypoactive Sexual Desire Disorder is a condition involving deficient or absent sexual thoughts and fantasies and marked reduced urges and desire for sexual activity. Distress is experienced as a result of the condition and many with the diagnosis may experience erectile and ejaculatory difficulties. Diagnosis is made on a more subjective level and involves determining if there is a significant discrepancy between expected and actual sexual desire based on age, social, and cultural variables. Psychiatric conditions (e.g., anxiety), substance abuse (e.g., with alcohol), and illness can diminish sexual desire. Approximately 40 percent of men aged 66 to 74 experience problems with sexual desire; however, accurate estimates of the disorder are lacking.

Premature (Early) Ejaculation involves persistent or recurrent ejaculation within one minute of sexual activity involving penetration along with a subjective sense that orgasm has occurred too early in the sexual act. Marked anxiety often accompanies this disorder, as does apprehension and a sense of lack of control. While this condition does occur in older men, greater incidence is reported in younger age groups.

EVALUATION OF SEXUAL DYSFUNCTION
The foundation of effective evaluation of sexual dysfunction is open and honest communication between the individual under examination and a medical (physician, nurse practitioner) or mental health (psychologist,

social worker, counselor) professional. Open communication is not always readily or easily achieved, especially with highly personal or potentially embarrassing information. The examining clinician should take an active role in pursuing concerns about sexual functioning and create an atmosphere whereby topics are examined directly and without judgment, using common vocabulary. Thorough examination may involve multiple clinicians (e.g., primary care physician, urologist or gynecologist, mental health professional) and should include a medical and psychiatric history, sexual and relationship histories, physical exam with special focus on neurologic, circulatory and endocrine systems, and appropriate lab studies. The presence and participation of the individual's sexual partner can often facilitate the evaluation.

TREATMENT OF SEXUAL DYSFUNCTION

As with evaluation, effective treatment of sexual dysfunction starts with open and direct communication. Education and reassurance regarding the normal effects of aging on sexuality may be enough to promote comfort and reduce anxiety in many older individuals. Sexual practices may be modified via education to facilitate more enjoyable and less problematic sexual functioning. For example, a woman with arthritis may be advised to try new sexual positions that require less exertion or minimize pain. Similarly, a couple might extend foreplay to allow the man more time to achieve an erection.

Many substances and medications are available to treat sexual dysfunctions, ranging from over-the-counter lubricants to counter genital dryness or tissue reduction to physician prescribed phosphodiesterase-5 inhibitors to treat erectile dysfunction (e.g., Sildenafil or Viagra among others). Hormonal therapy may play a greater role in treating dysfunction in older populations compared with other age groups. Consideration of the effects on sexual functioning of medications used for treating co-morbid illnesses should lead to frank discussion regarding health expectations and priorities. It is important that medications be prescribed by a physician knowledgeable of evidence-based treatment options and caution should be paramount if considering over-the-counter or unregulated substances for treatment. The same caution applies with recommendations from unlicensed practitioners. Surgical intervention, such as an implant for erectile dysfunction, is typically considered as a last resort for treatment, especially in older adults.

Psychotherapy and several psychologically based strategies have been found to be effective in treating sexual dysfunction. Addressing relationship factors such as communication styles and life stressors beyond sexuality often has collateral benefit in improving sexual functioning. Cognitive-behavioral treatment of depression and anxiety, involving modifying self-defeating thoughts and problematic behaviors has been found to reduce co-existing sexual symptoms. Exercises designed to reduce anxiety and promote relaxation and confidence in sexual performance may be recommended and taught in a systematic fashion to couples experiencing sexual difficulties. A well-researched technique, known as Sensate Focus, involving graduated sexual activity and stimulation, reduced focus on orgasm, and efforts to alleviate performance anxiety, has been found effective in older couples.

—*Paul F. Bell, Ph.D.*

See also: Medications; Men and aging; Reproductive changes, disabilities, and dysfunctions; Sexuality; Smoking; Stress and coping skills

For Further Information

Agronin, Marc. "Sexual Dysfunction in Older Adults." UpToDate, 24 Oct. 2017. www.uptodate.com/contents/sexual-dysfunction-in-older-adults. An internet resource providing descriptions of sexual dysfunction and information relating to medical diagnosis and treatment.

American Psychiatric Association. *Diagnostic and Statistical Manual of Mental Disorders*, 5th. ed., American Psychiatric Publishing, 2013. Provides diagnostic criteria and demographic data for the sexual disorders.

"Attitudes about Sexuality and Aging." *Harvard Health*, Harvard Medical School, Mar. 2017. www.health.harvard.edu/staying-healthy/attitudes-about-sexuality-and-aging. Online resource examining myths and realities relating to sexuality in older adults. Presents optimistic and realistic views of how sexual functioning changes with age.

McCarthy, Barry W., and Emily J. McCarthy. *Rekindling Desire*. 2nd ed., Routledge, 2014. Provides strategies and exercises to promote communications skills and enhance sexuality in couples. Uses case studies to facilitate understanding of and solutions to common sexual concerns and frustrations.

Price, Joan. *The Ultimate Guide to Sex after Fifty: How to Maintain—or Regain—a Spicy, Satisfying Sex Life.* Cleis P, 2014. Provides practical information and advice for achieving a satisfying sex through the life span after age fifty.

SEXUALITY

Relevant Issues: Health and medicine, psychology, sociology, values

Significance: The study of sexuality among senior citizens is a growing field of interest as people are healthier and living longer, and those over the age of 65 are a fast-increasing segment of the world population. Sexual activity is now considered as a normal function of aging and an area of active research.

Our current social narrative is that 60 is the new 40, 70 is the new 50, and 80 is the new 60. Images of youthful, active, and attractive seniors bombard our advertisements. Sexually appealing images sell images of Viagra, which create and sustain erection. All put pressure on not acknowledging what really happens with aging and sexuality. Most people don't think about older people and sex until they themselves get old. What is the truth about sexuality and aging?

The Boomer Generation, which is comprised of those born from 1946-1964, are now senior citizens. They have been through the sexual revolution of 1960s, including the advent of the birth control pill in 1960, the rise of Viagra in 1998, and the introduction of the Internet and social media. Individuals in their 50s and 60s are in many ways different from those in their 70s, 80s, and 90s, and, therefore, should not be lumped together as one "senior group." There are roughly 46 million seniors in the United States today.

THE CHANGING PHYSIOLOGY OF AGING AND SEXUALITY FOR BOTH SEXES

There is no doubt that aging is an uphill battle. Although the field of medicine continues to offer improvements and aides, the progression of ageing is inevitable. The Age Lab at MIT has created AGNES, or the sudden aging suit to simulate the experience of aging. "These include yellow glasses, which mimic the yellowing of the ocular lens that comes with age. A boxer's neck-strengthening harness reduces the mobility of the cervical spine and makes it harder to retain one's posture. Bands around the elbows, wrists, and knees gave the impression of stiffness. Gloves added to the picture, reducing tactile acuity while addressing resistance to finger movements" (Coughlin, *The Longevity Economy*; 173). With age, everything is an effort. The suit helps people appreciate the ease of movement that comes with youth.

Besides the stiffness, lack of mobility and aches, the volume of serious diseases increases. These include arthritis, diabetes, cancer, heart disease, and cognitive decline. All of the above have sexual repercussions. Most adults are on medicine. Some of these, including antidepressants, stimulants, blood pressure meds, and antihistamines can interfere with sexual response.

WOMEN AND PHYSIOLOGICAL CHANGES

The onset of menopause is usually between 45-65. Known as "change of life," it is marked by the ending of both menstruation and the ability to get pregnant, and, most importantly, the production of female hormone estrogen ends. Estrogen keeps the vagina moisturized, elastic, and supplied with blood, which leads to engorgement and orgasm. The depletion of estrogen and other symptoms of menopause can negatively affect a woman's sexuality by causing vaginal dryness, decrease in libido, and a decrease in sensation and orgasm. Some women experience pain and vaginal atrophy.

Many women choose Hormone Replacement Therapy (HRT) to counteract these symptoms; though these treatments are FDA approved, there is still controversy surrounding their use. Other women use natural supplements, and some do nothing. This is a personal and medical decision.

There are many lubricants on the market. Hormonal topical creams and vaginal inserts are available by prescription. Pharmaceutical companies are working to create a female Viagra. So far, only Addyi has been FDA approved. Addyi changes brain chemistry to increase sex drive or the desire to have sex. Unlike Viagra, which is taken as needed, Addyi must be taken daily. It does not guarantee the ability to achieve orgasm. There are some side effects to be aware of and use requires strict medical supervision.

Professionals often recommend various vibrators and sex toys for women who have issues with desire, arousal, and orgasm. Vibrators may do the trick, but over time create a lack of sensitivity to human touch, which may affect relationships.

MEN AND PHYSIOLOGICAL CHANGES

Like women, men undergo a physiological mid-life change called Andropause. This is the slow but continuous decline of testosterone production throughout a man's remaining lifetime.

These changes directly affect sexual function. Symptoms include the decrease of psychogenic erections that do not require physical stimulation (fantasies, mental images). Men will now need physical stimulation to have an erection and when they get an erection they will have difficulty holding it. Some men are upset about the decrease in volume in ejaculations. Feelings of shame generally accompany this new erectile dysfunction (ED). Men may also develop body image and ego problems due to the loss of hair, muscle tone, and physical strength. There have been groundbreaking medical advances to combat these issues.

Viagra, Cialis, and Levitra are popular medications. These drugs must be used under strict doctor supervision and cannot be mixed casually with other medicines or the use of alcohol. Surgical pumps and implants are also available. Another option is testosterone therapy.

Many older men are watching porn, which is easily available through the Internet in the privacy of their homes. Men (and women) should be aware of the legalities of ethical porn: It must be between consenting adults of legal age (over 18). These criteria are hard to discern while casually exploring porn sites, and seniors could find themselves unknowingly in trouble, especially with sites that use teens or the word young as a seduction. Child porn is under the legal age of 18.

OPTIMISTIC NEW, OLDER, "COOLER" IDEAS FOR SEXUALITY IN LATER YEARS

The MIT AGELAB has discovered that seniors dislike the use of the word old and do not respond positively to it. They prefer adjectives like cool, amazing, and fun (Coughlin). Whatever it is called, we must create a theory of sexual life span developmental psychology. As physiological and emotional maturity progresses, the definition of sex must evolve to include the sexual self, the erotic self, the sensual self, and the intimacy self.

The journey of sexual development is lonely for most seniors because the societal narrative is not up to date. Many are living with standards for themselves from the "good old days." For those who can accept the new realities, many options exist.

Sexologist Lawrence Siegel suggests that in lifetime sexual development terms, seniors often revert to a stage similar to adolescence. This stage is marked by kissing and heavy petting. Holding hands, hugging, cuddling, lying next to each other, and perhaps kissing can be all that is needed for closeness. This non-penetrative sex was given the name outercourse by Dr. Marty Klein. In his book Let Me Count the Ways: Discovering Great Sex without Intercourse, he offers many creative ideas for seniors to try.

Both women and men mourn the loss of the spontaneous desire of their youth. It is now believed that Desire can be cultivated during sexual activity. All that's needed to start is Willingness. This is quite a liberating concept for older adults. There is an emerging movement about techniques that intensify the sexual, sensual, erotic experience that can help seniors be more responsive.

POSITIVE ATTITUDES AND BEHAVIORS THAT WORK

1. Be present! Discipline yourself to be totally in the moment.
2. Turn off distracting thoughts during sex. Whether it be trivial rumination about your day or something more important, it is critical to focus on the moment.
3. Whether it is critical self-judgment about yourself or your partner's performance, negative judgment is a killer of enjoyment.
4. Be playful; don't be too serious.
5. Do not be solely focused on performance or orgasm.
6. Get comfortable talking and communicating about sex in a loving manner.

TECHNIQUES FOR ACCESSING YOUR EROTIC NATURE FOR BOTH MEN AND WOMEN

1. Erotic Mindfulness: The intention of this technique is to get in tune with the sensations of your body without distractions. The goal is to more intensely experience sensual pleasure. Dr. Lori Brotto gives a full program of exercises in her book Better Sex Through Mindfulness.

2. Sensate Focus: Weiner and Avery-Clark offer a mindful, structured program of progressive touching from non-genital, to exploring the entire boy, to coitus in their book Sensate Focus and Sex Therapy...the Illustrated Manual. It can be helpful for both couples and individuals.

3. Nicole Daedone teaches the art of slow sex in her book Slow Sex: The Art and Craft of the Female Orgasm. One of her tips is very slow, soft stroking of the upper left quadrant of the clitoris for 15 minutes. Women who thought they were "dead" were surprised at how "alive" they could get.

4. Andrew Goldstein, MD, and Marianne Brandon, PhD, teach a broader program for sexual preparedness and sexual health in Reclaiming Desire: 4 Keys to Finding your Lost Libido. Their program encompasses physical health including hormone adjustments and adaptations to physical difficulties such as arthritis. It also emphasizes emotional resilience, intellectual stimulation, and spiritual practice. Dr. Goldstein is the founder of the comprehensive Sexual Wellness Center in Maryland and New York.

SENSUALITY FOR SENIORS

Taking time to indulge the sensual self whether alone or with a partner can be a satisfying and relaxing experience. Being sensual involves the pleasure of developing all 5 senses: seeing, hearing, feeling, tasting, and smelling. Whether it be an aromatic candle, sexy music, or massage can all contribute to the experience. Many sensuality workshops are available online, where one learn to get in touch with and awaken one's sensual self.

FINDING A PARTNER

Many seniors find themselves alone due to death of a partner, divorce, or other circumstances. Whether with the same partner, a new partner, or alone, seniors are seeking connection. Many new opportunities for meeting others have emerged.

Obviously the Internet offers many dating sites, which advertise romance or marriage. Seniors can benefit from help navigating the roller coaster of high hopes, exaggerated profiles, and rejection. For the resilient, connections can be made.

Many seniors find themselves not attracted to prospects. Instead of giving up on a possibly good person Dr. Bonnie Eaker Weil suggests a 30 second kiss and 30 second hug to get the oxytocin going in her book *Make Up Don't Break Up: Getting the Magic Going*. Thus a possible relationship with an otherwise good match can be saved. Dr. Ruth Westheimer gives many good tips for safe use of the Internet and other ways to meet people in *Dr. Ruth's Sex After 50: Revving up the Romance Passion, and Excitement!*

Many seniors just feel lonely and want connection and platonic friends. Not everyone is seeking romance. Some seniors want to meet others in the hope of finding someone to talk to, watch TV and movies with, and accompany them on trips. Honesty of intention is the best policy.

There is a growing trend for seniors to downsize and move into 55+ communities. One attraction to this lifestyle is the increased opportunities for activities and connection.

Some older men and women look for casual hook-ups on sites like Tinder and Craig's List. STIs are becoming more common among seniors due to unprotected sex.

THE DREAM TEAM

All of the above is not easy. There is little information out there geared to seniors and most seniors are embarrassed to talk about sex and intimacy. Professionals are often not trained in this area.

Sexologist Ricky Siegel suggests building your own Dream Team of support. This includes a Gynecologist or Urologist trained in Sexual Health and a qualified Sex Therapist to guide your process and help you feel comfortable talking about sex.

Additionally, Pelvic Floor Physical Therapists are able to do manual physical therapy to the vulva area, which increases blood flow and flexibility in soft muscles of the area.

They also assist men with issues of early ejaculation and pain.

A regular massage therapist can help aging people keep their body supple, while a relationship therapist can help seniors navigate the complications of relationships.

LGBTQ+ OLDER ADULTS

The LGBTQ+ (lesbian, gay, bisexual, transgender and queer) population, which now includes around 3

HOW TO TALK TO SENIORS ABOUT SEXUAL HEALTH

How Do They Feel?

Seniors may find aspects of age-related changes to their sexual health challenging. Bodily changes can make sex seem difficult or unappealing. Because seniors become more easily fatigued than younger adults, they may despair at being unable to perform exactly as they did in their younger years. They may suffer from lack of self-esteem, worrying that they are unattractive or unsatisfying to their partner. At the same time, older adults—like anyone else—want to be desired. This can cause frustration, anxiety, and even depression. A senior's other health issues, or those of their partner, can also take time, energy, and focus away from relationship matters. This stress can lead to a loss of important feelings of closeness and intimacy.

On the other hand, many seniors take advantage of the opportunity to enjoy an active sex life. A more mature perspective on life and relationships can lead to a sense of freedom and fulfillment. Those who learn of treatments for common sexual problems can be excited and relieved to be able to enjoy sexual activity again. For women especially, moving past menopause often brings a new surge of energy and self-acceptance. The lack of worrying about getting pregnant can also be liberating. However, some older adults may tend to not be aware of or ignore guidelines regarding safe sex.

How Do I Start The Conversation?

When you raise the topic of sexual health with seniors, it is important that you do so in a respectful way and are reasonably informed about the topic yourself. If your approach is seen as rude, intrusive, overbearing, or uninformed, it will likely be ignored or resisted. There may be specific issues you feel are important to focus on depending on an individual's situation:

- Being proactive about sexual health, including regular doctor checkups
- Safe sex and STDs
- Normal aging changes versus illnesses or other conditions
- Remedies and treatments, and consulting a doctor or therapist
- Maintaining closeness and connection with a partner

Discussions can be had one-on-one or in a group setting, depending on comfort level. For many people, sexual health is a very private and sensitive subject, so special care should be taken not to upset. For some caregivers, it might be best to hold a group lecture or talk, with a question-and-answer session as appropriate. This provides seniors with general information in a nonthreatening way, and personal issues can be addressed later. For other caregivers or family members, engaging in a frank but respectful conversation may be more appropriate. If the senior is reluctant to discuss the subject, you might try relating a story of someone else who successfully dealt with a sexual health issue. Use gentle questions to better understand the person's situation and steer the discussion toward possible solutions.

In all cases, actively listen to seniors and be empathetic to their point of view. If their responses indicate a lack of knowledge, gently supply information or suggest reading material or other resources. Make it clear that talking to their health-care practitioner will be helpful. However, avoid being judgmental or telling them what they "should" or "must" do. Instead, support them in their own efforts to address personal sexual health concerns. Your efforts at effective communication will also help establish a framework for how they can effectively communicate with doctors or partners. Sexual health includes a major psychological component, so keeping older adults comfortable and fostering self-esteem throughout the discussion is beneficial.

Your conversation can also highlight how seniors can be proactive in taking care of their general health, which will, in turn, positively affect their sexual health. Encourage them to boost energy levels by participating in physical exercise and eating a healthy diet.

—Leah Jacob

million people in the United States, faces more problems due to discrimination and lack of children.

Social connection is key to counteract isolation. Help is more available in locations that have a large LBGTQ population. However the new addition of Gender Studies at many universities and training institutes gives hope for more resources in the future.

NURSING HOMES AND DEMENTIA

Many nursing homes and dementia facilities are grappling with issues of sexuality amongst their population. Issues of consent and competence are in the forefront. However, these facilities are gravitating toward providing more opportunities for privacy and closeness. Increased dialogue about sexual feelings and expression would help residents.

Sexual activity later in life is better viewed on a continuum of sexual development throughout the lifespan. As physiological, mental, and emotional maturity progress, the definition of sexual behavior evolves into what is realistic and practical. A more expanded view would put more emphasis on intimacy, erotic and sensual experiences, and feelings of closeness. This is a divergence from the focus on performance and orgasm. Because our culture discourages the discussion of senior sexuality, this journey can often be lonely and discouraging. For those who accept the reality with positivity, many options exist. A support team of Sexual Health professionals can help in this uphill battle.

—*Cathleen Jo Faruque and Bonnie Kellen, PsyD*

See also: Ageism; Change: Women, Aging, and the Menopause, The; Cohabitation; Communication; LGBTQ+; Loneliness; Marriage; Men and aging; Menopause; Psychiatry, geriatric; Reproductive changes, disabilities, and dysfunctions; Sexual dysfunction; Social ties; Stereotypes; Widows and widowers; Women and aging

For Further Information

Brotto, Lori A., PhD. *Better Sex Through Mindfulness.* Greystone Books, 2018. In this accessible, relatable book, Brotto explores the various reasons for sexual problems, such as stress and incessant multitasking, and tells the stories of many of the women she has treated over the years.

Goldstein, Andrew MD, and Marianne Brandon, PhD. *Reclaiming Desire: 4 Keys to Finding Your Lost Libido.* Rodale, 2009. Presents the holistic approach used to successfully treat women with low libido.

Snyder, Stephen, MD. *Love Worth Making: How to Have Ridiculously Great Sex in a Long-Lasting Relationship.* St. Martin's P, 2018. This acclaimed, paradigm-shifting guide turns traditional sex therapy inside-out to reveal the hidden rules for great sex.

Westheimer, Ruth K. *Dr. Ruth's Sex after 50: Revving Up the Romance, Passion, and Excitement!* Quill Driver Books, 2006. Westheimer, world-famous sex therapist, guides the reader through the physical and emotional challenges of sex after 50, revving up the romance, passion and excitement.

SHEEHY, GAIL

Born: November 25, 1937; Mamaroneck, New York
Relevant Issues: Family, health and medicine, psychology, sociology
Significance: Sheehy is the author of widely read self-help books dealing with midlife crises and passage through life stages, particularly middle age through menopause and beyond.

Gail Sheehy won many awards during her career as a journalist and had authored 17 books by 2019. Sheehy's most popular published works are *Passages: Predictable Crises of Adult Life* (1974), *The Silent Passage: Menopause* (1992), and *New Passages: Mapping Your Life Across Time* (1995). A survey conducted in 1991 for the Library of Congress on the most influential books in people's lives listed Passages as ninth.

In The Silent Passage, Sheehy discusses what she calls one of the few remaining taboos in modern society. She states that she was surprised to find out how little had been written about menopause but came to realize that in earlier times, before about 1800, men and women infrequently lived into the menopausal years, as the average lifespan rarely exceeded 30 years.

Sheehy was criticized for not taking into account the existing body of work on the subject. According to *Washington Post* reviewer Diana Morgan, "Sheehy focuses excessively on her own experiences in the book. The reader is told an astounding amount about the angst of Gail Sheehy." Barbara Ehrenreich, noted feminist author and *New York Times Review* contributor, applauded Sheehy for meeting the challenge of putting "the Change" on public view. Ehrenreich took exception to descriptions of the menopause as "an almost invariably volatile, frightening experience" and stated that Sheehy's book "actually supports a far less alarmist view."

New Passages began as an effort to revise *Passages*, but Sheehy soon realized that an entirely new book was needed. Cheryl Lavin, *Chicago Tribune* contributor, wrote that, "Sheehy wandered into a revolution of life cycles. People were taking longer to grow up and longer to die." Lavin reported, "Sheehy said men move from competing to connecting, while women graduate from pleasing others to realizing their own goals." Sheehy told Lavin that she intended *New Passages* to be a wake-up call to help people see themselves as they are, celebrate that they have a second adulthood, and get on with planning and enjoying it.

Nancy Matsumoto of *People Magazine* challenged the author to speak to the charges that Sheehy had shied away from dealing with the problems associated with growing older. Sheehy replied that, "Getting yourself into the second adulthood is not easy. It is about allowing yourself to experience this little psychic death and not trying to deny that you're moving into another stage. But society has always focused on the deficits, not on the gains." Sheehy argued that the gains far outweigh the losses.

Sheehy had many experiences abroad as a journalist throughout her career. She was in Thailand writing a story on Cambodian refugees for the *New York Times Magazine* when she first met her adopted daughter, Mohm, who was eleven and had been orphaned at age six by the Khmer Rouge. She became the subject of Sheehy's seventh book, *Spirit of Survival* (1986). Sheehy believed that Mohm's story offers lessons of self-help for every-day misfortunes. "Above all Mohm reminds us we have the power to prevail," Sheehy wrote. Both Mohm and Sheehy's biological daughter, Maura, became writers.

Sheehy also wrote many articles for many magazines, including such as *New York Magazine* and *Vanity Fair*, as she took part in a style revolution characterized as "the New Journalism" by Tom Wolfe (also known as creative non-fiction), which used dialogue, scene-setting, and intense detail. Sheehy also wrote character studies of many important people, including Hillary Clinton, George H.W. Bush, George W. Bush, Margaret Thatcher, Anwar Sadat, and Mikhail Gorbachev.

—*Virginiae Blackmon*
Updated by Bruce E. Johansen, PhD

See also: Aging: Biological, psychological, and sociocultural perspectives; Men and aging; Menopause; Middle age; Midlife crisis; Women and aging

For Further Information
Sheehy, Gail. *Daring: My Passages: A Memoir*. Reprint ed., William Morrow, 2015. Sheehy returns with her inspiring memoir—a chronicle of her trials and triumphs as a groundbreaking "girl" journalist in the 1960s, to iconic guide for women and men seeking to have it all, to one of the premier political profilers of modern times.
———. *New Passages: Mapping Lives across Time*. Ballantine Books, 1996. Sheehy discovers and maps out a completely new frontier—a Second Adulthood in middle life.
———. *Passages: Predictable Crises of Adult Life*. Bantam Books, 1976. Gail Sheehy's brilliant road map of adult life shows the inevitable personality and sexual changes we go through in our 20s, 30s, 40s, and beyond.
———. *The Silent Passage: Menopause*. 6th ed., Pocket Books, 2010. Candid, enlightening, inspiring, and witty, with the latest information on everything from early menopause to Chinese medicine and natural remedies.

SHEPHERD'S CENTERS

Relevant Issues: psychology, recreation, values
Significance: Shepherd's Centers are interfaith, community based organizations created to help older adults live happy and healthy lives.

The mission of the Shepherd's Centers of America is to make aging meaningful. They strive to empower the elderly by encouraging personal growth through life-long learning, healthy living, volunteering, and social enrichment.

Shepherd's Centers were founded in 1972 by Elbert Cole, a minister. As more people were living well past the age of retirement, he saw a need for programs to promote positive aging. The first Shepherd's Center was opened in Kansas City, MO, but they can now be found across the United States. Individual centers are run as separate, non-profit organizations, and each has an independent Board of Trustees. Although the original

Shepherd's Center was funded by a government grant, centers now rely on donations and dues. Each center establishes the cost of membership (generally less than $100 per year). Scholarships are available for people who are not able to afford the programming.

Because the centers are designed to make life better for senior citizens, all programs are designed by older adults. The goal is to empower senior citizens to shape their own experiences in a way that is meaningful to them and to allow older people to take care of each other and to give back to their communities.

FOUR AREAS OF PROGRAMMING

The Shepherd's Centers offer programming in four areas: Adventures in Learning, Healthy Living, Social Enrichment, and Volunteering. The Adventures in Learning component offers college-like courses and workshops that are taught by retired persons or community experts. They cover a wide range of topics including computer technology, current events, foreign languages, hobbies, crime scene investigation, and more based on the interests of the people in the community. Across all topics, the focus is on a passion for life-long learning.

The programming in Healthy Living is about health and wellness in the aging population. These programs include everything from exercise classes to instruction on nutrition to health screenings. The focus of the health programs is on maintaining health and preventing problems. As part of their health and wellness initiatives, the Shephard's Centers also provide support to the caregivers of the elderly by establishing support groups for them and providing a respite from care with their Breaktime Club.

The Social Enrichment programming encourages the elderly to engage in enjoyable activities that they find meaningful and that allow them to establish and maintain friendships. The specific programs are chosen by the older adults rather than by the staff to ensure that the activities are desirable to the group they are intended to serve. Activities range from short trips to parties and dances.

The fourth area of programming, Volunteering, provides opportunities for older adults to give back to their communities while also having fun and staying actively engaged. People can volunteer to instruct Adventures in Learning classes, provide transportation to others, work in the office, or work in the community helping people of all.

SUPPORT SERVICES

Shepherd's Centers also offer support services for senior citizens that allow them to live safely and independently for longer. The most frequently provided service is transportation. Many older persons wish to remain in their own homes, but they are no longer able or willing to drive themselves. Volunteers can drive people to medical appointments, to get groceries, or to social events. This transportation is provided at no or low cost. Drivers are also willing to assist their passengers with getting out of the house and into the car if needed. Other services include visits or calls, handyman services, shopping, and advocacy.

—*Monica L. McCoy, PhD*

See also: Adult education; Creativity; Exercise and fitness; Leisure activities; Religion; Senior citizen centers; Social ties; Transportation issues; Volunteering

For Further Information

Cole, Gene. "Rev. Dr. Elbert C. Cole, Jr." RootsWeb, Ancestry.com, 2011. sites.rootsweb.com/~mostodd2/history/stod-settlers/cole/elbertjr.htm. A brief biography of Elbert Cole, Jr., the founder of Shepherd's Centers, written by his son.

Koenig, Harold G. "Shepherds Centers: Helping Elderly Help Themselves." *Journal of the American Geriatrics Society*, vol. 34, no. 1, Jan. 1986, p. 73. EBSCOhost, doi:10.1111/j.1532-5415.1986.tb06343.x. Koenig explains the purpose and impact of Shepherd's Centers after a four-day visit.

Shepherd's Centers of America, www.shepherdcenters.org/.

SHOOTIST, THE (FILM)

Director: Don Siegel
Cast: John Wayne, Lauren Bacall, Ron Howard
Date: Released in 1976
Relevant Issues: Culture, death, media, values
Significance: This film depicts the last days of an aging Western gunfighter who has discovered that he is terminally ill with cancer.

In *The Shootist*, John Wayne plays the part of an aging gunfighter John Bernard Books. The film covers the last weeks of this man's life as he tries to reconcile his past glory with the reality that his life is rapidly approaching its end.

The Shootist opens with actual scenes from Wayne's early film career, and the audience is able to observe how Books (and Wayne) has aged over the course of four decades. Visiting the town doctor, Books learns that he is terminally ill; he wishes only to avoid suffering as death nears. Among the questions with which Books must deal, however, is whether his life has been worthwhile. He has no family, and while his life had no shortage of adventure, he wonders about the legacy that he is leaving behind.

Books arranges to spend his last days in the home of a widow, Bond Rogers (Lauren Bacall), and her teenage son Gillom (Ron Howard). The widow and son display ambivalent feelings toward their tenant; Gillom is enthralled by the presence of a famous gunfighter, while Bond has mixed emotions for the same reason. Still, she cannot avoid pitying the man. Eventually, all feelings are reconciled. Books dies a hero's death, and Gillom realizes the futility of a gunfighter's life.

Wayne's character, although placed specifically in a Western setting of the late nineteenth century, exhibits many feelings that are common among the terminally ill, such as the desire to not suffer, worries about dying alone, and doubts about whether one's life has been worthwhile. Ironically, Wayne himself was diagnosed with stomach cancer shortly after completion of this motion picture. He died from the disease in 1979.

—*Richard Adler*

See also: Cancer; Death and dying; Death anxiety; Terminal illness.

SIBLING RELATIONSHIPS

Relevant Issues: Death, demographics, family, psychology

Significance: Brothers and sisters occupy an important position in the lives of many older adults, and sibling relationships will increase in significance as the baby boomers reach older ages.

Siblings are assumed to be offspring of the same parents, thereby sharing, on average, 50 percent of the same genes. Most adult sibling research is limited to biological and adopted siblings. Little is known at this time about adult stepsiblings or half siblings who share one biological parent and quasi siblings with different biological parents living together. Less is known about fictive siblings who achieve sibling status by formal ritual. The steadily increasing rate of divorce and remarriage will undoubtedly affect sibling relationships. With the increase in blended families through remarriage, there will be more half siblings and stepsiblings. For divorced older people who do not remarry, sibling interaction may become more important than when they were married. The degree of commitment to these new and varied relationships is unknown at this time.

The sibling relationship is unique. Siblings share the same biological heritage, cultural heritage, and family history. They have a relationship that can last a lifetime, and they are members of the same generation.

ROLE OF SIBLINGS IN LATER LIFE

Sibling relationships assume, or reassume, critical importance in the lives of older adults. After young adult siblings leave home to establish their own life, the relationship between them often goes underground until they are older. For many older adults, siblings are the only surviving support system. The nature of sibling relationships also changes over the life course. Sibling ties may be strong among children, then become weaker as jobs, marriage, and parenting make demands on time and energy. During the middle years, siblings may live far apart and have little in common in terms of values and interests. Later life events like the departure of children from the home, retirement, and widowhood often bring siblings closer together. Older adults often mention the importance of their brothers and sisters, and as people age, the sibling bond becomes even more important. Siblings often provide support to each other and are a source of psychological well-being in old age.

Sometimes siblings become closer when they have to plan for an aging parent. Caring for their parents can renew and enhance sibling relationships. The siblings have to refocus their attention on their family of origin. Role and power reversals occur. When there is more than one adult child in the family, caring for parents has an impact on all siblings. Siblings who may have little contact find themselves in more frequent contact as they coordinate care arrangements. Caring for ailing parents does not always enhance relationships among older adult siblings. The stress of the caregiving and the parents' illness may break through the veneer of politeness covering the anger that underlies many sibling relationships.

Siblings may also care for each other as they grow older, although more likely, they only provide emotional support. Siblings can function as an insurance policy for older adults. The demographics of the American family are changing caregiving patterns. The growth in the number of single elders and the geographic mobility of adult children increase the need for siblings to be part of each other's social support systems. Research results are mixed in the area of siblings as caregivers for each other. In one study of persons aged fifty-five and older, the majority of respondents felt that their siblings would help them in a crisis, although only 25 percent had actually received such help. Illness often reconstitutes the sibling social support network. One widow explained how her sisters pitched in when her husband became sick. Having peer or same generational status was found to give siblings more empathy for and identification with their ailing brothers and sisters. Some research concluded that for some older adult siblings, giving or receiving help was distressful.

SIBLINGS IN CONFLICT

Past tensions and family feuds can keep siblings in conflict. If parents have kept their children in emotional bondage by withholding approval and love, children compete for affection and become alienated from each other. In such families, adult siblings may be unable to reconcile until one or both parents die. Instead, they may continue to replay earlier sibling rivalries in their old age. Gender differences in sibling conflict are interesting. Women express more conflict about sisters than men express about brothers. High levels of conflict between sisters have been attributed to the greater intensity of feeling in the relationship. Sister-to-sister expressions of conflict may also be a result of cultural devaluation of female characteristics, which women themselves have internalized. Women, however, devalued brothers as well as sisters, suggesting a gender difference in expression of strong feelings.

Overall, older persons express lower negative ratings of siblings than younger persons. This is perhaps due to the successful completion of the developmental task of resolving sibling conflict in old age. The older adult years can provide siblings who have been estranged from each other with a rich opportunity to move toward reconciliation. Even older adult siblings who have had especially close relationships often find that the later years can be a time of increased closeness and sharing. It is at this time that many older adult siblings rediscover each other as travel companions, as a source of emotional support, and as fellow travelers back into the land of family memories and nostalgia.

INFLUENCE OF FAMILY SIZE AND GENDER

The nature of sibling relationships is partly determined by the size and gender composition of the sibling group. A brother whose siblings include a sister is more likely to be close to his siblings than one who has only brothers.

The bond between sisters is closest, and sisters are more likely to take care of each other. For example, a seventy-five-year-old widow left her children in the East when her husband died and returned to her Ohio hometown to be near her two sisters. The three sold their own homes, bought a home together, and pooled their possessions and other resources. When one of the sisters became ill, they hired an aide to provide some daily care. And because all the sisters pitched in, no single individual had to bear a large burden.

Men's ties to their siblings are likely to be of longer duration than any other relationship in their lives, especially in families in which children are closely spaced. Because of divorce, men may become outsiders in their family of procreation, and as a result, siblings may play an increasingly important role in men's lives as they grow older.

DEATH OF SIBLINGS

The first death among older adult siblings has a profound effect on each sibling. It is a break in the mental and emotional armor that protects them from their own sense of mortality. Most research emphasis has been placed on the impact of the death of parents of older adults. The first and later deaths of siblings remove or reduce any chance for siblings who are emotionally distanced from each other to resolve their differences. Each death also removes one more member of the childhood memory bank. Another person with whom early family experiences were shared is gone forever.

Sibling sharing of memories can serve as a buffer for some older adults as they struggle with the more difficult aspects of aging. As older adult siblings begin to die, the sibling structure changes profoundly. Younger members in a large family can become the oldest, or the youngest can become the only child at the death of the last older sibling.

TRENDS

Current demographic trends will affect these relationships in future decades. As more couples remain childless or have only one or two children, siblings will become even more important supports. Greater longevity and better health among the current middle-aged cohort imply greater availability of living siblings in the future. This is a particularly salient issue for baby boomers who are rapidly approaching sixty-five years of age. This group tends to have more siblings than children as potential support providers. However, reduced fertility rates in the current period will mean that later cohorts will have fewer siblings on whom to rely.

—*Peggy Shifflett*

See also: Caregiving; Childlessness; Communication; Family relationships; Friendship; Social ties

For Further Information

Degges-White, Suzanne. *Sisters and Brothers for Life.* Rowman & Littlefield, 2017. Examining such factors as the early family constellation, birth order, cultural diversity, and family communication patterns, Degges-White illustrates how sibling relationships can affect so many other areas of our lives, and considers how adult sibling conflict, rivalry, abuse, and loss influence our lives.

Goldfarb, Anna. "How to Maintain Sibling Relationships." *The New York Times,* 8 May 2018. www.nytimes.com/2018/05/08/smarter-living/how-to-maintain-sibling-relationships.html. A collection of advice, using input from experts, on how to improve relationships with siblings in adulthood.

Greif, Geoffrey L, and Michael E. Woolley. *Adult Sibling Relationships.* Columbia U P, 2016. With in-depth case studies of more than 260 siblings over the age of forty and interviews with experts on mental health and family interaction, this book offers vital direction for traversing the emotional terrain of adult sibling relations.

Henig, Robin Marantz. "Your Adult Siblings May Be the Secret to a Long, Happy Life." NPR, National Public Radio, 27 Nov. 2014. www.npr.org/sections/health-shots/2014/11/27/366789136/your-adult-siblings-may-be-the-secret-to-a- long-happy-life. Henig describes her relationship with her own younger brother, as well as reviews current studies and statistics that explore the benefits and downsides of sibling relationships in adult life.

Soysal, F. Selda Öz. "A Study on Sibling Relationships, Life Satisfaction and Loneliness Level of Adolescents." *Journal of Education and Training Studies,* vol. 4, no. 4, 2016. doi:10.11114/jets.v4i4.1240. This study examines the relation between sibling relationships, life satisfaction, and the loneliness level of adolescents with regard to gender, order of birth, and sibling dyads.

SINGLEHOOD

Relevant Issues: Family, psychology

Significance: People who have never married often experience a level of satisfaction in many aspects of late adulthood equal to that of married people; both groups tend to experience greater satisfaction than do their divorced and widowed agemates.

Although the vast majority of adults in all societies marry at some point in their lives, a small number of individuals reach old age having never married. Once known as "avowed bachelors" or "aging spinsters," this group of elders is now referred to as never-married or ever-single people, or lifelong singles. Popular myths depict this group of older, never-married adults as being unhappy, regretful, and even bitter. Society expects adults to fulfill certain roles as they go through the life span, and people who do not marry are typically viewed as shirking social responsibility or missing out on some of life's pleasures.

Popular wisdom and gerontological research concur that married people fare better than unmarried people throughout life, especially in late adulthood when they enjoy the benefits of better health, wealth, and happiness than their unmarried counterparts. However, the question arises over what aspects of married life contribute to this outcome. Is it the presence of a spouse in later years? Is it because married people have not experienced the negative consequences of being widowed or divorced? A closer examination of lifelong single people in their later years has provided compelling support for the latter.

LIFELONG SINGLES AND HEALTH

Several studies have divided older single people into four categories: divorced, widowed, separated, and never married. When comparisons are made among these groups, those who have never married report having the best health and fewest disabilities than those in the other three groups. Older adults who have never married also have the lowest incidence of suicide and report higher levels of mental health than the divorced and separated elders.

Even though never-married individuals enjoy better mental and physical health than those who are divorced, widowed, and separated, they are more apt to spend the later years of their lives living in nursing homes. This does not necessarily reflect a sudden decline in health for the lifelong single elders, but rather a lack of traditional caregiving options. When an older person can no longer live independently, the first option is to remain at home and be cared for by a healthier spouse. If no spouse is available, the second option is to remain at home and be cared for by a son or daughter. A person who has never married usually does not have these options and, as a result, enters assisted living facilities or nursing homes at a younger age and in better health than older adults who have spouses or children.

LIFELONG SINGLES AND WEALTH

Most of the information on lifelong singles in late adulthood comes from studies of women. The major reason for this is simply that older women outnumber older men in almost every category, and lifelong singles are no exception.

Women who have never married achieve more in their careers than women who marry. They have more education and advance further and more quickly in their jobs. One reason for this is that lifelong single women typically work steadily throughout their career years and do not take time off for childbearing and child rearing. In addition, women who have never married seldom have children to support and educate or the unexpected financial responsibilities of single parenthood after divorce or widowhood. Furthermore, women who have never married are more apt than other women to plan for retirement. With high and steady incomes during early and middle adulthood, no dependents, and the opportunity to focus most of their time and energy on their careers, women who have never married tend to go into retirement with solid assets and good pensions.

Although never-married women have higher incomes in retirement than divorced or separated women, they have lower incomes than widowed women who are collecting pensions from their late husband's earnings because of the income differential between equally qualified men and women that was common and substantial in decades past. Formerly married women with histories of low wages, and those who did not work at all, can collect retirement benefits based on their late husbands' higher wages. In spite of having lower incomes than widows, lifelong single women report equal satisfaction with their retirement incomes, while divorced and separated women report significantly less satisfaction with this aspect of their retirement years.

LIFELONG SINGLES AND HAPPINESS

The happiness and life satisfaction of married couples has been studied across the life span. General findings have been that early adulthood is a happy time for couples, middle adulthood is a little more difficult, and the later years bring renewed happiness and life satisfaction. One of the major causes of the middle adulthood dip in happiness is children. Couples with no children report more stable levels of happiness and life satisfaction across the life span.

When taken as a group, men and women who have never married are happier than married people in early adulthood and less happy in late adulthood. However, when the happiness levels of men and women are considered separately, older never-married women are significantly happier than their male counterparts. In fact, comparing never-married women with married women in later years shows little difference in happiness levels, while never-married men are significantly less happy than their married counterparts.

Another important factor in the happiness of older adults is the presence or absence of social support, which is defined as having people in one's life in whom one may confide and from whom one receives caring, positive attention. The typical source of social support for adults is a spouse, and those who have lost spouses through divorce or widowhood report lower levels of life satisfaction and adjustment.

Studies of people who do not marry, especially women, show that they maintain close ties with their parents during early and middle adulthood, often being the primary caregivers of elderly parents. They also have close relationships with their siblings throughout adulthood and foster close relationships with nieces and nephews. Furthermore, the lifelong single person often has close and long-term friendships with people they consider family, relationship sociologists refer to as "Fictive kin." Lifelong single women report less loneliness than divorced or widowed women in late adulthood, and they give indications of satisfaction with their social support equal to that of married women. Apparently, the relationships lifelong singles cultivate throughout adulthood provide social support in the later years similar to that enjoyed by married couples. In contrast, it seems that married people do not seek out these additional sources of social support during early and middle adulthood, and if they are widowed or divorced, they experience more social isolation than the lifelong single person.

In general, it seems that marriage is the best life situation for older adults who chose to marry, and singlehood is the best life situation for older adults who chose not to marry. Problems arise when those who chose to marry find themselves living alone for reasons beyond their control, such as the death of their spouse or divorce.

—*Barbara R. Bjorklund*

See also: Divorce; Facility and institutional care; Family relationships; Marriage; Men and aging; Retirement; Social ties; Widows and widowers; Women and aging

For Further Information

Kislev, Elyakim. *Happy Singlehood: The Rising Acceptance and Celebration of Solo Living.* U of California P, 2019. Based on personal interviews, quantitative analysis, and extensive review of singles' writings and literature, Kislev uncovers groundbreaking insights on how unmarried people create satisfying lives in a world where social structures and policies are still designed to favor marriage.

Tamborini, Christopher R. "The Never-Married in Old Age: Projections and Concerns for the Near Future." *Social Security Bulletin*, vol. 67, no. 2, 2007. This article focuses on a growing yet understudied subgroup of the elderly in the United States: the never-married and assesses how never-married persons fare during retirement.

SKIN CANCER

Relevant Issues: Health and medicine
Significance: The skin is the most common site of cancer in older light-skinned residents of North America.
Key Terms:

keratosis: an area of skin marked by overgrowth of horny tissue

melanin: a dark brown to black pigment occurring in the hair, skin, and iris of the eye in people and animals; it is responsible for tanning of skin exposed to sunlight

melanoblast: a cell that originates from the neural crest and differentiates into a pigment cell

melanocyte: a mature melanin-forming cell, especially in the skin

The largest organ in the body, the skin is the body's interface with the physical and chemical constituents of the external world, many of which are harmful and can cause cancer in the long term. Human skin is composed of two layers: The outer, protective epidermis covers a deeper layer called the dermis. The basal layer of the epidermis adjacent to the dermis contains a number of specialized cells, melanoblasts and melanocytes, that produce the pigment melanin, which gives the skin its color. The dermis contains blood and lymphatic vessels, sensory nerve endings, and specialized structures such as sweat glands, sebaceous glands, and hair follicles. Epidermal cancers are overwhelmingly more common than cancers of the dermal components (nonepithelial skin cancers). The common types of epidermal cancers are discussed here.

TYPES AND CAUSES OF SKIN CANCER

Of the many different varieties of skin cancer, the three most common are basal cell carcinomas, squamous cell carcinomas, and melanomas or malignant melanomas. The first two behave in a distinctly less aggressive fashion than the last and are generally discussed under the rubric nonmelanoma skin cancers.

Skin cancers are not inherited, although conditions favoring skin cancer formation are. Because external or internal irritants take considerable time to result in cancer, skin cancers are often seen in aging populations. The most common cause of skin cancer production is the sun's ultraviolet (UV) rays. Vertical rays of the sun are particularly dangerous, as the atmospheric ozone layer can screen out considerable portions of the UV rays. Equatorial latitudes and the sun exposure between 10 A.M. and 3 P.M. are particularly potent in causing skin cancer. UV rays are also reflected by sheets of water or snow and from sandy beaches. The effect of the sun's rays is mainly on the melanoblasts in the basal layer of the skin. Natural pigmentation of the skin is the best protection against the UV rays. Hence, skin cancers are significantly more prevalent in light-skinned individuals.

Other, rare causes of skin cancer include chronic non-healing scars from injuries or burns and prolonged exposure to arsenicals, as in a contaminated water supply. Some forms of medical treatment can also be carcinogenic: Special types of X-rays, hydroxyurea derivatives used in the treatment of myeloproliferative disorders, and immunosuppression for organ transplantation can all increase the incidence of nonmelanoma skin cancers.

INCIDENCE

Basal cell carcinomas and squamous cell carcinomas are the most common type of skin cancers in the United States and also the most easily treated. In 2019, the American Cancer Society estimates that 5.4 million cases of basal and squamous cell skin cancers are diagnosed in the United States. These numbers keep rising due to longer life expectancy, improvements in diagnosis, and more sun exposure. The death rate from these cancers is estimated at 2,000 per year. While melanoma is less common, accounting for only one percent of skin cancers, it is the most frequent cause of death from skin cancer in the United States. The rates of melanoma have also been rising and the American Cancer Society estimates that in 2019, 96,480 individuals will be diagnosed with melanoma. The death rate from melanoma is estimated at 7,230 per year. Age increases the risk of melanoma; the average age of diagnosis is 63.

NONMELANOMA SKIN CANCERS

The skin shows a number of changes with increasing age. Of these, superficial flaky lesions called solar or actinic keratoses on the sun-exposed skin of the head and neck and extremities, especially the backs of the hands, are considered to be premalignant, or precursors of later basal cell carcinomas and squamous cell carcinomas. These cancers arise in skin as a result of chronic sun exposure. Other rare precursor conditions include abnormal lack of pigmentation, such as that found in xeroderma pigmentosa, albinism, and Bowen's disease.

In North America, basal cell carcinomas are about four times more common than squamous cell carcinomas. Basal cell carcinomas are especially common on the head and neck and may have a number of different appearances. Generally, they are pearly, discrete plaques in the skin with a long history of slow growth. They may be pigmented (and, therefore, can be mistaken for melanoma) or ulcerated with serpiginous edges (sometimes called a rodent ulcer). Long-neglected basal cell carcinomas can produce monstrous local deformities. They rarely spread to distant organs (metastasize) and are quite amenable to the standard treatment modalities.

Squamous cell carcinomas are the less common but more threatening nonmelanoma skin cancers. Arising on nonexposed as well as sun-exposed skin, they are usually red, ulcerated, and raised above the skin, although clinical differentiation between them and basal cell carcinomas is usually impossible. If they are neglected, a number of them will proceed to the local and then distant lymph nodes and even to distant viscera, such as the lungs.

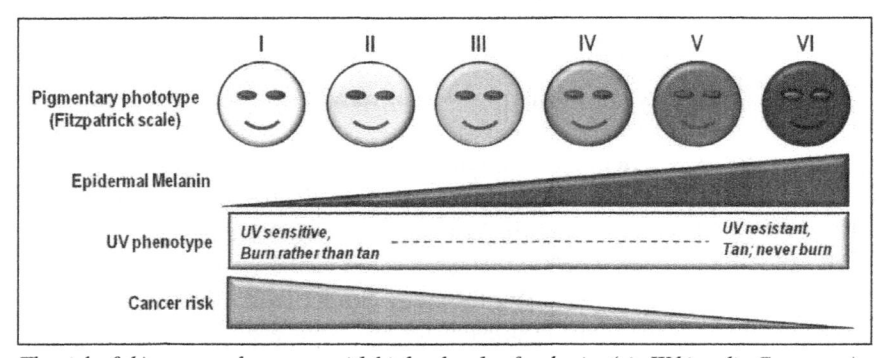

The risk of skin cancer decreases with higher levels of melanin. (via Wikimedia Commons)

Cancers arising on burn scars (Marjolin's ulcer) are often squamous cell carcinomas. This type of skin cancer is eminently curable with early surgical excision.

MALIGNANT MELANOMAS

Melanomatous skin cancers arise from the melanoblasts in the epidermis. These cancers are more common in light-skinned people, especially those with light-colored or blond hair, blue or green eyes, and of Celtic descent. Malignant melanomas are the most rapidly increasing type of cancer in the United States. Acute intensive sunburn, particularly in children or teenagers, is thought to cause these cancers in later life.

Melanomas are seen at ages earlier than nonmelanoma skin cancers. Four clinical types are recognized, based on appearance, both clinical and histological, and the natural history of the disease: superficial spreading melanoma, nodular-type melanoma, acral lentiginous-type melanoma, and lentigo maligna.

Superficial spreading melanoma is the most common type (50 to 70 percent). These malignant cells spread horizontally along the dermal-epidermal plane, with little tendency to penetrate the dermis. Thus, they are distant from the lymphatic and venous channels thought to be necessary for distant spread. The peak incidence is in the fourth and fifth decades of life, and common sites are on the legs and backs of white women and the upper backs of white men.

Nodular-type melanoma is less common (15 to 30 percent) but considerably more dangerous than superficial spreading melanoma. The cells proliferate in a vertical plane. Therefore, they form nodules on the skin and also invade the dermis. Their propensity to spread (and hence their potential lethality) has been shown to relate to the depth to which they penetrate both by histological layer and by measured thickness.

These two types constitute the great majority of melanomas. Clinically, melanomas have a variegated appearance with varying shades of brown and black in the lesion, which is generally more than 6 millimeters in diameter. The colored patch may be in the plane of skin or raised even into the nodules. Its margins or borders are uneven. The lesions often arise spontaneously and progress relatively rapidly; they may occasionally rise on preexisting moles that suddenly change their appearance and start to grow. Some ulcerate, and others itch. In advanced cases, evidence of distant spread may be manifested by enlargement of draining lymph nodes or symptoms related to distant viscera.

Acral lentiginous-type melanomas (2 to 5 percent) are seen in the palms, soles, and under the nails of the hands and feet. This type is often seen in African Americans and generally appears in the seventh decade of life. Nail apparatus melanoma starts off as a flat, variegated, black patch that destroys the nail and soon becomes nodular. These lesions are particularly invasive.

Lentigo maligna (Hutchison's freckle) or lentigo maligna melanomas (1 to 2 percent) appear as broad, brown, and irregular patches on the sun-exposed skin of older persons. After a prolonged indolent course of many years, they start to proliferate rapidly and take on the characteristic appearance and lethality of nodular melanoma.

SOME SPECIAL CONSIDERATIONS

Immunosuppression in transplant patients causes cancers at various sites, including melanoma. The rate and site seem to be genetically influenced. According to C. S. Ong, A. M. Keogh, and colleagues, among light-skinned heart transplant patients in Australia, 31 percent developed nonmelanoma skin cancers after ten years and 43 percent developed them after twenty years; squamous cell carcinomas were three times more common than basal cell carcinomas. As reported by H. Kishikawa, Y. Ichikawa, and colleagues, among renal transplant patients in Japan, the new cancer rate was much lower, 3.9 percent at ten years and 13.9 percent at twenty years, and mainly in the digestive tract and not on the skin.

Genetic influences undoubtedly play a part in melanoma development and spread, though the exact relationship is currently unclear. Melanomas are often associated with defective p53 tumor suppressor genes (also seen in other cancers). The HLA-DR4 phenotype is associated with an increased risk of both melanomas and basal cell carcinomas.

DIAGNOSIS AND TREATMENT

Exact identification of the type of lesion is essential for appropriate treatment, follow-up, and prognosis of skin cancer patients. Therefore, it is essential to do a biopsy of any lesion that cannot be excised with an adequate margin. Microscopic examination is generally adequate, although more sophisticated methods such as staining for tumor-specific markers have to be used.

Surgical excision is the current preferred treatment for both nonmelanoma skin cancers and melanomas. A special combination of excision and chemosurgery (Moh's technique) may be used under special circumstances. Excisions of nonmelanoma skin cancers must be complete, with adequate and clear margins. Early surgery cures almost all basal cell carcinomas and over 95 percent of squamous cell carcinomas. Radiation therapy is effective in treating nonmelanoma skin cancers when surgery is refused or is impossible.

For melanomas, the width and depth of the excision are dependent on the thickness of the lesion. According to W. H. McCarthy and H. M. Shaw, for a thin melanoma, a 0.5 centimeter margin is probably adequate; deeper penetration requires a 1 to 3 centimeter margin of excision. The results of surgical treatment of melanomas have significantly improved in recent years. A near 100 percent cure can be expected with early superficial spreading melanomas. Nodular-type melanomas that are still limited to local tissues can be cured in 60 to 80 percent of patients. The modern technique of mapping sentinel lymph nodes to determine if there has been spread to the lymphatic system (in the absence of clinical findings) allows early clearance of affected nodes. With metastasis to the local lymph nodes, however, the cure rate drops to around 30 percent. With generalized spread to the visceral, a cure is unattainable by current methods.

No specific chemotherapeutic drugs are currently useful against nonmelanoma skin cancers. For advanced stages of melanoma, other therapies are used in the treatment of this disease. Immunotherapy stimulates the individual's own immune system to attack the cancer cells while targeted therapies identify different parts of the melanoma cells in the body and slow the growth of the cancer. Chemotherapy is not first-line treatment for advanced cancer but may be used if immunotherapy and targeted therapy are ineffective in order to help relieve symptoms. All of these therapies have significant side effects.

PREVENTION

Of the inciting causes of skin cancer, the one that is easiest to control is solar UV rays. Nonmelanoma skin cancers are caused by long-term or chronic exposure to these rays. They can be avoided by leaving as little of skin exposed as possible when outside. Skin that cannot be covered should be protected with repeated applications of a sunscreen with a sun-protecting factor (SPF) of at least 30 against both UVA and UVB rays. The practice of sunbathing not only ages skin but also increases the possibility of skin cancers, especially if exposure is to the vertical solar rays between 10 A.M. and 4 P.M. (Such sun protection does not decrease the important formation of vitamin D analogues by the skin.) Tanning beds emit both UVA and UVB rays and are not recommended.

The key to the prevention of skin cancer in middle and old age is caution in youth. Acute significant sunburn in children is particularly conducive to malignant melanomas in later life. It is, therefore, important to protect children from this type of exposure, especially on playing fields, beaches, and on hiking trips. While parents should be aware of this, children also need to be taught the dangers of exposure to UV rays. Use of clothing, hats, and sunglasses are other protective measures against the harmful effects of UV rays that should be employed at an early age.

Finally, recognition of the health hazards of ozone depletion is needed by the business and manufacturing communities, lawmakers, and the public. Skin cancers, both nonmelanoma skin cancers and melanomas, in older adults are among the many unwelcome legacies of this human assault on the environment.

—*Ranès C. Chakravorty*
Updated by Mary E. Dietmann, EdD, APRN, CNS

See also: Cancer; Skin changes and disorders

For Further Information

Agnew, Karen L., et al. *Fast Facts: Skin Cancer.* Revised 2nd ed. Karger Publishers, 2015. Written by three international experts in skin cancer treatment to equip health-care professionals with the necessary skills to save lives.

Dong, Haidong, and Svetomir N. Markovic. *The Basics of Cancer Immunotherapy.* Springer International Publishing, 2018. The patient-friendly, concise, easy-to-understand, and up-to-date knowledge presented in this book will inform patients about the benefits and risks of cancer immunotherapy, and help them and their care providers to understand how immunotherapy would control their unique disease.

Forest, Chris. *What You Need to Know about Cancer.* Capstone P, 2016. Clear, concise information breaks down the disease, the experience of having it, or relating to someone who has cancer. Be inspired by true stories from youths who have experienced cancer in their own lives, and how they fought this disease.

Garcovich, Simone, et al. "Skin Cancer Epidemics in the Elderly as An Emerging Issue in Geriatric Oncology." *Aging and Disease*, vol. 8, no. 5, 1 Oct. 2017, pp. 643-61. doi:10.14336/ad.2017.0503. Reviews the recent evidence on the scope and problem of skin cancer in the elderly population as well as age-related variations in its clinical management, highlighting the potential role of a geriatric approach in optimizing dermato-oncological care.

Halloran, Laurel. "Here Comes the Sun: Addressing Skin Cancer." *The Journal for Nurse Practitioners*, vol. 10, no. 6, June 2014, pp. 439-40. doi:10.1016/j.nurpra.2014.03.005. Provides advice for nurses dealing with skin cancer diagnoses and patients.

Kogler, Peter. *Skin Cancer: America's Most Common Cancer.* Lucent, 2019. Through engaging text, augmented with full-color photographs, quotes from experts, and detailed charts, readers learn about the newest data and research pertaining to skin cancer as well as the steps they can take to reduce their risk of developing it.

Shahrokni, Armin, et al. "How We Care for an Older Patient with Cancer." *Journal of Oncology Practice*, vol. 13, no. 2, 1 Feb. 2017, pp. 95-102. doi:10.1200/jop.2016.017608. Describes how the Geriatrics Service at Memorial Sloan Kettering Cancer Center approaches an older patient with colon cancer from presentation to the end of life, show the importance of GA at the various stages of cancer treatment, and how predictive models are used to tailor the treatment.

SKIN CHANGES AND DISORDERS

Relevant Issues: Health and medicine

Significance: Changes in skin and hair are the most visible signs of aging; skin changes predispose the elderly to develop age-related skin disorders.

Structurally, the skin is composed of three layers: the outer epidermis, the middle dermis, and the underlying hypodermis or subcutaneous layer. Specialized cells in the skin include keratinocytes, which produce keratin, a fibrous, horny material that acts as a protective, mechanical shield. Melanocytes produce melanin, the substance that gives the skin its color tones and acts as a screen to protect the body from ultraviolet rays. Langerhans cells in the skin are part of the immune system and protect the body against harmful substances. The appendages of the skin include the eccrine and apocrine sweat glands, sebaceous glands, nails, and hair.

Functionally, skin acts as a barrier that provides protection against loss of body fluid, trauma, and microbes and other harmful agents. Skin also assists in the regulation of body temperature, secretes sweat and sebum, participates in the synthesis of vitamin D, and contains sensory receptors to touch, pain, and temperature.

THE EFFECTS OF AGING

All skin structures and functions are adversely affected by the aging process. Skin changes occur because of intrinsic factors related to inevitable tissue aging, as well as extrinsic factors, primarily exposure to ultraviolet light. Skin damage caused by ultraviolet light is referred to as photodamage, while skin change caused by ultraviolet rays is referred to as photoaging or dermatoheliosis. The extent of change to the epidermis and dermis is related to the cumulative effects of the aging process and sun exposure. Chronically sun-exposed skin looks leathery, thickened, and deeply creased. A comparison can be made between the sun-exposed skin of the face and the covered skin over the buttock. Overall, melanocytes decrease in number with age, leaving the skin more sensitive to ultraviolet rays. Darker skin has more protective melanocytes and, therefore, shows less damage from the sun's ultraviolet rays. The development of many noncancerous (benign) and cancerous (malignant) skin lesions is related to the effects of ultraviolet rays.

Cigarette smoking contributes to an aged appearance of the skin. Characteristic skin changes associated with smoking include "purse-string" wrinkles around the lip border and increased wrinkles over the face. Skin changes correlate to length and quantity of smoking (pack years).

Changes occur in the structure of all layers of the skin with age. As cell reproduction in the epidermis declines, the skin layer becomes less dense, and the skin will appear thinner. In the very old, the skin looks like parchment; the fragile, thinner skin is easily torn. Superficial blood vessels are more prominent, and easy bruising occurs because the small blood vessels lose the support originally provided by the connective tissue and subcutaneous pad. The blood vessels are more easily traumatized, resulting in irregular-shaped, purplish, superficial hemorrhages of various sizes called actinic or senile purpura, which can last for several weeks. These purpuric areas can occur spontaneously from the leakage of superficial capillaries. Senile purpura are frequently seen on the hands and forearms. The area of attachment between the epidermis and dermis decreases with age, enabling the skin to tear more easily with shearing force.

Other age-related changes include a decrease in the function of the sebaceous and sweat glands located within the skin. The sebum produced by the sebaceous glands lubricates the hair follicle and, to a lesser degree, lubricates the skin. A decline in function results in a diminished production of oil and drier skin. Sebum has antimicrobial properties, so the decrease makes the skin surface more vulnerable to infection. The decline in sweat production contributes to dryness of the skin. Drier skin with less perspiration results in a condition called xerosis. The exact cause of xerosis is unknown, but it is typically, and commonly, seen in the elderly. The skin is rough, dry, and flaky. The dryness causes skin to itch (pruritus). Low humidity, harsh soaps, hot baths, rough clothing, and exposure to sun can compound the itchiness. Scratching can cause breaks in the skin that can become infected. With less sweat production, the cooling mechanism of perspiration and evaporation is lost or diminished. This increases the risk of hyperthermia or heat stroke in the elderly.

Structural changes in the collagen and elastic fibers of the dermis of the skin cause a loss of suppleness and elasticity. The skin becomes progressively more inelastic and lax, resulting in wrinkling and sagging. Facial wrinkling begins as early as the second decade of life as a result of repeated muscle movement associated with facial expressions. These wrinkles can be seen around the eyes and mouth and over the forehead as aging occurs. Additional fine, diffuse wrinkles appear over the skin with the loss of moisture and elasticity of the dermal layer and the decrease in the subcutaneous or fatty layer of the skin. A decrease in the elasticity and turgor also results in loose or drooping skin seen most obviously under the chin, along the jaw, beneath the eyes, and in the earlobes.

The lax, loose skin can result in overlapping folds, creating intertriginous areas where two skin surfaces are in constant contact. One such area is the corner of the mouth, where the loose skin from the cheek and upper lip overlaps the lower, outer lip. Overlapping is exaggerated in those individuals who are edentulous (without teeth). Other intertriginous areas are under the breasts and in the groin area. Moisture collects where skin surfaces overlap; this creates an environment conducive to skin breakdown and the development of skin infections.

Age changes cause the barrier functions of the skin to be less effective, and the elderly are more prone to develop contact dermatitis caused by sensitivity to such substances as leather goods, certain metals, and formaldehyde in clothing fabric. A decrease in Langerhans cells leads to a decline in immune response by the skin and an increased risk for skin infection. The elderly are also more prone to photosensitivity reactions when exposed to the sun. Photosensitivity is a side effect of a number of medications frequently taken by older adults.

Nerve endings for pain and temperature perception that are located in the skin decline with age. The decrease in function can lead to frostbite and burns. Once injury to the skin occurs, tissue repair and healing will be a slower process in the elderly, partly because of the decreased vascularity of the dermis and decreased cell reproduction. This is true of all wound healing; the process takes longer in the elderly, and wound separation is more likely to occur.

With a decrease in the subcutaneous layer, which serves as a "padding" or "cushion," bony prominences and joints appear more conspicuous, sharper, and more angular; at the same time, hollows around the bony skeleton deepen. These changes are apparent over the upper chest, shoulders, and neck. Because of the loss of padding, the elderly are more likely to sustain injuries from a fall, and bedridden elderly are more prone to developing pressure ulcers (bed sores) over bony prominences. As the subcutaneous fat pad also serves as insulation, other consequences of loss of the subcutaneous layer are feeling cold more easily and vulnerability to hypothermia.

With age, skin color appears less uniform and more blotchy. Functioning melanocytes do not spread evenly, so areas of hyperpigmentation and hypopigmentation occur. These changes are generally related to photodamage and are more apparent in fair-complexioned individuals. Increased freckling and lentigo are common. Senile or solar lentigines, also called age spots or liver spots, are round, flat, brown areas of various sizes with well-defined borders. They occur in chronically sun-exposed areas, usually over the face and back of the hands and wrists. Lentigo appear during the middle decades of life, and the number and size increase with age. Whitish, depigmented patches, termed pseudoscars, appear as well.

Senile or cherry angiomas are tiny, red, slightly raised lesions that turn brown with age. Cherry angiomas are vascular in origin. They appear over the trunk and arms in midlife and increase with age. Telangiectasias, which are small, superficial, dilated blood vessels, are frequently seen over the nose, cheeks, and thighs.

A decrease in melanocytes results in the graying of the hair. The age of onset for graying is typically in the thirties, although darkly pigmented individuals begin graying approximately one decade later. A decline in sebaceous oil production causes the hair to feel coarser and to look less shiny. The rate of hair growth declines. Although more pronounced in men, scalp hair in both men and women becomes sparser with increased age. There is an increase in coarse facial hair in women and an increase in nasal, ear, and eyebrow hair in men. With aging, nails thicken, take on a yellowish color, and develop heavy vertical ridges. The nail plate becomes more brittle and can split or peel. Changes in the toenails are more apparent than in fingernails. Thickening of the toenails can make them difficult to trim. An inability to keep the feet and nails clean can lead to fungal infections of the toenails.

SKIN DISORDERS

Senile or seborrheic keratosis is a common, pigmented skin growth that usually first appears in middle age. They develop from the keratin-containing cells of the skin; increased melanocytes give them their dark color. Keratoses are yellow-brown to black, raised, wart-like lesions that become darker and larger over time. They vary in size and have a sharp border, and most appear to be set on top of the skin surface. Sun exposure does not seem to be a factor in their development, as they appear on covered body surfaces, such as the back. It is not clear what factors do contribute to their development, but there appears to be a familial tendency. Seborrheic keratoses originally appear as small, flat, tan areas. They most commonly develop on the trunk, face, scalp, and neck, and increase in number with age. They can appear singularly or in profusion over the body. Dermatosis papulosa nigra is a form of seborrheic keratosis seen in darkly pigmented individuals. These lesions are small and raised and may be pedunculated. Multiple lesions develop over the face and neck. Seborrheic keratoses are benign growths, creating a cosmetic rather than a medical problem. The growths can be removed with cryotherapy, electrodesiccation, or laser therapy.

Actinic or solar keratoses, unlike seborrheic keratoses, are precancerous. They appear as tannish-red or pigmented, roughened or scaly patches on sun-exposed areas, such as the hands, forearms, face, bald scalp, and ears. Solar keratoses are treated with cryotherapy, fluoroplex cream, or laser therapy. Cutaneous horns, which develop from one type of actinic keratoses, are skin-colored, hard projections of keratinized skin. They vary in size from a few millimeters to several millimeters and usually grow on the hands or forehead. Although usually benign, in some cases the base can be cancerous, so removal and biopsy is usually recommended.

Skin tags or acrochordons are also more common with increasing age. They are soft, skin-colored or pigmented, pedunculated growths that develop frequently on the neck, axilla, inner thigh, and other areas of friction. Skin tags are small, usually 1 to 3 millimeters. They can appear singly or in large numbers. Skin tags present no health problem and are easily removed. Keratoacanthoma is a skin-colored elevation of the skin with a central area of keratin. These lesions develop rapidly, usually on sun-exposed areas in individuals over fifty years of age, and resolve spontaneously over a few months. Because they closely resemble squamous cell carcinomas, a biopsy is indicated.

Sebaceous gland hyperplasia frequently occurs on the forehead and nose. The lesion appears as a yellow, slightly raised area with a central depression, ranging in

> **SENIOR TALK:**
>
> **How Do You Feel About Bruising?**
> You may feel concerned or anxious when you notice your body bruising easily. You might be worried that it's a sign of a serious illness, or you might have no idea where the bruises came from. It can be relieving to speak to your doctor or dermatologist and learn that bruising is often a normal part of the aging process. If you have a particular concern, such as a long-lasting bruise or many sudden bruises with no obvious cause, consult a doctor right away. They can advise you regarding the type of bruising and possible underlying health problems. If you're concerned that medications are contributing to your bruising, a doctor can recommend dose adjustments or alternatives.
>
> It's common to feel self-conscious about bruises if they're on exposed areas of your body. Rest assured that many other adults also experience bruising. You may choose to wear clothing or makeup to cover your bruises. However, you should not hide bruising from your doctor. Your doctor needs to know about the condition to treat any underlying causes. This is especially important if you're experiencing falls or other injuries that might be preventable, such as elder abuse.
>
> —*Leah Jacob*

size from 1 to 3 millimeters. It is important to differentiate these benign lesions from basal cell carcinoma. Sebaceous hyperplasia is most often the result of chronic sun damage. Sun damage can also lead to solar elastosis, a condition characterized by a thickening of the fibers in the dermal layer. Other features of sun-damaged skin are nodularity, comedones or blackhead, ruddiness, and telangiectasias. Treatment generally includes topical tretinoin (Retin A).

Although herpes zoster (shingles) can occur at any age, the vast majority of cases occur in those over forty years of age, perhaps because of the decline in immune system functioning with age. In a significant number of elderly persons, postherpetic neuralgia or pain persists after the herpes lesions have healed. The pain can continue for months or indefinitely.

Although two malignant skin cancers, basal cell and squamous cell carcinomas, commonly occur in the elderly, they rarely metastasize beyond the site of origin. Both types occur more often in males and in fair-skinned individuals.

Skin manifestations can occur with systemic medical disorders. One common example in the elderly is the skin changes that occur in the lower extremities resulting from circulatory problems. When venous blood drainage from the lower extremities is slowed, increased blood pressure in the venous system results (venous insufficiency). The increased pressure causes leakage from the blood vessels, which creates edema or fluid accumulation in the tissue. If the condition persists, the skin becomes tight, red, and scaly. The condition is referred to a stasis dermatitis or gravitational eczema. Hyperpigmentation develops over the anterior, lower leg from iron in the red blood cells being deposited in the tissue, a condition referred to as hemosiderosis. A chronic situation of decreased circulation and edema can result in skin breakdown or ulcer formation. Leg ulcers can also be the result of decreased arterial blood flow.

Regardless of the amount of earlier sun damage, all individuals benefit from using sunscreen and protective clothing when they are exposed to the sun's rays. Totally avoiding sun exposure during midday is recommended. Moisturizers provide temporary relief from skin dryness. Mild soaps and bath oil clean the skin without further drying. Closely trimmed fingernails are less likely to cause abrasions if itching results in scratching. Adding humidity to the environment during the winter increases comfort. It is important to report any new, unusual, or changing skin lesions to a primary health-care provider.

—*Roberta Tierney*

See also: Age spots; Aging process; Cancer; Cosmetic surgery; Face lifts; Gray hair; Hair growth; Hair loss and baldness; Skin cancer; Smoking; Temperature regulation and sensitivity; Wrinkles

For Further Information

Blume-Peytavi, Ulrike, et al. "Age-Associated Skin Conditions and Diseases: Current Perspectives and Future Options." *The Gerontologist*, vol. 56, no. Suppl 2, 2016. doi:10.1093/geront/gnw003. Describes the main gaps and challenges associated with skin aging and argues why a public health approach is needed.

Dyer, Joseph M., and Richard A. Miller. "Chronic Skin Fragility of Aging." *Journal of Clinical and Aesthetic Dermatology*, vol. 11, no. 1, Jan. 2018, pp. 13-18. www.ncbi.nlm.nih.gov/pmc/articles/PMC5788262/. In this review, the authors explore the risk factors, pathogenetic mechanisms, clinical expression, and evidence-based therapies reported for chronic skin fragility due to aging.

Farage, Miranda A., et al. "Characteristics of the Aging Skin." *Advances in Wound Care*, vol. 2, no. 1, 2013, pp. 5-10. doi:10.1089/wound.2011.0356.

Linos, Eleni, et al. "Geriatric Dermatology—A Framework for Caring for Older Patients with Skin Disease." *JAMA Dermatology*, vol. 154, no. 7, 2018, p. 757. doi:10.1001/jamadermatol.2018.0286. The authors present unique considerations for the care of older persons with skin disease and describe central principles of geriatric science that allow for more appropriate care for this rapidly expanding segment of the population.

"Skin Care and Aging." National Institute on Aging, U.S. Department of Health and Human Services, 1 Oct. 2017. www.nia.nih.gov/health/skin-care-and-aging. General information on several skin related changes due to age.

SKIPPED-GENERATION PARENTING

Relevant Issues: Demographics, family

Significance: Grandparents who are raising their grandchildren have specific stresses that result from child rearing; support services can assist them with providing care.

While grandparents have always been a source of support in child rearing, the contemporary practice of providing primary care for their grandchildren can present older people with stressful family issues and need for support. In situations where a child permanently or temporarily loses a parent, the grandparent typically becomes the next available care provider in the family. While some grandparents may care for only one child, others raise several children who may range in age from infancy to late adolescence. Some grandchildren live with their grandparents for a time-limited period, such as a prison sentence, while others will be raised by their grandparents until adulthood.

Grandparenthood is a role that is not exclusively held by people in later life. Grandparents who are in their late thirties are not uncommon. Yet, many grandparents who are raising their grandchildren are past the usual age of child rearing, such as their fifties, sixties, or seventies. These older grandparents may have a difficult time readjusting to their caregiving role. In addition, these older adults are beginning to experience some age-related changes that can compromise their ability to provide care.

FAMILY ISSUES

Grandparents who are in midlife or later life may be experiencing the physical, social, and economic changes associated with the aging process. These age-related changes can compound the usual stresses that are associated with raising children. Grandparents often describe the physical exertion that is required in caring for younger children. The consequence ranges from "feeling run down" to exacerbating an existing health problem such as hypertension or diabetes. In addition, the time expended in child rearing leaves fewer hours for the grandparents to spend in other activities. Grandparents may eliminate positive health practices, such as exercising and sleeping, which also takes a negative toll on physical health.

There are also social costs related to caregiving. The child-rearing role can decrease the quality of the grandparents' marriage and other social relationships. One stressful aspect can be a lack of opportunities to spend time as a couple or with friends. The outcome can be a sense of isolation or loneliness for the grandparents.

The nature of the relationship with the parent of the child can also create tension within the family. A drug-addicted parent, for example, may reappear for a time and temporarily reunite with their children. This "sometimes parenting" can be frustrating and confusing for the children and create an additional strain around the caregiving relationship with the grandparent.

The relationship with the child's parent can also have an emotional price for the grandparents, who may feel a sense of guilt over the problems experienced by their own son or daughter. At the same time, they may struggle to continue hoping that their son or daughter can overcome his or her problems by being granted parole or overcoming an addiction. The outcome can be a confusing set of loyalties for the grandparents—being divided between having hope for their own son or daughter and feeling a sense of responsibility for their grandchildren.

As many of these grandparents have passed their own child-rearing years, the question of parenting competence also rises. Contemporary youths face different social situations and pressures—including violence in school, gangs, sexual relationships, drugs, and the prevalence of social media—than those existing when many grandparents raised their own children. Grandparents may not possess the knowledge or experience to know how to guide their grandchildren through these difficult issues.

The economics of child rearing can also present a stressor for these grandparents. While skipped-generation families are found in all income and racial groups, a disproportionate number are in low-income, African American families. These grandparents often have more limited financial resources to support a child. In addition, many of these child-care arrangements are informal; therefore, the family does not receive the social welfare benefits, such as cash subsidies or allowances, that may be available in formal custodial or guardianship situations.

Grandparents also report positive experiences in raising their grandchildren. For some, this opportunity is one that allows them a second chance to rectify mistakes that they may have made with their own children. A strong motivator is that the grandparent is able to keep the child out of the foster care system and provide a home with family members. In spite of the physical, social, and emotional consequences, the grandparents would feel worse if their grandchildren were raised by nonfamily care providers.

SUPPORT PROGRAMS

Because of the demands of raising a grandchild, several communities have instituted support programs for grandparents. Many such programs are aimed at decreasing isolation of the caregivers by helping them make contact with others of the same family form. Support groups may be sponsored by schools, churches, or other child welfare organizations for this purpose. These groups provide grandparents with a social outlet and an opportunity to discuss their experiences with others who share similar situations.

Respite care is another support program that can assist grandparents. Respite is a brief period of relief from the responsibilities of child rearing. This type of support can provide grandparents with an opportunity to spend time with their spouses or on themselves. This relief can come from someone taking care of the children within the household or from a group, such as an outing for the children to a community event.

Grandparents may also benefit from education on child development and social issues. Education groups can address a number of topics that help grandparents learn more about their grandchildren's social development. Particular topics may range from dealing with unmanageable behaviors of the grandchildren to contemporary social pressures such as sexual relationships, drugs, and violence. These sessions can provide information and opportunities for grandparents to build different parenting styles.

One area in which grandparents may need particular assistance is legal issues. There are often questions about terminating parental rights and gaining legal custody of the grandchildren. This process is one that is very emotional and complicated for grandparents. In addition, other legal issues need to be pursued carefully, such as estate planning and drafting a will. Often, legal issues come to attention in the case of a crisis, such as the health problem of a grandchild, when there is no formalized process to gain legal consent from the grandparents. To the greatest extent possible, grandparents should be aided in considering the legal action that needs to be taken prior to the occurrence of an emergency.

Children who are being raised in skipped-generation families may exhibit challenging child-rearing issues. Many of the children who are in the care of their grandparents have been through traumatic experiences with their parents. These backgrounds include physical or sexual abuse, neglect, or abandonment. In addition, the health status of the mother, especially if she had an addiction or was HIV-positive, can contribute to the health and mental health problems of the children. Because of such early life experiences, these children may present challenging behaviors to the grandparents, such as detachment, overdependency, or oppositional behaviors. Grandparents who have these experiences with their grandchild may need to have intensive support from a child mental health or guidance agency.

SUMMARY

The number of grandparents who are primary care providers of their grandchildren is on the rise. Many grandparents in these roles are past the period of caregiving for their own children and are experiencing some age-related changes that can add stress to child rearing. As these family forms increase in frequency, various programs will be constructed to help and support these families. Demographics suggest that an even-greater array of these types of services may be needed in the United States as the older population continues to expand.

—*Nancy P. Kropf*

See also: African Americans; Caregiving; Family relationships; Grandparenthood; Parenthood

For Further Information

Garrison, Gary. *Raising Grandkids: Inside Skipped-Generation Families*. U of Regina P, 2018. Collecting together stories from grandparents and reflecting on his own experience as an older caregiver to his stepchildren, Garrison paints a compassionate yet compelling picture of the joys, fears, and passions that drive some grandparents to put their later lives on hold to raise their children's children.

Hayslip, Bert, et al. "Grandparents Raising Grandchildren: What Have We Learned Over the Past Decade?" *The Gerontologist*, vol. 59, no. 3, 2017. doi:10.1093/geront/gnx106. In this manuscript, the authors update the literature over the last decade in addressing several new content areas that have emerged in the grandfamilies literature, along with issues that are still important to understanding grandparents raising their grandchildren today.

Moore, Susan, and Doreen Rosenthal. *Grandparenting: Contemporary Perspectives*. Routledge, 2017. Moore and Rosenthal draw on quantitative and qualitative, experimental, survey, observation and case study research, including unique data on grandfathers. They examine how people respond to the challenges and possibilities of grandparenting, and how this influences intergenerational relationships and adapting to growing older. The book provides a comprehensive, up-to-date evidence base for students in health, sociology and psychology and those interested in gerontology and the life span.

Scommegna, Paola. "More U.S. Children Raised by Grandparents." Population Reference Bureau, 26 Mar. 2012. www.prb.org/us-children-grandparents/.

Shakya, Holly Baker, et al. "Family Well-Being Concerns of Grandparents in Skipped Generation Families." *Journal of Gerontological Social Work*, vol. 55, no. 1, 2012, pp. 39-54. doi:10.1080/01634372.2011.620072. Co-resident grandparents who are responsible for raising their grandchildren completed surveys, focus groups, or individual interviews.

SLEEP CHANGES AND DISTURBANCES

Relevant Issues: Biology, health and medicine, psychology

Significance: A sizable proportion of the elderly report sleep disturbances, which can lead to problems in daytime functioning and dissatisfaction with quality of life.

The reasons why people sleep, like the reasons why people age, are not well known. Many researchers believe that sleep serves a restorative function. Indeed, it appears that sleep is necessary to keep the brain functioning normally; sleep deprivation can lead to distortions in perception and cognition. Rapid eye movement (REM) sleep is apparently necessary for brain development and learning. Whatever its function, sleep is irresistible and universal in all vertebrates.

STAGES OF SLEEP

There are several well-known stages that occur during a typical night's sleep. These stages are distinguished primarily by the electrical activity of the brain, as measured by an electroencephalogram (EEG), that occurs during each stage. These EEG recordings are in the form of wave activity and are described according to the frequency and amplitude of the wave. While awake but relaxed, a person's EEG will show electrical activity characterized by medium-frequency (8 to 12 hertz) and low-amplitude waves. Such activity is called alpha activity. When awake and alert, an individual's EEG activity will consist of beta activity—irregular, low-amplitude waves of 13 to 30 hertz.

During sleep, a person's EEG record will show regular movement among various stages, each characterized by a particular pattern of electrical activity. After becoming drowsy and falling asleep, a person enters stage 1 sleep, characterized by the presence of brain waves of 3.5 to 7.5 hertz. Approximately ten minutes later, the sleeper will enter stage 2 sleep, which consists of wave activity whose overall frequency is less than in stage 1. There will also be brief bouts of 12- to 14-hertz wave activity called sleep spindles during this stage. Stage 3 sleep, which follows about ten minutes after the onset of stage 2, consists of brain wave activity that has a lower frequency, but higher amplitude. The same is true for stage 4. Both stage 3 and stage 4 are considered deep sleep, or slow-wave sleep, and are characterized by the presence of bursts of very high amplitude delta activity (brain waves less that 3.5 hertz).

Approximately ninety minutes after the onset of sleep, the EEG pattern undergoes a drastic change in appearance. The waveform is indicative of a person who is awake. Other measurements (such as respiration and heart rate) also suggest that the person is awake. In spite of these measures, the person is still asleep but has entered a stage called REM sleep, named for the rapid eye movements that accompany this stage. An additional feature of REM sleep is the occurrence of dreaming. During a typical night's sleep, a person will experience four to five regular cycles of REM and non-REM sleep.

SLEEP CHANGES WITH AGE

Sleep problems are reported in approximately 40 percent of the elderly population and can result from a number of causes. For example, the changes seen in sleep might be the result of a normal aging process. They might also be secondary to a medical or psychiatric condition, or they might be the result of poor sleep hygiene. Sleep hygiene includes, among other factors, sleep schedule, bedroom acoustics and lighting, daytime napping, dietary habits, exercise (or lack of), exposure to daylight, and use of alcohol and caffeine. Each of these can affect the quality of an individual's sleep.

In general, older individuals experience a number of age-related changes in their sleep patterns. Included among these changes are spending more time in bed, spending less time asleep, decreased sleep efficiency (spending less time in stages 2, 3, and 4, but more time in stage 1), and taking more time to fall asleep. Research suggests that much of this change in sleep quality is not accounted for by medical or psychiatric problems. Some sleep disturbances are affected by diseases (such as dementia), which increase in prevalence with age; however, most research suggests that when health factors are controlled for, the prevalence of sleep complaints in the elderly are less than previously thought.

Sleep disorders that are age-related include sleep-related breathing disturbance (SRBD), or sleep apnea, and periodic leg movement during sleep (PLMS), or nocturnal myoclonus. However, it is not clear whether the presence of SRBD or PLMS has any debilitating effect on daytime functioning in the elderly, so the clinical significance of these disorders is questionable.

A disproportionate number of prescriptions for sedatives are given to the elderly who complain of poor sleep quality. These sedatives, while perhaps useful for the transient relief of sleep disorders, have limited useful-

Complications of Insomnia

Psychological
- Lower performance
- Slowed reaction time
- Risk of depression
- Risk of anxiety disorder

Poor immune system function

Other:
Overweight or obesity

High blood pressure

Risk of heart disease

Risk of diabetes

> **SENIOR TALK:**
>
> **How Do You Feel About Sleep Changes?**
> The effects of insomnia, being unable to sleep, can create intense emotions. We need our sleep to feel well emotionally and physically. Depression and anxiety are common causes of insomnia or sometimes sleeping too much (hypersomnia). At the same time, insomnia can also cause us to feel depressed. Hypersomnia can likewise create feelings of fatigue, drowsiness, or agitation during the day. Stress can prevent us from sleeping, and we can also feel stressed because we are not getting enough rest. We may suffer from a shortened attention span, memory problems, and difficulty concentrating or engaging meaningfully in enjoyable activities. Chronic sleep problems also contribute to such major health problems as obesity, heart disease, and diabetes.
>
> When we are unable to fall asleep, or if we wake during the night and lie in bed tossing and turning, we can feel demoralized and frustrated. It is often at these moments in the dark that our minds start to wander, and we feel especially vulnerable, anxious, or afraid. We may feel frustrated about our inability to sleep. At these times, if we have been trying to fall asleep for an extended period, it is usually helpful to get out of bed and try to do something calming for a short time. You might choose to listen to a relaxing piece of music or to read something inspirational. Once we break the pattern of frustration or anxiety, we are in a better position to return to bed, calmer and ready to submit to sleep.
>
> *—Leah Jacob*

ness for the chronic treatment of sleep disturbances. Tolerance develops, and the administration of these drugs, ironically, can worsen the quality of sleep in those individuals already experiencing sleep disturbances.

CIRCADIAN RHYTHMS

Sleep is clearly a behavior that follows a rhythmic pattern. Not only does an individual cycle between sleep and wakefulness during a twenty-four-hour period, but also sleep itself follows a regular pattern of REM and non-REM sleep during the night. Research suggests that some of the disturbances in sleep seen with age are the result of changes in circadian rhythms. However, these changes in circadian rhythmicity and sleep quality with age might be reversible.

Circadian rhythms are regulated by the brain structures (the suprachiasmatic nucleus and the pineal gland) and neurochemicals (serotonin and melatonin) that make up the circadian system. This system regulates a number of physiological and behavioral functions, including body temperature and hormonal rhythms, in addition to the sleep-wakefulness rhythm. Age-related changes in the circadian system include a decrease in amplitude (the range of changes between the maximum and minimum values) and an advance in phase (a specific measuring point linked to a particular clock time). The most consistently reported change with age is diminished amplitude (reduced release of melatonin), which affects sleep quality by decreasing time spent sleeping during the night. This reduction in sleep quality can result in impaired alertness and performance the following day. Phase shifting results in a particular phase (for example, temperature regulation) occurring earlier according to clock time. For example, older adults regularly go to bed earlier than younger adults, and this change in behavior might be a function of an earlier phase of the body temperature rhythm. Declines in body temperature are a cue for sleeping, and if these declines occur earlier in the evening, a change in sleeping behavior could follow.

These changes in rhythmicity might result from a number of factors, including decreases in the sensitivity of the eye to light, changes in the biochemistry or structure of key sites in the circadian system, and reduction in exposure to light in the elderly. It has also been found that there are reductions in the release of melatonin, a hormone with soporific qualities. If reduced light and reductions in melatonin underlie the changes in the circadian system that occur with age, it is possible that these changes can be attenuated with therapy. Phototherapy and exogenous administration of melatonin are examples of therapies that might restore circadian rhythmicity and improve the overall quality of sleep in aging individuals.

Sleep changes with age can result from a number of causes. Some of these disturbances might be secondary to other medical or psychiatric problems; some are caused primarily by aging itself. In addition, judgment of sleep quality is, in many ways, a subjective appraisal. Disruption of sleep during the night might be very troubling for one individual but merely annoying for another. For these reasons, a careful examination of the overall health of the aging individual, as well as that individual's sleep hygiene, are necessary in any evaluation of sleep disturbance. The growth in the number of sleep laboratories and sleep disorder clinics in the United States has made such evaluations more feasible than in the past.

—Kevin S. Seybold

See also: Aging: Biological, psychological, and sociocultural perspectives; Aging process; Brain changes and disorders; Circadian rhythms; Depression; Medications; Menopause; Overmedication; Temperature regulation and sensitivity

For Further Information

"Aging Changes in Sleep." *MedlinePlus*, U.S. National Library of Medicine, 12 July 2017. medlineplus.gov/ency/article/004018.htm. General information on sleep changes that come with aging.

Li, Junxin, et al. "Sleep in Normal Aging." *Sleep Medicine Clinics*, vol. 13, no. 1, 2018, pp. 1-11. doi:10.1016/j.jsmc.2017.09.001. This article describes age-related changes in sleep, circadian rhythms, and sleep-related hormones.

Suzuki, Keisuke, et al. "Sleep Disorders in the Elderly: Diagnosis and Management." *Journal of General and Family Medicine*, vol. 18, no. 2, 2017, pp. 61-71. doi:10.1002/jgf2.27. Reviews sleep disorders commonly observed in the elderly and describes their diagnosis and management.

SMOKING

Relevant Issues: Death, health and medicine
Significance: Smoking poses important health risks that are significantly decreased by smoking cessation, even in older age.

Smoking is the main avoidable cause of death in the United States and many other developed nations. More than 10 percent of North Americans over the age of sixty-five smoke cigarettes, putting themselves and those with whom they live at risk for significant health problems. These risks appear to increase both with age and with the number of years of smoking, as well as the number of cigarettes smoked per day. After World War II, more women began smoking. Because the diseases related to smoking usually take several years to develop, only in the last part of the twentieth century did rates of smoking-related diseases among women began to approach those of men. On the other hand, research indicates that smoking cessation appears to be beneficial, even in a person who has smoked for many years.

THE HEALTH EFFECTS OF SMOKING

Cigarette smoking has long been known to have adverse effects. The adverse effects began to receive significantly after 1963, when the U.S. Surgeon General issued a detailed report linking smoking with ill health. Smokers get more wrinkles than nonsmokers, so they tend to look older than their chronological ages. They also are more likely to develop gum disease and lose teeth, adding to the changes related to eating, such as alterations in sense of smell and taste, that are normal as people age. Loss of teeth leads to difficulty chewing, which in turn leads to difficulties with digestion. Most people who lose teeth eventually develop loss of the bone that should support their teeth, making it increasingly difficult to fit dentures.

Smokers are ten times more likely to get lung cancer than nonsmokers. Lung cancer is now the number-one cause of cancer death in women, as well as in men. In addition to lung cancer, smokers have a higher incidence of cancers of the head and neck, esophagus, colon, rectum, kidney, bladder, and cervix. Smokers are twenty times more likely to have a heart attack than nonsmokers. In older people, the major risk factor for disease of the coronary arteries is hypertension, but smoking is still significant, especially when combined with other risk factors for heart disease, such as diabetes or high cholesterol. Smoking and diabetes are also the two most important risk factors for diseases of the veins and arteries of the lower leg. Those who continue to smoke once these diseases develop are much more likely to require limb amputation than those who quit. Smokers may develop chronic obstructive pulmonary disease (COPD), which includes emphysema and chronic bronchitis, and are eighteen times more likely than nonsmokers to die of diseases of the lungs other than cancer. Older smokers also show decreases in muscle strength, agility, coordination, gait, and balance. The changes in these areas make them seem five years older than their actual age.

Smoking also long has been associated with peptic ulcer disease. In addition, smoking makes the symptoms of many diseases worse or increases the risk of complications in patients with allergies, diabetes, hypertension, and vascular disease. Male smokers are at greater risk of experiencing sexual impotence. Female smokers tend to experience an earlier menopause and are at increased risk for hip fracture than nonsmokers. Smokers are more likely to develop glaucoma than nonsmokers. Studies completed in 1996 indicated an increased risk with smoking for macular degeneration, the leading cause of blindness in older adults. The evidence is mixed on smoking and Alzheimer's disease, but a 1998 study contradicted earlier work and found that the risk is greater in smokers than nonsmokers. Finally, smokers are at greater risk of death or injury caused by cigarette-related fires.

SMOKING AND MEDICATIONS

Cigarette smoking tends to speed up the processes in the liver for breaking down, using, and eliminating medications, both nonprescription and prescription. This means that medications may not perform as expected in the body. Smokers may need to take medications more frequently or in greater doses than nonsmokers, so it is important for health-care providers to know whether a person smokes. The drugs known to be affected by smoking include sedatives, narcotic and synthetic narcotic painkillers, certain antidepressants, anticoagulant medications, asthma medications, and beta blockers. These changes are of particular concern in the older population for a number of reasons. First, older people (whether smokers or nonsmokers) tend to need more medications than younger people. With each additional drug taken, the risk of serious drug interaction and other adverse effects increases. Secondly, changes in body composition and function that alter the metabolism of drugs come with age, making medication use somewhat riskier in older persons, in terms of adverse effects and complications. The additional changes associated with smoking increase these risks significantly.

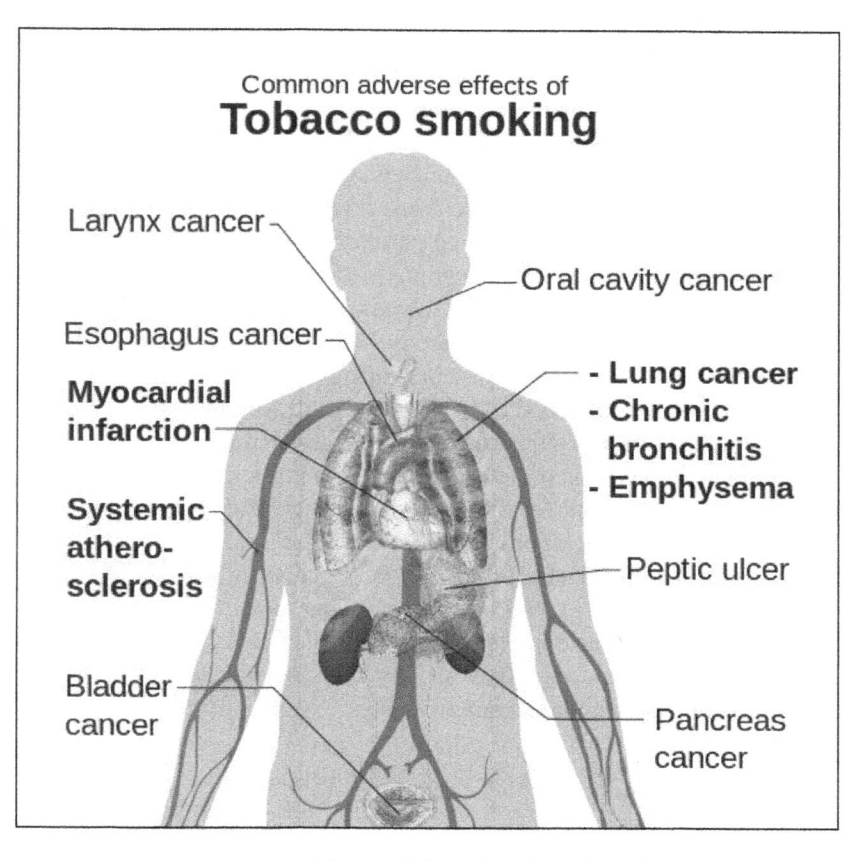

The dangers of passive smoking are well documented. The effects seem to be more harmful in children than in adults, but adults who are affected are at increased risk for cancer, heart disease, noncancerous lung diseases, and allergies.

THE BENEFITS OF SMOKING CESSATION

Numerous studies have shown that smoking cessation has health benefits in as little as one year, such as reducing the risk of heart attack and coronary artery disease. Within two years of smoking cessation, the risks of stroke and diseases of the blood vessels in the lower leg are reduced as well. Even though chronic lung disease is not reversible, those who quit smoking slow the decline in lung function considerably. Risks for cancers also decrease significantly with smoking cessation and are similar to the cancer risk for nonsmokers in ten to thirteen years. These findings indicate that it is worthwhile even for older people to give up smoking.

Because nicotine (which is inhaled through smoking) is an addictive chemical, it may be difficult to quit, particularly after years of cigarette use. Most smokers have to stop several times before quitting permanently. Setting a quit date, attending support group meetings, taking it one day at a time, undergoing hypnosis, making a contract with a friend or a health-care provider, substituting carrot sticks for cigarettes, increasing exercise (particularly swimming), and breathing deeply all seem to be helpful techniques. Nicotine replacement systems are available in the United States on a nonprescription basis, but it is important for older people, particularly those with health problems or whom are taking multiple medications, to consult a health-care professional prior to using them. It is also important that anyone using these aids stop smoking completely. It is possible to get a toxic dose, perhaps even a fatal one, by smoking and using nicotine replacement simultaneously.

—*Rebecca Lovell Scott*
Updated by Bruce E. Johansen, PhD

See also: Cancer; Dental disorders; Emphysema; Fractures and broken bones; Glaucoma; Heart attacks; Macular degeneration; Medications; Osteoporosis; Respiratory changes and disorders; Sexual dysfunction; Skin changes and disorders; Strokes; Vision changes and disorders; Wrinkles

For Further Information

Gao, Kaiye, et al. "The Life-Course Impact of Smoking on Hypertension, Myocardial Infarction and Respiratory Diseases." *Scientific Reports*, vol. 7, no. 1, 28 June 2017. doi:10.1038/s41598-017-04552-5. Examines the impact of smoking on respiratory diseases, hypertension and myocardial infarction, with a focus from a life-course perspective.

"How Smoking Can Affect the Elderly: Updated for 2019." AgingInPlace, 3 Dec. 2018. www.aginginplace.org/how-smoking-can-affect-the-elderly/. Starts with statistics on older smokers, then discusses the harmful effects on older adults' health as well as possible cessation techniques.

Kleykamp, Bethea A., and Stephen J. Heishman. "The Older Smoker." *JAMA*, vol. 306, no. 8, 12 Sept. 2013. doi:10.1001/jama.2011.1221. Considers that older smokers will be an increasing proportion of the patient population and that these smokers might require modification of treatment for smoking cessation.

Pirie, Kirstin, et al. "The 21st Century Hazards of Smoking and Benefits of Stopping: A Prospective Study of One Million Women in the UK." *The Lancet*, vol. 381, no. 9861, 2013, pp. 133-41. doi:10.1016/s0140-6736(12)61720-6. This study analyzes 1·3 million UK women were recruited from 1996-2001 and resurveyed postally about 3 and 8 years later.

"Quitting Smoking for Older Adults." National Institute on Aging, U.S. Department of Health and Human Services, 17 Jan. 2019. www.nia.nih.gov/health/quitting-smoking-older-adults. A collection of information and resources designed to assist older adults to quit smoking.

SOCIAL MEDIA

Relevant Issues: Demographics, social media, social well-being, isolation,

Significance: Social media accessed through the Internet may have many benefits for older adults as well as risks.

As the number of American ages 65 and older continues to increase, so does the number of that group who are accessing the Internet. In 2017, the U.S. Census Bureau reported that the number of persons in the United States ages 65 and older on July 1, 2015, was 47.8 million, growing 1.6 million from 2014. They also reported that in 2015, 35.3 million seniors ages 65 and older responded to an American Community Survey that they had computers in their homes. In 2014, that number was 32.9 million. The Pew Research Center reported that Internet use in this age group increased 150 percent during the years 2009 to 2011. Seventy-one percent of the elderly reported they went online daily.

Technology and the Internet offer many benefit for seniors, especially those who are homebound or find leaving home challenging, such as seniors with chronic illness and increasing physical limitations. Although they may not drive any more or have transportation readily available, they can shop from home without leaving their residence with returns usually picked up at their door when prearranged. Many places of worship offer live and recorded broadcasts online. Seniors can find information about personal interests or their health and attend webinar or classes on the Internet. Health-care providers are more likely to communicate with patients through an online presence than in the past. Seniors can access government sites such as the Social Security Administration to read more about programs available, request a social security card replacement, or update their personal information without going to an office. Once comfortable with accessing the Internet, they can discover how useful this tool can be to improving various aspects of their lives including social interactions.

SOCIAL MEDIA PLATFORMS

One of the fastest growing interests of the age 65 and older group who access the Internet is social media. The Pew Research Center reported that 34 percent of people ages 65 and older use social media. Some of the social media platforms preferred by seniors include Facebook, Instagram, YouTube, Pinterest, and Twitter. Some seniors who are still working or even retired may enjoy staying in touch with work friends through the LinkedIn platform. Social media can bridge the intergenerational gap with children and grandchildren for improved relationships regardless of geographic location.

Facebook allows a broad and diverse platform for seniors with a fairly easy set up process. They can reconnect with people from the past such as high school or college friends. Facebook has a video calling application called FaceTime where seniors can see the person they are calling in real time, a good way to visit face to face with family or friends with a smart phone. Older adults can join interest groups such as cooking, diet, or exercise groups or even play games. Whatever the interest or hobby, Facebook usually has a group to match it. Seniors can visit the pages of friends and family to see photos and learn what's going on in their lives. They can share the same on their own Facebook page. If interested, they can organize an event such as a family reunion and publish it for those interesting in attending.

RESOURCES FOR OLDER ADULTS

Computer classes may be available at senior centers or through AARP chapters. There older adults can learn how to use the Internet alongside peers with instructors who have experience with this population. They can set up an e-mail account to stay in touch with family and friends or subscribe to blogs. Classes on social media may include help to set up an account such as a Facebook page. Instructors can demonstrate how to upload pictures to share with others through social media such as Instagram.

Classes are also available online for those unable to attend in person. Several universities and professional groups provide education through use of a computer, tablet, or smartphone and Internet—often for free or a small fee. The YouTube online channel offers many videos on diverse topics including how to use various platforms of social media.

BENEFITS OF SOCIAL MEDIA

Participating in social media allows seniors the opportunity to extend their social interactions outside the home. Many research studies have confirmed that social relationships play a valuable part of elder health and psychological wellness. With social media, seniors can connect with friend and family and create community even when unable to be part of their local community due to their limitations. With the high degree of isolation and depression that can accompany aging and compromised health, social media may be one way to combat these often devastating conditions. Studies have shown that seniors trained in use of social media had improved cognitive skills and slowed decline. Clearly social media can be a boost to the lives of many older adults.

RISKS OF SOCIAL MEDIA

Risks to online sharing and use of social media can be managed best by awareness and user actions. For example, privacy is an issue that requires the user to set guidelines at the site and limit who can see the person's information. Using strong passwords is a must to online use. Seniors should choose their friends carefully when using social media like Facebook and remember it is acceptable to decline a friend request from someone they do not know. Also seniors should be careful to not share certain personal information such as their address, birthdate, or social security number as identity theft can occur. They should avoid posting vacation plans or pictures that could alert someone their home is likely empty. Scammers are as prevalent online as in any setting so they should avoid clicking on any site unless familiar with it. Seniors should never give out bank account or credit card information to unknown or insecure online sites that can appear in the thread on Facebook as advertisements. If ever any doubt, the senior should check with a reliable person such as a family member before proceeding with online social media.

One other risk is addiction to the Internet and social media platforms. The Internet with all it can offer can also be overwhelming and become an obsession so other activities of daily living and relationships are ignored. Social media should not take the place of in-person interactions nor time spent in developing healthy behaviors such as exercise and pursuing interests or hobbies.

—*Marylane Wade Koch, MSN, RN*

See also: Adult education; Communication; Fraud against the elderly; Friendship; Leisure activities; Loneliness; Social ties

For Further Information

Anderson, Monica, and Andrew Perrin. "Technology Use Among Seniors" Pew Research Center, 17 May 2017. www.pewinternet.org/2017/05/17/technology-use-among-seniors/. Discusses and provides data about technology use among those ages 65 years and older.

"Computers and Internet Use" Profile America Facts for Features: Older America Month, May 2017, United States Census Bureau, 27 Mar. 2017. www.census.gov/content/dam/Census/newsroom/facts-for-features/2017/cb17-ff08.pd. Provides information and statistics about various relevant topics to celebrate adults 65 year and older.

Dunham, Nancy. "A+ for Elearning" AARP, 28 Feb. 2017. www.aarp.org/home-family/personal-technology/info-2017/online-education-courses.html. Author discussed how she found her Zen class online and the benefits of online education.

"Identity Theft and Social Media: What You Need to Know." *Retirement Living*, 11 June 2019. www.retirementliving.com/identity-theft-and-social-media. Details how to stay safe when using social media to avoid identity theft.

Saur, Alissa. "The Benefits of Social Media Use for Seniors" Leisure Care Retirement Resources, 3 Aug. 2018. www.leisurecare.com/resources/benefits-of-social-media-for-seniors/. Lists six benefits of social medial use for seniors and describes each.

The 2018 Guide to Best Technology Resources and Tools for Seniors, Institute on Aging. www.ioaging.org/the-2018-guide-to-best-technology-resources-and-tools-for-seniors#resources-for-socialization-and-support. General discussion of technology application to seniors with specific links for further information.

Thompson, Dennis. "Social Media for Seniors" *Everyday Health*, 7 Feb. 2014. www.everydayhealth.com/news/social-media-seniors/. Encouraging website for seniors with interest in social media. Includes description of the social media sites Facebook, Twitter, Pinterest, LinkedIn, and Google+.

SOCIAL SECURITY

Relevant Issues: Demographics, economics, law, work
Significance: Social Security provides protection against income losses that can accompany the disability, death, or old age of working persons.

The Old-Age, Survivors, and Disability Insurance (OASDI) programs, commonly known as Social Security, provide monthly benefits to retired and disabled workers, their dependents, and survivors. In 2017, 67 million Americans were receiving benefits from programs under the Social Security Administration. Of those, about 5.5 million were people who were newly awarded benefits that year. Women comprised 55 percent of the adult Social Security beneficiaries. The average age of disabled worker beneficiaries was 54.5, and 86 percent of persons receiving Supplemental Security Income (SSI) were disabled or blind.

A fact sheet was released by the Social Security Administration with beneficiary data from the month of December 2018. Retired workers numbered 43.7 million with an average monthly benefit of $1,461 for a total of $64 billion expenditure. Their dependents numbered at 3.1 million for an additional cost of $2.3 billion. Disabled workers numbered 8.5 million with an average monthly benefit of $1,234 or a total of $10.5 billion with 1.6 million dependents adding $0.6 billion in expenditures. Survivors numbered 6 million for an expenditure of $7 billion. This means that in 2019 over 64 million Americans will receive Social Security benefits that total over one trillion dollars.

The OASDI programs have been the subject of public concern in large part due to anticipated costs associated with the growing and increasing life expectancy of the elderly population. In 1995, 12.5 percent of the total U.S. population was sixty-five years of age and over increasing to 14.9 percent or 47.8 million in 2015. By 2035, the number of U.S. elderly is expected to reach over 79 million. By 2060 that number is projected to be

98.2 million or one in four residents with about 19.7 million of those being age 85 or older. This increase is primarily attributed to the aging of millions of baby boomers, those born between 1946 and 1964. Life expectancy increased from 72.5 years for men and 79.3 years for women in 1996 to an average of 78.6, or 76.1 for men and 81.1 for women in 2017. Federal expenditures for the OASDI programs increased from $11 billion in 1960 to $117.1 billion in 1980 to $301.1 billion in 1993 to $1 trillion in 2017. Social Security continues to be a major source of income for older adults with social security benefits totaling 33 percent of their income. About 48 percent of married couples and 69 percent of unmarried persons rely on social security for 50 percent of their income while 21 percent of married couples and 44 percent of unmarried person rely on their Social Security check as 90 percent of their income.

THE DEVELOPMENT OF SOCIAL SECURITY IN THE UNITED STATES

Old age benefits were provided for retired workers in the original Social Security Act of 1935, which covered only workers in commerce and industry, then about 40 percent of the workforce. The 1935 act provided monthly benefits to retired workers sixty-five years of age and over and a lump sum death benefit to the estate of these workers. In 1939 benefits were extended to dependents of retired workers (wives sixty-five years of age and older and children under sixteen) and to survivors of deceased workers (widows sixty-five years of age and older, mothers caring for an eligible child, children under the age of sixteen, and dependent parents). In 1956 benefits were further extended to disabled workers fifty to sixty-four years of age and to the disabled children over the age of eighteen of retired, disabled, or deceased workers, if they became disabled before they were eighteen (changed to disabled before the age of twenty-two in 1973). Benefits for disabled workers under fifty years of age were provided in 1960. The Medicare insurance program was created in 1965. As a result of the Social Security amendments of 1972, monthly cash OASDI benefits have been automatically adjusted since 1975 to keep pace with inflation.

Social Security was originally conceived as one leg of a three-legged income stool for retirees. Personal savings and private pensions were the two other legs, and both of these were expected to constitute the major portion of retirement income. That view was challenged by a 1975 Advisory Council, which saw Social Security as the nation's primary pension plan, providing more retirement income than private savings.

BENEFITS

Benefits can be paid to workers and their dependents or survivors if workers have worked long enough in covered employment to be "insured" for these benefits. Insured status is determined by a formula applied to workers' average monthly earnings indexed to the increase in average annual wages. The formula includes the highest 35 years of earnings. If the applicant does not have 35 years of earnings, the years without earnings will count as zero. The Social Security website offers a retirement estimator tool to estimate retirement payment benefits at www.ssa.gov/benefits/retirement/estimator.html. This is only an estimate and can change based on

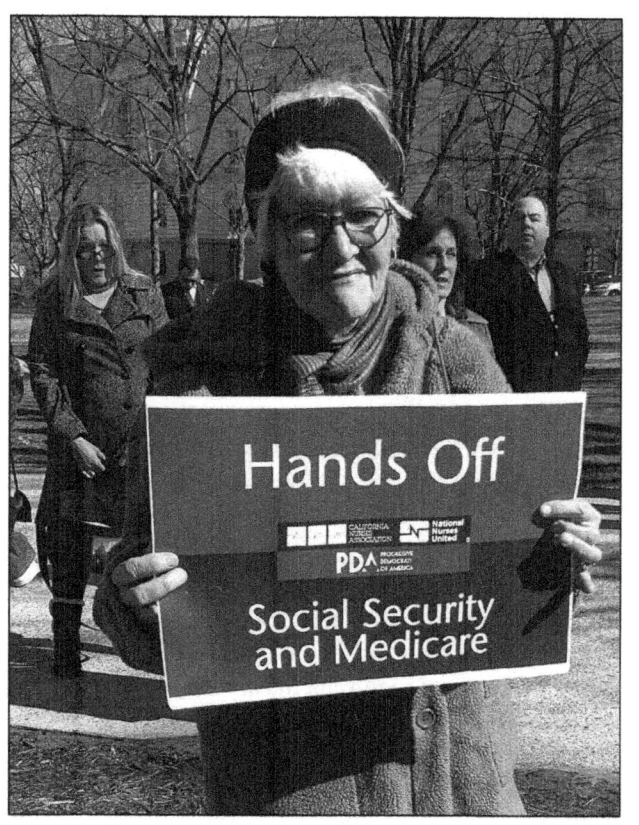

A nurse of National Nurses United holds a sign in support of Social Security at a rally in Senate Park, Washington D.C., 2013. (via Wikimedia Commons)

increased or decreased future earnings, cost of living adjustments, or military service, work with the railroad, or pensions where Social Security taxes were not paid. Also, the law governing benefits may be amended as needed.

Family Benefits Workers must be at least sixty-two years old to be eligible for retirement benefits. There is no minimum age requirement for disability benefits. A benefit is payable to a retiree, spouse or ex-spouse of a retired or disabled worker when a currently married spouse is at least sixty-two years old; is caring for one or more of the worker's entitled children who are disabled or have not reached the age of sixteen; or when a divorced spouse is at least sixty-two, is not married, and the marriage lasted at least ten years before the divorce became final. A divorced spouse may be entitled independently of the worker's retirement if both the worker and divorced spouse are sixty-two years of age and if the divorce has been final for at least two years. To learn more about family benefits and stay current on any changes in this law, visit the Social security website area on Benefits for your Family (www.ssa.gov/planners/retire/applying7.html).

SURVIVOR BENEFITS

When a worker dies, widows, widowers (including divorced widows and widowers), children, and dependent parents may be eligible for survivor benefits. Specific guidelines address each of these areas online at the Social Security website section on survivors. (www.ssa.gov/planners/survivors/). A 16-page downloadable booklet is also available to review the details of how to qualify and how to apply for survivor benefits (www.ssa.gov/pubs/EN-05-10084.pdf).

DISABILITY BENEFITS

The Social Security Administration offers two disability benefit programs: Social Security Disability and Supplemental Security Income (SSI). For most applicants, the medical requirements are the same. Other areas of consideration are work and education history. To learn more and make an application, visit "Benefits Planner" on the Social Security Administrations website (www.ssa.gov/planners/disability/).

ADDITIONAL EARNED INCOME

Social Security law also reduces benefits for nondisabled recipients who earn income from work above a certain amount. In 2019 recipients under the age of full retirement can earn up to $17,640 a year in wages or self-employment income without having their benefits reduced. For earnings above this amount, recipients under full retirement age will lose $1 of benefits for each $2 of earnings above the annual limit. However, in the last year before full retirement eligibility, the worker can earn up to $46, 920 and lose $1 of benefits for each $3 of earnings. The earnings limit does not apply to recipients after they reach full retirement age. The earnings limits rise each year indexed to the rise in average wages in the economy. At issue is the extent to which the incentive structure of Social Security encourages retirement (discourages work) for those under age seventy. Research has shown that labor force participation rates of older workers, particularly men, have decreased over the past several decades, but the influence of Social Security compared to other factors on this trend remains questionable.

Applicants are encouraged to access the "Benefits Planner" section of the Social Security Administration website (www.ssa.gov/planners/) to find specific areas of information regarding retirement, disability, survivors, and calculators. Using this site will assist in staying up to date with current laws and guidelines for Social Security benefits. Applications for Social Security benefits can be initiated up to four months before the benefits will start. Contact the Social Security Administration through their website, www.socialsecurity.gov or call the automated service at 1-800-772-1213 or the TTY number 1-800-325-0778 if applicant is deaf or hard of hearing.

THE FINANCING MECHANISM OF SOCIAL SECURITY

There has been much debate about how financially sound Social Security is. The Fast Facts about Figures About Social Security 2018 publication describes social security as a pay-as-you-go program with the primary source of OASDI revenue being payroll tax paid by covered workers used to pay benefits for current recipients. This section on how social security is financed includes graphs about sources and use of revenue. In 2017 OASDI had $996.6 billion in revenues with 87.7

percent from payroll taxation and reimbursements from the General Fund of the Treasury and 3.8 percent from income tax on Social Security benefits. The remaining 8.5 percent was interest from government bonds held by trust funds. In 2017, assets increased due to total income exceeding expenditures for paying out benefits and covering administrative expenses.

However, the current demographics challenge the future financial security of Social Security. The 2018 Trustee report predicts the number of retirees will increase quickly with continued retirement of the post World War II baby boomers. Within 50 years the number of retired workers will likely double. In addition, with people living longer and fewer babies being born, the Trustees estimate the ratio of workers paying taxes to those receiving benefits will fall from 2.8 to 1 in 2017 to 2.2 to 1 by 2033. They further project that pattern of the 2010 tax and noninterest income's inability to cover the program costs will continue for another 75 years or more unless changes are made. On the positive side, the Trustees believe that redemption of the trust fund assets will allow full benefit payments until 2033.

The long-term financial outlook of Social Security is not encouraging. In 2018 The Trustees predicted that the reserves from the OASI and DI trust funds will be totally depleted by 2034 with the payroll taxes and other income insufficient to cover the program costs at about 79 percent. Over the next 75 years that shortfall is estimated at 2.84 percent.

A continuing issue is the extent to which all retirees come to rely on Social Security as a larger share of total income, thereby becoming increasingly dependent on workers whose proportionately shrinking take-home pay must also meet workers' own financial obligations. The debate over Social Security reform promises to be lively, as workers seek to maximize their take-home pay and elders seek to protect their economic wellbeing.

—*Richard K. Caputo*
Updated by Marylane Wade Koch

See also: Baby boomers; Disabilities; Dual-income couples; Health care; Health insurance; Life expectancy; Medicare; Pensions; Poverty; Retirement; Retirement planning; Townsend movement

For Further Information

"Benefits Planner." Social Security Administration. www.ssa.gov/planners/. Has separate areas of information for retirement, disability, survivors, and calculators. Use this to stay up to date with current laws and guidelines for Social Security benefits.

"Fact Sheet: Social Security 2018-2019." Social Security Administration. www.ssa.gov/news/press/factsheets/basicfact-alt.pdf. Offers key interesting facts about Social Security in the years 2018-2019.

"Fast Facts and Figures about Social Security, 2018." Social Security Administration, Office of Retirement and Disability and Office of Research, Evaluation, and Statistics. Sept. 2018. www.ssa.gov/policy/docs/chartbooks/fast_facts/2018/fast_facts18.pdf. Designed to address the most frequently asked questions concerning the SSA's programs with basic data about Social Security and Supplemental Security Income.

Jeffery, Terrance. "Social Security Spending Tops $1 Trillion for the First Time." *CNS News*, 25 Oct. 2017. www.cnsnews.com/news/article/terence-p-jeffrey/social-security-administration-spending-tops-1-trillion-first-time. Compares money spent by various government department with that spent by SS administration on OASDI and SSI.

"Spouse and Children." AARP, American Association of Retired Persons. www.aarp.org/retirement/social-security/questions-answers/spouse-dependents/?intcmp=AE-SSRC-QA-SPSCH#/. Addresses frequently asked questions about benefits for spouse and children.

"Survivor's Benefits." Social Security Administration. www.ssa.gov/pubs/EN-05-10084.pdf. Downloadable 16-page booklet explaining survivor benefits and application process.

"Your Retirement Checklist." Social Security Administration. www.ssa.gov/pubs/EN-05-10377.pdf. Addresses frequently asked questions about Social Security retirement to keep applicants informed and updated.

SOCIAL TIES

Relevant Issues: Culture, family, sociology, values
Significance: AS the link not only between social ties and social well-being but also health and emotional stability is further established, research is increasingly focusing on social ties and aging.

Age plays a basic role in determining how societies are structured or organized. It influences the allocation of social resources and social roles which, in turn, influence the patterns of everyday living. The patterns and networks of social ties, for instance, differ for persons at various stages of their life. As the everyday activities of children differ from adults, so the pattern of daily life for the elderly tends to differ from that of either children or nonelderly adults.

The role of social ties and social networks is of particular importance in defining the aging process. Considerable research has indicated that the way people live—how and with whom they interact day after day—significantly affects everything from their health to their mental, emotional, and economic well-being. The types and quality of social ties an individual maintains with others are paramount. These ties involve contacts of all sorts with family, friends, and acquaintances. The social ties and the networks they represent provide a certain level of support, both emotionally and practically.

To have a significant and supportive network of social relationships means individuals are interconnected through a number of meaningful and ongoing social ties. The ties themselves, rather than the attributes of the individuals in the network, are most important. To be immersed in a web of group affiliations is the very basis of social, emotional, and practical support. Someone who is isolated and experiencing problems will not receive support to the same extent as individuals who are engaged in a wide range of significant social ties. For instance, family, friends, and acquaintances may help ensure compliance with a treatment regimen by reminding the elderly to take their medicine on time or by arranging for transportation to the doctor's office or a clinic.

Social networks are intimately interconnected with life events and life changes, both positively (weddings, births, and anniversaries) and negatively (deaths, divorces, and the loss of a job). Potentially disruptive life changes such as the death of a spouse and being forced to move or forced to retire—events that regularly confront the elderly—represent the disruption or termination of social ties. Social networks are apparently "coping recourses" that can serve as a buffer to the stressful impact of such life changes. When social ties are disrupted, the "adaptive energy" of the participants diminishes and their ability to cope with changing circumstances lessens, as does their ability to alter their social milieu. This is an especially difficult challenge for the elderly living in fast-paced, rapidly changing societies such as contemporary America where change is seldom easy to anticipate or handle.

Although the link between social ties and aging is well established, a number of unanswered questions remain. Why do stressful events call forth such differing outcomes in individuals with similarly structured social networks? Short-lived problems, chronic problems, minor problems, and acute problems can all be produced in similarly situated individuals by the same stressful event. Is the quality of relationships more important than the quantity of relationships? In studying situations in which the elderly receive support, some of their social ties provide support while others are not supportive. How does the configuration or structure of their social networks affect the level of support for the elderly? Is the effect of either social support or of increasing isolation cumulative? Although social ties influence health and illness, to what extent does prior illness influence the configuration of an individual's social networks? The inability to meaningfully participate in a network of social relationships may be primarily due to an individual's health status. As health continues to deteriorate, isolation usually increases, which in turn may contribute to further deterioration in health status.

A particularly interesting question concerns the relative importance of strong ties and weak ties for the elderly. Research suggests that strong ties (defined as close, intimate, and emotionally significant) and weak ties (those less intimate, less emotionally significant, and more often task-oriented) play somewhat different roles in the lives of the elderly. After the death of a spouse, for example, the emotional support needed by the widow or widower is usually most effectively provided through strong ties to close family and friends. As the widow or widower begins to adjust to their new life and look to the future, their less intimate and less emotionally significant or weak ties may be more useful in providing them with valuable information, ideas, and contacts. The importance of weak ties is seen in their potential to foster social cohesion through expanding social networks as a conduit to influence, information, and social mobility and as the basis for community and political organizing.

Although the relationship between social ties and aging is complex and further examination is needed, the importance of social ties for the elderly is undeniable. People who have frequent and meaningful contacts with neighbors, friends, family, or organizational associates report "being happy" more frequently. People need social ties to fulfill numerous basic, practical needs. Although different people have different needs depending on their personal circumstances, the elderly in particular have needs that must be met through social contacts. These include obtaining help when ill, locating and acquiring medical assistance, shopping, house cleaning, borrowing money, and other types of caretaking.

CROSS-CULTURAL DIFFERENCES IN AGING
In addition to the differing patterns of age-related activities and expectations within a society, the social activities and social roles performed by the elderly also differ from one society to another. In some societies, aging enhances prestige and social standing while in other societies aging depreciates prestige and social standing. In some societies, the elderly are assigned and perform functional roles that contribute to the well-being of the group. In these societies, the elderly maintain their employment, continue to work, and generally remain active in a variety of social roles. In other societies, the elderly systematically relinquish socially valued positions such as their job and other formal positions, including being officers and active members in a variety of organizations and associations. These differing patterns are modified by such factors as social class, gender, and physical and psychological capabilities.

In those societies where the status of the elderly is depreciated, the loss of formal roles means the elderly move into informal or what are referred to as tenuous social roles. In such settings, the elderly find themselves drawn into such activities as caring for children, storytelling, preparing food, and mending, washing, and ironing clothing. Such roles typically exclude the elderly from many areas of social life. This, in turn, diminishes their network of meaningful social ties, which can have a variety of negative outcomes for the elderly, including the loss of social value as well as social identity. The absence of meaningful roles and relationships means older people not only tend to experience the loss of social identity but isolation and withdrawal as well. This contributes to the elderly suffering from diminished social integration, which in turn furthers the decline in the breadth and strength of their social ties.

In extreme cases, particularly where the conditions of life are difficult, such as in harsh climates and where the very survival of society or the group is questionable, the sick and very old have been abandoned to die. Examples from the past can be found among nomadic groups such as the Lapps of northern Europe and the Hopi Indians of the southwest United States. In contrast, where aging contributes to social standing, the elderly are seen as having greater wisdom based on their having lived a long life and having accumulated a wealth of experiences. In these societies the elderly are often in the mainstream or the very core of social life. This is seen in both the respect and deference they receive as well as the richness of their social ties which, in one way or another, link them in meaningful ways to a wide range of significant others.

Having briefly reviewed the diversity of expectations, roles, and relationships characterizing aging cross-culturally, it is necessary to identify the sociocultural trends that affect the elderly in the modern Western world, including the United States. This requires examining not only the trends, but their impact on the process of aging, and their significance for understanding social ties and aging.

SOCIOCULTURAL TRENDS AND AGING
A wide range of significant political, economic, and cultural trends have unfolded in the modern Western world in recent years. Many if not most of these trends have contributed to redefining the process of aging, including the pattern of social ties among the elderly. With the evolution from a traditional agrarian to industrial and eventually to postindustrial or information-based society, the size of the core or nuclear family, composed of husband and wife and children, if any, has declined dramatically.

Having large numbers of children was commonplace and economically viable when America was largely a nation of farmers, for many hands were needed to work the fields. The advent of industrialization and subsequently the postindustrial society, coupled with inflation, rendered having children less economically feasible. Smaller families mean fewer children to assist parents and grandparents as they age. The decline of the larger or extended family (where contact with nieces, nephews, cousins, and other distant relatives is less regular, frequent, and meaningful), the fast pace of modern life, increased geographic mobility with family members often living and working some distance from one another, and the appearance of two-working-parent families have contributed to the elderly increasingly turning to social service personnel rather than family members as care givers who assist with shopping, transportation, health, and housekeeping needs.

The "senior boom" America is experiencing, in which both the total number of elderly and the overall percentage of the elderly in America's population have increased, has affected society in many ways, not the least of which is the quantity and quality as well as the types of social ties the elderly experience. Although millions of elderly Americans are self-sufficient, live at home, and continue to actively participate in the life of society, millions of others face difficult physical, mental, emotional, and financial problems. Many struggle to remain in their homes. For those whose families cannot or choose not to be caregivers to their elderly relatives, a variety of programs, both public and private, exist to assist many elderly people to remain in their homes. These programs include meal delivery, in-home health services, in-home social visitations, and transportation assistance for the elderly.

One of the fastest growing segments of the population is the very-old, those over seventy-five years of age. As the baby boomers age, the number of old people, generally, and the very old, in particular, will continue to expand. The role of modern medicine and medical technology, coupled with improved sanitation, are major contributors to increased longevity. This has and will continue to place increasing demands on society to provide the necessary resources to care for the elderly. Not only will in-home social services expand, but the need for specialized facilities to care for those elderly who require additional care and can no longer live alone will continue to increase. In addition, the need for nursing homes and centers for the aged where various social service and health-care personnel provide differing levels of care from residential to skilled nursing will grow. Clearly, the living arrangements of the aged exert a considerable influence on their social ties. Those who live in specialized facilities for the elderly, particularly when they are no longer mobile, usually experience diminished contact with the non-elderly.

CONCLUSION

Although there is much that is not well understood about the relationship between the process of aging and social ties, much is known. The aged, like all human beings, are most appropriately thought of in holistic terms. That is, they are simultaneously physical beings, social beings, and emotional beings. The significance of social ties in everyday life is seen in the fact that the patterns, extensiveness, and strength of the social ties of the elderly are linked to their social well-being, which in turn is related to both their physical and emotional well-being. This is not only the case for the elderly, but is characteristic of each stage in the process of aging.

There is a definite pattern to the process of aging; however, the elderly are clearly not as homogeneous a category as many people believe. Stereotypes about the elderly, however misinformed they might be, persist in many societies including the United States. Common thinking and attitudes toward the elderly portray them as dependent, submissive, isolated, and often abused. While this is true for many, others are independent, definitely not submissive, actively integrated and involved in a wide range of social activities, and not abused. Many others represent various combinations of these traits.

The aged are truly a diverse group. Even their ages vary dramatically. Being ninety is far different than being sixty or seventy. Social class, gender, and racial and ethnic differences among the elderly are as consequential as for other age categories. One constant factor surrounding social ties and aging is that both, in addition to their relationship, are dynamic. As societies change, so the process of aging changes, which then feeds back and influences the society of which it is a part.

—*Charles E. Marske*

See also: Abandonment; Caregiving; Childlessness; Cohabitation; Communication; Death of a child; Death of parents; Divorce; Empty nest syndrome; Family relationships; Friendship; Full nest; Leisure activities; Loneliness; Marriage; Mentoring; Neglect; Parenthood; Personality changes; Remarriage; Retirement communities; Senior citizen centers; Sexuality; Sibling

HOW TO TALK TO SENIORS ABOUT STAYING SOCIAL

How Do They Feel?

Some older adults intentionally cut off social interactions, for example after the loss of a spouse or due to a medical condition they see as embarrassing. For some people this is normal, though for others it may be a sign of depression. However, many others become isolated for reasons other than choice. Seniors often prefer to live alone in order to maintain their independence, but this can become lonely. Decreased mobility and declining health may affect their ability or desire to go out, and they might find themselves doing activities that keep them housebound.

Seniors may long for the liveliness of social encounters and the warmth of friendships, especially if they previously enjoyed an active social life. Many older adults prefer to see people face to face, and might regret the decline in such interactions. They may resist using other forms of communication, such as computers and video chatting. Being isolated or lonely can lead to feelings of sadness, despondency, frustration, resentment, and depression.

Some seniors are proactive in finding ways to stay socially engaged. Others may they feel challenged or overwhelmed by arranging social activities. They may benefit from speaking to other seniors in the same position to get ideas or find resources. A social worker or health-care practitioner may be a useful source of information. Seniors who remain socially active often feel better emotionally, cognitively and physically. Speaking to others, sharing news and common interests, and smiling and laughing together boosts a sense of belonging and promotes feelings of self-worth. Social arrangements also have the benefit of drawing attention away from health issues and other concerns.

How Do I Start The Conversation?

How you start the conversation with seniors about staying social will depend on their personality and circumstances. Some seniors may be eager to find all means possible to have social interactions and activities, whereas others may be reluctant. No matter how you approach the conversation, the senior should be actively involved. The best conversations will be held as discussions to find out what your senior enjoys and what type of social interactions work best for them. It will not be productive to impose your ideas of enjoyable social activity on them. Instead, use their favorite pastime as a starting point and discuss ways in which they could become more engaged.

You might help them investigate the different types of social activities available in their area. Depending on their physical ability and state of health, you can make suggestions accordingly. You may also want to ask them about the biggest challenges they face in maintaining an active social life. Work together to find out ways you can help make it easier for them.

You may decide to discuss the health benefits of staying social with your senior, especially if they are reluctant to make plans to socialize. You should approach this discussion with sensitivity, perhaps using an interesting article or video presentation to raise the topic. You could highlight how the mental stimulation of using language and social skills have positive effects on cognitive and emotional health. Try to keep the conversation positive and discuss the numerous possibilities available for arranging social activities that they will enjoy.

In some cases seniors may be open to using technology to stay social. You can arrange for someone (such as a family member, friend, volunteer, or professional) to show them how to use a computer, tablet, or smartphone to set up and access video chats, an e-mail account, instant messaging applications, or social media. As they find the activities that are best suited to their needs and desires, your nonjudgmental support will be greatly helpful. Your senior will then be able to enjoy how staying socially active enhances their life.

—Leah Jacob

relationships; Skipped-generation parenting; Sports participation

For Further Information

Atchley, Robert C. *Social Forces and Aging: An Introduction to Social Gerontology*. 11th ed. Belmont, Calif.: Wadsworth, 2009. A thorough overview of the social aspects of aging. Social ties and aging are touched upon through the examination of numerous topics.

Bonifas, Robin P. *Bullying among Older Adults: How to Recognize and Address an Unseen Epidemic*. Health Professions P, Inc., 2016. Filled with practical resources and examples, this book offers effective interventions, including empathy and civility training, empowerment strategies, bystander interventions, and more.

Luong, Gloria, et al. "Better with Age: Social Relationships across Adulthood." *Journal of Social and Personal Relationships*, vol. 28, no. 1, 2010, pp. 9-23. doi:10.1177/0265407510391362. This paper integrates current developmental research to explain why social relationships are generally more positive with age.

Qualls, Sarah Honn. "What Social Relationships Can Do for Health." *Generations*, 2014. This article provides a brief overview of key findings on health and positive social relationships and reviews the powerful negative effects on health of negative social interactions.

Rook, Karen S., and Susan T. Charles. "Close Social Ties and Health in Later Life: Strengths and Vulnerabilities." *American Psychologist*, vol. 72, no. 6, 2017, pp. 567-577. doi:10.1037/amp0000104. Studies the positive and negative effects that social relationships have on the health and well-being of older adults.

SPORTS PARTICIPATION

Relevant Issues: Culture, psychology, recreation, sociology

Significance: Participation in recreational and competitive sports provides an avenue for socialization while enhancing self-efficacy and improving overall health.

Baby boomers are currently the largest segment of our population. With improved medical care, people are not only living longer, healthier lives—they are engaging in active sports, volunteering, going back to school and developing new relationships. Recreational activities and sports participation are options available for older adults to meet the need to be more active for optimal health. The negativism previously associated with aging has been deemphasized as more middle-aged and older adults become involved in physical activity and sports participation.

FACTORS AFFECTING RECREATIONAL PATTERNS

Several factors are associated with an older adult choosing to be active in recreational pursuits. In the past, generation of family members lived together (within one residence/ under one roof), but in recent years an increasing number of adults are living by themselves either in the nursing homes, assisted living facilities or senior living communities. Many do not want to live in these facilities, thus a few retirement facilities have changed the level of care based on individual needs.

Although many people accept the health benefits of exercise, only a small minority of adults meet the minimum daily physical activity recommendations as participation decreases with age. Younger and middle-aged adults with positive attitudes toward aging and activity continue to be active, productive older adults as long as they remain healthy. Recreational preferences are also based upon past experiences established earlier in life. If the experiences were enjoyable and the opportunity to continue participation are present, the older individual is likely to continue his or her activities. Those individuals who have the support and encouragement of a "significant other" or caretaker will be the most successful in accomplishing their recreational goals.

On the other hand, older adults who were brought up with preconceived notions that people must slow down as they age will not be very active. In addition, those who were brought up with a strong "work ethic" tend to have a difficult time engaging in leisure activities unless there is a specific purpose behind the action (other than simple enjoyment). Oftentimes, the reason why many do not participate in recreational activities and sports programs is because they themselves internalize negative stereotypes and attitudes towards exertion.

Other reasons for not participating can be due to poor environmental planning, poor maintenance, or safety issues regarding facilities. A recreational facility must be in a safe, easily accessible location. Faucets in showers need to be large enough to enable arthritic hands to turn the shower on and off. Asphalt walking paths should be covered with crushed bark to absorb moisture and reduce slippery surfaces. Swimming pool ladders should be a height that requires a minimum of shoulder strength, and nonskid mats and handrails should be placed in and around the pool and shower areas.

Being more active means a greater risk for incurring an activity-related injury. However, 2018 Department of Health and Human Services issued its 2nd edition book on Physical Activity Guidelines for Americans indicating substantial health benefits from regular physical activity. Being active makes it easier to perform activities of daily living, decrease risk of falls, preserve function and mobility (leading them to be independent longer), which is key in preventing and managing chronic diseases, lowers risk of psychological disorder and provides opportunities for social engagement & interactions. Sports that have the lowest risk of injury include walking, swimming, dancing, Tai Chi, golf, tennis, volleyball, and softball. Activities such as yoga and Tai Chi are good options for older adults because they focus on body awareness and flexibility rather than strength and speed. Other activities that are popular for both middle-aged and older adults include hiking, cycling, fishing, and bowling.

SPORTS PARTICIPATION CHOICES

When choosing a sport, several factors need to be considered. First is sport category preference. There are three general sports categories: individual sports that can be performed alone (walking, running, swimming); dual sports that require a partner (racquet sports); and team sports that require more than two players (basketball, softball). Second, the individual's fitness level must be taken into consideration. Although many sports can accommodate a range of fitness levels, certain ones, such as squash, handball, and downhill skiing, require high levels of physical fitness. Third, if expense is an issue, activities that cost the most money are ones requiring special fees and equipment rentals (or purchases) such as golf and skiing.

Adults tend to be more self-conscious when learning a new sport skill. If an older adult becomes socially embarrassed because he or she was unable to execute a simple athletic movement, he or she will be less likely to attempt that sport again. Therefore, to reduce the anxiety of new-sport participation, the new sport chosen should have similar motor skills already learned from an earlier activity. For instance if an individual used to play softball, those same motor skills can be applied to tennis doubles. The hand-eye coordination and arm strength will transfer and having a partner will lessen the intensity of the activity. It is also suggested that novice participants start off in a low-pressure situation—for instance, golfing during off-peak times.

SPORTS PROGRAMS

The thrill of victory has been shown to be significantly related to aging, especially among the seventy-to eighty-nine-year-old age group, thereby contradicting the stereotypical impression that interest in competition declines with aging. A tremendous surge of interest in the master's athletic competition occurred beginning in the late 1970s. A "master athlete" is any individual who exceeds a minimum age requirement and competes in a given sporting event. Several specialized senior and master's athletic competitions are held at the regional, national, and international levels; they are sponsored by sporting goods manufacturers, health care systems, and communities.

In an attempt to meet this need, a variety of recreational club memberships have been formed. Organizations such as the National Senior Game Association, at nsga.com and the American Association of Retired Persons (AARP), at www.aarp.org, have set up computer websites to access senior-oriented sports and leisure activities. The United States Tennis Association (USTA) sponsors tennis programs for older adults.

Well-known athletic competitions include the World Masters Championships and the World Veterans Games, both track and field competitions, and the World Masters Swimming Championships. However, the most widely known master competition in the United States is the National Senior Game Association, formerly known as the Senior Olympics. The first Senior Olympics took place in 1987 and attracted 2,500 people. Within the last 20 years, the Senior Olympics has developed to now accommodate the more than 20,000 athletes throughout an ever increasing list of athletic events.

These events, include archery, badminton, basketball, cycling, pickleball, power walk, race walk, racquetball, road race, shuffleboard, softball, swimming, tennis and table tennis, triathlon & tri relay, track and field and volleyball as well as less strenuous events such as bowling, golf, horseshoes, and shuffleboard. The minimum age to compete is fifty years, and the events are divided into age groups with five year intervals. While awards are given for first, second, and third place (gold, silver, and bronze medals), a major emphasis is placed on participation to encourage all adults to exercise regularly for better health, happiness, and productivity. The most important reasons given by older adults for participation in the National Senior Game Association were enjoyment of the activity, the sense of accomplishment, the thrill of competition, and winning. Information about National Senior Game Association events can be obtained by contacting NSGA, PO BOX 5630, Clearwater, FL 33758; Email: nsga@NSGA.com or www.nsga.com.

—Bonita L. Marks
Updated by Anubhav Agarwal, MD

See also: Exercise and fitness; Injuries among older adults; Leisure activities; Reaction time; Safety issues; Social ties

For Further Information

Baker, Joseph, et al. "Sport Participation and Positive Development in Older Persons." *European Review of Aging and Physical Activity*, vol. 7, no. 1, 2009, pp. 3-12. doi:10.1007/s11556-009-0054-9. This discussion highlights the inherent paradox of sport participation—that it has the potential to provide considerable positive growth but also the potential for significant negative consequences.

Chen, Chiehfeng, et al. "Factors Influencing Interest in Recreational Sports Participation and Its Rural-Urban Disparity." *Plos One*, vol. 12, no. 5, 2017. doi:10.1371/journal.pone.0178052. This study sets out to gain a more comprehensive understanding of the behavioral and socioeconomic factors influencing interest in recreational sports participation in Taiwan, as well as to evaluate the effect of any urban-rural divide.

Gayman, Amy M., et al. "Is Sport Good for Older Adults? A Systematic Review of Psychosocial Outcomes of Older Adults' Sport Participation." *International Review of Sport and Exercise Psychology*, vol. 10, no. 1, 2016, pp. 164-85. doi:10.1080/1750984x.2016.1199046. A mixed studies systematic review to identify psychosocial outcomes of sport for adults over age 65 and to determine whether sport provides psychosocial outcomes that are distinct from other forms of physical activity.

Jenkin, Claire R., et al. "Sport for Adults Aged 50+ Years: Participation Benefits and Barriers." *Journal of Aging and Physical Activity*, vol. 26, no. 3, 2018, pp. 363-71. doi:10.1123/japa.2017-0092. This qualitative study explores the benefits and barriers regarding older adult community sport participation, from the perspective of national sporting organizations, in addition to older adult sport club and non-sport club members, across eight focus group interviews.

Kim, Amy Chan Hyung, et al. "Psychological and Social Outcomes of Sport Participation for Older Adults: A Systematic Review." *Ageing and Society*, 28 Feb. 2019, pp. 1-21. doi:10.1017/s0144686x19000175. This article provides the results of a systematic review of the psychological and social outcomes of sport participation for older adults.

Sibel, Arslan. "Factors Affecting Recreation Preferences and Expectations of Disabled Adult Learners." *Educational Research and Reviews*, vol. 9, no. 20, 2014, pp. 975-80. doi:10.5897/err2014.1917. This study determines factors effective on recreation preferences and expectations of the disabled individuals who utilize from the recreation services offered by the Ankara Metropolitan Municipality.

STEREOTYPES

Relevant Issues: Culture, media, psychology, sociology
Significance: Stereotypes about the elderly are widely shared and are capable of affecting interpersonal relationships as well as self-image.

Age is culturally defined. Most cultures, including that of the United States, define age chronologically, while others define age in terms of accomplishments. While all cultures differentiate between children and adults, some cultures (for example, the United States) utilize many more categories. Each age category has its own socially prescribed roles based on the respective beliefs and stereotypes associated with it. Age categories, together with their accompanying beliefs and stereotypes, are subject to change; as life expectancy increases, the designation of old age tends to change accordingly.

In the United States, the recognized age categories are infancy (birth to about age two), childhood (ages two to twelve), adolescence (ages twelve to eighteen), and adulthood, which is subdivided into young, middle, and old age. Since the advent of Social Security in the 1930s, sixty-five, which was the usual age for retirement, has been commonly identified with old age. Gerontologists have since subdivided this category into young-old (ages sixty-five through seventy-five), middle-old (ages seventy-five through eighty-four), and old-old (age eighty-five and over). Aging occurs biologically (organs, bodily functions, and systems), psychologically (personality, perceptions, and mental functions), and socially (roles, relationships, and stereotypes).

MEANING, FUNCTIONS, AND CONSEQUENCES

The word "stereotype" comes from a Greek word meaning "hard core." Stereotype has come to mean a set of largely static and oversimplified ideas about a group or social category. These ideas may be either positive or negative but usually include both types. Stereotypes may arise from personal contact with members of a group or social category, but more commonly they are learned through socialization. They are taught—directly or indirectly—in homes, schools, churches, other groups, and mass media. These stereotypes can be held and shared regarding groups and social categories of people with whom personal contact has never been made.

The primary function of stereotypes is to reduce uncertainty by simplifying reality and allowing people to live in a complex world without the necessity of dealing with individual differences. Thus, when individuals are identified with a particular group or social category (such as the elderly), they are assumed to possess certain characteristics and are treated accordingly. This situation may result in a self-fulfilling prophecy wherein the elderly are admonished to "act their age" as defined by society. Sometimes, elderly individuals accept the role expected of them because, they believe, it is natural and inevitable.

One consequence of negative stereotypes regarding the elderly is "ageism," a term coin by Robert N. Butler, the former director of the National Institute on Aging. Like racism and sexism, ageism is an ideology of superiority and inferiority that results in prejudice and discrimination aimed at the elderly. Stereotypes are problematic because they influence people's behavior toward the elderly. They not only affect interpersonal relations but also are capable of affecting social policies and even elderly individuals' sense of self. Beliefs that the elderly are physically and mentally impaired led to the passage of laws requiring mandatory retirement and a proliferation of nursing homes that were little more than warehouses where residents waited to die.

Even positive stereotypes can have negative consequences. For example, voters and legislators who believe that the elderly are independent and financially well off are unlikely to support public aid, which is viewed as unnecessary. Also, the belief that grandparents are exceptionally good with children and have free time to do what they want has resulted in using elderly retired parents for free babysitting. Finally, stereotypes that portray the elderly as religious, trusting, and helpful make them frequent targets for unscrupulous individuals who want to defraud them of their life savings.

COMMONLY HELD STEREOTYPES

Stereotypes of the elderly fall mainly into three categories: physical, psychological, and social. Common physical stereotypes include gray hair, balding, wrinkled skin, false teeth, poor eyesight, hearing impairment, gnarled hands, and impotence. Psychological stereotypes include memory loss, forgetfulness, irritability, feelings of isolation, lower self-esteem, and lack of interest in sex. Social stereotypes include being old-fashioned, living on a low income, needing nursing care, being dependent on family members, being poor drivers, and proving to be unproductive or unreliable workers.

A youth-oriented culture such as that found in the United States tends to have more negative than positive stereotypes regarding the elderly. This is compounded by the fact that in the United States, a person's social identity, worth, and status are all tied to employment, and employment declines with age. In a study to determine how older workers were perceived, perspective business managers indicated a belief that older workers (age sixty) were lower than younger workers (age thirty) in efficiency, motivation, productivity, ability to work under pressure, and creativity. They believed, however, that older workers were higher in dependability, trustworthiness, and reliability and were less likely to miss work for personal reasons. In reality, data show both high productivity and low rates of absenteeism among older workers. Because of the strong cultural emphasis on work and productivity, retired Americans are sometimes reticent to admit that they are no longer employed and often identify themselves with their past occupation or profession.

Another study testing the accuracy of commonly held stereotypes found that the elderly are believed to have high levels of poor health, poverty, fear of crime, feelings of not being needed, loneliness, and isolation. In addition, they are believed to lack friends, have little or nothing to do, and have been forced to retire. Although the study found that these characteristics did exist to some degree, they were not true of the majority of elderly persons. Thus, stereotypes often persist even when there is evidence to the contrary. Elderly individuals who exhibit the expected traits are seen as proof of the stereotype, whereas the individuals who do not exhibit that trait are considered exceptions, regardless of their number.

Some positive stereotypes are that old people are wise and experienced, do not like handouts, are good with children (especially grandchildren), are willing to help, and are concerned for family. Politicians also see the elderly as conservative and politically active, which makes them important constituents.

—*Philip E. Lampe*

See also: Age discrimination; Ageism; Aging: Biological, psychological, and sociocultural perspectives; Aging: Historical perspective; Aging process; Cultural views of aging; Employment; Golden Girls, The; Humor; Loneliness; Over the hill; Retirement; Sexuality; Wisdom

For Further Information

Carlson, Kristy J, et al. "Stereotypes of Older Adults: Development and Evaluation of an Updated Stereotype Content and Strength Survey." *The Gerontologist*, 2019. doi:10.1093/geront/gnz061. The authors analyze the Stereotype Content and Strength Survey (SCSS) designed to update assessment tools commonly used to measure stereotypes of older adults.

Carmona, Marie Jose. "Battling Stereotypes Against Older People." Inequality.org, Institute for Policy Studies, 29 May 2019. inequality.org/research/battling-stereotypes-older-people/. Discusses the movement in Spain of older people pushing for decent state pensions.

Nelson, Todd D. *Ageism: Stereotyping and Prejudice against Older Persons*. MIT P, 2004. This volume presents the current thinking on age stereotyping, prejudice, and discrimination by researchers in gerontology, psychology, sociology, and communication.

STONES

Relevant Issues: Health and medicine

Significance: While there is no evidence of increased incidence of urinary stones with advancing age, stones of the biliary tract (cholelithiasis) do rise with age, affecting approximately 33 percent of the U.S. population over seventy years old.

Stones, or calculi, are hard deposits of material in the body associated with urine and bile. Unlike the typical calcium-based composition of kidney and ureter stones, bladder stones are most often composed of uric acid (a byproduct of protein metabolism) or struvite (a result of chronic urinary infection). Gallstones contain very little calcium; they are primarily composed of cholesterol.

KIDNEY AND URINARY TRACT STONES

Kidney stones or stones in the urinary tract affect 5 to 10 percent of the general population of the United States. The likelihood of a person to form a stone for the first time in their life decreases with advancing age. In people who have a prior history of urinary stone formation, however, the incidence, recurrence, and severity of urinary stone disease is similar between the geriatric and younger population. The composition of urinary stones in the older population is no different from those found in younger patients; however, the underlying urinary abnormality leading to the stone formation is different. More frequently, urinary stones in the elderly are caused by high uric acid levels and low citrate levels in the urine. Similar difficulties in the disposal of protein metabolites can lead to gouty arthritis.

The symptoms that accompany urinary stone disease are dependent on the location of the stone, the size of the stone, how long the stone has been present, whether infection is associated with the stone, and the degree of obstruction to urinary flow caused by the stone. Urine, which is produced by the kidneys, located beneath the ribs of the back, is collected into a structure just outside the kidney known as the renal pelvis. From the renal pelvis, urine passes into a thin narrow tube called the ureter and travels a relatively long distance to the urinary bladder. It is easy to envision how a stone traveling along such a narrow, long tube can get stuck and dam the further flow of urine.

Stones caught in the renal pelvis, prior to entry into the ureter, generally cause an intermittent, sharp pain in the back or side. Stones that pass into the ureter can cause pain in the back as well as points distant to the urinary system (the groin, the lower abdomen, and the testicle and penis in men); this phenomenon is known as referred pain. Occasionally, stones in the lowest portion of the ureters will cause pain only with urination or produce the desire to urinate frequently but only in small amounts. Often, blood not visible to the naked eye can be found in the urine with a simple chemical dipstick or by looking at the urine under a microscope, both easily accomplished in most doctors' offices.

Several radiological tests can be performed to pinpoint the location of a stone lodged in the urinary tract. An intravenous pyelogram (IVP) is a series of X rays performed following the administration of a dye into the patient's vein. This dye is concentrated in the urine and can be visualized as it travels through the urinary tract. High-frequency sound waves, or ultrasound, can determine if obstruction is present in the kidneys but will frequently miss stones lodged in the ureters. A computed tomography (CT) scan is similar to an IVP but uses advanced computer technology to visualize better all contents of the body. Although the CT scan is the most sensitive test for the detection of urinary stones, certain situations may necessitate the use of different tests. Frequently, people with poor renal function cannot receive the X-ray dye because of its potential harmful effects on the kidneys. A CT scan without contrast or ultrasound will frequently be performed in this situation.

Treatment of any stone depends on the location of the stone, its size, the time it has been in place, and any complicating issues such as infection. The methods for treatment are broad, and the specific means by which a stone is removed is often debated among the experts in this field. Some stones—especially if they are small, cause no pain, and are not significantly obstructing—are

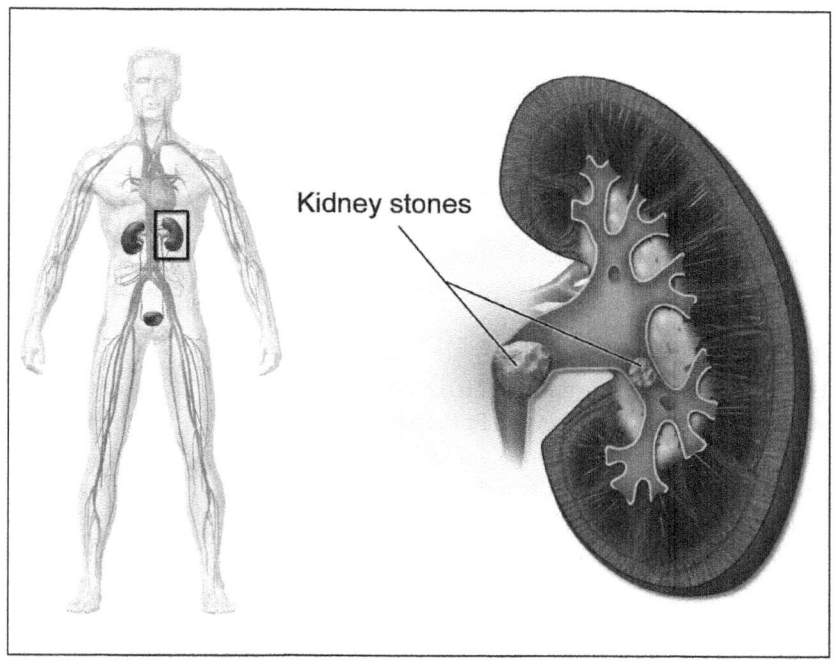

Stones form in the kidney when minerals in urine are at high concentration. Risk factors include high urine calcium levels; obesity; certain foods; some medications; calcium supplements; hyperparathyroidism; gout and not drinking enough fluids. (via Wikimedia Commons)

given a chance to pass on their own, a treatment termed watchful waiting. The most frequent non-invasive means to treat a small stone located in the urinary tract above the pelvic bone is extracorporeal shock wave lithotripsy (ESWL). This procedure involves the use of high-energy sound waves created by a machine outside the body and focused through the skin onto the stone. These sound waves break the stone into fine sand, which passes in the urine without symptoms. This is frequently the best method to deal with stones in elderly patients who have other medical problems that can make surgical means of removing a stone risky. Endoscopic removal of a stone involves the use of small telescopes passed into the urinary tract either through the urethra or through the back directly into the kidney. Different means of fragmenting the stone into smaller pieces for direct removal are then employed through the telescopes. This method is highly successful and often used for larger stones. Like ESWL, this low-invasive, endoscopic means of removing the stone places minimal stress on the elderly patient with other medical problems.

The development of these minimally invasive procedures for stone removal has led to a significant decrease in the need for open surgery. Nevertheless, there are special situations when an open surgical procedure may be the first reasonable option for the elderly patient with a urinary stone. These situations include abnormal urinary tract anatomy, concurrent urinary tract pathology other than the stone, or the failure of less invasive means to remove the stone.

BLADDER STONES

Bladder stones are found much less frequently than stones in the kidney and ureter. Perhaps the most famous person to have suffered from bladder stones is Benjamin Franklin, who reportedly stood on his head to urinate. Throughout the world, bladder stones are almost exclusively a disease of the older, male population. They are most frequently found in association with enlargement of the prostate that obstructs the bladder's ability to empty and allows these stones to crystallize in the urine. Other causes of bladder stone formation should be excluded, such as a narrowed urethra, an abnormal pouching of the bladder, a chronic urinary infection, or a neurologic dysfunction leading to poor bladder emptying.

Symptoms of a bladder stone are pain in the lower abdomen that worsens with movement, intermittent blockage of the urinary stream, a weak urine stream, increased frequency of urination often associated with a strong and urgent need to void, recurrent urinary tract infections, or blood in the urine. Definitive diagnosis of a stone can be made with a simple X ray of the abdomen alone; however, the physician will often need to perform additional tests, including a direct look into the bladder.

Treatment is very successful and appropriate for the elderly. As with stones of the kidney and ureter, a bladder stone often can be endoscopically removed using small telescopes. Most bladder stones, however, are removed with open surgery. Paramount to the successful treatment of a bladder stone is the treatment of the underlying cause for its formation, which frequently dictates the method of removal. Whether endoscopic or open surgery is chosen, both are generally well tolerated by elderly patients even if significant other medical problems exist.

GALLSTONES

The biliary system stores bile formed in the liver and delivers it to the intestines following a meal, aiding in the digestion of fat and the absorption of certain vitamins. The gallbladder is a blind-ending pouch that comes off of the bile duct as it courses from the liver to the small intestine. After consumption of a fatty meal, its muscle-lined wall contracts to release bile into the intestine. Stones can form in the gallbladder and can cause pain or infection when lodged in the bile duct or common hepatic (liver) duct. If a stone causes blockage and infection, the patient can become very sick and require emergency medical care.

Diseases affecting the gallbladder and bile ducts occur commonly in the elderly. By the age of seventy, stones in the gallbladder and bile duct represent the most frequently occurring disorder affecting this organ system. The symptoms associated with stones in the gallbladder or bile duct are numerous and depend on the location and size of the stone and whether there is an associated infection. Often, patients complain of pain in the right upper part of the abdomen. This pain often occurs after the consumption of a fatty meal, which causes the gallbladder to contract and release its bile. Fever, sweats, and chills may accompany the pain if there is infection present. Jaundice, a yellowish discoloring of the skin, may occur if the common bile duct or hepatic duct becomes obstructed with a gallstone. As with stones in the urinary tract, it is the blockage of flow of bile from the gallbladder that leads to the symptoms. Elderly patients who appear jaundiced may not always be suffering from gallstones, especially if there is no associated pain. Other diseases of the liver and biliary system, such as cirrhosis of the liver or hepatitis, will also cause jaundice and are frequently found in the elderly.

Unlike kidney stones, gallstones are frequently not visible on plain X-ray examination of the abdomen. Despite their hard nature, gallstones contain very little calcium. They are primarily composed of cholesterol which, unlike calcium, is not dense enough to be visible on an X-ray. Ultrasound examination of the liver and gallbladder is almost always the first test ordered by a physician who is suspicious that a patient may have a gallstone. To determine if obstruction of the bile duct is present, a physician can also use nuclear medicine studies, which uses a radioactive material concentrated by the gallbladder, similar to the concentration of X-ray dye used in the diagnosis of kidney stones. On occasion, the diagnosis of a gallstone lodged in the bile duct requires the placement of a telescope into the patient's stomach and intestine and direct visualization of the common bile duct's entry into the intestine.

Treatment of symptomatic gallstones almost always involves surgery using lighted telescopes passed either directly into the abdomen (laparoscopes) or through the stomach and intestine (endoscopes), or open surgery. Unlike the removal of kidney and bladder stones, which most often merely involves the removal of the actual stone and not the kidney, ureter, or bladder, treatment of gallstones usually also involves the removal of the gallbladder itself. The loss of this unpaired organ often does not lead to significant digestive problems, though in the elderly loose, foul-smelling bowel movements may result from the altered digestion of fats.

The choice of surgical approach again depends on whether an infection is associated with the stone, how severe the symptoms are, whether any liver dysfunction is associated with the stone, and the overall health of the patient. Gallstones not causing symptoms are generally not removed. Patients with diabetes mellitus and other complicating medical conditions are dealt with in a more cautious manner and often undergo surgery to remove the gallstone and gallbladder even if symptoms do not exist.

—*John F. Ward and Prodromos G. Borboroglu*

See also: Gastrointestinal changes and disorders; Gout; Nutrition; Urinary disorders

For Further Information

"Bladder Stones." Mayo Clinic, Mayo Foundation for Medical Education and Research, 16 Aug. 2019. www.mayoclinic.org/diseases-conditions/bladder-stones/symptoms-causes/syc-20354339. General information on bladder stones.

Lieske, John C., et al. "Stone Composition as a Function of Age and Sex." *Clinical Journal of the American Society of Nephrology*, vol. 9, no. 12, 2014, pp. 2,141-46. doi:10.2215/cjn.05660614. In this study, the authors examine the distribution of stone types from the Mayo Clinic Metals Laboratory to determine stone composition.

Lopushinsky, Steven R, and David R Urbach. "Gallstone Disease in the Elderly: Diagnosis and Management." *Aging Health*, vol. 1, no. 3, 2005, pp. 441-47. doi:10.2217/1745509x.1.3.441. This article reviews the diagnosis and management of patients with different clinical presentations of gallstone disease, with special emphasis on the role of age in the decision-making process.

Nassar, Yousef, and Seth Richter. "Management of Complicated Gallstones in the Elderly: Comparing Surgical and Non-Surgical Treatment Options." *Gastroenterology Report*, vol. 7, no. 3, 2019, pp. 205-11. doi:10.1093/gastro/goy046. This study evaluates the differences in clinical outcomes of endoscopic retrograde cholangiopancreatography (ERCP), ERCP followed by cholecystectomy (EC) and percutaneous aspiration (PA) in the elderly population with choledocholithiasis.

STRESS AND COPING SKILLS

Relevant Issues: Family, health and medicine, psychology

Significance: Understanding stress and coping across the life span has both practical and empirical implications. Greater awareness of the impact of stress on health, along with methods of reducing its harmful effects can promote wellness in all age groups, including older adults.

Much of what is known about the physiological effects of stress on the body came from animal researchers in the early 1930s. Findings suggest that emotional experiences, such as pain and fear, act as a mobilizing force by producing physiological changes in the body (such as increased adrenal gland output) to help an organism ward off the threat and take action. The general adaptation syndrome is a model explaining the body's response to stress that involves three stages: alarm, resistance, and exhaustion. Stress across a short period is adaptive; however, with prolonged exposure to a threat and commensurate bodily alterations, it could be harmful. Important parallels apply to humans and the stress process: Stress affects health by overcoming capacities for adaptation; there are individual differences in each person's abilities to adjust to stress; and daily stressors, even when experienced as transitory and mild in intensity, can have negative effects on the health of the mind and body.

Research examining the effects of stress and physical health, mental health, and immune functioning has yielded mixed results and identified a large range of responses that individuals may exhibit under similar circumstances. Additional evidence suggests that individual coping strategies, levels of resilience, and access to supportive resources play significant roles in adapting to stress and serve as buffers to potential associated adverse consequences. In older adults, these findings have particular importance because changes in health, financial status, and access to social and familial support are commonly associated with aging.

STRESS AMONG OLDER ADULTS

Despite experiencing a number of significant life changes associated with aging, older adults report lower perceived stress than younger adults. Stressful events most commonly reported by older adults include death of a spouse, retirement, illness or hospitalization, and decreased income. Each of these high frequency events involves role losses of some type for older adults. Additionally, they are inextricably related to other life circumstances of an individual, such as their social relationships. For example, while the death of a spouse involves grief and psychological distress, this experience may also result in decreased number of friends and diminished income. Although the impact of other daily stressors associated with aging, such as loneliness, boredom, and loss of physical abilities such as vision, hearing, balance, and mobility may not be recognized as apparent life events, they too can strain the coping resources of individuals. Research on stress has identified links with high blood pressure, weakened immune system, anxiety, depression, insomnia, indigestion, and increased risk for heart disease.

COPING WITH STRESS

The coping process involves the behaviors and actions that an individual engages to manage stress. Research indicates that there are marked individual differences in how people manage stressful situations and, as would be expected, the extent to which they are successful. Coping strategies may also vary as developmental changes associated with aging occur across the lifespan, and as a function of the particular stressful situation (e.g., health problems, retirement) one is trying to manage

Age-related coping has been conceptualized in several different ways by researchers. The developmental interpretation suggests that there are real changes in how people cope as they age. The underlying implication is that changes in coping result from developmental change and is not solely determined by environmental circumstances. Some research suggests that older adults regress or become less sophisticated in their coping as they age, resulting in decreased effectiveness. Others research indicates that individuals become more mature in their coping as they age, frequently utilizing humor, distancing, reflective thought, and other comparatively more effective strategies.

A contextual interpretation of how people change in coping postulates that age differences occur because of changing life contexts and demands with age. This interpretation promotes examining the person-environment interactions r to better understand coping. For example, knowing the age, available social resources, and type of stress are all critical to gain an appreciation of the coping strategy employed.

A third interpretation focuses on examination of the historical experiences and birth cohort (group) to which an individual belongs to identify how that individual may cope. For example, differences in expectations regarding pain relief, identification and expression of emotions, and thresholds for seeking assistance may exist among alternate generational cohorts. Other research has identified marked gender differences, with men becoming more passive in strategies used and women becoming more aggressive as they age.

A body of research has identified normative differences in the types of stresses experienced by younger and older adults. For the younger sample, the majority of stressors revolved around financial problems, work, taking care of the household, and dealing with personal problems and family; for older adults, health issues and lack of ability to carry out everyday tasks as easily as before predominated. Not surprisingly, the younger sample appraised their stressful circumstances as more changeable and reported a greater sense of control over the situations compared to older adults. This pattern was reflected in the predominant types of coping strategies reported by younger and older adults. Younger adults used more problem-focused strategies (seeking social support, planned problem solving), whereas older adults more frequently engaged in emotion-focused coping (distancing, acceptance, positive reappraisal).

Other researchers, however, found fewer age differences among alternate age groups and more stability to coping approaches. Part of this disagreement may be because of differences in research design. Despite differences in research methods, it appears that research supports the contextual interpretation of age differences in coping. That is, age differences in coping are a function of what situation people cope with and how they interpret the stressful circumstance rather than just the presence of stage-related developmental changes through which all individuals progress.

Several coping strategies have been found to be employed across age groups including by older adults. These include direct and indirect strategies, and efforts toward building and maintaining personal, psychological, social, physical, and mental care.

Direct coping strategies include confronting the source of stress, changing the interpretation of stress, and changing oneself. Confronting the source of stress might involve identifying and directly addressing problems with a spouse, family member, or living circumstance. Changing the interpretation of stress may require reappraising goals (e.g., due to physical limitations), acknowledging vulnerabilities, modifying expectations, and engaging in self-reinforcement (e.g., in adapting to altered roles associated with retirement). Changing oneself in response to stress can include identifying stressors, self-monitoring responses (e.g., effects on mood, anger, sleep), committing to act on problems or identified helpful responses, and acquiring or enhancing coping strategies (e.g., through mindfulness training, physical therapy, or continuing education).

Effective indirect coping strategies may include learning relaxation techniques (e.g., yoga), engaging in exercise, taking medications (e.g., antidepressants), and keeping a healthy diet. Less effective or even problematic coping strategies may involve substance use or abuse, adopting the "sick" role, excessive reliance on defense mechanisms (e.g., denial), and engaging in escape, avoidance, or isolation.

Developing and maintaining a personal care plan in effort to cope with stress in older adulthood may include keeping a balanced perspective regarding psychological, spiritual, social, physical, and mental factors. Psychological and spiritual considerations include efforts at self-awareness of stressors and the responses they elicit, maintaining spiritual practices, pursuing relaxation activities, seeking contact with nature, and finding humor in life. Social considerations may involve maintaining established healthy relationships and support systems when possible and developing new ones when necessary, seeking help when needed, and engaging in social (e.g., political) action. Physical considerations include strength and fitness building activities, healthy nutrition and diet, and restorative sleep habits. Mental considerations may involve pursuing continuing education and ongoing skill development, especially with increasing life spans and correspondent longer retirement periods, and engaging in challenging, purposeful, and useful cognitive exercises.

—Karen Kopera-Frye and Richard Wiscott
Updated by Paul F. Bell, Ph.D.

See also: Death and dying; Death anxiety; Death of a child; Death of parents; Depression; Divorce; Grief; Heart attacks; Hospitalization; Loneliness; Memory loss; Psychiatry, geriatric; Relocation; Retirement; Social ties; Widows and widowers

For Further Information

Kabat-Zinn, J. *Full Catastrophe Living (Revised Edition): Using the Wisdom of Your Body and Mind to Face Stress, Pain, and Illness Paperback.* Bantam Books, 2013. A practical guide employing mind-body approaches to reduce and cope with stress and promote well-being and healing. Utilizes evidence-based strategies to build resilience and alleviate pain and suffering.

Leland, J. *Happiness Is a Choice You Make: Lessons from a Year Among the Oldest Old.* Farrar, Straus, Giroux, 2018. A collection of lessons on how to live well while aging and the power individuals have in influencing happiness, effective coping, and wellbeing in the face of life's challenges. An optimistic and insightful accounting of the richness and contentment that can be found in the late stages of life derived from the wisdom of six individuals over the age of 85.

STROKES

Relevant Issues: Health and medicine

Significance: Strokes are characterized by decreased blood flow to the brain, often due to an obstruction or bleed. Strokes are a leading cause of death and long-term disability early recognition and treatment of a stroke is critical.

Key Terms:

embolic stroke: when a blood clot that forms elsewhere in the body breaks loose and travels to the brain via the bloodstream

hemorrhagic stroke: when a weakened blood vessel ruptures and spills blood into brain tissue

thrombotic stroke: when a blood clot forms and blocks blood flow through the artery in which it formed

According to the United States Center for Disease Control, more than 750,000 people in the United States experience a stroke each year. Strokes are one of the leading causes of death in those over sixty-five. Strokes have devastating physical, financial, emotional, and social effects that impact the entire family.

A stroke is defined most simply as an interruption in the blood supply to the brain. When the brain does not get enough oxygen, brain cells die and leave permanent damage. This can occur because of an obstruction in blood flow or a bleed. A transient ischemic attack (TIA) can be a precursor to stroke. TIAs occur when the brain lacks sufficient oxygen and causes a temporary deficit, such as slurred speech, difficulties with vision, weakness or numbness in the face or extremities, loss of balance, or altered consciousness. However, the effects of a TIA last no more than twenty-four hours and resolve entirely without intervention. Although these may be considered "miniature" or "temporary" strokes, TIA should be taken seriously as a possibility of developing a full stroke later in life.

CAUSES AND RISK FACTORS

There are several common causes of stroke. Strokes can be caused by clots, hemorrhage, narrowing of vessels, and high blood pressure. The most common cause of stroke is a thrombus, a clot that forms in the brain (thrombotic), resulting in a thrombotic stroke. Narrowing of vessels can also lead to lack of oxygen to the brain. Such narrowing is often related to arteriosclerosis, or fatty deposits along the vessel walls. These vessels may include the intracerebral arteries (the arteries in the head), but can also include the carotid artery (in the neck). Clots can also come from other parts of the body (embolic), resulting in an embolic stroke. For example, a blood clot in the heart can break off and travel to the brain, causing an occlusion. This type of clot is called an embolus. A hemorrhagic stroke results when a weakened blood vessel leaks or bursts. This is most commonly caused by elevated blood pressure, deposition of cerebral amyloid (CAA), aneurysms or vascular malformations, or a combination of these risk factors.

There are several factors that put a person more at risk for stroke. Some of these can be controlled and others cannot. Stroke risk increases with age. Men generally experience more strokes than women; after menopause, however, the numbers are more equal. African Americans, especially African American men with heart disease, have more strokes than Caucasians. Finally, a family history of strokes also increases the risk.

The risk factors that can be controlled are many. These include high blood pressure (also called hypertension), high cholesterol, heart disease, diabetes, smoking, obesity, a sedentary lifestyle, and stress. If treated, risk of stroke can be reduced. Prevention of stroke centers on making changes related to these factors.

WARNING SIGNS AND EFFECTS

It is essential that elderly individuals be aware of the warning signs of stroke. Knowing these symptoms can help a person decide when to seek help and can provide a better chance for recovery. These include numbness or tingling in the face, arms, or legs; difficulty speaking; headache; blurred or other disturbed vision; dizziness; loss of consciousness; and sudden weakness or paralysis (often affecting just one side of the body). A simple mnemonic commonly used by the National Stroke Association and American Heart Association is F.A.S.T.: Face drooping, arm weakness, speech changes, and time. If any of these signs are manifested in an older person, they should immediately seek medical treatment.

The effects of strokes are numerous and vary from person to person. No one can predict the exact effect of a stroke, as the deficits seen depend on the area of damage within the brain. Although small strokes may result in full or near-full recovery, larger strokes may result in more profound deficits.

Speech. Patients who have suffered a stroke may not be able to speak or may have trouble understanding what is said to them. These types of problems with the use of language are referred to as aphasia. The muscles involved with speech and swallowing are closely related, so individuals may experience deficits in both of these areas. Certain swallowing problems may lead to aspiration and subsequent pneumonia. Thus, a speech therapy evaluation is often needed for any individuals exhibiting problems with eating, swallowing, or speech. Dietary modifications may be necessary for the person to swallow safely. If a patient is unable to swallow for prolonged periods of time, they may need a nasogastric (NG) or feeding tube to help them get nutrition.

Senses. Other problems can affect such senses as sight and touch perception. Visual problems may range from blurred vision to double vision to partial or total blindness. Patients may also have loss of touch and have subsequent numbness or not be able to recognize part of the world or part of their body (neglect).

Motor. Patients who have had a stroke often suffer from hemiparesis, or one-sided unilateral weakness that affects the opposite side of the body from where the stroke was. These symptoms may require long-term rehabilitation and may cause significant impairment in activities of daily living such as dressing, eating, and bathing.

Some deficits are more common with right- and left-sided brain damage. Those with a left-sided stroke (right-sided weakness) tend to have swallowing problems and may require a feeding tube for some time after the stroke. They generally have a slow and cautious behavior style and may be fearful when learning new tasks. Those with a right-sided stroke (left-sided weakness) tend to be more impulsive and may not acknowledge that anything is wrong with them. They pose a safety risk to themselves by overestimating their abilities and have a high rate of falls. Disabilities in those with a right-sided stroke may be less obvious to others but nonetheless put the person at risk for injury.

TREATMENT

When a patient is suspected of having a stroke, the most critical point of information is the "Last Known Well". This timepoint describes the last time a patient was last known completely normal. Often, patients who wake up with strokes will have a last known well of the night

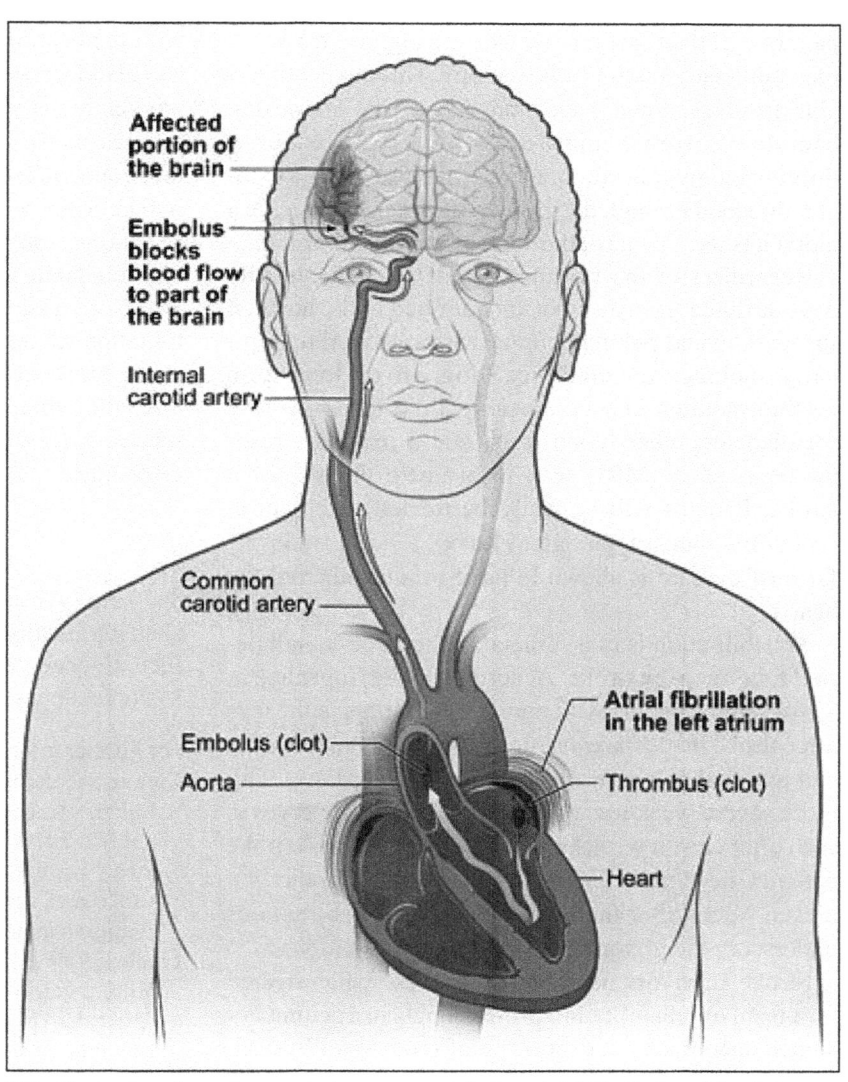

This illustration shows how a stroke can occur during atrial fibrilation. blood clot can form in the left atrium of the heart. If a piece of the clot breaks off and travels to an artery in the brain, it can block blood flow through the artery. The lack of blood flow to the portion of the brain fed by the artery causes a stroke. (via National Heart Lung and Blood In-

before. This is important as it describes the treatment course—patients who are within a certain time window are eligible for certain therapies.

Patients who are brought to the hospital after stroke-like symptoms will be given a computed tomography (CT) scan to evaluate for signs of blood. Patients who have had a hemorrhagic, or bleeding, stroke, will be admitted to the hospital for blood pressure control and blood pressure monitoring and are not eligible for acute intervention. Patients who do NOT have signs of a bleed and who are within 3 hours (now 4.5 for certain patients) of their last known well are eligible for tissue plasminogen activator (tPA) therapy. This medication is able to break down a clot, but has a risk of causing bleeds. Patients may also be eligible for a thrombectomy procedure, which involves using a catheter threaded through the groin to the brain, to retrieve a clot if it is seen in one of the large arteries in the brain.

Regardless of the treatment modality, patients who have suffered from a stroke are admitted to the hospital for workup and risk reduction treatment. Workup typically includes an electrocardiogram or long-term rhythm monitor, echocardiogram, lipid levels, testing for diabetes, other blood tests, and a magnetic resonance imaging (MRI) scan to evaluate the size of a stroke. Patients will typically be treated with aspirin (with or without clopidogrel/Plavix), a statin, and warfarin (if the clot is shown to have originated from the heart).

Rehabilitation is most crucial in the three-month period following the stroke. According to the Copenhagen Stroke Study, people with minimal weakness in the legs after stroke made maximal progress within three weeks and minimal progress after nine weeks. For those with more severe weakness or paralysis, little recovery was seen after eleven weeks. Overall, however, most stroke patients did recover the ability to walk within the first eleven weeks after the stroke. These research findings underscore the importance of early rehabilitation.

Stroke survivors have better recovery when treated by a team of rehabilitation professionals in a setting designed specifically for this type of recovery. Physical, occupational, and speech therapy (if needed) should begin in the hospital as soon as possible. Physical therapy focuses on lower extremity strengthening, helping the person learn exercises for the legs and regain walking skills. Occupational therapy centers attention on use of the arms and hands to perform key life activities, such as dressing, bathing, and eating. The occupational therapist also assists the person in resuming home management skills, such as doing laundry and cooking, as well as in reentering the community with a physical limitation. The speech therapist, also called a speech-language pathologist, assists patients in regaining speech, relearning skills that may be impaired because of memory problems or aphasia, and setting up an appropriate diet. Nurses in inpatient rehabilitation help patients with medication schedules, nutrition, skin care, bowel and bladder retraining, and family education. The social worker helps patients and families connect with resources in the community, work out insurance problems, and make discharge plans. The patient's physician will help diagnose and treat medical problems and complications, and a psychologist or psychiatrist is generally available for counseling with the person and the family, if needed. Together, this interdisciplinary rehabilitation team helps patients and families achieve their goals. Most patients get better outcomes if transferred to a rehabilitation unit or center soon after the stroke to receive more intensive therapy with the goal of home discharge.

—*Kristen L. Easton*
Updated by Derrick Cheng, BSc

See also: African Americans; Arteriosclerosis; Brain changes and disorders; Communication; Hypertension; Incontinence; Mobility problems; Personality changes; Vision changes and disorders

For Further Information

Corrao, Salvatore, et al. "Cognitive Impairment and Stroke in Elderly Patients." *Vascular Health and Risk Management*, vol. 12, 2016, pp. 105-16. doi:10.2147/vhrm.s75306. Reviews current knowledge about the interaction between stroke and vascular risk factors and the development of cognitive impairment and dementia.

Lindley, Richard I. "Stroke Prevention in the Very Elderly." *Stroke*, vol. 49, no. 3, 2018, pp. 796-802. doi:10.1161/strokeaha.117.017952. Discusses prevention methods for stroke in older adults.

Lui, Siew Kwaon, and Minh Ha Nguyen. "Elderly Stroke Rehabilitation: Overcoming the Complications and Its Associated Challenges." *Current Gerontology and Geriatrics Research*, vol. 2018, 27 June 2018, pp. 1-9. doi:10.1155/2018/9853837. This review summarizes the consequences of stroke in the elderly, predictors of stroke rehabilitation outcomes, role of rehabilitation in neuronal recovery, importance of stroke rehabilitation units, and types of rehabilitation resources and services available in Singapore.

"Stroke." National Institute on Aging, U.S. Department of Health and Human Services, 16 May 2017. www.nia.nih.gov/health/stroke. General information on stroke.

Taylor, Jill Bolte. *My Stroke of Insight: A Brain Scientist's Personal Journey.* Penguin Books, 2016. Taylor provides a valuable recovery guide for those touched by brain injury and an inspiring testimony that inner peace is accessible to anyone.

SUICIDE

Relevant Issues: Death, health and medicine, violence
Significance: Suicide rates are increasing across every state in the United States since 1999 and currently is a major public health concern.

Suicide is the 10th leading cause of death in the United States. Between the years of 2001 and 2017 the total suicide rate in the United States increased 31 percent from 10.7 to 14.0 per 100,000 population. In 2017, there were approximately 1,400,000 suicide attempts and 47,173 deaths secondary to suicide. The rate of suicide is highest among adults between 45 and 54 years of age and followed by older adults 85 years and older. In 2015, suicide cost the United States $69 billion dollars in health-care expenses.

GROUP DIFFERENCES

Suicide rates among older adults vary by gender. Men are likely to complete suicide more often than women, although women attempt suicide more often than men. The most common proposed reason from the "gender paradox" is the choice of suicide method. Men are much more likely to use violent methods of suicide, particularly firearms, than women are. Other possible theories are associated with males having more impulsive, self-destructive, high-risk behavior and worse social support systems. Most common suicide methods used by men were firearm (56 percent), suffocation including hanging (27.7 percent), and poisoning (9 percent). Among females, the most common methods of suicide were poisoning (31.4 percent) and firearm (31.2 percent).

Suicide rates among older adults also vary by ethnicity. Among the most prominent ethnic groups, the suicide rate is highest among American Indian/Alaska Native, followed by white males. Much lower rates were found among African Americans, Asian Americans, and Pacific Islanders. Other group differences in suicide exist as well. At all ages, suicide is higher among single, separated/divorced, or widowed persons as compared to married individuals.

RISK FACTORS FOR SUICIDE IN LATE LIFE

Major psychiatric disorders, such as depression, schizophrenia spectrum, anxiety disorders, and substance abuse, are the most important risk factors for suicide in older adults. Affective illness was the most common psychiatric disorder affecting 54 percent to 87 percent of older adults. However, 54 percent of people who die by suicide may not have a known mental health condition. Usually older adults who are successfully diagnosed with a psychiatric disorder are able to respond well to treatment and in some cases even better than younger adults.

Studies show that personality disorders and traits as hostility, timidity, rigid personality, independent style may be associated with late-life suicide rate. Hopelessness also plays a critical predictor in eventual suicide.

Chronic physical illness is another risk factor for suicide among older adults. Overall, the risk for suicide is 1.5 to 4 times higher if a person has a chronic disease. In one study, 94 percent of older suicides had physical problems at the time of death, and 57 percent had seen a healthcare professional in the previous thirty days.

The illnesses most frequently cited were diseases of the central nervous system (especially dementia), HIV/AIDS, Huntington's disease, malignancies, cardiopulmonary conditions, spinal cord injury, and urogenital diseases. The prospect of living many years with chronic pain or disability and subsequently becoming dependent upon the health care-system or family members may be especially difficult for older persons who have traditionally achieved an independent lifestyle. The association between chronic illnesses and suicide may also be partially secondary to depression (chronic illnesses can cause depression and depression increases the risk for suicide).

A previous history of suicide attempt is a risk factor for suicide. Among all age groups, those who attempt suicide once are more likely to try again than those who have never attempted suicide. Previous history may be especially risky for older individuals because they have fewer failed suicide attempts than younger people. Other risk factors include stressful life events, lack of social support, significantly functional impairment, bereavement, and financial stressors. High risk of suicide is also present in small subgroups such as military veterans, LGBTQ community, and persons with autism.

ASSESSMENT AND INTERVENTION

Asking simple, open-ended questions is recommended for evaluating suicide risk. A direct question such as, "Have you ever thought of hurting or killing yourself?" can convey understanding and the willingness to take a person seriously. This does not provoke people to become suicidal and most people will answer truthfully. Another useful method to assess suicide risk is through standardized screening tools, such as the Geriatric Depression Scale (GDS), the Columbia-Suicide Severity Rating Scale (C-SSRS), the Suicide Assessment Five-Step Evaluation and Triage (SAFE-T), and the Patient Health Questionnaire (PHQ-2), which is a two-question depression screen, and if positive, the PHQ-9 may be added. If someone reveals suicidal thinking or plans, follow-up questions should be about specifics. Does the person have a concrete plan? Does he or she have the means to carry out the plan? For example, does the person have a gun and know how to use it? When a person is suicidal, he or she will need a referral to a mental health professional, medication, and/or hospitalization; the care option will depend on the specific circumstances relating to the individual's needs.

Mental health professionals who are treating a suicidal person may incorporate a comprehensive approach including, stabilization and safety of the individual along with assessment of risk factors, on-going treatment, problem-solving and coping skills. The professional may violate confidentiality if the person is of imminent harm to self or others.

During the acute phase, admission to inpatient setting or involuntary commitment may be required to warrant individual safety. Treatment overall focuses on treating the underlying disease, decreasing suffering and increasing coping skills. Once the acute phase is resolved the clinician can begin to address long-standing problems. A no-suicide, no-harm agreement can be useful, and the clinician will often elicit help from the suicidal person's social support system. Evidence-based interventions include cognitive behavioral therapy for suicide prevention, non-demand caring contacts, dialectical behavioral therapy, restructuring strategies, techniques for regulating emotions, structured problem-solving therapies and/or medications.

PREVENTION

Prevention requires a comprehensive approach from the individual, family, and community. The goal is to decrease factors that increase risk of suicide and to increase factors that develop resilience. Effective prevention strategies include education about suicide, adequate training for healthcare professionals, decrease access to suicide methods (firearms, substance abuse), and decreasing the quantity of over-the-counter medications.

Educating health care providers and the general public about risk factors for suicide in older adults may reduce the conditions that can lead to suicide.

EUTHANASIA

Euthanasia is the deliberate ending of a person's life to relieve pain and suffering. This contrasts with physician-assisted suicide, in which the patient self-administers a lethal dose of a drug that was prescribed by a physician who knew that its purpose was to induce death. One piece of evidence that attitudes in the United States toward euthanasia have become more positive is the acceptance of living wills, in which individuals decree that no heroic procedures or exceptional life-sustaining measures be employed in the event of their incapacitation.

The prototype of the older adult suicide is a widower who is retired and lives alone. He is isolated from family and friends and is not active in church, community, or other social activities. He feels lonely, depressed, and helpless to do anything about his situation, and he may have other psychiatric problems as well. Though not terminally ill or in debilitating pain, he has recently seen a physician. He feels hopeless about the future and finds no meaning in his existence. He has turned to alcohol or other drugs to drown his sorrows. He has family member(s) who have committed suicide. He has attempted suicide in the past and has thought about suicide recently. He has a gun in his home.

Though the myth is otherwise, the overwhelming majority of people who are terminally ill fight for life to the end. Only 2 to 4 percent of suicides occur in the context of terminal illness. A request for death comes from a person who is desperate, whether he or she is medically ill. In such cases, a comprehensive psychiatric assessment should include inquiring into the source of the person's desperation. It should also include trying to relieve this source. Older individuals who are informed of acute, potentially fatal medical conditions may express angry preoccupation with suicide and request assistance in carrying out these wishes. The majority are motivated primarily by dread of what will happen to them, rather than by current pain or suffering. They fear debilitating pain, dependency on others, loss of dignity, the side effects of medical treatment, burdening of their family and friends, and death itself. Those who are medically ill may not know what to expect. When they can express their fears, their request for euthanasia may quickly disappear.

Sociologists note that argument about the right to suicide and assisted suicide for the older adult is a symbol of society's devaluation of old age. Ageism results in easy acceptance of the concepts of euthanasia, rational suicide, and assisted suicide. It creates a society in which suicide is not only expected but also demanded of all who might be a burden.

—Lillian M. Range
Updated by Ecler Jaqua, MD and Miriam E. Schwartz, MD, PhD

See also: Death and dying; Depression; Euthanasia; Living wills; Men and aging; Terminal illness; Widows and widowers

For Further Information

Conejero, Ismael, et al. "Suicide in Older Adults: Current Perspectives." *Clinical Interventions in Aging*, vol. 13, 2018, pp. 691-99. doi:10.2147/cia.s130670. Provides a critical evaluation of recent findings concerning specific risk factors for suicidal thoughts and behaviors among older people.

Conwell, Yeates, et al. "Suicide in Older Adults." *Psychiatric Clinics of North America*, vol. 34, no. 2, 2011, pp. 451-68. doi:10.1016/j.psc.2011.02.002. Reviews the evidence for factors that place older adults at risk for suicide or protect them from it.

Jahn, Danielle R. "Suicide Risk in Older Adults: The Role and Responsibility of Primary Care." *Journal of Clinical Outcomes Management*, vol. 24, no. 4, Apr. 2017. Reviews the literature and good clinical practices to provide primary care practitioners with the knowledge required to identify and address older adult suicide risk in their practice.

Koo, Yu Wen, et al. "Profiles by Suicide Methods: an Analysis of Older Adults." *Aging & Mental Health*, vol. 23, no. 3, 2017, pp. 385-91. doi:10.1080/13607863.2017.1411884. Investigates choice of suicide method in individuals aged 65 years and over.

"Suicide Rising across the US." CDC, Centers for Disease Control and Prevention. www.cdc.gov/vitalsigns/suicide/. General information on suicide statistics and advice on intervention.

"Suicide Statistics." AFSP, 16 Apr. 2019. afsp.org/about-suicide/suicide-statistics/. Current statistics on suicide in the United States.

SUNSET BOULEVARD (FILM)

Director: Billy Wilder

Cast: Gloria Swanson, William Holden, Erich Von Stroheim

Date: Released in 1950

Relevant Issues: Media, psychology, values

Significance: This satiric film explores the consequences of false values that make it impossible for a formerly glamorous film star to accept both her own aging and changing times.

Sunset Boulevard is largely set in the Hollywood home of the faded silent screen star Norma Desmond (played by silent screen star Gloria Swanson). After the advent of talking pictures, the imperious Norma retreated to her sumptuous but decaying mansion, living in almost complete isolation. The illusion that she is still a popular star is sustained by her devoted butler, Max Von Mayer-ling (Erich Von Stroheim), who is Norma's first husband and her former director. Living in the glory days of her past, the aging Norma is unable to acknowledge that time has gone by—she still hopes to return to the big screen with a script in which she will portray the seductive biblical temptress Salome.

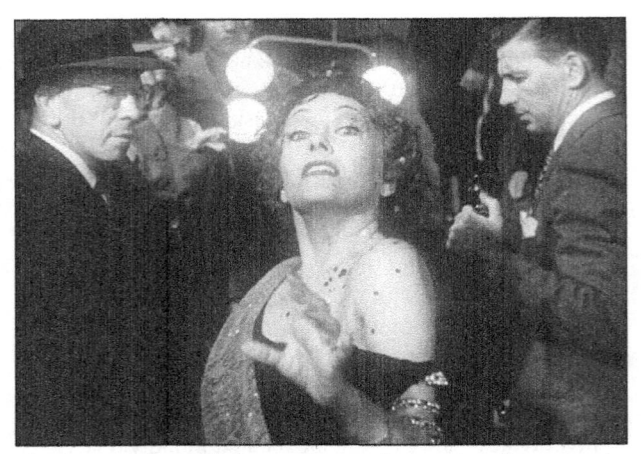

The famous "I'm ready for my close-up" scene from Sunset Boulevard. (via Wikimedia Commons)

Hoping that he will rejuvenate her professionally and personally, Norma employs young, good looking screenwriter Joe Gillis (William Holden) to work with her on the script. Pressed by his creditors and pitying Norma's desperation and neediness, Gillis also agrees to become her kept man. As Norma becomes increasingly overbearing and possessive, Gillis breaks off with her and, in a moment of bitterness, reveals the devastating fact that both she and her screenplay have been rejected by the film industry that had once celebrated her as a great star. Haggard and despairing, Norma shoots him with the gun that she had intended to use on herself. Placed under arrest, Norma walks down her staircase to a waiting squad car in a state of utter self-deception, convinced that she is performing the role of the bewitching Salome for her admiring fans.

Sunset Boulevard won Academy Awards for Best Screenplay, Best Art Direction, Best Set Decoration, and Best Score. It was adapted into a musical play by composer Andrew Lloyd Webber in 1993.

—*Margaret Boe Birns*

See also: Age discrimination; Ageism; Beauty; Women and aging

TELL ME A RIDDLE (BOOK)
Author: Tillie Olsen
Date: Published in 1961
Relevant Issues: Death, family, psychology, values

Significance: Olsen's novella powerfully delineates the last life stage of a Russian Jewish immigrant who defies conventional expectations for older women as she struggles to find her individual voice.

Readers of all ages respond to Tillie Olsen's poignant story of one woman's late-life anguish and struggle. The main character, Eva, is larger than her roles of wife and mother but constrained by them in ways that become intolerable in the last year and a half of her life. An orator in the 1905 Russian Revolution, she rebels against her husband's plan to move them to a senior residence. Angry, tired of sacrificing for others, and intent on solitude, Eva wants "never again to be forced to move to the rhythm of others." She refuses to be a sweet grandmother who tells riddles to amuse her grandchildren. Metastasized cancer heightens her withdrawal.

Olsen richly details Eva's painful dying as thoughts of past and present stream through her consciousness,

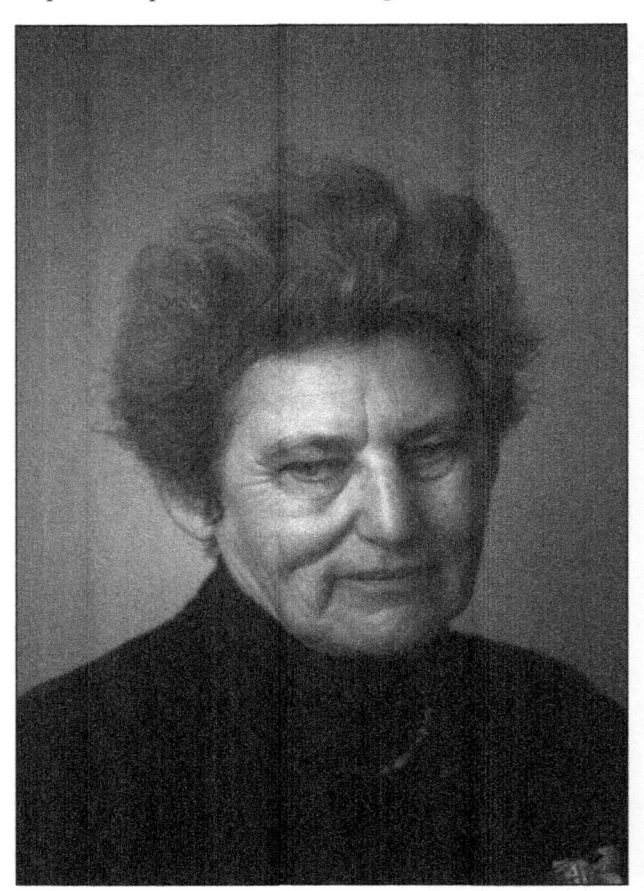

Tillie Olsen in her 60's. (via Wikimedia Commons)

and she accepts devoted nursing from a granddaughter. She reaches out to her husband in a gesture of reconciliation. Although Eva dies with parts of herself unfulfilled, giving the story a somber tone, Olsen also expresses faith in human endurance and family ties and hope in rebellion against confining roles. The novella illuminates the capacity for change in old age, even in unpromising circumstances, and suggests that the search for life's meaning is truly lifelong.

—Margaret Cruikshank

See also: Cancer; Death and dying; Family relationships; Grandparenthood; Loneliness; Old age; Women and aging

TEMPERATURE REGULATION AND SENSITIVITY

Relevant Issues: Health and medicine

Significance: The human body functions efficiently and comfortably within a very narrow temperature range; aging can decrease the body's ability to tolerate extremes of environmental temperatures.

Normal internal (core) body temperature is around 37 degrees Celsius (98.6 degrees Fahrenheit). Core temperatures below 35 degrees Celsius (95 degrees Fahrenheit) are considered abnormally cold (hypothermia), while temperatures above 38.3 degrees Celsius (101 degrees Fahrenheit) are too hot (hyperthermia) for normal function. Thermoregulation, the monitoring and controlling of body temperatures, is primarily coordinated by the hypothalamus, located in the brain. The process of thermoregulation becomes active when air temperature rises above or drops below approximately 22 degrees Celsius (72 degrees Fahrenheit), depending on the relative humidity.

Tolerance of cool temperatures increases with body size, body fat, and muscle mass. The body also has two active strategies to maintain body temperature in cool environments: reducing heat loss or increasing internal body temperature. Body heat is normally lost through the skin's surface. Blood vessels in the skin can narrow with cold temperatures and decrease blood flow, thus reducing heat loss. Shivering, which involves contraction of muscles, can rapidly raise metabolism and body temperature. Inactive older people tend to lose muscle mass with aging, thus decreasing the ability to raise body metabolism and temperature. In addition, elderly people are usually not able to contract skin vessels as efficiently as the young, thus decreasing their ability to minimize heat losses.

Increased blood flow to the skin and sweating are the two primary body changes involved in reducing body temperature, thus preventing hyperthermia. Widening of skin blood vessels, increased blood flow from the heart, and redistribution of blood flow from the intestines, kidneys, and other organs can increase blood flow to the skin. Widening of skin blood vessels does not occur as efficiently in older people as it does in the young. In addition, the ability to increase blood flow from the heart and redistribute blood flow from vital organs to the skin can decrease with aging. Sweating also decreases with aging, possibly because of the increased sun damage to the skin over time. Hydration status also influences both sweating and the ability to redistribute blood flow to the skin. Older people tend to be less hydrated than the young, further decreasing their ability to thermo-regulate in hot environments.

Illnesses and a sedentary lifestyle are considered the greatest threats to thermoregulation in the elderly. Therefore, a healthy and active lifestyle is probably the best way to preserve thermoregulatory functions with aging. Proper nutrition helps reduce dehydration and overheating, while sunscreens may help preserve the structural functions of the skin, which are vital for thermoregulation. Appropriate clothing can also help with thermoregulation. Research suggests that postmenopausal women taking estrogen maintain better hydration status and have improved functions of the skin, which helps with thermoregulation.

—Laurence M. Katz

See also: Aging process; Menopause; Skin changes and disorders

For Further Information

"Aging Changes in Vital Signs." *MedlinePlus*, U.S. National Library of Medicine, 12 July 2018. medlineplus.gov/ency/article/004019.htm. Describes how vital signs change with age, including body temperature.

Blatteis, Clark M. "Age-Dependent Changes in Temperature Regulation: A Mini Review." *Gerontology*, vol. 58, no. 4, 2012, pp. 289-95. doi:10.1159/000333148. Describes the principal, age-associated changes in physiological functions that could affect the ability of seniors to maintain their body temperature when exposed to hot or cold environments.

TERMINAL ILLNESS

Relevant Issues: Death, health and medicine, law, psychology

Significance: Many controversial issues surround what determines when a disease process is terminal and the resulting choices and options for care.

A terminal illness is an illness that can be expected to cause the diagnosed person to die given the expected trajectory of the disease. Examples of terminal illness may include late stage dementia, kidney or liver failure, terminal cancer, or progressive neurologic conditions such as Amyotrophic lateral sclerosis (ALS), also known as motor neurone disease (MND) or Lou Gehrig's disease.

When an individual is diagnosed as terminally ill, his or her social status changes radically. These patients may suffer from a loss of identity, reduced social or family support, anxiety, depression, and existential or religious fears about dying. However, the process of dying has been well studied, and there is an increased understanding among geriatric or palliative care medical providers that terminally ill patients can still live fulfilling lives with minimized suffering if appropriate resources are utilized.

STAGES OF DYING

Elisabeth Kübler-Ross, the Swiss-born psychiatrist who did extensive work with the dying, described five distinct stages through which many terminally ill patients pass. In 1969, she wrote that each stage acts as a defense mechanism against the fear of death. The stages she described are not universal, and do not necessarily follow a set order, but they provide a framework to describe the developmental changes of a dying person.

The first of Kübler-Ross's stages is known as denial. When first learning of a terminal illness, the patient registers shock and disbelief. The individual may argue with the physician that a wrong diagnosis has been made and that the laboratory reports are in error. The patient may demand a second opinion and perhaps a third and fourth. Usually, this stage is relatively short unless the family members also continue to deny the illness. The second stage of dying in this framework is anger. The diagnosed terminally ill patient may fret, "Why me? What did I do to deserve this?" The person may strike out verbally at family, friends or health professionals. Sometimes, the person may blame himself or herself for some indulgent habit. The person's anger may also be unfocused. He or she may be irritable, complaining, and a challenge for others. The third stage is bargaining. During this stage, the dying person often makes deals with a higher power, even if they did not have prior religious affiliation. Alternative medicines, herbs, faith healers, vitamin supplements, and experimental drugs are explored by the dying individual. Almost anything is acceptable to postpone death. The fourth stage is depression. The dying person withdraws from friends and family to mourn losses of capabilities and relationships. Death is recognized as inevitable, and the feelings of loss are often overwhelming. The fifth stage of dying in the Kübler-Ross model is acceptance. No longer agitated or seeking sympathy, the dying individual is often tired and weak and spends the day sleeping, resting, and reminiscing with only one or two close people.

Since Kübler-Ross, many other researchers have attempted to more accurately describe the dying process—particularly E. Mansell Pattison, who defined three stages of the living-dying interval in 1977. Pattison's stages are acute, chronic, and terminal. In the acute stage, individuals face the knowledge of their imminent death and may react with anxiety, denial, or anger. In the chronic phases, individuals begin to confront their fears of dying, such as loneliness and pain. They also deal with fears of what will happen after death. The final or terminal phase signals the end of hope and the beginning of withdrawal from the outside world upon realization of the inevitability of death. The goal of treatment for the dying, according to Pattison, is to help them cope with the first phase, help them live through the second, and move them toward the third.

RIGHTS OF THE DYING

The process of dying takes a great deal of physical and mental energy. Sedatives, painkillers, and some treatments can further reduce energy and cause disorientation and diminishing capabilities. As strength decreases, the dying are progressively less able to carry out activities of daily living. They become very vulnerable. Family members and health professionals must advocate for the dying person to ensure their rights are not violated. The following are some of these rights.

Patients have the right to open communication about death. Because individuals commonly deny that they are dying in the early stages, it can be useful for a medical provider to inform them first that their condition is serious and to allow them to ask more questions as they are ready to hear it. Knowledge of impending death allows dying persons to complete certain tasks before dying and to close their life in accordance with personal wishes. Additionally, full awareness of impending death allows an individual to make responsible decisions, such as where to die and what treatments to allow.

The terminally ill have the right to a painless death, to the greatest extent possible, if that is in accordance with their wishes. A common fear among the terminally ill, especially the elderly, is that their death will be painful. Patients considering suicide most often cite fear of prolonged suffering and painful death as a reason. Pain is more than just an unpleasant physical sensation. It may impair function, lead to fear and anxiety, interfere with social relationships, and cause spiritual distress.

Patients benefit from having been given "permission" to discuss their feelings about pain. They may have to unlearn reluctance stemming from previous encounters with unsympathetic or uninformed clinicians. Sometimes the terminally ill feel they must be brave or put on a front to help ease their family's distress. Pain can isolate patients, especially when they must hide it from others, and isolation in itself increases the risk of depression and suicide.

Health professionals should work cooperatively with a dying patient, because the patient is the best judge of his own pain and desires for pain relief. Medical providers with specialty training in palliative care are experts in symptom management, and can be a useful resource if a physician is having difficulty controlling pain or navigating the possible side effects of pain medication. Palliative care experts are also trained to consider non-pharmacologic methods of pain control, as well as treating pain as a complex psychosocial issue. Some patients' pain may be poorly controlled because they are having a spiritual crisis or are feeling isolated from family, and palliative care providers are trained to incorporate social workers, chaplains, and therapists into their treatment plans.

Terminally ill people have the right to as much control over environment as possible. Because the dying so often experience loss of control over their environment and declining health, it is imperative that family and health professionals allow the dying person as much control as possible, even in little things. Allowing patients some choice over meals, visiting hours, roommates, frequency of nursing interruptions, and medical treatments can greatly enhance their feelings of autonomy. This right to environmental control extends to a dying person's wishes for visitors. One possible source of great fear for the dying person is abandonment at the time of death. They fear that they will die alone. A high proportion of elders may spend their dying interval without a concerned person to help make medical decisions or advocate adequate medical treatment.

The dying, like other patients, have the right to have all medical treatments fully explained. This includes a description of the prognosis and methods of treatment, as well as the potential risks, benefits, and side effects. Individuals also have the right to refuse treatment for their illness and to seek out alternative medicine, even those not condoned by the medical profession. The terminally ill have the right to seek quality of life over quantity of hours. Patients have the right to refuse all heroic, artificial efforts to sustain life. These issues are best spelled out in a living will. Living wills are advance directives that express the desires of competent adults regarding terminal care, life-sustaining measures, and other issues pertaining to their dying and death.

UNDERSTANDING THE PATIENT SELF-DETERMINATION ACT

On December 1, 1991, the Patient Self-Determination Act (PSDA), a federal law enacted to ensure patient rights, went into effect. This law required Medicare- and Medicaid-certified hospitals, nursing homes, home health agencies, hospices, and health maintenance organizations to implement procedures to increase public awareness regarding the rights of patients to make treatment choices. The law was particularly concerned with advance directives, documents specifying the type of treatment individuals want or do not want under serious medical conditions in which they might be unable to communicate their wishes to the physician.

Advance directives include two distinct forms: a living will and a durable power of attorney for health care. Living wills, which may vary from state to state, outline the medical care individuals want if they become unable to make their own decisions. A durable power of attorney for health care, on the other hand, designates another person to act as an "agent" or a "proxy" in making medical decisions if the individual becomes unable to do so. Healthcare proxies, however, are not always perfect executors of patients' wishes. In one study, family members named as surrogates were asked for their view of patients' preferences on resuscitation. The surrogates correctly guessed what the patients (who were chronically ill, but still competent) wanted only 68 percent to 88 percent of the time. The study, however, pointed out a likely cause for surrogates' misunderstanding: lack of discussion. Patients by and large simply assumed their families and physicians would know what they wanted. For this reason, it is important to encourage discussions regarding your wishes at the end of life with your chosen healthcare proxy. Directives that include information on the patient's attitudes on life, health, and health care eliminate guessing. The medical directive should ask what the goals of treatment in various clinical situations should be (for example, to prolong life, to provide comfort). Such information helps the proxy and health care professionals because the question is not always "What do you want to do with the ventilator?" but "What does quality of life mean to you?" Clinicians and ethicists in recent years have increasingly come to view artificial nutrition (tube feedings) and hydration (intravenous fluids) as medical treatment rather than as food and water. As such, they may be withdrawn, much like a ventilator. A family may not share that view, however, even if withdrawal of artificial nutrition and hydration is consistent with the terminally ill person's wishes. Health care professionals must support the family by telling them that they are not "starving" the person but that these invasive procedures are only prolonging the dying process without curative powers.

The burden of responsibility needs to be removed from the shoulders of family members, who may feel a duty to make sure caregivers continue treatment. Clergy and other support people need to be available to help the family deal with any lingering doubts. More often than not, however, families react to the change of focus from cure to ensuring a comfortable death not with guilt but with relief, especially when the patient's wishes have been respected—that, in some measure, the dying person has been allowed to face death on his or her own terms.

KNOWING EACH STATE'S LAWS

States vary in their acceptance of living wills; there may even be variation among agencies as to the conditions under which this document will be entered into the medical record. In most states, at least one physician (and sometimes two) must certify that the patient is terminally ill before an advance directive can be fulfilled. But in Idaho, a patient does not have to be terminally ill or permanently unconscious for the living will to be fulfilled. Rather, the individual must be a qualified patient: someone who is of sound mind and eighteen years of age or older.

—Maxine M. McCue
Updated by Patrick Richardson, MSN

See also: Acquired immunodeficiency syndrome (AIDS); Breast cancer; Cancer; Communication; Death and dying; Death anxiety; Death of a child; Death of parents; Depression; Durable power of attorney; Funerals; Grief; Health care; Kübler-Ross, Elizabeth; Living wills; Medications; Prostate cancer; Psychiatry, geriatric; Skin cancer; Suicide; Widows and widowers

For Further Information

Campos-Calderón, C., et al. "Interventions and Decision-Making at the End of Life: The Effect of Establishing the Terminal Illness Situation." *BMC Palliative Care*, vol. 15, no. 1, 2016. doi:10.1186/s12904-016-0162-z. This study analyzes the health interventions performed and decisions made in the last days of life in patients with advanced oncological and non-oncological illness to ascertain whether identifying the patient's terminal illness situation has any effect on these decisions.

Clark, Katherine. "Care at the Very End-of-Life: Dying Cancer Patients and Their Chosen Family's Needs." *Cancers*, vol. 9, no. 12, 2017, p. 11. doi:10.3390/cancers9020011. This non-systematic review summarizes the symptoms most feared by people imminently facing death. Also explores the incidence and management of problems that may affect the dying person which are most feared by their family.

Kyota, Ayumi, and Kiyoko Kanda. "How to Come to Terms with Facing Death: A Qualitative Study Examining the Experiences of Patients with Terminal Cancer." *BMC Palliative Care*, vol. 18, no. 33, 2019. doi:10.1186/s12904-019-0417-6. This study explores how terminal cancer patients who have not clearly expressed a depressed mood or intense grief manage their feelings associated with anxiety and depression.

Mayo Clinic Staff. "Terminal Illness: Supporting a Terminally Ill Loved One." Mayo Clinic, Mayo Foundation for Medical Education and Research, 16 Nov. 2018. www.mayoclinic.org/healthy-lifestyle/end-of-life/in-depth/grief/art-20047491. Offers advice on how to offer support and deal with grief in the face of terminal illness.

Maytal, Guy, and Theodore A. Stern. "The Desire for Death in the Setting of Terminal Illness: A Case Discussion." The Primary Care Companion to *The Journal of Clinical Psychiatry*, vol. 8, no. 5, 2006, pp. 299-305. doi:10.4088/pcc.v08n0507. This report presents the case of a patient with terminal illness who expressed a desire to hasten his death. The authors discuss the meaning of the request and several possible interventions.

Warren, Karen J. "I Just Learned That I Have a Terminal Illness: Now What?" Psychology Today, Sussex Publishers, 21 Mar. 2018. www.psychologytoday.com/us/blog/naked-truth/201803/i-just-learned-i-have-terminal-illness-now-what. Karen Warren tells her personal story of dealing with terminal illness and offers 7 steps for the patient who has recently been diagnosed with a terminal illness.

THIS CHAIR ROCKS: A MANIFESTO AGAINST AGEISM (BOOK)

Writer: Ashton Applewhite
Date: 2016
Relevant Issues: Culture, demographics, economics, family, health and medicine, law, marriage and dating, media, psychology, sociology, values, work
Significance: Applewhite asserts that discrimination against the aging, or ageism, affects everyone, including the young. She calls for an end to any kind of discrimination against older adults and points out the details of how ageism insinuates itself into every aspect of life.

SUMMARY

Applewhite's book *This Chair Rocks: A Manifesto Against Ageism* follows the author along her journey as a baby boomer believing that becoming old was the end of life as she knew it into "old age," where she realizes that she has been duped. She documents how she fell into believing the myths about aging that the media pushes—that wrinkles should be eliminated, grey hair should be colored, and bald heads should be covered with hair. She shows how our culture perpetuates the ideas that older people have frail minds and bodies that just can't compete with the young in the working world or in the bedroom. She uncovers how ageism developed throughout history and how it becomes a self-fulfilling prophecy—if you believe you are old, you are. She pushes the agenda of "age equality," where age would not be allowed as a marker for judgment just as race, sex, gender, or any other type of discrimination is not allowed. The book offers suggestions of how to "push back" against ageism.

CRITICAL RECEPTION

This Chair Rocks: A Manifesto Against Ageism received high praise from critics from the moment it was published. Critics praised the amount of research that Applegate performed to write her book along with her lively, upbeat, entertaining and practical voice. It was nominated by the *Washington Post* Book World's staff as one of the "100 Best Books to Read at Any Age," and was a Best Book in *Publisher's Weekly*. *Forbes* called Applewhite one of the "Forty Women to Watch Over 40." She has been called the champion and activist for anti-ageism.

—*Marianne Moss Madsen, MS*

See also: Ageism; Age discrimination; Age Discrimination Act of 1975; Age Discrimination in Employment Act of 1967; Baby boomers; Stereotypes

THYROID DISORDERS

Relevant Issues: Biology, health and medicine
Significance: Normal functioning of the thyroid gland is essential for overall health; thyroid disorders can cause significant illness and are often difficult to diagnose in elderly individuals.

More than 20 million people have some form of thyroid disease and almost two-thirds of that number is unaware of their affliction. More women than men develop thyroid disease, with the disease affecting one in eight women. Thyroid disease often occurs in women immediately after pregnancy or menopause. Abnormal function of the thyroid gland leading to thyroid disorders causes multiple symptoms in the elderly that are often overlooked in determining a diagnosis. Fluttering of the heart, severe constipation, being overly sleepy, unexplained weight loss or gain, hearing loss and tremors can all be symptoms of thyroid disorders in the elderly. Because these symptoms often mimic other diseases found with aging, diagnosis may be delayed. When these symptoms appear, thyroid disorders should be added to the list of diseases evaluated, especially with a family history of the disease or previous radiation therapy near the gland. The thyroid gland is one of several organs or glands that compose the endocrine system. Endocrine glands produce substances, called hormones, which are released into the bloodstream and distributed throughout the body, where they act upon specific target tissues or organs. Hormones control most of the chemical reactions of the body.

The thyroid gland is a butterfly-shaped organ located in the neck just in front of the trachea (windpipe) and just below the larynx (voice box). It produces two principal hormones, triiodothyronine (T3) and thyroxine (T4), which act on most tissues of the body by increasing metabolic rate. The thyroid gland is stimulated to produce T3 and T4 by a hormone called thyroid-stimulating hormone (TSH) generated by the pituitary gland, which is located in the brain and known as the master gland.

With aging, the thyroid gland atrophies or shrinks somewhat but it continues to function adequately and remains sensitive to the stimulating effect of TSH from the pituitary gland. In elderly people, the most important thyroid disorders are hypothyroidism and hyperthyroidism.

Hypothyroidism is a deficient production of T3 and T4 by the thyroid gland. It is the most common thyroid disorder, occurring in 2 to 5 percent of those aged sixty-five and older. It is much more common in women than men and more common in institutionalized rather than community-living elderly people. The main causes of hypothyroidism in adults are damage to the thyroid gland from radiation therapy, surgical removal of the gland (for cancer treatment), Hashimoto's disease (a disorder in which a person's immune system erroneously attacks the thyroid gland and destroys it), and other unknown (idiopathic) causes. Iodine deficiency is another cause for hypothyroidism, though this is rarely a problem in the United States as iodine from foods and iodized salt is readily available.

The classic symptoms of hypothyroidism typically develop slowly over months or years and include a low metabolic rate, cold intolerance, tiredness, and lack of energy. Elderly people commonly develop nonspecific symptoms such as depression, mental confusion, constipation, loss of appetite, and weight gain, making diagnosis of hypothyroidism difficult. Although its diagnosis may be tricky, treatment of hypothyroidism is readily accomplished by giving supplemental thyroid hormone in pill form.

Hyperthyroidism is an excess production of thyroid hormone. The most common causes of hyperthyroidism

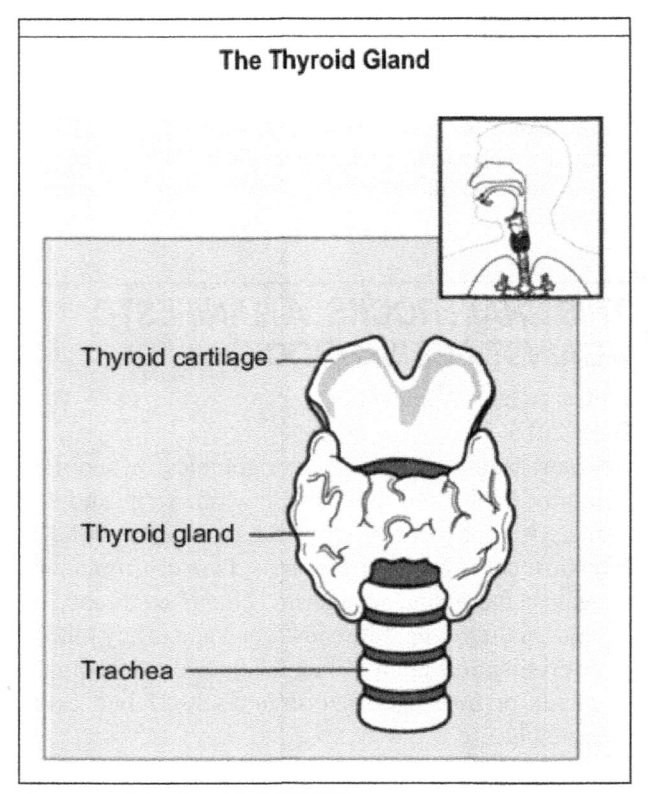

Anatomy of the thyroid. © EBSCO

are Graves' disease (in which the immune system produces substances that act like TSH and stimulate the thyroid gland to overproduce T3 and T4) and thyroid tumors or nodules that secrete excess thyroid hormone. Typical symptoms of hyperthyroidism include increased metabolic rate, heat intolerance, increased appetite, weight loss, rapid heart rate, restlessness, and goiter (enlarged thyroid gland). In the elderly, hyperthyroidism often is confused with other disorders related to gastrointestinal, cardiac, muscular, or psychiatric function and is easily misdiagnosed. Treatments for hyperthyroidism include surgical removal of the thyroid gland and the use of radioactive iodine and other drugs.

Thyroid disorders are relatively common, frequently misdiagnosed in the elderly, and easily treated. Early detection and treatment can spare elderly individuals unnecessary suffering and disability.

—*William J. Ryan*
Updated by Patricia Stanfill Edens, RN, PhD, FACHE

See also: Illnesses among older adults; Weight loss and gain.

For Further Information

Barbesino, Giuseppe. "Thyroid Function Changes in the Elderly and Their Relationship to Cardiovascular Health: A Mini-Review." *Gerontology*, vol. 65, no. 1, Jan. 2019, pp. 1-8. doi:10.1159/000490911. This review summarizes the most recent large population studies analyzing thyroid changes with aging and interprets their effects on cardiovascular health in the elderly.

Calsolaro, Valeria, et al. "Hypothyroidism in the Elderly: Who Should Be Treated and How?" *Journal of the Endocrine Society*, vol. 3, no. 1, 19 Nov. 2018, pp. 146-58. doi:10.1210/js.2018-00207. Evaluates the state of the art on hypothyroidism in the elderly with special focus on the effect on cognition and the cardiovascular system function. Also summarizes recommendations for a correct diagnostic workup and therapeutic approach, with special attention to the presence of frailty, comorbidities, and poly therapy.

"Endocrine Diseases." National Institute of Diabetes and Digestive and Kidney Diseases, U.S. Department of Health and Human Services. www.niddk.nih.gov/health-information/endocrine-diseases. A collection of resources on endocrine disorders, including links to Hashimoto's Disease, hyperthyroidism, and hypothyroidism.

Kyle, Emily, and Nadine Greeff. *The 30-Minute Thyroid Cookbook*. Rockridge P, 2018. Offers quick recipe solutions to manage hypothyroid and Hashimoto's symptoms, so that you can get in and out of the kitchen and back to your life.

Leng, Owain, and Salman Razvi. "Hypothyroidism in the Older Population." *Thyroid Research*, vol. 12, no. 1, 8 Feb. 2019. doi:10.1186/s13044-019-0063-3. Reviews the current literature pertaining to hypothyroidism with a special emphasis on the older individual and assesses the risk/benefit impact of contemporary management on outcomes in this age group.

Myers, Amy. *The Thyroid Connection*. Little, Brown and Company, 2016. Complete with advice on diet and nutrition, supplements, exercise, stress relief, and sleep, *The Thyroid Connection* is the ultimate roadmap back to your happiest, healthiest self. Dr. Myers, originally misdiagnosed herself, understands the struggles of thyroid dysfunction firsthand.

"Older Patients and Thyroid Disease." American Thyroid Association. www.thyroid.org/thyroid-disease-older-patient/. Explains how thyroid disorders affect older adults.

TOWNSEND MOVEMENT

Date: Launched in September, 1933
Relevant Issues: Economics, sociology, work
Significance: A movement to design an old-age pension plan, the Townsend movement attempted to end the Great Depression of the 1930s and bring about a general economic recovery.

In response to his own desperate situation and the general collapse of the American economy during the Great Depression, Francis Everett Townsend (1867-1960) developed a plan that was intended to assist elderly Americans directly and to stimulate an economic recovery throughout the United States. In September 1933, Townsend announced a pension plan that would eliminate the economic distress being experienced by senior citizens and provide the U.S. economy with an influx of capital. He proposed that all Americans age sixty and older who had been citizens for at least five years receive $200 monthly for the remainder of their lives on the condition that they spend it within thirty-five days of receiving it. To finance this twenty-billion-dollar pension scheme, a 2 percent sales tax on all transactions would be imposed. Townsend maintained that his plan would restore confidence in the American economy and family-based values.

Within ninety days of his announcement, Townsend's proposal was transformed into a major social movement. Local and regional Townsend clubs were established, and The Townsend National Weekly began publishing in 1934. Although his plan was denounced by economists and officials in the administration of President Franklin D. Roosevelt, Townsend continued to attract support during 1935. Townsend entered into an anti-Roosevelt coalition with the Share Our Wealth Society, founded by Louisiana governor Huey P. Long, and the National Union for Social Justice of the reactionary, anti-Semitic priest Charles E. Coughlin. Their Union Party failed to achieve a credible level of support in the 1936 election. The movement collapsed with the gradual economic recovery of the late 1930s.

—*William T. Walker*

See also: Advocacy; Pensions; Poverty; Social Security

For Further Information

"The Townsend Plan Movement." Social Security Administration. www.ssa.gov/history/towns5.html. General background information on the Townsend Plan.

TRANSPORTATION ISSUES

Relevant Issues: Culture, demographics
Significance: The elderly have the same need for transportation as younger people; however, most American communities fail to provide adequate transportation services for the aged.

Whether people can maintain independence in their communities as they age depends, in part, on their access to the goods, services, and social contacts necessary for a good quality of life. This access relies largely on whether they have transportation choices that serve their personal mobility needs and preferences. For the older adult who chooses to maintain an independent residence, reliable transportation is the link between home and a variety of social and medical services. Several factors can complicate the older adult's access to transportation.

Although many older adults retain their own automobiles, declining vision and other physical impairments may affect their ability to drive. To compensate, they may simply limit their driving to essential trips, which may be made only during the day and only in good weather. As the cost of maintaining a rarely used vehicle mounts, the older adult may opt to rely on others to provide transportation, which can severely limit the older person's lifestyle.

The trend of building accommodations for the elderly in outlying areas, inconveniently located away from stores, hospitals, and other vital services, further complicates transportation needs. Older adults who no longer have the use of their automobiles may find themselves relying on public transportation to access vital services. With public transportation options decreasing nationwide, it is clear that society is unable to meet this growing need. Where public transportation is available, the older adult's ability to take advantage of it is severely restricted by its high cost, limited access, or inconvenient scheduling.

The availability of a support network is sometimes a decisive factor when making a choice among a selection of transportation arrangements. Some communities have a wide variety of formal services available. Friends, family, and church or other organizations are all potential sources of transportation. Unpaid caregivers provide aid to more than 1 million noninstitutionalized older adults. Three-fourths of the community-living elderly who need assistance get help only from family or friends. Almost three-quarters of unpaid caregivers are middle-aged women, and approximately one-half of the caregivers reside with the care recipient.

TRANSPORTATION SERVICES

Older people are often given discounts for bus, taxicab, subway, and train services. Commissions or offices on aging, health departments, departments of social services, and local chapters of the American Red Cross are often able to direct people to services accommodating wheelchairs and other special needs. Various health and medical facilities provide transportation for people using their services. For example, nursing homes may provide transportation for their residents to dentists, physicians, and rehabilitation services. Health services for the aged are provided by health departments, hospital clinics, and private practitioners. These providers may also assist the elderly in obtaining transportation and financial assistance for their health care. A variety of life-care communities, villages, mobile home parks, and apartment complexes, specifically designed for older people, include transportation services for residents to health services and recreational activities.

Surveys have examined sociocultural and quality-of-life variables as they affect use of health care and transportation services. Most respondents reported their health status as poor or very poor, and more than one-half had no medical care during the preceding six months despite the presence of multiple physical symptoms. Social isolation from family or neighborhood support systems exacerbated problems with transportation, and most of the elderly people relied on public transportation to gain access to health services. Public transportation services posed additional barriers to health care use, including fear of making trips alone within the complex urban transportation system.

Mobility for the elderly means having access to the goods, services, and social interactions that are necessary to independent living. A standard measure of mobility is the number of trips that people make away from their homes. Mobility may be affected by numerous factors, including emotional and physical health, economic well-being, and the ease or difficulty in getting around one's community. However, little research has been done on how older people themselves perceive their transportation options or the reduced mobility that accompanies old age.

CORRECTING TRANSPORTATION PROBLEMS

Key questions emerged from the report's findings that require further research about how best to meet the transportation needs of people age seventy-five and older. These questions include: To what degree is the reduced mobility of older people dependent on personal health status? To what degree is reduced mobility dependent on external barriers, such as crime or limited community transportation resources? How do older people perceive public transportation as an alternative to the automobile? Is the level of mobility of older drivers sufficient to assure access to the goods, services, and social contacts necessary to independent living? Are older drivers satisfied with their level of mobility? Do they simply prefer or need less mobility, or do they accept reduced mobility as part of getting old? Are nondrivers as immobile as these data suggest? How do they connect to their communities? Do they have sufficient access to the goods, services, and social contacts necessary to independent living? Do the families and friends of older people believe that they can meet the mobility needs of older people?

Because the majority of people rely on driving themselves well into their later years, public policies should support maximizing the capacity for safe driving through the life span. These policies include improvement of road design and signage, regulation of drivers on the basis of individual functional ability and driving record, and automobile design that addresses the needs of an aging population.

The fact that one-quarter of the seventy-five and older population are nondrivers means that federal, state, and local governments must identify and support transportation options designed to meet currently unmet transportation needs. These policies would be most useful if they were founded on the habits, preferences, and attitudes of older people to increase the likelihood that older people will use and be satisfied with their transportation choices. Zoning laws, transportation planning, regulation of public transportation, and allocation of federal funds for transportation services all have an impact on the short-term and long-term ability of people of all ages to connect with their communities and to maintain independence throughout their lives.

Other surveys have attempted to understand the needs of physically handicapped and elderly people and to recommend appropriate operational and physical changes within the system to meet these needs. The secondary intent of such studies is often to bring about public awareness of the mobility problems of the physically limited and the elderly.

Transportation and the quality of available health care are major problems for rural senior citizens because of the lack of rural public transportation. Although 30 percent of the population of the United States lives in such areas, only about 1 percent of the capitol federal investment and annual operating moneys spent on public transportation are allocated to help meet rural needs.

TRANSPORTATION PLANNING

Communities develop planning guides designed to aid service agencies in their choices for setting up transportation services for the elderly. Alternatives to actual service include special buses for the elderly. This service may be provided directly by the coordinating agency and may include such vehicles as specially equipped vans, school buses, and station wagons. Another alternative is the reduced fare program whereby older adults may ride existing public transit at a reduced fare.

In some communities, buses provide scheduled trips to such destinations as grocery stores, medical appointments, and community centers. For many, buses are the vital link to a variety of activities, including doctor visits. Door-to-door and curb-to-curb service is often available. Most buses are wheelchair accessible. Some entrepreneurs have established businesses focused on the needs of the elderly that provide multidimensional services, including transportation, bill paying, and assisted-living options.

All evidence suggests that the elderly population will continue to depend on the private car to give them freedom, independence, and choice—as do younger travelers. It seems unlikely that other modes or options can provide anywhere near the level of mobility that the elderly want or need. Almost three-fourths of those over age sixty-five live in suburban or rural areas, where transit and paratransit options are inherently impractical or costly. These elderly individuals make choices about doctors, hospitals, friends, and social and recreational options based on their lifelong access to the car. When they can no longer drive or receive rides, their mobility will drop, and they may have to make drastic changes in their life network to be able to access just a few necessary services.

Those concerned with the use of medical services by the elderly population must focus not only on transportation but also on other variables that create the need for a car. Transportation needs are clearly linked to where and how medical and social services are made available. As the aging population grows, medical and human service agencies are likely to make an effort to make their programs accessible to the elderly population rather than simply locating their facilities where they please and assuming that elderly people or transportation planners will somehow deal with the resulting loss of mobility.

—*Jane Cross Norman*

See also: AARP; Discounts; Driving; Facility and institutional care; Mobility problems; Vacations and travel; Wheelchair use

For Further Information

Cothron, Anna Lea, et al. "Aging and Transportation as a Necessity." Aging Today, American Society on Aging, 2018. www.asaging.org/blog/aging-and-transportation-necessity. Discusses programs in Tennessee designed to assist seniors with transportation.

Dickerson, Anne E., et al. "Transportation and Aging: An Updated Research Agenda to Advance Safe Mobility among Older Adults Transitioning from Driving to Non-Driving." *The Gerontologist*, vol. 59, no. 2, 2017, pp. 215-21. doi:10.1093/geront/gnx120. In this article, the authors review what is currently known about two areas relevant to safe mobility for older drivers: the process of transitioning to non-driving and the maintenance of mobility after driving has ceased. They identify future research in these areas.

National Aging and Disability Transportation Center. www.nadtc.org/. The NADTC works to promote the availability and accessibility of transportation options for older adults, people with disabilities and caregivers.

TRAVEL. *See* VACATIONS AND TRAVEL.

TRIP TO BOUNTIFUL, THE (FILM)

Director: Peter Masterson
Cast: Geraldine Page, John Heard, Rebecca De Mornay
Date: Released in 1985
Relevant Issues: Death, family
Significance: In this film, an elderly woman's trip home serves as a type of life review and preparation for death.

A life review can be important in late adulthood as a way of reaching ego integrity. In the film *The Trip to Bountiful*, which takes place in the 1940s, this life review is represented in the main character's desire to return to her home in the town of Bountiful, Texas. Carrie Watts (played by Geraldine Page) is an elderly woman who now lives with her son and daughter-in-law in Houston. Carrie feels driven to take a trip to Bountiful to see her old home and friends before she dies. The trip serves as an opportunity for the aging woman to remember her past and become better prepared for her future.

When she arrives in Bountiful, she realizes how it has changed during the twenty years she has been away. Everyone has either moved or died, and the town consists of just a few empty buildings. Nevertheless, Carrie feels at home as she arrives at the house in which she was raised. Being in Bountiful makes her feel safe, at peace, ready to return to her son's home in Houston—ready, eventually, for death.

Based on the 1953 play by Horton Foote, who also wrote the screenplay, *The Trip to Bountiful* is a moving drama about searching for peace by returning home. Page won an Academy Award for her portrayal of Carrie Watts. Throughout the film, the hymn "Softly and Tenderly" provides musical support for the theme. The hymn includes these words in the chorus: "Come home, come home. Ye who are weary, come home." Going home can be a powerful drive for those who are tired and in need of peace. Carrie found that peace during her trip to Bountiful.

—*Kevin S. Seybold*

See also: Death and dying; Death anxiety; Women and aging

TRUSTS

Relevant Issues: Death, family, law

Significance: A trust—an entity enabling people to pass title to property to others during their lifetime or at death—can be used to implement many estate-planning techniques.

Trusts are often referred to as gifts with strings attached: instructions and conditions given to the trustee as to whom, how, and when property contained in the trust can be distributed. Trusts can be cancelled or changed during the lifetime of the settlor or grantor (creator of the trust) so long as he or she remains competent.

CHARACTERISTICS OF A TRUST

A trust is a legal entity in which one person or corporation holds property for the benefit of another under written instructions and directives. A trustee (holder of the property for another's benefit) can be either an individual or a bank or other corporate institution. Banks generally have a trust department to administer assets held in trust in exchange for payment of a fee, usually based on a percentage of the value of the trust's assets (corpus). Using a bank or other corporate entity eliminates the need to name a successor trustee to act upon the death, resignation, or incompetence of the original trustee. In other circumstances, however, where a close friend or family member is named trustee, it is a good idea to name a successor. If there are minor children, a guardian and successor guardian should be named.

The settlor owns equitable title to the trust corpus: the right to use, possess, and enjoy the property; the trustee owns bare legal title (property in the name of the trust). Trustees are fiduciaries and have entered into a trust relationship with the settlor—the ultimate duty imposed by law. Trustees are absolutely mandated to follow instructions of the settlor, to exercise good judgment, responsibility, and objectivity. If this duty is breached, trustees can be sued for breach of fiduciary duty.

Trusts cannot last forever. The rule against perpetuities limits the length of a trust, generally specifying that a trust can last no longer than the lifetime of the beneficiary alive at the time the trust was created plus twenty-one years.

TYPES OF TRUSTS

The inter-vivos trust (also called a living trust) can be structured so that settlors retain the right to change or terminate the trust during their lifetime. This type of trust is revocable; those that cannot be changed are irrevocable. In the revocable trust, settlors give what is owned to whomever they wish, whenever they wish, subsequent to death; terms and requirements about how the property passes can be spelled out. Settlors can control, coordinate, and distribute all property interests during their lifetime and at death. The inter-vivos trust ensures privacy on death or incapacity because probate is not required. It is easy to create and maintain, and it can be changed or amended at the will of the settlor. For these reasons, the inter-vivos trust is often referred to as a will substitute. Property not placed in trust during the settlor's lifetime can still be placed in trust after death through use of a "pour-over will" stating that any property not in trust will pass to the trust (pour over to it) after death.

A testamentary trust created in a valid will is not operative until death. The testamentary trust is never created to benefit the settlor and is subject to probate. A marital trust provides benefits to a surviving spouse. Testamentary trusts are often set up as A-B trusts when a married couple is involved and when their combined estate may be taxable. The single trust is divided into two trusts (A and B) at the death of the first spouse. The deceased spouse's share flows into the B trust, containing flexible and discretionary provisions. The surviving spouse's share and the remaining share of the deceased spouse, if any, is placed into the A, or survivor's, trust (also called the marital trust). The surviving spouse normally has complete control over the A trust. This manner of dividing trust corpus may result in considerable tax savings, depending on the size of the estate.

Qualified terminable interest property (Q-TIP) trusts provide for children from different marriages. The marital deduction allows spouses to leave entire estates to each other without paying taxes. If there are children from other marriages, settlors might prefer that their biological children receive more from their estate than their current spouse's children from a previous marriage. The Q-TIP trust allows one to leave property in trust for one's spouse; after the spouse's death, it goes to whomever the settlor specifies.

Totten trusts are accounts at commercial banks or savings and loans that are registered "A in trust for B." It is presumed that the account belongs to the adult named as trustee unless the trust was irrevocable. On the death of the adult trustee, the account proceeds would belong to the minor beneficiaries but would be controlled by the local probate court on behalf of the minor until he or she reaches adulthood. This should be distinguished from a Uniform Gifts to Minors Act account, where an adult is named as custodian to manage the account until the minor reaches adulthood; in a savings account trust at a savings and loan, a minor can deposit or withdraw at will with no liability to the savings and loan.

Children's trusts are irrevocable trusts used to make gifts to children or grandchildren, providing for their future education and benefit. Appreciated assets are removed from the testator's estate and placed into the children's trust, where they will continue to grow. This is another tax-saving technique because the asset is taken from the estate of the testator and placed in a separate trust for the benefit of another, thus reducing the amount of testator's taxable estate. One caveat is that testators should not name themselves as trustee of the children's trust to ensure that the property will not be included in their taxable estate.

Prior to 1976, it was possible to avoid federal estate tax when property passed to future generations by means of a generation-skipping trust. In this situation, a settlor creates a trust funded at the settlor's death. His or her spouse receives all income and principal as needed. At the spouse's death, the children receive all income and principal as needed. At the children's death, the principal passes to the grandchildren. Another variation specifies that the settlor can mandate that on the death of his or her spouse, the property passes directly to the grandchildren, bypassing the children and bypassing estate tax on these transfers. The Tax Reform Act of 1976 subjected generation skipping assets to federal estate tax on the deaths of the beneficiaries of the generation-skipping trust. The Tax Reform Act of 1986 subjects an estate to double tax—the normal estate tax at the settlor's death and the generation-skipping tax at the death of the skipped individual. Exemptions from estate tax under current law nevertheless make this trust advantageous to the very wealthy.

Discretionary trusts contain provisions under which trustees can distribute the income and principal among various beneficiaries, or control disbursements to a single beneficiary, as they see fit. Spendthrift trusts can be set up for people whom the settlor believes would not be able to manage their own affairs because of their extravagance, immaturity, or mental incompetency. Support trusts direct the trustee to spend only as much income and principal as needed for the education and support of the beneficiary. Charitable remainder trusts are irrevocable. The settlor gives up control of appreciated assets placed in trust. In so doing, the settlor receives current tax deductions and a lifetime income without paying gift tax or capital gains tax. Assets can also be used for donation to private foundations rather than a public charity.

A grantor trust is a valuable estate planning device that can save estate and/or gift taxes and pass substantial assets to future generations. Estate tax is imposed for the privilege of passing assets to beneficiaries after the death of the settler; gift taxes provide for transfer of assets during one's lifetime. The estate tax rates in the United States can be as high as 40 percent for estates larger than $1 million and up. In order to pay less, it is advisable to make substantial gifts during one's lifetime ($15,000 per person as of 2019) with no limit as to how many gifts are made. Gifts to charities are tax free regardless of the amount so long as the gift is made directly to the charity.

—*Marcia J. Weiss*

See also: Estates and inheritance; Living trusts; Wills and bequests

For Further Information
Andersen, Roger W., and Susan N. Gary. *Understanding Trusts and Estates.* 6th ed., Carolina Academic P, 2018. Examples, charts, cross-references among similar concepts, and frameworks for analyzing problem areas all combine to give students the tools to deepen their understanding.
Barrow, Mary L. *The Savvy Client's Guide to Trusts: Is a Trust Right for You?* Savvy Client P, 2018. In this second volume in the Savvy Client Series, Barrow answers questions about trusts in a practical, easy-to-understand way.
"What Is A Trust"? Fidelity. www.fidelity.com/life-events/estate-planning/trusts. Explanations of several different kinds of trusts.
"What Is Required of an Executor"? ElderLawAnswers. 26 Feb. 2019. www.elderlawanswers.com/what-is-required-of-an-executor-6434. A step-by-step guide for those who find themselves as an executor of a trust.

URINARY DISORDERS

Relevant Issues: Biology, health and medicine
Significance: Decreases in the functional efficiency of the kidneys are associated with a number of diseases and pathological conditions; urinary disorders are among the leading causes of death in the elderly.

As a by-product of its everyday activities, the human body produces wastes that must be eliminated. A number of organs excrete cellular wastes: the skin, lungs, large intestine, liver, and kidneys. Of these organs, the kidneys are, by far, the most important for maintaining the body in a healthy state. Kidney failure is fatal unless treatment is initiated promptly.

The two kidneys are the major organs of the urinary system; they are located on either side of the spine just below the rib cage. The urinary system is composed of two ureters, which pass from the kidneys to the urinary bladder, and the urethra, which moves the urine from the bladder to outside of the body. Kidneys are the major excretory organs, but other organs have excretory function as well. For example, along with excreting carbon dioxide, the lungs may also excrete ammonia. The liver and skin also excrete metabolic wastes.

KIDNEY FUNCTION

The functional unit of the kidney is the nephron; each kidney contains about 1 million of them. The nephron is an exquisitely designed structure. It consists of a glomerulus, a ball of capillaries designed to act as a filter through which a fluid is separated from the blood and passes into Bowman's capsule, an expanded chamber in the kidney that surrounds the capillaries. Under normal conditions, the fluid is free of cells and larger molecules, and consists of mostly water and certain small molecules, including urea, a waste product of metabolism. The fluid that enters the kidneys is mostly water, and large amounts would be eliminated in the urine if nothing further was done in the kidneys. In a typical person, some 200 quarts of fluid pass into the kidneys each day, but only about 2 quarts end up being eliminated as urine. Most of the water that passes into the kidneys is reabsorbed back into the blood stream, as are most of the small molecules, including glucose. There are well over 100 miles of filtering units and tubules in the kidneys to keep substances at normal levels in the body.

Although there is a decrease in the number of nephrons with the aging process, a decrease can also occur with certain diseases. However, kidneys have a considerable reserve capacity and can function at a level many times greater than under normal conditions. It is estimated that a person may live successfully with a 60 to 80 percent loss of their nephrons. In some cases, people can be born with only one kidney and never know it.

The kidneys produce urine but perform several other important functions to help maintain the chemical constancy of the blood by regulating both the volume and specific composition of body fluids. To accomplish this regulation function, about 1,700 quarts of blood, representing about 25 percent of the blood pumped by the heart into the aorta, passes through the kidneys of an average person every day.

Ureters drain urine, produced in the kidneys, into the urinary bladder, which is the temporary holding site for urine. The urinary bladder also functions in the process of elimination (also known as urination or micturition). The bladder is a hollow, baglike structure that, under normal conditions, holds between 300 and 500 milliliters of urine. Both voluntary and involuntary nerves control bladder functions. As the bladder begins to fill with urine, sensory receptors in the bladder wall are stimulated. Typically, a person has been toilet trained, and bladder control is usually voluntary; however, some elderly people may experience a loss of voluntary bladder control. Incontinence is the inability to retain urine until an appropriate time and place can be found for elimination. Urinary incontinence may be of considerable importance among the elderly and may be a problem in 10 percent of the population over sixty-five. It is especially common in older women but occurs in men as well.

Given the amount of blood that passes through the kidneys each day, it is evident that most of the fluid must be reabsorbed back into the bloodstream to conserve it from being eliminated in the urine. The process of water reabsorption is controlled by several hormones. One, the antidiuretic hormone (ADH), is produced in the pituitary gland. ADH acts on the distal tubules in the kidneys by increasing the rate of water reabsorption, thereby reducing urinary output. Certain diseases can interfere with the production of ADH. A form of diabetes called diabetes insipidus leads to inadequate amounts of ADH. Affected people may produce gallons of dilute urine each day.

Kidney function is critical for life, and a complete loss of functioning brings death within just a few weeks. Serious kidney problems or renal failure may be caused by severe infections, an immune reaction to antibiotics, or a sudden and significant decrease in blood flow. Some impairment of kidney function may be related to the processes of normal aging.

CHANGES WITH NORMAL AGING PROCESSES
Although several anatomical and physiological changes occur in the kidneys as a result of aging, they can continue to function well enough to maintain a homeostatic balance and keep the proper salt and water balances. Problems are likely to arise when conditions outside of the normal range, such as disease or excessive stress, place additional demands on the system.

The kidneys are dependent on an adequate blood supply for normal functioning. A decrease in blood to the kidneys may be caused by several conditions. In general, cardiac output tends to fall with age. The heart puts out less blood, and the proportion going to the kidneys also decreases. In young adults, 25 percent of the blood pumped by the heart reaches and is processed by the kidneys. A noticeable decrease is evident by forty to fifty years of age; by the age of seventy to eighty, blood flow to the kidneys may be one-half of what it was at age twenty. Ultimately, the decreased blood flow results in less efficient functioning of the kidneys.

Additional changes that further compound the problems caused by decreased blood flow take place in the kidneys themselves. Of the two million nephrons present in the kidneys of young adults, up to one-half will be lost by the age of seventy to seventy-five. Those nephrons that remain show degenerative changes that result in decreased functioning. The detection of large

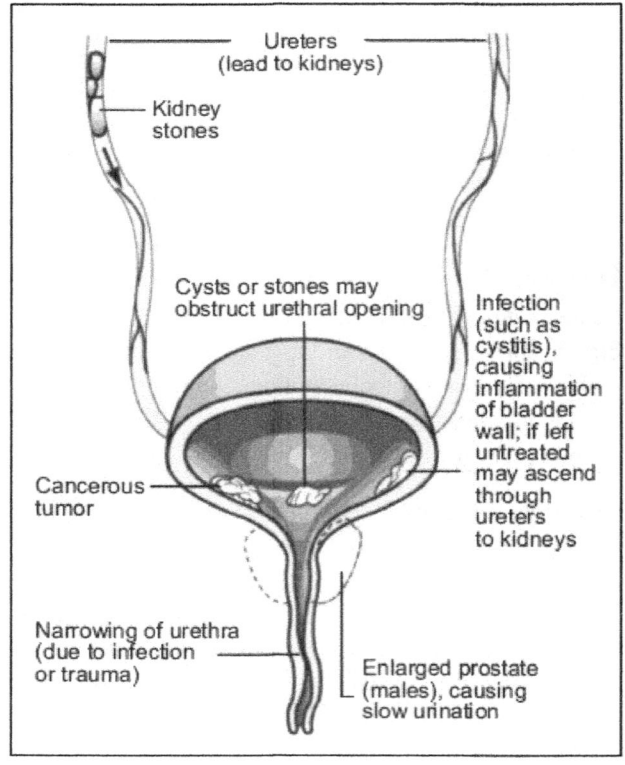

In addition to the variety of infections that may attack the urinary system, urinary disorders may be caused by cancerous tumors, cysts, stones that cause obstruction, reactions to trauma, and in

molecules—such as proteins, red blood cells, white blood cells, and glucose—in the urine during a urinalysis are indicative of some sort of disease or malfunction in the urinary tract.

In addition to changes in blood flow to the kidneys and a decrease in the functional efficiency of cells in the kidneys, problems can occur in the actual structures of the lower portion of the urinary tract. Loss of muscular tone with age may affect functioning of the ureters, bladder, and urethra. People may experience incomplete and difficult emptying of the bladder if there is a sufficient decrease in muscle tone. There also is a tendency for bladder capacity to decline in older people to less than one-half of that of young adults. Some older people may, therefore, experience more frequent and urgent urination.

CHANGES WITH DISEASE CONDITIONS

Diseases of the urinary tract occur in young and middle-age adults; in specific cases, they may be even more common in these age groups than in the elderly. However, a number of urinary system disorders are age related and are likely to have more severe symptoms and outcomes; of special significance to the elderly are infections (including cystitis, pyelonephritis, and glomerulonephritis), kidney stones, cancers, incontinence, and renal failure.

The National Kidney Foundation has provided a list of symptoms that are warning signs of kidney disease: burning or difficulty during urination; more frequent urination, particularly at night; passage of bloody urine; puffiness around eyes and swelling of hands and feet, especially in children; pain in the small of the back just below the ribs; and high blood pressure. However, some diseases can be present without any overt symptoms, and other types of tests are required for diagnosis. As a part of an annual physical checkup, routine urine and blood analysis can detect many forms of kidney disease. Accurate diagnosis is essential, as the type of treatment and outlook for recovery depend upon the nature of the disease and its early detection.

Kidney stones, or renal calculi, are small when they first form, not much bigger than the size of a grain of sand. They form when crystals of salt become concentrated in the urine and, as long as they remain small, will usually wash out with the urine. However, if water reabsorption by the kidneys is high and the volume of urine is low, the stones will grow and may become stuck in the ureter as urine passes from the kidneys to the bladder. The pain produced by the stones irritating the ureter is extreme. If large enough, the stones can actually block the ureter and may cause a backing-up and flooding of the kidneys. Bleeding may occur from the irritation of the walls of the ureter, the condition being one of the reasons for the appearance of blood in the urine.

A number of factors are associated with the formation of stones. Atypical diets can shift the acid-base composition of the urine. If the pH shifts to either extreme, stones can form. Excessive loss of water or inadequate water consumption may concentrate the urine, creating an environment conducive to forming crystals. Kidney infections and a lack of exercise or situations of extreme inactivity also can contribute to the process. Overlying all of these factors is the observation that kidney stones tend to run in families, indicating that there is likely a genetic component. Prevention and treatment may involve procedures to ensure good dietary practices, adequate water intake, and an exercise program. Conventional surgery and ultrasonic techniques may be required to break up and dislodge the stones.

An urgency to urinate, burning and pain during urination, and a need to urinate frequently, which may require getting up several times during the night, are symptoms of a urinary tract infection (UTI). Infections may occur in the kidneys, bladder, and lower urinary tract. They can be chronic and are often difficult to cure. Urinary tract infections are more common in women than in men and are most likely caused by the shorter urethra of females and its anatomical placement. Infection of the urinary bladder is known as cystitis and, in addition to causing an urgency of urination and pain on urinating, may produce pain in the lower abdominal region. Patients are asked to drink large amounts of water to increase their frequency of urination; antibiotics may be required to control the bacterial infection. Infections of the lower urinary tract may spread to the kidneys, possibly damaging them and, more critically, possibly leading to kidney failure. In addition, bacteria may spread to other parts of the body and cause other types of severe complications.

Bacterial infection of the kidneys is known as pyelonephritis or nephritis. The chronic form is more

> **SENIOR TALK:**
>
> **How Do You Feel About Urinary Tract Infections?**
> Urinary Tract Infections (UTIs) can cause considerable discomfort and pain. The symptoms may make you feel upset, frustrated, or even depressed, especially if you aren't sure of the cause. Understanding the condition and informing your doctor of your symptoms will help ease your mind. You may also be anxious about what may happen if you have a serious UTI. Knowing that a spreading infection can cause kidney damage and other complications can be frightening. This may be especially true if you have recurrent UTIs or an existing medical condition that puts you at higher risk of infection. However, you can take comfort in the fact that UTIs are highly treatable. Be sure to monitor your health and keep you doctor informed. Although it may be bothersome to keep track of a prescribed course of antibiotics, know that such treatment is important and seek assistance if you have trouble managing.
>
> In some older people, the only visible UTI symptoms may be confusion, agitation, or other mental changes. If you or those close to you notice such changes, it's important to get a diagnosis right away. Otherwise these symptoms might be mistaken for an early stage of dementia or other condition. Feelings of dizziness can also cause falls, a significant health concern for seniors.
>
> —*Leah Jacob*

common in the elderly than is the acute form. Either form can lead to kidney failure and cause waste products to accumulate in the blood. If untreated, toxic substances will continue to accumulate, possibly resulting in death.

Although it is not a fatal disorder, urinary incontinence is a major physiological, psychological, health, and social problem among the elderly. Incontinence is almost twice as common in women as in men; the incidence may approach 50 percent or higher among the elderly. There are several types and causes of incontinence, making diagnosis and treatment difficult. Incontinence may be caused by certain drugs or medications. Exercise, sneezing, and even laughing may induce what is known as stress incontinence. Loss of mobility and psychiatric disorders can also lead to incontinence. Depending on the diagnosis of the cause, treatment might include exercise, drug therapy, counseling, and behavioral modification.

The prostate is a small gland found only in males; it is one of the sexual accessory glands that functions in reproduction. Its secretions contribute to the seminal fluid and probably assist in the activation of sperm. The prostate surrounds the urethra just as it leaves the urinary bladder; certain conditions that affect it can have serious consequences for the functioning of the urinary system. Any disorder of the prostate that leads to an increase in size may interfere with the passage of urine through the urethra. Extreme cases may even cause a complete obstruction of urine flow. Partial obstruction, if prolonged, can lead to bladder and kidney damage. Although the precise cause is not known, prostate enlargement (benign prostatic hypertrophy) is common among aging men and may require treatment if urine flow is impeded.

Cancerous growths, or carcinomas, may occur at various sites throughout the urinary system, including the kidneys, bladder, and prostate gland. Prostate cancer is the most common cancer in men and, although usually not fatal, is still the third leading cancer that causes death in men. Bladder cancer is also more common in males, and its incidence may be related to smoking or exposure to certain types of chemicals, especially aniline dyes. In the case of all types of cancer, early detection is critical so that treatment can be effected before it has spread (metastasized) to other sites.

—*Donald J. Nash*

See also: Diabetes; Heart changes and disorders; Incontinence; Prostate cancer; Prostate enlargement; Stones

For Further Information

Alpay, Yesim, et al. "Urinary Tract Infections in the Geriatric Patients." *Pakistan Journal of Medical Sciences*, vol. 34, no. 1, 2018. doi:10.12669/pjms.341.14013. This study investigates clinical findings, diagnostic approaches, complicating factors, prognosis, causative microorganisms and antimicrobial susceptibility in geriatric patients diagnosed with UTI.

"Bladder Health for Older Adults." National Institute on Aging, U.S. Department of Health and Human Services, 16 May 2017. www.nia.nih.gov/health/bladder-health-older-adults. General information on different urinary conditions.

Chu, Christine M., and Jerry L. Lowder. "Diagnosis and Treatment of Urinary Tract Infections across Age Groups." *American Journal of Obstetrics and Gynecology*, vol. 219, no. 1, 2018, pp. 40-51. doi:10.1016/j.ajog.2017.12.231. In this review, the authors explore the evidence behind the use of signs, symptoms, and urinary testing in prediction of UTIs in women across age groups.

Gibson, W., and A. Wagg. "New Horizons: Urinary Incontinence in Older People." *Age and Ageing*, vol. 43, no. 2, 2014, pp. 157-63. doi:10.1093/ageing/aft214. This review examines recent developments in research into the aetiology, physiology, pathology and treatment of urinary incontinence and lower urinary tract symptoms in older people.

Mayne, Sean, et al. "The Scientific Evidence for a Potential Link between Confusion and Urinary Tract Infection in the Elderly Is Still Confusing—a Systematic Literature Review." *BMC Geriatrics*, vol. 19, no. 1, 2019. doi:10.1186/s12877-019-1049-7. A systematic review of the literature was conducted assessing the association between confusion and UTI in the elderly.

VACATIONS AND TRAVEL

Relevant Issues: Culture, economics, recreation, values

Significance: The freedom to explore vacation and travel options is one of the benefits of aging; the options taken largely depend on habits acquired over a lifetime.

The desire to see new parts of the world and extend cultural horizons is a large part of the impulse that sends people of all ages on exploratory voyages. This impulse can be of particular importance to those older citizens who have fulfilled their familial obligations, achieved some financial security, and acquired leisure time to devote to travel. This age group is a growing market for travel opportunities of all kinds.

TRAVEL AND VACATION CHOICES

Travel by seniors can take many forms and satisfy a variety of needs. One choice that must be made is whether to travel alone, with a companion, or in a group. Seniors might also decide to combine travel with some kind of cultural or educational venture. A further choice is whether to travel abroad or to rediscover one's own county, state, country, or continent. Some seniors travel independently, perhaps in a vehicle leased or purchased for that purpose or on scheduled mass transportation, while others seek the services of a professional tour operator. In addition, a wide range of accommodation may be considered, from providing one's own shelter to renting a cabin, engaging in a home or apartment exchange, or staying in a luxurious hotel or resort.

The travel choices that seniors make will depend on a variety of factors, including lifestyle, physical condition, kind of experience sought, and personal preference. No matter where the older traveler decides to go, a wide variety of travel books can help in deciding how to get there, what to see and do upon arrival, where to stay, and what or where to eat. Increasing numbers of shops catering to the needs of the traveler exist, often owned by people glad to share their knowledge and experience. Most countries, and many tourists destinations, have offices or agencies that provide free brochures upon request.

FOREIGN TRAVEL

Many factors might motivate senior travel to countries abroad, including curiosity about people and cultures different from one's own; the desire to see and photograph beautiful landscapes, visit famous art and archaeology museums, or explore fabled cities; an interest in attending sporting events, visiting summer festivals of music and the arts, or trying new cuisines in their natural setting. The older traveler might also develop an interest in discovering or connecting with family roots or wish to try out recently acquired language skills. The novelty of this kind of travel, particularly for those whose lives have been devoted to caring for family and pursuing a career, may be one of its most compelling features. Whether one is naturally gregarious or solitary, foreign travel affords many opportunities to expand awareness of the world.

People who engage in travel, particularly abroad, are often divided into one of two categories: travelers or tourists. Although any person may partake of both worlds, there is a difference in how these two categories are perceived and, sometimes, treated. For the tourist, the hazards and uncertainties of the journey are kept to a bare minimum, while the comforts of home are, if not guaranteed, at least provided in some measure. Many tour operators provide older people with food, lodging, sightseeing, and recreation that is predictable and not too unlike the daily routine of home. The tour operator arranges transportation, makes hotel and other reservations, organizes sightseeing expeditions, chooses restaurants, and sets up a timetable, presumably on the basis of past satisfactory experience with similar age groups. An itinerary is delivered that meets the desires of the clientele for safety, comfort, cleanliness, and order.

This type of group travel arrangement is often promoted for older people because of their ability to pay the concomitant higher price and to allay their anxiety about traveling in countries where language, money, time, food habits, and living standards may be different from that to which they are accustomed. Quite often, these package tours are small group expeditions that may be targeted to a particular age, sex, occupation, or socioeconomic category. For the older first-time tourist, this may be a wise option, because it removes some of the anxiety-causing elements of solo travel.

Among the chief joys of travel are the associated experiences of planning the trip, often in considerable detail, and in reminiscing about it after the trip or vacation is over. The highlights of the trip may be shared with friends and family through photographs or slides, video recordings, or stories about the inevitable mishaps that occur. Although the predictability of guided tourism may be tempting, there is much to be said for the extra involvement of planning one's own itinerary.

Youth hostels, in spite of their name, are open in most countries to all ages. These are among the most cost-effective lodging choices for international travelers. If the older traveler has a spirit of adventure, likes to meet people of all ages and backgrounds, and does not expect too much in the way of creature comfort, youth hostels offer a good deal. When planning to engage in this more adventurous style of travel, however, it is important to invest in some of the basic necessities of any traveler: good walking shoes, plastic zippered bags, antidiarrheal medicine, photocopies of medical prescriptions, a Swiss Army knife, a pocket flashlight, and spare batteries. When planning to travel by rail, a bottle of mineral water is essential. For those seniors who prefer a higher level of comfort, however, there are many privately owned pensions and inns that offer comfort and hospitality but still provide amenities that the older traveler might prefer. It is wise to pack as little as possible, as carrying unnecessary baggage can make traveling much more exhausting than it has to be. A medical examination before setting out on a long trip is a wise idea, as not all medicines are readily available abroad; any prescriptions should be renewed and purchased beforehand.

Tourists planning to travel by rail in Europe have the advantage of being able to purchase numerous rail passes that make train travel there quite affordable. They must be purchased before arrival in Europe, however. This feature is enhanced by the ease of accessing rail timetables, and even purchasing rail passes, on the Internet.

SECURITY MEASURES

A frequent concern of older travelers is personal security. Although almost everyone who travels frequently has some stories to tell of untoward occurrences, from purse snatching to loss of personal possessions, commonsense precautions will alleviate most of these concerns. It is wise to conceal large amounts of convertible currency in a money belt worn next to the body and to carry travelers' checks separately from the receipt so that they can be replaced if lost or stolen. Passports should also be worn next to the body, as replacing a lost or stolen passport can be a time-consuming and exasperating experience. Copies of the front page of the passport, address book, and a list of all credit card account numbers should also be made and stored separately from the items themselves. A small purse slung over the shoulder that hugs the body is preferable to a large one that hangs loosely from the arm.

These security precautions repay the small effort they take to lessen the impact of an unfortunate incident. The traveler usually wants to view travel as an opportunity to make new friends, and an undue concern about security should not be allowed to limit the inevitable and welcome opportunities for interpersonal relations. A supply of visiting cards may come in handy when making new friends on the road.

MONEY, COMMUNICATION, AND EDUCATIONAL TRAVEL

A real boon to the modern traveler is the automatic teller machine (ATM), available virtually everywhere, which makes carrying large amounts of cash unnecessary. It is wise to check with one's own bank before traveling abroad to make sure that the personal code and type of machine can be used in other countries. Credit cards can be useful when traveling as exchange rates are often more favorable via a credit card than at a currency exchange office, many of which charge high commissions. They also obviate the need for carrying large amounts of cash.

Another concern of older travelers is in knowing how to find out whether everything is going well back home. Although it is possible to call a neighbor or family member from abroad, one must keep in mind the time difference and the cost of international telephone calls. It might be easier and cheaper to arrange to connect with home via the Internet. A number of Internet sites provide free electronic mail (e-mail), which can be accessed for sending and receiving messages while traveling. Once the account and logon information has been set up, preferably before leaving, one can then correspond on the road with friends or family, which can be important for peace of mind. Special Internet cafes, often called cyber cafes, exist all over the world. They are usually inexpensive and service-oriented, and they can provide assistance for new users. Many libraries, particularly in the United States and Canada, also provide this service, sometimes at no charge. In fact, the plethora of websites facilitating travel planning of all kinds make the Internet a basic resource for older persons who do not want unanticipated surprises while traveling.

Opportunities for extending educational horizons can be found through many programs that provide travel opportunities, both in one's own country and abroad. A program that caters to seniors in particular is called Road Scholar. This program is conducted through universities and colleges throughout North America. Courses ranging from nuclear physics to Sufi dancing and Russian literature are offered in attractive college settings. Dormitory space and food are provided, and opportunities to meet like-minded older people are abundant. Many foreign universities promote similar programs, particularly in the summer months when dormitory space is available, and tourism is an objective. For those who feel that education is a lifelong enterprise, these options should be seriously considered.

TRANSPORTATION

Senior travel in the United States and Canada, particularly by citizens of those countries, may differ considerably from travel overseas. A large market exists for recreational vehicles (RVs), many quite luxurious, that make it possible to travel in comfort and to bring items from home that are felt to be necessary, as well as to travel with pets. For many people, the ease of movement and flexibility of planning make this type of travel very attractive. Well-marked RV parks in scenic areas and a wide variety of public parks throughout North America are features that attract travelers from all over the world.

On the other hand, the poorly developed land transportation system for mass transit on the North American continent, particularly the United States, hampers the kind of unencumbered travel possible in other countries, especially those in Europe. In the United States, some form of private automotive transport is almost a necessity, whereas trains and buses serve tourists well in Europe and much of Asia and South America. For those wishing or needing to rely on public transportation in North America, however, there are special discount fares for senior citizens on Amtrak trains and on the Canadian rail system. Perhaps the best travel bargain for those over sixty-two in the United States, where air transport over vast distances is often needed, is a booklet of four senior airfare coupons, each for a single flight anywhere within the United States. They are sold by all the major airlines and are inexpensive.

VACATION HOMES AND TIME SHARES

Some older persons who like to encounter new places but do not like to feel uprooted prefer to set up home exchanges, to buy a vacation house, or to purchase shares in a time share resort. Each of these options has its advantages and limitations. A caveat on time shares is to avoid those who lurk at tropical resorts and lure unsuspecting tourists to high-pressure sales rooms. One should investigate purchasing a vacation home or time share as carefully as any other major purchase, because such a choice may limit one's freedom to travel elsewhere. A number of home exchange organizations exist, easily found in most travel guides or at various Internet sites.

CONCLUSION

The travel industry is the world's largest economic enterprise. Although much has been written about the colonial aspects of travel and its association with class, privilege, and economic disparity, observation indicates that the desire to travel, to see new places, and to meet new people is almost a universal human trait. Although the comforts of home may beckon, the lure of the unknown has an equally persuasive attraction. The freedom to travel that comes with retirement and increasing age is a powerful palliative to the much-touted discomforts of growing older.

—*Gloria Fulton*

See also: AARP; Adult education; Communication; Discounts; Early retirement; Friendship; Harry and Tonto; Housing; Leisure activities; Pets; Relocation; Retirement; Social ties; Transportation issues; Vaccines

For Further Information

Road Scholar. www.roadscholar.org/. Alongside renowned experts, participants experience in-depth and behind-the-scenes learning opportunities by land and by sea on travel adventures designed for boomers and beyond.

"Safe Travel Tips for Older Adults." HealthInAging.org. American Geriatrics Society, June 2019. www.healthinaging.org/tools-and-tips/safe-travel-tips-older-adults. Tips for seniors to promote safety and well-being while traveling.

"Senior Travel & Vacations: Elderly Travel Groups, Tours & Clubs." SeniorLiving.org. www.seniorliving.org/travel/. Provides advice on senior travelling as well as links to popular travel groups and clubs.

"Seniors and Travel." AgingInPlace.org, 20 Nov. 2018. www.aginginplace.org/seniors-and-travel/. Tips for ground, air, and water travel, as well as advice on things to do before vacation.

VACCINES

Relevant Issues: Health and medicine

Significance: Routine immunization of older adults can reduce the risk of complications and death from some of the common infections against which vaccines are available.

As age increases, the body's ability to counter infections successfully is reduced, which results in increased rates of complications and death. Pneumonia and influenza are among the leading causes of death in older adults against which effective vaccines are available. Data suggest, however, that immunizations are underused in older adults even though many infections and death can be prevented by the proper use of these vaccines. Some of the common reasons for underutilization include practitioners' limited knowledge of specific recommendations, poor documentation of vaccination records, inadequate reimbursement, patients' reluctance or refusal to be vaccinated, and poorly developed and insufficiently promoted programs for immunizing adults.

The use of routine vaccination in older adults not only decreases complications and death but also is highly cost effective. Each vaccine is administered according to its own guidelines, depending on the length of time that the immunity lasts or depending on the frequency with which the offending organism changes its properties, thus requiring new vaccine(s). Some of these vaccines require periodic boosters, which are added doses of vaccines to amplify the immune response of the body. Based on the current guidelines, all older adults should get influenza, pneumococcal, shingles, diphtheria (Td), and tetanus, diphtheria and pertussis (Tdap) vaccines.

INFLUENZA

Influenza virus, which is commonly referred to as flu, begins with fever, sore throat, dry cough, fatigue and muscle aches, and usually lasts less than a week. Antiviral medications can be used to treat and prevent influenza virus. There are four antiviral medications that act against both influenza A and B: oseltamivir phosphate (Tamiflu), inhaled zanamivir (Relenza), intravenous Peramivir (Rapivab), and oral baloxavir marboxil (Xofluza). Adults over 65 years old are more susceptible to the complications of influenza virus. The flu virus is associated with 70-90 percent of flu-related deaths and 50-70 percent of hospitalizations. Adults 65 years and older can receive regular flu vaccines approved for their age, but there are two influenza vaccines specific for this population: high dose flu vaccine and adjuvanted flu vaccine. Both vaccines are associated with high antibody production. The vaccine is 40-60 percent effective in preventing illness in older adults and even if they get the disease, the vaccine will reduce the rates of complication and death. It must be given each year because the virus that causes influenza changes its protein components each year, making the previous vaccine ineffective. The vaccine is manufactured based on the predictions of the most likely viruses to circulate during the upcoming influenza season.

Influenza vaccine cannot cause the disease, as is commonly believed, because it is made from inactive virus. It should ideally be given by the end of October; however, it may be offered throughout the flu season. The vaccine causes antibody production against the influenza virus, and it takes about two to four weeks to reach protective levels. It is important that older persons should be vaccinated earlier in the fall so that the body can produce sufficient antibody levels in time for the influenza season, which begins in October and ends in May, with most cases happening between late December and early March. Generally the vaccine is quite safe, but it may cause low-grade fever, muscle aches, and fatigue that may last for one to two days. Persons with known allergies to egg products who have only experienced hives after exposure should get any recommended influenza vaccine. Persons who reported more severe reactions like respiratory distress, angioedema, lightheadedness, recurrent vomiting or required emergent interventions should also get any recommended influenza vaccine, but should be given under supervision by a medical provider. Recombinant Influenza Vaccine (RIV) is a vaccine made without eggs and, if available, it is an option for adults 18 years and older. Influenza vaccine should not be given in persons with life-threatening allergies to a component of the vaccine. Persons with history of Guillain-Barré syndrome (GBS) six weeks after receiving the influenza vaccine have a higher risk for recurrent GBS and should avoid the vaccine, if they have low risk(s) for influenza complications. Persons who are currently ill (moderate to severe illness) with or without fever should wait until full recovery before receiving the flu vaccine.

PNEUMOCOCCAL VACCINES

Pneumonia is usually caused by bacteria called Streptococcus pneumonia or pneumococci. It results in fever, chills, cough, phlegm, shortness of breath, weakness, and lethargy. Patients generally appear ill, and unless treated with appropriate antibiotics in a timely manner, they may have serious complications including sepsis (infection present in the blood and in various organs of the body) and potentially death. Pneumococci also cause bacteremia, meningitis, otitis media and sinusitis. Approximately 400,000 hospitalizations in the United States are a result from pneumococcal pneumonia, with higher rates among the older adults.

There are two types of pneumococcal vaccine for older adults 65 years and older: PCV13 (Pneumococcal conjugated vaccine) and PPSV23 (Pneumococcal polysaccharide vaccine). Per the Centers for Disease Control and Prevention (CDC), both immunizations are recommended for adults in two groups who have not previously received the vaccine: (1) 65 years or older and (2) 19 years or older with certain medical conditions such as diabetes mellitus, alcoholism, and chronic heart, lung or liver disease. The PPSV23 vaccine can be given to those 65 years or older even if they have previously been immunized. The CDC reference for guidelines in immunization of older adults have further details regarding the timing of vaccinations and specific instructions when individuals have certain medical conditions.

Most healthy adults develop protection within two to three weeks of vaccination. The PPSV23 is effective in about two-thirds of the adult population but is somewhat less effective in older adults with chronic diseases and immunodeficiency.

Side effects of both pneumococcal vaccines include soreness, swelling and redness at the site of injection. Fever, chills, headache, nausea, vomiting and muscle aches are less common, but may also occur.

Contraindications include severe allergic reaction to a previous pneumococcal vaccine or to a component of the vaccine. Persons with more serious illness with or without fever should wait until full recovery from their illness before receiving the pneumococcal vaccine.

TETANUS, DIPHTHERIA AND PERTUSSIS (TDAP)

Tetanus, diphtheria and pertussis (Tdap) are discussed together because the Tdap vaccine is usually given as a combination. Tetanus is caused by a bacteria called Clostridium tetani. Spores of this organism, which are present in the soil, enter through a wound and, in an unimmunized individual, cause tetanus. The patient usually has slight pain and tingling at the site of wound followed by muscle spasms throughout the body. Most cases occur in those over the age of 60 and almost exclusively in persons who are unimmunized or inadequately immunized. About 40 percent of the patients who develop tetanus die from this disease.

Diphtheria is caused by Corynebacterium diphtheriae, which usually attacks the respiratory system. It causes runny nose, sore throat, fever, and fatigue and can cause serious heart and nervous system complications unless treated adequately with appropriate antibiotics. The few cases that occur each year are in unimmunized patients. As many as 84 percent of those over the age of 60 lack adequate immunity to diphtheria.

Pertussis or whooping cough is a contagious respiratory disease that causes severe coughing spells followed by a high-pitched "whooping" sound while taking a breath after the cough. Bordetella pertussis primarily affects infants who are not completely immunized and adults whose immunity has faded.

The vaccine for tetanus, diphtheria, and pertussis (Tdap) are available as a combination; the majority of individuals receive these shots as part of their childhood immunization. Every individual, regardless of whether he or she received immunization during childhood or adulthood, should receive a booster dose every 10 years due to fading protective levels.

Adults 19 years and older who never received Tdap vaccine, which is usually given between 11-12 years old should get a dose that may replace the 10-year Td booster. However, the Tdap vaccine can be given at any time after the most recent tetanus, diphtheria (Td) vaccine. The Tdap vaccine is only required once in a lifetime with Td booster every 10 years. Td vaccine is also recommended for wound management, if the last Td booster was more than five years ago.

Side effects are mild and include soreness and redness at the site of injection. A contraindication to the Tdap vaccine is a serious allergic reaction to the previous dose or to a vaccine component. Persons with history of Guillain-Barré syndrome (GBS) six weeks after receiving the tetanus toxoid-containing vaccine should discuss the risks and benefits of having the vaccine with their medical provider. Persons who are currently ill (moderate to severe illness) with or without fever should wait until full recovery before receding the Tdap vaccine.

SHINGLES

Shingles is a painful rash caused by the varicella-zoster virus (the same virus that causes chickenpox). The rash contains blisters and develops in the affected side of the body. The blisters develop scabs in 7-10 days and usually the pain lasts for a few weeks. The most common complication is post-herpetic neuralgia (PHN), a severe pain in the site of the rash that persists for months to years after rash resolves. Older adults are most commonly affected with PHN and their pain is more severe.

People can only develop shingles if they had chickenpox in the past, but not everybody who had chickenpox will develop shingles. The chickenpox virus stays inactive in the nerve tissue of the brain and spine; when the virus is reactivated, it causes shingles. People who did not have chickenpox cannot get shingles, but they can develop chickenpox.

There are two vaccines approved for shingles, Zostavax and Shingrix. The Zostavax is a live vaccine usually given to adults 60 years and older. Protection from shingles with Zostavax lasts approximately 5 years and can decrease the risk of shingles and PHN by 50 to 60 percent. Contraindications include life-threatening reaction to a vaccine component, primary or acquired immunodeficiency, cancer, organ transplant, daily corticosteroid therapy, immunomodulatory therapy, HIV and fever of 101.3oF or higher.

Shingrix is an inactive recombinant vaccine recommended to adults 50 years and older. It is the newest and preferred vaccine requiring two doses. The second dose should be given between 2 to 6 months after the first dose. If Zostavax was administered in the past, Shingrix can be given at least 8 weeks after the Zostavax. In adults 70 years and older, Shingrix is approximately 90 percent effective against shingles and PHN.

Contraindications include life-threatening reaction to a vaccine component, negative immunity for varicella zoster virus (people need the varicella zoster virus vaccine series instead of the shingles vaccine), use of specific antiviral medications 24 hours before the vaccine, current acute episode of shingles, severe acute illness, and fever of 101.3oF or higher.

SPECIAL SITUATIONS

In addition to the above vaccines, older individuals may need additional vaccines depending on their level of

> **SENIOR TALK:**
>
> **How Do You Feel About Vaccinations?**
>
> Getting vaccinations as an adult is often a topic of discussion. You may have heard friends or colleagues talking about whether they are getting a particular vaccination (especially the seasonal flu shot) or not. You may even know or have heard of some people who are opposed to vaccination altogether and claim it's unsafe. This may be confusing as you try to decide what to do. Everyone has a unique medical history and background, and your doctor is your best guide regarding the right vaccinations for you. It's important to be aware of allergies and medical conditions that may make you unfit for certain vaccines. However, it's also important to know that vaccines as a whole are not dangerous. Claims that they cause autism, for example, have no scientific basis.
>
> It's common to feel nervous about any potential side effects of a vaccine. Knowing that you're receiving a form of a disease-causing organism, even a dead or weakened one, can be disconcerting. Speak to your doctor or another trusted health-care professional and share your concerns in order to be fully informed. This can help to alleviate anxiety or the sometimes overwhelming feeling of making decisions about your health. Knowing which vaccines are safe and recommended for you, and receiving them, can help you feel better about your overall health outlook.
>
> —Leah Jacob

risk, which is based on their lifestyle, pre-existing diseases, occupation, or travel. These include hepatitis A and B, measles, mumps, rubella, and chickenpox vaccines. It is important to carefully review the immunization history for persons planning to travel outside the United States. Depending on the area to which they are traveling and the presence of diseases in those regions, they may require poliomyelitis, typhoid fever, cholera, Japanese encephalitis, meningococcus, or rabies vaccines.

—*Shawkat Dhanani*
Updated by Ecler Jaqua, MD and Miriam E. Schwartz, MD, PhD

See also: Health care; Illnesses among older adults; Influenza; Medications; Pneumonia; Vacations and travel

For Further Information

Booy, Robert, and Paul Van Buynder. "Pneumococcal Vaccination in Older Persons: Where Are We Today"? *Pneumonia*, vol. 10, no. 1, 5 Jan. 2018. doi:10.1186/s41479-017-0045-y. This review examines differences in pneumonia vaccine recommendations from several countries and proposes a new way forward.

"Components of Vaccines." Institute for Vaccine Safety, John Hopkins Bloomberg School of Public Health, 8 Apr. 2019. vaccinesafety.edu/components.htm. Provides a list of vaccines including information on manufacturers, dosage, schedule, and storage.

Doherty, T. Mark, et al. "Vaccination Programs for Older Adults in an Era of Demographic Change." *European Geriatric Medicine*, vol. 9, no. 3, 19 Mar. 2018, pp. 289-300. doi:10.1007/s41999-018-0040-8. This paper summarizes some of the challenges and opportunities due to the increasing burden of infectious diseases in an aging population.

"There Are Vaccines You Need as an Adult." Centers for Disease Control and Prevention, National Center for Immunization and Respiratory Diseases, 2 Mar. 2016. www.cdc.gov/vaccines/adults/. General information on which vaccines older adults need and how to get them.

VANCE V. BRADLEY

Date: Decided on February 22, 1979
Relevant Issues: Law, values, work
Significance: The U.S. Supreme Court decided that mandatory retirement at age sixty for U.S. Foreign Service officers does not violate equal protection under the Fifth Amendment, nor does mandatory retirement constitute age discrimination under the Constitution.

Vance v. Bradley involved Holbrook Bradley and several other productive Foreign Service officers who were forced to retire at age sixty in accordance with Section 632 of the Foreign Service Act passed by Congress in 1932. Bradley sued the federal government, claiming that Congress and the State Department had violated the equal protection component of the Constitution's Fifth Amendment due process of law clause. By requiring the retirement, at age sixty, of able Foreign Service officers but not those in the Civil Service, Congress had made an unconstitutional, discriminatory distinction. A three-judge federal district court upheld Bradley's complaint, noting that little evidence was presented by the government to support its legal argument. Employees aged sixty and over were not shown to be less able, competent, productive, or dependable than younger Foreign Service officers.

On direct appeal by Secretary of State Cyrus Vance and others, the U.S. Supreme Court reversed the lower court decision. Eight members of the U.S. Supreme Court ruled that Congress did not deny equal protection of the law when it required mandatory retirement for Foreign Service officers. Congress sought to assure the professional competence and mental and physical reliability of the diplomatic corps that serves overseas under hardship conditions. Moreover, compulsory retirement at age sixty creates predictable opportunities for promotion and, thus, stimulates superior performance and enhances morale among junior Foreign Service personnel. Those above sixty are sufficiently old and less capable than younger persons of confronting the rigors of overseas duty.

It is constitutionally permissible to place a high value on the proper conduct of U.S. foreign policy, to subject Foreign Service officers to an earlier retirement age than occurs in the Civil Service, and to assure that promotion opportunities would be available among the limited number of Foreign Service officers. The goal of maintaining a competent Foreign Service is rationally related to the means of mandatory retirement at age sixty. In 1978, Congress repealed the mandatory retirement age for Civil Service personnel (5 percent of those who serve abroad) but left untouched mandatory retirement for those under the Foreign Service system, 60 percent of whom serve overseas at any given time.

Justice Thurgood Marshall dissented and argued that the Court should afford those terminated by age a heightened level of judicial scrutiny110 and protection. The prevalence of age discrimination in American society should require government to show a substantial relationship between a mandatory retirement system and actual governmental objectives. The federal government failed to provide evidence that it has encountered age-related problems with Foreign Service officers age sixty and over, and federal officials failed to show that forced retirement that affects one's livelihood and dignity boosts productivity.

—*Steve J. Mazurana*

See also: Age discrimination; Age Discrimination Act of 1975; Age Discrimination in Employment Act of 1967; Employment; Johnson v. Mayor and City Council of Baltimore, Massachusetts Board of Retirement v. Murgia; Mandatory retirement; Retirement

VARICOSE VEINS

Relevant Issues: Health and medicine

Significance: Although varicose veins can occur at any time, they are particularly predominant among the elderly; 50 percent of all individuals can expect to develop varicose veins by the age of fifty.

Key Terms:

endovenous thermal ablation: a newer technique that uses a laser or high-frequency radio waves to create intense local heat in the varicose vein or incompetent vein

sclerotherapy: the treatment of varicose blood vessels by the injection of an irritant that causes inflammation, coagulation of blood, and narrowing of the blood vessel wall

vein stripping: a surgical procedure done under general or local anesthetic to aid in the treatment of varicose veins; the surgery involves making incisions (usually the groin and medial thigh), followed by insertion of a special metal or plastic wire into the vein; the vein is attached to the wire and then pulled out from the body

The main task of normal leg veins is to return blood to the heart and lungs. This is difficult because the blood must be pushed upward, against the constant force of gravity. The force that propels the blood up the leg comes from the contraction of the calf muscles surrounding the deep veins that occurs during the act of walking. This forward momentum is quickly lost as gravity pulls the blood back down; however, one-way valves attached to the inside of the vein wall allow blood to pass up the leg freely, then close before the blood can be pulled back down. With each step taken, the column of blood moves up the leg until it eventually reaches the heart.

DAMAGE TO THE VALVES

The system works well until one of the valves fails. It is unclear why valves fail. It may be due to one or more causes. Valves may fail because of congenital defect or because of damage from venous thrombosis (blood clots in the veins of the leg). Valves may fail because of increased intra-abdominal pressure, as with pregnancy or obesity. Women are at an increased risk of developing varicose veins. As one ages, long periods of standing or straining eventually cause even normal veins to become stretched out and dilated, causing the valve leaflets to close improperly. When the vein valves do not close correctly, blood leaks backward, placing extra pressure on the valve beneath it. This increased pressure causes the vein to become dilated and twisted. Such veins are said to be "varicose." If this vein is near the skin, they will bulge out and become visible. These unsightly veins become more pronounced while standing and disappear or become less noticeable when lying down.

Once damaged, the valve cannot repair itself. The increased pressure continues to damage valve after valve until the small bump eventually becomes a large, bluish rope. Varicose veins are frequently accompanied by an aching sensation or a feeling of heaviness in the legs. There can also be cramping, throbbing and/or a feeling of restlessness in the legs. These symptoms are aggravated by sitting or standing. People who must be on their feet all day usually experience severe discomfort. As the condition worsens, the legs and feet swell. These symptoms, which are often absent upon arising from bed in the morning, usually become more severe as the day progresses. Elevating the legs can give relief.

POSSIBLE COMPLICATIONS

Although varicose veins are embarrassing and sometimes painful, they are not always a serious condition. Most people experience only minor inconvenience from them. However, if allowed to progress, varicose veins may lead to more serious conditions. One of the most common—and most serious—of these complications is a blood clot within the varicose vein. As long as blood is moving quickly in a vessel, it is very difficult for it to clot. When a vein becomes varicose, the dilated portion of the vein allows blood to pool. If blood stagnates, it can become a solid mass of blood called a thrombus, or a blood clot. This blood clot may continue to grow up the vein. It can fill the entire vein from the foot to the groin and enter the deep veins of the leg.

A clot in a deep vein is a potentially life-threatening condition, as it may break loose, pass through the heart, and lodge in the arteries that take blood to the lungs. This condition is referred to as a pulmonary embolism. If this happens, and the blood clot is small, the patient

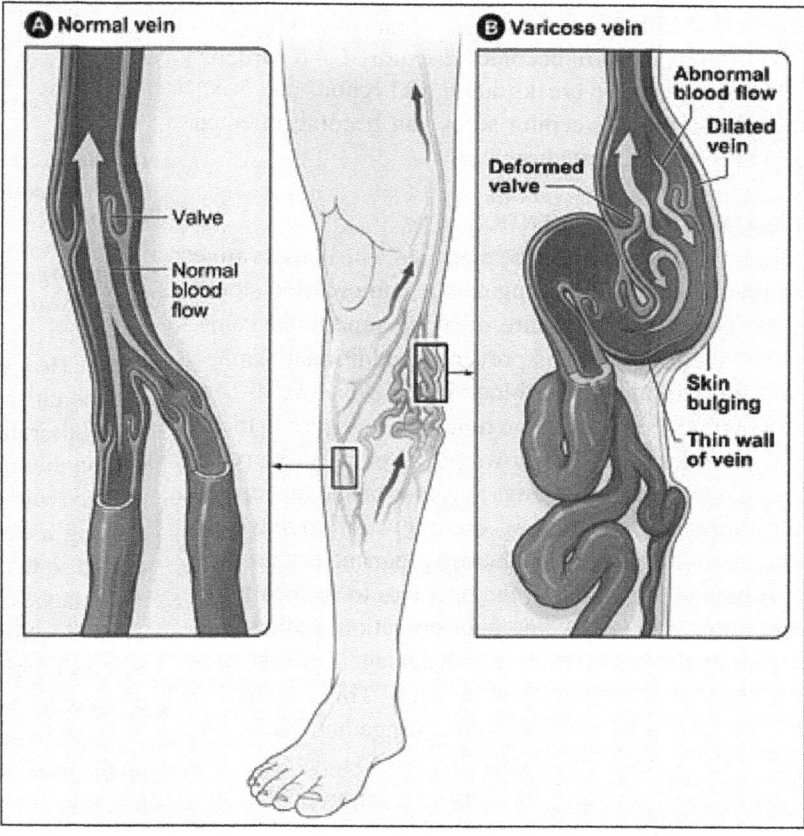

The illustration shows how a varicose vein forms in a leg. Figure A shows a normal vein with a working valve and normal blood flow. Figure B shows a varicose vein with a deformed valve, abnormal blood flow, and thin, stretched walls. The middle image shows where varicose veins might appear in a leg. (via National Heart Lung and Blood Institute)

experiences shortness of breath and chest pain. If the clot that breaks loose is big and lodges in a larger lung artery, it can result in sudden death. Blood clots limited to the superficial veins (near the skin) are far less likely to break loose and result in a major pulmonary embolism. The symptoms of clot in the superficial veins are pain and redness directly over the vein involved. The varicose vein may also become hard. This is called a superficial cord. As the clot grows, the redness, pain, and cord move up the leg. This is a serious condition and requires immediate medical attention.

Other complications associated with varicose veins relate to the impact of having increased venous pressure in the legs over a long period of time. When the valves are working, the pressure in the tissue at the ankle is kept at a low level. When varicose veins are severe, the pressure in the tissue can becomes so high that blood flow to the skin decreases. If this occurs over a long period of time, the skin becomes discolored and hardens. Ultimately, the skin breaks down, and venous ulcers occur. These open, weeping sores can become infected and become a chronic problem.

TREATMENT AND PREVENTION

Minor varicose veins can be managed with conservative treatment using well-fitting elastic compression stockings. These place pressure over the superficial veins, giving them support and preventing additional damage to them. This also forces blood into the deep veins. Assuming the deep veins have functioning valves in them, this provides relief and slows progression of the problem. Compression stockings may also be the first option for those who cannot or do not wish to have an interventional therapy, including pregnant women.

A popular approach in the past was to surgically remove the damaged vein. This operation, called vein stripping, removes the veins with damaged valves, forcing blood to go through healthy veins. This can resolve the symptoms of varicose veins altogether. However, other veins may eventually become varicose. Even though the technique for surgical stripping has improved, it is now considered the third line of interventional therapy for most varicose veins.

The first line or recommended interventional therapy is endovenous thermal ablation. A small tube (catheter) is inserted into the vein (endovenous) under local anes-

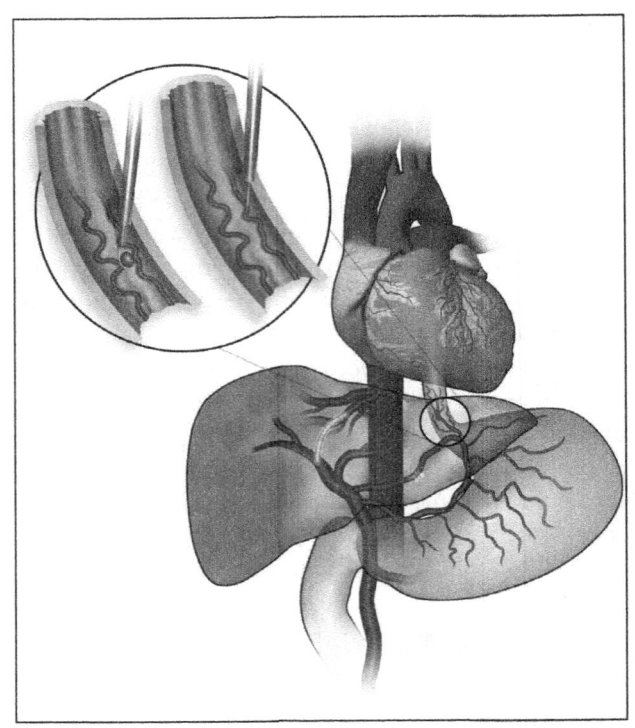

Injecting the unwanted veins with a sclerosing solution causes the target vein to immediately shrink, and then dissolve over a period of weeks as the body naturally absorbs the treated vein. Sclerotherapy is a non-invasive procedure taking only about 10 minutes to perform. The downtime is minimal, in comparison to a more invasive varicose vein surgery. (via Wikimedia Commons)

thesia. Heat (thermal), either by laser or radio waves is used to close (ablation) the varicose vein.

Another intervention to get rid of varicose veins is injection therapy, or sclerotherapy, in which the patient is injected with a material that irritates the varicose vein, causing a clot to form in it. The clot is carefully controlled so that it stays only in the vein being treated. The clot attaches to the vein wall, causing the vein to shrink. This shrinking of the vein makes it seem to disappear. Sclerotherapy is not appropriate in more serious cases of varicose veins.

There is nothing that can be done to change congenital or inherited factors that cause varicose veins. There are, however, simple measures that can prevent the development of varicose veins before they occur or can slow their progression once they have developed. These preventive measures all have a common theme: avoiding long periods of sitting or standing and keeping the calf muscle active. Doctors advise people who must sit or stand for any length of time to flex and relax their calf muscles by pulling their feet up and pushing them back down. This keeps the blood moving and keeps it from pooling. Other measures include breaking up long periods of inactivity by walking a few minutes every hour, elevating the legs from time to time, and wearing loose clothing that does not restrict blood flow. Other measures are to avoid elevated intra-abdominal pressure. One recommendation would be by maintaining a healthy weight. Increased intra-abdominal pressure can also come from straining with constipation. Therefore, some doctors may recommend eating a high-fiber diet to minimize straining during difficult bowel movements.

—Steven R. Talbot
Updated by Linda Roethel, MD, FAAFP

See also: Aging process; Cosmetic surgery; Health care

For Further Information

Argyriou, Christos, et al. "The Effectiveness of Various Interventions versus Standard Stripping in Patients with Varicose Veins in Terms of Quality of Life." *Phlebology: The Journal of Venous Disease*, vol. 33, no. 7, Aug. 2018, pp. 439-50. doi:10.1177/0268355517720307. Compares the effects of various therapeutic strategies among patients with varicose veins.

Cronenwett, Jack L., and K. W. Johnston. *Rutherford's Vascular Surgery.* 8th ed., 2-vol. set, Elsevier Saunders, 2014. Published in association with the Society for Vascular Surgery, Rutherford's Vascular Surgery presents state-of-the-art updates on all aspects of vascular health care. Extensively revised by many new authors to meet the needs of surgeons, interventionalists, and vascular medicine specialists, this medical reference book incorporates medical, endovascular and surgical treatment, as well as diagnostic techniques, decision making and fundamental vascular biology.

Jacobs, Benjamin N., et al. "Pathophysiology of Varicose Veins." *Journal of Vascular Surgery: Venous and Lymphatic Disorders*, vol. 5, no. 3, May 2017, pp. 460-67. doi:10.1016/j.jvsv.2016.12.014. Provides the most current understanding of the hemodynamic and cellular and molecular processes that underlie the development of varicose veins.

Raetz, Jaqueline, et al. "Varicose Veins: Diagnosis and Treatment." *American Family Physician*, vol. 99, no. 11, 1 June 2019, pp. 682-88. Reviews current information and techniques for diagnosing and treating varicose veins.

"Varicose Veins." MedlinePlus, U.S. National Library of Medicine, 8 Apr. 2019. medlineplus.gov/varicoseveins.html. General information on varicose veins.

VETERANS

Relevant Issues: Culture, demographics, health and medicine, psychology, sociology

Significance: A new generation of veterans is entering their senior years. As the earlier generation of World War II veterans passes, the baby boomer generation, including veterans of the Vietnam War and later wars, enters social systems. These veterans often have different needs, both physically and mentally, from previous veteran populations that society (including health care) needs to meet.

The typical older veteran is no longer someone who served proudly in World War II, returning home to a hero's welcome. Veterans from the Vietnam War and later are now becoming a major part of the aging population. The injuries, both mental and physical, that are caused by modern warfare make this population one that has special needs.

DEMOGRAPHICS

The median age of all veterans is 64. There are over 9 million veterans in the United States that are over the age of 65. The face of the aging veteran is changing as more and more women and people of color enter the senior veteran population. An older veteran is more likely to be better educated than past aging veterans. They are also more likely to have had a higher income during their working years than the general population and the previous population of veterans. The share of the general population who are veterans is dropping, coinciding with the drop in active-duty personnel.

HEALTH-CARE ISSUES

This population enters their senior years with a different set of health-care issues than previously seen. Veterans from the Vietnam War and later wars such as the Gulf War are more likely to suffer from issues such as post-traumatic stress syndrome (PTSD), drug and alcohol addiction, HIV infection, and a variety of physical and neurological issues caused by chemical warfare,

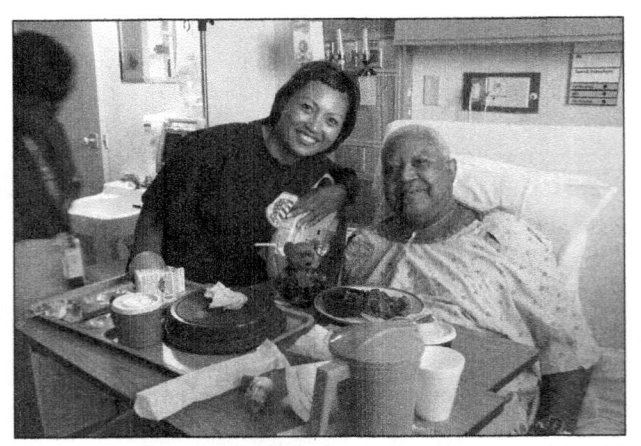

Chief Hospital Corpsman (Select) Jonnalynn Cummings visits with Air Force veteran Leon Gilbert at Chicago's Westside VA Hospital during Chicago CPO Pride Day. (via Wikimedia Commons)

such as Agent Orange used in Vietnam. Veterans of the Vietnam War era and later are also more likely to suffer from issues such as homelessness and abusive relationships. These issues, combined with the diseases that already come with aging such as heart disease, diabetes, and cognitive decline, combine to create a complex and difficult health-care picture for these veterans.

One large, ongoing study that provides information about veterans and their health as they age is the Veterans Aging Cohort Study (VACS). It was specifically started to study the effects of HIV infection on the aging population but has expanded to include an in-depth representation of all veterans.

—*Marianne Moss Madsen, MS*

For Further Information

"American Veterans by the Numbers." Infoplease, Sandbox Networks, Inc., 2016. www.infoplease.com/american-veterans-numbers. Data on how many veterans live in the United States, where they served, their race, ethnicity, and more.

Justice, Amy C., et al. "Veterans Aging Cohort Study (VACS)." *Medical Care*, vol. 44, no. suppl. 2, 2006. doi:10.1097/01.mlr.0000223741.02074.66. Provides background and context for analyses based upon VACS data, including study design and rationale as well as its basic protocol and the baseline characteristics of the enrolled sample.

Pruchno, Rachel. "Veterans Aging." *The Gerontologist*, vol. 56, no. 1, 2016, pp. 1-4. doi:10.1093/geront/gnv671. The 15 articles in this Special Issue highlight the salient role that serving in the military has for veterans and their families. The articles teach us that wartime experiences are complex and that many hidden variables associated with wartime experiences affect the aging process.

VIRTUES OF AGING, THE (BOOK)

Author: Jimmy Carter
Date: Published in 1998
Relevant Issues: Family, health and medicine, religion, work
Significance: Carter's book emphasizes the importance of quality of life rather than quantity of years or possessions for senior citizens.

In *The Virtues of Aging* (1998), former president Jimmy Carter reveals his philosophy of aging; the book is an inspirational autobiographical account that he prepared as a guide for how the elderly can seek an improved lifestyle. He addresses the social, physical, and emotional aspects of aging and encourages readers to welcome opportunities that being elderly offers them.

Carter, writing in his seventies, describes the despair he felt when he lost the 1980 presidential election. He endured a personal crisis, feeling hopeless about the future. Gradually, he became involved in new projects and realized that aging did not require him to cease activity. Retirement enabled him to have time to grow spiritually

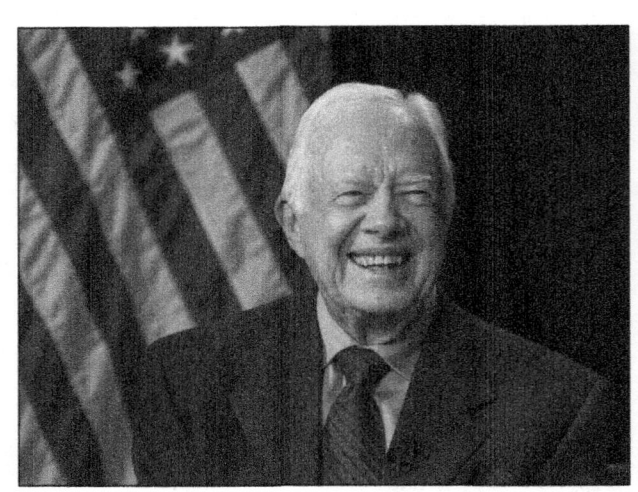

On March 22, 2019, Carter gained the distinction of being the nation's longest-lived president, when he surpassed the lifespan of George H. W. Bush, who was 94 years, 171 days of age when he died in November 2018; both men were born in 1924. (via Wikimedia Commons)

and intellectually and to explore previously unconsidered options.

Carter describes how attitudes toward retired Americans changed during the twentieth century, comparing different generations, cultural perceptions of work, and the establishment of government policies for the elderly. Carter laments that ageism exists. He cites statistics showing that life spans are increasing, resulting in longer retirements and greater numbers of senior citizens. Carter urges the elderly to accept the challenges and changes presented by aging and advises people to seek knowledge and plan for the future, especially regarding financial decisions. He provides exercise and nutritional tips to offset physical limitations caused by aging. Carter believes senior citizens should volunteer, sharing their talents to improve their communities.

Love for self and others is Carter's main theme. He discusses aged mentors who have influenced him. He explains how his spirituality has enhanced his happiness as he has aged and how he hopes to enlighten others with his awareness of aging as a positive experience to be savored.

—*Elizabeth D. Schafer*

See also: Religion; Successful aging; Volunteering

VISION CHANGES AND DISORDERS

Relevant Issues: Biology, health and medicine
Significance: The eye is a highly specialized and intricate organ; many of the normal biological changes associated with aging affect the structure and function of the eye, resulting in changes in vision and increased occurrence of eye diseases.

The job of the eye is to gather visual information and transmit these images to the brain, where they are synthesized into a meaningful picture of one's surroundings. These images provide information for balance, direction, and safety. Vision also plays a role in intellectual development and learning through activities such as reading and writing. The eye develops through an involved process in which it must be properly positioned, supplied with nutrients through blood circulation, supported with bone and fat, moved by an intricate set of muscles, and directed by a complex set of nerves. The proper functioning of the eye is so important to human life that the eye is serviced by four major nerves that arise from the brain.

Light enters the eye through an adjustable opening called the iris. The iris is the part of the eye that determines a person's eye color. In the middle of the iris is a black hole, called the pupil, which is made larger or smaller depending on the availability of light. In bright sunlight, the iris contracts and makes the pupil opening very small, limiting the amount of light that enters the eye. In dim light or at night, the iris creates a very large pupil opening in order to gather as much light as possible. The part of the eye that is responsible for focusing the light is the lens, a transparent cover over the iris and pupil. The lens focuses the light on an area at the back of the eye called the retina, where special cells called photoreceptors process the light information and send it to the brain. To focus light properly, the lens must be flexible and able to elongate or shorten. The front of the eye is completely covered by the transparent cornea. A series of six muscles moves the eye from side to side, up and down, and inward and outward.

NORMAL AGE-RELATED CHANGES IN THE EYE

The eye is supported and cushioned in the eye socket, or orbital, by a layer of fat called orbital fat. As a person ages, this fat breaks down and degenerates, and the eye may appear sunken or hollow. A second change that is easily observed is the loss of tone and elasticity of the skin and muscle that surrounds the eye. The skin around the eye loses the ability to stretch and snap back into shape, much like the elastic in an old pair of underwear. The result is that the skin above the eye tends to fold over the upper eyelid. Sometimes this extra fold of skin can increase the pressure on the eye or reduce overhead vision.

The retina is also affected by the aging process. The cells of the retina, the photoreceptor cells that receive the light information and transmit it to the brain, are gradually lost over time and are not replaced. Also, the blood supply to the periphery (outer parts) of the retina decreases. This decrease in blood supply means that cells in the outer portion of the eye are not receiving as much nourishment from the blood. Sometimes a loss of peripheral vision, the ability to see things coming from the sides of the field of vision, results from this decrease in blood supply. All the arteries and veins that supply the eye with blood become narrower, or sclerosed, with age, just like all the other arteries and veins of the body. The macular area of the retina—the area of the retina that is responsible for the sharpest, central sight—collects the end products of the aging and dying photoreceptors.

Many changes also occur with the outer components of the eye. The most obvious change is the hardening of the lens, causing an inability to focus objects that are close to the eye. The inability to see near objects (presbyopia) affects all individuals and usually begins around age forty-five. People who had completely normal sight will require reading glasses to correct this, while people who are nearsighted often need bifocals.

The lens also becomes less transparent or more opaque. Sometimes this loss of transparency results from changes in lens proteins caused by exposure to ultraviolet (UV) light over time. The lens becomes brownish-orange or yellow in appearance. The yellowing causes changes in color vision; for instance, the perception of different shades of blue is more difficult because the yellowish color filters out blue light (like wearing a yellow pair of sunglasses) and allows more red and yellow light to enter the eye. This gradual loss of transparency of the lens can also lead to cataracts.

The eye is filled with a watery, gelatinous substance called the vitreous humor. The vitreous humor may collect particles of debris that can be seen by the individual as "floaters" that occasionally cross the field of vision. The vitreous humor may become more watery and less gelatinous over time. This causes the gel to shrink, and it can become detached from the retina, resulting in visual impairment.

With age, the cornea of the eye can lose its natural transparency and become more opaque, much like the lens does. Additionally, deposits of fats and lipids may accumulate in a circular ring bordering the cornea, known as the arcus senilis. Often decreased tear flow, or dry eye, becomes a problem with age. As tears are important for keeping the surface (cornea) of the eye well lubricated, the outside of the eye can become damaged from being too dry.

The pupil itself changes with age as well. It loses its ability to quickly accommodate, or change in response to, differences in the brightness or dimness or light. The pupil generally becomes smaller as a person ages, giving the individual an increased depth of focus in the central field of view but reducing the total size of the visual field.

AGE-RELATED PERCEPTUAL CHANGES IN VISION

Because of the many physical changes of the eye with age, the individual will experience perceptual changes in vision. For instance, dark adaptation becomes more difficult because the pupil is less able to respond to changes in light brightness. Glare becomes a significant problem. Glare reduces the ability of all individuals to see because it creates a scattering of light that reduces the sensitivity of the viewed objects. Although people of all ages are affected by glare, this scattering is even more pronounced in older individuals who have much yellowing of the lens and cornea. Headlights from oncoming cars, for example, can literally blind the aged driver.

Visual acuity—the ability to see small objects under normal lighting and contrast—also may suffer with age. As the pupil opening is smaller (thus letting less light into the eye) and the lens and cornea are less transparent (thus scattering the light that does reach the eye), acuity decreases significantly with age. For every thirteen years of life, the amount of light needed for the eye to function properly increases twofold because of the changes in the pupil, lens, and cornea. More light is needed for such tasks as reading and writing; this condition is sometimes called night blindness. This reduction in acuity may decrease visual performance in unfamiliar environments as insignificant objects become distracting. Also, the person will experience changes in color vision as already described, having more difficulty perceiving blues that are filtered out by the increasingly opaque lenses.

AGE-RELATED EYE DISEASES

One of the most common reasons for loss of sight in the elderly is age-related macular degeneration (ARMD), also known as senile macular degeneration. The macula is the part of the retina where most of the photoreceptor cells are located. The macula is responsible for the sharp, central line of vision; when a person looks directly at an object, the macula is the part of the retina that collects the light information and transmits it to the brain. People who stare too long at a solar eclipse destroy their sight because the intense light damages the macula.

There are two types of macular degeneration: dry and wet. Dry macular degeneration is caused by a decrease in the nutrient supply reaching the macular tissue. This is usually caused by a loss of blood vessels supplying this region of the eye. Vision loss from this type of macular degeneration is generally slow and less severe than the vision loss associated with wet macular degeneration. Often diet (eating foods rich in vitamins A, C, and E or taking ocular vitamin supplements) can slow or prevent dry macular degeneration.

Wet macular degeneration is more serious, and the vision loss occurs more rapidly than with dry macular degeneration. With wet macular degeneration, waste products fail to be transported away from the retina. This results in an increase in fluid within the macula, and this fluid can accumulate in small pools. The pools of fluid stimulate the growth of small, weak blood vessels, which can hemorrhage (rupture) and cause vision loss. This type of macular degeneration is usually treated by laser surgery to seal off small vessels, keeping them from growing into the pools of fluid.

Some of the risk factors that seem to be associated with macular degeneration not only include age but also include smoking in males; a family history of the macular degeneration; light-colored eyes; a history of heart disease; a history of recurrent, severe respiratory infections; and a decrease in hand grip strength. All of these factors do not directly contribute to macular degeneration, but they are associated with an increased risk of the disease.

A second age-related eye disease is glaucoma. Approximately 1 percent of all people over age forty have glaucoma. Glaucoma is an increase in pressure within the eye. This increase can be caused by overproduction of fluid by the eye or failure to drain eye fluid properly. The most common kind of glaucoma results from blockage of the fluid drainage system of the eye. The optic nerve that transmits the information collected by the photoreceptor cells to the brain is particularly sensitive to this increase in pressure. The increased pressure will damage the nerve and will ultimately cause blindness if the condition is not treated.

Early symptoms of glaucoma are very hard to detect, and the pressure from fluid buildup can stay high for many years, causing the optic nerve to atrophy. The central vision of the eye is the last to be lost from glaucoma. Undiagnosed glaucoma results in approximately five thousand new cases of blindness each year in the United States. In the population over age seventy, glaucoma is one of the top three causes of blindness. Factors that increase the risk of developing glaucoma include smoking, stress, consuming large quantities of alcohol, high blood pressure, and prolonged use of steroid medication. The nerve damage from glaucoma is irreversible, but the disease can be slowed and vision loss prevented or lessened through medications.

Cataract, or lens opacity, can develop any time from infancy to adulthood. The most common cataracts are age-related and often occur after age fifty. Although cataracts can result from a variety of causes, such as injury to the eye or toxins, most age-related cataracts result from the gradual decrease in transparency of the lens that happens with age. Cataracts are removed surgically when vision loss causes difficulty in performing daily activities, such as reading or watching television. Medications, particularly the prolonged use of steroids, may cause cataracts. Systemic illnesses, such as diabetes, can also cause cataracts. Symptoms of cataracts include blurred vision that is often noticed when reading or driving. Other symptoms include double vision, a decrease in the ability to judge distances, and increased sensitivity to glare.

A final common eye disease among older individuals is diabetic retinopathy. This condition affects diabetics and results from the weakening of the small blood vessels that nourish the retina; it is the leading cause of blindness in individuals aged twenty to seventy-four. These weakened vessels can be damaged, leading to hemorrhage. New, weaker vessels may try to grow into the area of the hemorrhage and result in the formation of scar tissue. This scar tissue may eventually lead to retinal detachment and vision loss. Unless the macula is affected by this scar tissue, the diabetic will be unaware of the disease process. Therefore, diabetic patients should have annual eye examinations to screen for this problem. Patients with diabetic retinopathy do benefit from early intervention, such as laser treatment to seal leaky blood vessels and prevent fluid buildup.

> **SENIOR TALK:**
>
> **How Do You Feel About Vision Loss?**
>
> A certain degree of vision loss is a normal aspect of aging and can often be corrected with glasses or contact lenses. When the vision loss is acute or severe, however, it can have a profound effect on your daily life. Many people who experience such vision loss feel depressed or afraid. They may be unsure how to deal with the new reality. They may become withdrawn given the challenges presented by reduced vision. Some people feel embarrassed by their vision problems. This has a direct impact on our social lives and active involvement in community, with a negative effect on our overall well-being and quality of life. Speaking to a social worker or therapist who specializes in aging and/or vision loss can help you develop coping strategies.
>
> When our independence is threatened due to vision loss, our attitude plays a significant role in how we cope with the challenge. Maintaining a positive attitude can help you find the best way of adjusting. For example, if vision loss becomes severe, our ability to drive may be threatened. Not being able to drive anymore due to impaired vision can strip us of our independence. Being told to stop driving and to hand over the keys feels very disempowering. It also raises a number of practical concerns. However, making a proactive decision to stop driving can make it easier to graciously accept that staying safe on the road is paramount.
>
> —*Leah Jacob*

A healthy lifestyle that includes a well-balanced diet is essential to visual health throughout the life span. The diet should be low in fats and salts but high in dietary fiber. Supplementing the diet with vitamins A, C, and E provides some protection against eye degeneration, and the diet should include plenty of water. Maintaining normal body weight, not smoking, and limiting alcoholic intake will also benefit eye health. As with all medical problems, early diagnosis of eye diseases is key to successful treatment; individuals are advised to have regular eye exams to screen for glaucoma, age-related macular degeneration, and other eye diseases.

—*P. Michele Arduengo*

See also: Aging: Biological, psychological, and sociocultural perspectives; Aging process; Cataracts; Diabetes; Glaucoma; Macular degeneration; Nearsightedness; Reading glasses

For Further Information

"Age-Related Eye Diseases and Conditions." National Eye Institute, National Institutes of Health. nei.nih.gov/healthy eyes/aging_eye. General information and resources about several age-related vision disorders.

Deloss, Denton J., et al. "Improving Vision Among Older Adults." *Psychological Science*, vol. 26, no. 4, 2015, pp. 456-66. doi:10.1177/0956797614567510. Examines whether a perceptual-learning task could be used to improve age-related declines in contrast sensitivity.

Magnus, Eva, and Kjersti Vik. "Older Adults Recently Diagnosed with Age-Related Vision Loss: Readjusting to Everyday Life." *Activities, Adaptation & Aging*, vol. 40, no. 4, 2016, pp. 296-319. doi:10.1080/01924788.2016.1231460. This study aims to explore how older adults recently diagnosed with age-related vision loss experience and readjust to their new everyday lives.

Owsley, Cynthia. "Aging and Vision." *Vision Research*, vol. 51, no. 13, 2011, pp. 1,610-22. doi:10.1016/j.visres.2010.10.020. This article summarizes and reviews research on aging and vision over the past 25 years.

Saftari, Liana Nafisa, and Oh-Sang Kwon. "Ageing Vision and Falls: A Review." *Journal of Physiological Anthropology*, vol. 37, no. 1, 2018. doi:10.1186/s40101-018-0170-1. This article reviews existing studies regarding visual risk factors for falls and the effect of ageing vision on falls. It then presents a group of phenomena such as vection and sensory reweighting that provide information on how visual motion signals are used to maintain balance.

VITAMINS AND MINERALS

Relevant Issues: Health and medicine

Significance: As the body ages, it utilizes vitamins and minerals less efficiently, placing the elderly at risk for nutritional deficiencies.

Vitamins are micronutrients that function as coenzymes, which are at the foundation of all bodily functions. Recommendations for vitamin and mineral requirements are issued by the Food and Nutrition Board of the National Research Council (NRC), National Academy of Sciences (NAS). The daily value (DV) has replaced the recommended dietary (or daily) allowance (RDA), which is still commonly used. Because the body becomes less efficient at using nutrients as it ages, the older population is at risk for several vitamin deficiencies; standard DVs may not fully meet their micronutrient needs.

VITAMINS A AND B

Vitamin A is an immune system booster that protects against diseases of the respiratory system and gastrointestinal system and decreases the risk of cancer and heart disease. An antioxidant, it destroys free radicals that may make the body more susceptible to cancer, cardiovascular disease, arthritis, and signs of aging. Beta carotene is the plant precursor of vitamin A, which enables the body to make active vitamin A. The requirement for beta carotene may increase with age. It is possible that beta carotene can reduce the incidence of eye disease associated with aging. The DV for vitamin A is 30 milligrams, or 5,000 international units (IU), although some nutritionists recommend 10,000 to 50,000 IU. The active form of vitamin A can cause adverse effects at a daily dosage of 50,000 IU, but it usually takes a dosage of 100,000 IU for a period of months to notice negative effects. Any adverse effects are reversible.

The B vitamins are useful in healing nerves and muscles. They enhance the immune system, ease the physiological wear of aging, and may alleviate mild depression, anxiety, and poor memory. Supplementation usually includes the entire B complex. As they work in concert, when individual B vitamins are recommended for a medical condition, additional amounts of the B complex should also be taken.

Vitamin B1 is called thiamine. Thiamine deficiency is common among the elderly; symptoms may include fatigue, depression, confusion, nervousness, memory loss, and numbness of hands and feet. The DV is only 1.4 milligrams for males and 1.1 milligrams for females, but nutritionists tend to recommend 25 to 300 milligrams. Vitamin B2, also known as riboflavin, may prevent or delay cataracts and is useful for neurological problems. Vitamin B3, which comes in the form of niacin and niacinamide, is helpful in treating circulatory problems, and large doses can cause the skin to flush. Pantothenic acid, formerly called vitamin B5, is important to nerve transmission and the immune system. It seems to protect against stress.

Vitamin B6 is one of the most widely utilized vitamins, but many studies have found the elderly to be deficient. Inadequate intake means poorer immune function and higher risk of heart attack in older people. The DV is 2.2 milligrams. Doses of one hundred times the DV can cause nerve damage, but it is reversible. Supplementation of 200 milligrams per day for more than one month can sometimes cause dependency and so should not be stopped abruptly.

Vitamin B12 (cobalamin) and folate deficiencies are common in the elderly. The DV is only 0.03 milligrams, but people over the age of sixty do not absorb vitamin B12 from foods as well as younger people; for this reason, the NAS recommends that older people take vitamin B12 supplements; 200 to 500 percent of the DV is recommended. Folic acid (also called folate) protects the heart and may help prevent colon cancer. The recommended DV is 4 to 12 milligrams.

VITAMINS C, D, AND E

Vitamin C plays a major role in maintaining the immune system, handling stress, and preventing cancer, and also functions as an antioxidant. Elderly, nonsmoking men have lower levels of vitamin C in blood plasma than young men with the same intake. The DV is only 60 milligrams, which may be too low; the National Institutes of Health (NIH) regards 200 milligrams as ideal. Many nutritionists suggest 200 to 500 milligrams. It is believed that supplementation of 120 to 180 milligrams lowers the risk of cancer and cataracts in the elderly. People with kidney problems are advised to consult with a qualified professional about vitamin C supplementation. Bioflavonoids are antioxidants that are present with vitamin C in citrus pulp. They strengthen capillary walls, which protects against black-and-blue marks and varicose veins.

Vitamin D in its active form is considered to be a hormone. It helps absorb calcium and metabolize phosphorus and contributes to bone density. Calcium and magnesium should be taken with vitamin D to treat the thinning bones of menopausal women. Although the human body can make vitamin D from sunshine, many elderly people may not be exposed to enough sun to get a sufficient dose. There is no DV, but most professionals regard 400 IU as a reasonable amount. Up to 1,000 IU appears to be safe, although most nutritionists advise against taking more than 800 IU.

Vitamin E is a powerful antioxidant that may slow aging by promoting cell vitality; it also protects the body against various carcinogens and toxins, and improves blood flow to the extremities. Vitamin E is possibly helpful in treating circulatory problems to which older people are more susceptible, such as angina, arteriosclerosis, thrombophlebitis, and intermittent claudication. It may even alleviate lipofuscin, commonly known as liver spots or age spots. The DV is 10 to 20 IU, but many researchers suggest 400 IU, and some cardiologists recommend 200 to 600 IU.

MINERALS

Some minerals are also essential to health, functioning like vitamins as coenzymes. In addition to building strong bones, calcium is important to white blood cells and helps ward off infections. Calcium also aids blood clotting, helps tired muscles, and also protects against high blood pressure. The DV is 800 milligrams, but 1,000 to 1,500 is recommended. Phosphorus contributes to the hardness of bones and plays a role in utilization of food. In most diets, phosphorus intake exceeds calcium intake, but nutritionists recommend as much calcium as phosphorus.

Zinc promotes a strong immune system and wound healing and helps prevent colds, but excess zinc interferes with absorption of copper; therefore, a zinc supplement should be taken with copper. One study found that zinc and selenium seemed to reduce infections in the elderly. Zinc is also helpful in treating the benign prostate enlargement common in older men. The decrease in taste that the elderly often experience may be alleviated by zinc supplementation. The DV for zinc is 15 milligrams, but some nutritionists suggest 22 to 50 milligrams. In one study, the zinc intake of elderly people was less than one-half the DV. Senile purpura (purple spots under the skin) may be caused by zinc deficiency. Copper is helpful in bone and heart health, blood sugar regulation, and iron absorption. The DV for copper is 2 milligrams. Copper deficiency is rare, but taking 1 milligram of copper for every 10 or 15 milligram of zinc will maintain the proper balance.

Selenium is an antioxidant synergistic with vitamin E; it may lower risk of prostatitis, lung, and colon cancer. Selenium deficiency may be associated with cardiovascular disease. A Finnish study of elderly people who were given selenium and vitamin E supplementation found improvement in mental states. The recommended DV is 1 milligram. Magnesium helps convert food into energy and is required for strong, healthy bones. It is linked to protection from diabetes, osteoporosis, atherosclerosis, and hypertension. The DV for magnesium is 400 milligrams. People with abnormal kidney function are advised to take magnesium supplements only under a physician's supervision.

Manganese is essential to many enzyme systems involved with metabolism and is required for proper functioning of the nerves. Manganese deficiency may affect the immune system and may play a role in glucose tolerance. There is no established DV, but the Food and Nutrition Board recommends 2.5 to 5 milligrams, and some nutritionists recommend 15 to 30 milligrams. Potassium is necessary for the fluid balance of cells, healthy skin, and stable blood pressure. Soft drinks contain large amounts of phosphorus, which depletes potassium. A potassium deficiency can cause a calcium deficiency. No DV has been established. Iron makes hemoglobin. Postmenopausal women need less iron. Only people with iron-deficiency anemia should take more than the DV, and some physicians suggest men avoid iron supplements.

—*William L. Reinshagen*

See also: Age spots; Antiaging treatments; Antioxidants; Cancer; Free radical theory of aging; Malnutrition; Nutrition; Osteoporosis; Prostate enlargement; Skin changes and disorders

For Further Information

Kritchevsky, Stephen B. "Nutrition and Healthy Aging." *The Journals of Gerontology Series A: Biological Sciences and Medical Sciences*, vol. 71, no. 10, 2016, pp. 1,303-05. doi:10.1093/gerona/glw165.

Ritchie, Christine, and Michi Yukawa. "Geriatric Nutrition: Nutritional Issues in Older Adults." *UpToDate*, 7 June 2019. www.uptodate.com/contents/geriatric-nutrition-nutritional-issues-in-older-adults. This article discusses assessment of nutrition in the older adult, as well as the etiology, evaluation, and treatment of weight loss, overnutrition, and specific common nutrient deficiencies.

"Vitamins and Minerals." National Institute on Aging, U.S. Department of Health and Human Services, 29 Apr. 2019.

www.nia.nih.gov/health/vitamins-and-minerals. General information and resources on key vitamins and minerals for people over age 50.

Ward, Elizabeth. "Addressing Nutritional Gaps with Multivitamin and Mineral Supplements." *Nutrition Journal*, vol. 13, no. 1, 2014. doi:10.1186/1475-2891-13-72. This article reviews the potential health benefits and risks of multivitamin and mineral supplements in several key areas, including cancer, cardiovascular disease, age-related eye disease, and cognition.

Wolfram, Taylor. "Special Nutrient Needs of Older Adults." *EatRight*, Academy of Nutrition and Dietetics, 23 May 2018. www.eatright.org/health/wellness/healthy-aging/special-nutrient-needs-of-older-adults. Brief description of the benefits of a few key vitamins and minerals.

VOLUNTEERING

Relevant Issues: Recreation, sociology, values, work

Significance: Volunteering provides many health benefits and gives older people an opportunity to participate in activities that they may not have been able to pursue when they were employed or raising a family.

Many Americans retire by the age of sixty, and almost all Americans have retired by the age of seventy. Yet the average American life expectancy is well beyond seventy; in fact, many people lead active, vital lives into their eighties and nineties. Thus, many retirees and people who spent their youth and middle years raising a family find that they have twenty or thirty years of free time. Some of these people choose to work at part-time jobs or in paid consulting positions. Others, however, turn to volunteer activities as a way to develop themselves, help their communities, and help their fellow citizens.

TYPES OF VOLUNTEER ACTIVITIES

Elderly Americans volunteer in a multitude of ways and in a wide variety of settings. Any community service position or profession can have a volunteer aspect to it. For example, many people volunteer in the public school systems. They do not serve in the professional capacity of classroom teacher, but they aid the classroom teachers by performing many tasks—such as grading papers, making photocopies, and keeping records—that the classroom teacher does not have time to complete. Also, many classroom volunteers tutor in subject areas and in basic skills such as reading and mathematics. In kindergarten and first- and second-grade classrooms, elderly volunteers sometimes read to children, thus helping the children to develop a love of reading and learning.

Older Americans may also volunteer to be on community councils and boards, such as town councils, boards of education, planning commissions, and other civic committees. Volunteers answer phones, edit newsletters, write reports, prepare press releases, organize fund-raising campaigns, and organize and train other volunteers. Older Americans make up many of the boards of directors of civic organizations across the United States, and they serve as officers for many of these organizations.

Many of the retirees who volunteer are also veterans. Often veterans are interested in helping other veterans; thus, they volunteer to perform nonprofessional services in veterans' hospitals throughout the United States. Other volunteers serve in nonprofessional positions, such as greeters and patient aides, in community hospitals. Libraries benefit from the services of older Americans who volunteer to shelve books, collect fines, check books in and out, and assist library patrons in locating reference materials. Children are the concern of many volunteers who regularly lead Boy Scout and Girl Scout trips and chaperon church youth groups on trips and at meetings.

Another area where volunteers have been especially helpful is in advocacy positions in the courts. Special volunteers, appointed as advocates by the courts, advocate for the rights of children who have to appear in court proceedings but who have no adult to advocate for their rights. These court-appointed advocates receive special training from the court system. Other groups, such as the indigent, the homeless, and the mentally impaired, also sometimes receive volunteer help from people who advocate for them. The homeless and the indigent are also the recipient of volunteer services in shelters, where much of the work, such as securing food and supplies, writing grants, meal preparation, and food service, is done by volunteers.

Many older Americans also volunteer in the private sector. Many people who have been successful in business serve as volunteer consultants, helping fledgling businesses and young entrepreneurs to become financially and personally successful. People retired from professions such as law, medicine, education, journalism, and engineering often choose to be volunteer mentors to young people who are entering, or who plan to enter, the profession from which the volunteer has retired. The retired professionals help the novices to understand how the profession works and how to avoid certain pitfalls that the professional life might present.

VALUE OF VOLUNTEERING

Volunteering has value for the person who volunteers, for the community as a whole, and for the people who are recipients of the volunteer services. There are enormous social, intellectual, emotional, and physical benefits for the older person who volunteers. Almost all volunteer activities require the volunteer to come into contact with other people. This contact helps the volunteer retain social bonds with others and assures that elderly people, whose family members may not live with them or even in the same community, do not become recluses. Volunteering helps the volunteer retain and develop intellectual functioning. Many volunteer activities, such as tutoring, require the volunteer to think and to solve problems, which keeps the elderly person mentally active.

Many volunteer activities also require volunteers to assume professional roles that they have never before assumed. As the volunteer thinks about the new role, adjusts to it, and considers its various aspects, he or she must exercise a type of mental flexibility. The ability to be mentally flexible keeps the mind active. There is evidence that elderly people who use their minds to engage in problem solving and who are flexible in their approach to life's problems live longer, healthier lives and are able to perform daily tasks further into old age than are people who do not attempt to problem solve or to perform mental tasks.

Volunteering contributes to the volunteer's emotional well-being. This is true for a variety of reasons. First, as has been mentioned, the person who volunteers makes social contacts. The social contacts themselves help volunteers feel more at ease in their environment and feel emotional satisfaction. Also, the knowledge that they have helped others is emotionally satisfying to nearly all volunteers. Finally, many volunteers do things that they would have liked to do at a younger age but were prevented from doing because they had to earn a living or care for a family. Thus, many older people find it satisfying to be able to fulfill their youthful dreams. Volunteering can also contribute to a person's physical well-being. Leaving the house, moving around, and meeting appointments may cause retirees to become more physically alert and more conscious of their physical health.

Volunteer services have great financial and social value to the communities in which they are performed. Each year, in every community across the United States, volunteers contribute literally thousands of service hours that the community would have to pay for if there were no volunteers. Beyond the financial value, these volunteer hours have enormous social value. Volunteer services help all citizens come together to work for the common good and for the survival of the community. No price tag could be put on the importance of citizens working for the common good. Citizens working together is what makes a community truly a community, rather than just a collection of houses, businesses, and public institutions.

Individuals who use volunteer services receive both general and specific value from these services. In general, the individuals receiving the services understand that they are part of a larger community that cares about their welfare and their future; the knowledge of this caring is important for the individuals' well-being. Also, individuals receive a multitude of specific good from volunteers—tutoring, counseling, meal preparation, disaster aide, transportation, and so forth. Specific services are important and often life-sustaining for the people who receive them.

Serving as a volunteer enriches the life of the volunteer, the life of the community in which the volunteer services are performed, and the lives of those who are recipients of the volunteer services. Some volunteers even go beyond the bounds of their own communities to perform work. Some older Americans join the Peace Corps and go to developing countries, where they teach, train farmers, serve in hospitals, and help local people develop businesses. Some retired medical personnel go to Africa, Eastern Europe, or Central America to help people who are victims of civil unrest. Others volunteer to help the Red Cross and other disaster relief agencies to get food and medical supplies to parts of the world where disaster has occurred.

—Annita Marie Ward

See also: Advocacy; Caregiving; Employment; Home services; Leisure activities; Mentoring; Retired and Senior Volunteer Program (RSVP); Retirement; Social ties; Virtues of Aging, The; Wisdom

For Further Information

Carr, Deborah. "Volunteering Among Older Adults: Life Course Correlates and Consequences." *The Journals of Gerontology: Series B*, vol. 73, no. 3, 2018, pp. 479-81. doi:10.1093/geronb/gbx179. The papers in this special section use sophisticated multi-wave data from large population-based surveys to document the ways that volunteering affects trajectories of physical, emotional, and cognitive well-being.

Dury, Sarah, et al. "To Volunteer or Not." *Nonprofit and Voluntary Sector Quarterly*, vol. 44, no. 6, 2014, pp. 1,107-28. doi:10.1177/0899764014556773. This study investigates whether potential volunteers, actual volunteers, and non-volunteers in later life are different from each other in terms of individual characteristics, resources, and social factors.

"How to Volunteer as a Senior." AgingInPlace.org, 27 Feb. 2019. www.aginginplace.org/how-to-volunteer-as-a-senior/. Discusses the benefits of volunteering on seniors and lists opportunities for those looking to start volunteering.

WALKERS. *See* CANES AND WALKERS.

WEIGHT LOSS AND GAIN

Relevant Issues: Biology, economics, health and medicine

Significance: Aging of the body causes many of its functions to slow down, altering body composition and resulting in changes in weight.

Aging is not merely the passage of time; it is the manifestation of biological events that occur over a span of time. Chronological age is a poor measure of aging; how many birthdays a person has celebrated does not reveal much about him or her. The changes seen with aging are highly individualized. Some of the changes that occur with advanced age are the result of genetic factors, others are the result of environment, and some are the result of lifestyle choices.

Gain or loss of weight with advancing age is partly attributable to all these factors with disease added to the mix, a more rapid loss or gain depending on the manifestation of the particular disease. Through most of the twentieth century, the progression of weight in both men and women followed a consistent pattern. Following adolescence, when maturation causes gains in weight, weight tends to stabilize for five to ten years. When middle age begins, weight increases to a maximum in men at about age fifty and in women at about age sixty-five. Afterward, there is a steady decline until around age eighty, where weight remains stable until death. There might be a dramatic decline in weight if the cause of death creates body wasting, as with cancer, but that loss is attributable to the disease process, not the aging process. In the 1990s, the U.S. population as a whole increased in weight, from youths through the elderly, but the chronological ages for weight changes seemed to remain stable. As more Americans live to one hundred years and beyond, research may find a second decline in weight noted after age eighty.

THE ROLE OF GENETICS

Genetic factors influencing weight occur through metabolic processes that affect body composition. Body composition is the relative amounts of lean mass, composed of more dense tissues such as bones and muscles, to fat mass, composed of less dense tissue or energy fat stores. The more dense the tissue present, the greater the weight of the person. Males have a higher level of the hormone testosterone, which result in denser bones, more muscle mass, larger organs, and less body fat. Their average weights are higher beginning at puberty and continuing throughout life. Females have higher levels of estrogen, a hormone that supports pregnancy, so they have relatively more body fat in addition to the smaller lean mass and thus lower average weights. This gender variation is about 10 pounds throughout life.

Some genetic variations exist among racial groups that also create similar differences for the sexes. African Americans tend to have more dense bones and a slightly higher percent of body fat. Mexican Americans, Pacific Islanders, and American Indians tend to have a higher percent of body fat, whereas Asian Americans generally have a lower percent body fat.

The genetics of aging and its effect on weight revolves around the control of metabolism and how nutrients are absorbed and digested. Metabolism is the sum of all the chemical events that occur in a living organism. The relationship to aging and weight is how the fuel that runs the body is stored and utilized. How quickly fuel is used is the metabolic rate. An analogy is gasoline consumption in a car, measured in miles per gallon. It is not unusual for consumption to decrease as a car gets older and is less efficient. Aging causes fuel to be used less efficiently, demonstrated by a drop in the metabolic rate. If calories taken in exceed what is needed by the body, then the excess is stored as body fat. If a person does not decrease caloric intake in conjunction with the decrease in metabolic rate, the result will be increased fat weight. Because of the concomitant decrease in lean tissue, the change in body composition might not affect body weight for a time, but it appears that at least in the United States, body fat is increasing at a faster rate than lean mass is decreasing, as demonstrated by the increase in obesity across the life span.

THE ROLE OF ENVIRONMENT

Several environmental factors can affect body weight, but probably the most influential is access to healthy food. In the elderly, low income is often associated with poor nutrition, especially in urban regions where food costs tend to be higher even for staples. When there are financial struggles, it is often likely that living situations are unfavorable as well. Regardless of age, lack of access to healthy food can cause unhealthy weight gain and weight loss. If an individual has a low income, oftentimes the neighborhood they live in isn't very safe to walk around or have adequate public transportation. It may also be possible that there is a food dessert, where access to grocery stores with fresh fruits and vegetables are not readily available. However, in at least one study of disease progression, the Baltimore Longitudinal Study on Aging found that the greater the body weight, the longer time until death during chronic illnesses. This would suggest that a slight excess of body fat may be protective in the elderly compared to being underweight. Elderly individuals whom become underweight are often facing many other factors that impact their health and ability to eat normally. This can put them at more risk of disease and illnesses.

Adequate protein intake is essential to maintaining lean mass. Often the most common protein food source, meat, is also the most expensive item on the grocery list. If the elderly person has not been educated of cheaper alternatives of protein such as eggs, vegetables, beans, lentils, nuts, or dairy products, the tendency is simply not to buy meat. Protein is not only important in building muscle and maintaining overall health, but it also helps satiate the person longer. Without protein they may be more likely to consume more carbohydrates or fats and can cause an increase in body weight. Conversely, this may also cause individuals to become malnourished and lose weight if are neither consuming enough protein or supplemental food items.

Unfortunately, lack of adequate protein affects not only lean mass, but also overall health. Many of the essential parts of the immune system are made of proteins as well as the enzymes that help in cellular function. Lack of both reduces the ability to adapt to environmental stressors and is one of the main reasons the elderly, especially those that are underweight and malnourished, to succumb to a viral disease such as pneumonia when a younger person would not.

Another environmental factor relates to the weather and temperature. There is a tendency for everyone, not only the elderly, to put on fat weight during the winter. Subcutaneous body fat helps insulate and regulate body temperature, so repeated exposure to cold causes an increase in body fat stores for more efficient regulation. In many people, it is probably not so much the temperature directly—the microclimate can be managed with clothing and shelter—but the tendency to be less active in inclement weather. If the calories eaten are not used for activity, they are stored as fat. There may also be a relationship to the economic issue: More financially stable retirees might move to a warmer climate or travel to one for the winter; if they remain, they can afford to join a health club to exercise. Any of these factors could mitigate the weather problem associated with weight.

THE ROLE OF LIFESTYLE

There may be a strong association between lifestyle and economics, but some lifestyle choices can be made independent of finances. As with genetics and environment, lifestyle can affect weight in either direction. Education probably has the greatest effect on lifestyle. For a person to make the choices necessary to optimize health, he or she needs to have been given the information necessary to make educated decisions.

Diseases that result from lifestyle choices became the largest cause of deaths in the early twentieth century. In the latter half of the century, researchers began to look more closely at the various factors that can affect health including weight. Obesity is a major modifiable risk factor that increases the risk of cardiovascular disease, diabetes, high blood pressure, hypertension, and high cholesterol. Together these diseases are termed metabolic syndrome, but not everyone whom is obese will have these complications or necessarily all four diseases. Despite this finding, the obesity rate in the American population continued to increase, especially in the 1990s. Research suggests that mortality and morbidity generally both decrease when weight, or more specifically fat, is kept within normal ranges. It is important to remember that it also depends where the fat is distributed in the body. It is more worrisome to have fat around the liver and the heart than the hip and thigh.

Maintaining a healthy weight or losing weight all come with a delicate balance of lifestyle choices that comprise of physical activity and healthy diet. The Center for Disease Control and Prevention (CDC) provides some guidelines and information for maintaining a healthy weight. It is important to have at least 150 minutes a week of moderate-intense aerobic activity, which include walking briskly, biking casually, light yard work, or actively playing with children. It is also important to have 75 minutes in the same week of vigorous-intensity aerobic activity, which include activities that make you breathe too hard and fast to have a conversation. For example, these include: running, jogging, jump roping, skiing, swimming laps, and most competitive sports (soccer, basketball, or football). Activity, both aerobic and strength training (such as weightlifting) have been shown to affect body composition and, in turn, health in all age groups. Studies of both men and women in their sixties, seventies, eighties, and even nineties have demonstrated similar effects across all age groups. Cardiovascular exercise can promote weight loss through decreasing body fat. Strength exercises can promote the body to build more muscle mass and stronger bones to, which promotes a faster metabolism and better body health. A healthy diet does not have to necessarily be expensive, but it does require mindfulness of what is going inside your body. It is important to limit caloric intake from items with added sugars, saturated fats, and high sodium. Instead eating a variety of calorically dense food across all food groups in the recommended amounts.

SUMMARY

It is clear that weight varies both throughout life as well as between individuals. When considering the effect of weight in older individuals, it seems safe to say that maintaining an ideal weight throughout life is optimum, and problems can arise with being either underweight or overweight. Genetics cannot be changed, so manipulating lifestyle and/or the environment is necessary to obtain this goal.

—*Wendy E. S. Repovich*
Updated by Shirley Kuan, RN

See also: Cancer; Exercise and fitness; Fat deposition; Malnutrition; Nutrition; Obesity; Thyroid disorders

For Further Information

Gaddey, Heidi L., and Kathryn Holder. "Unintentional Weight Loss in Older Adults." *American Family Physician*, vol. 89, no. 9, 1 May 2014, pp. 718-22. www.ncbi.nlm.nih.gov/pubmed/24784334. Discusses possible causes, evaluation and diagnosis, and treatment of unintentional weight loss in older adults.

Gill, Lydia E., et al. "Weight Management in Older Adults." *Current Obesity Reports*, vol. 4, no. 3, 2015, pp. 379-88. doi:10.1007/s13679-015-0161-z. This overview highlights the challenges and implications of measuring adiposity in older adults, the dangers and benefits of weight loss in this population, and provides an overview of the new Medicare Obesity Benefit.

Kritchevsky, Stephen B. "Taking Obesity in Older Adults Seriously." *The Journals of Gerontology: Series A*, vol. 73, no. 1, 2017, pp. 57-58. doi:10.1093/gerona/glx228. A review of the Haywood Paper, which presents the results of a randomized trial comparing exercise with dietary advice, exercise with a mildly hypocaloric diet, and exercise with a very low-calorie diet.

Nordqvist, Joseph. "Metabolically Healthy Obesity: All You Need to Know." Medical News Today, MediLexicon International, 18 Apr. 2017. www.medicalnewstoday.com/articles/265405.php. Discusses the basics of metabolically healthy obesity and calls for the need of more criteria to help define the condition.

Stenholm, Sari, et al. "Patterns of Weight Gain in Middle-Aged and Older US Adults, 1992-2010." *Epidemiology*, vol. 26, no. 2, 2015, pp. 165-68. doi:10.1097/ede.0000000000000228. Examines longitudinal changes in BMI in initially underweight, normal-weight, overweight, and obese U.S. men and women using individual-level repeat data from the Health and Retirement Study.

U.S. Department of Health and Human Services and U.S. Department of Agriculture. *2015-2020 Dietary Guidelines for Americans*. 8th ed. U.S. Department of Health and Human Services and U.S. Department of Agriculture, Dec. 2015.

WHEELCHAIR USE

Relevant Issues: Culture, health and medicine, recreation

Significance: The huge number of people in the United States who are of senior citizen status makes it likely that hundreds of thousands of elderly Americans will be using wheelchairs during the first decades of the twenty-first century. This pervasive wheelchair use will contribute to changes in cultural attitudes, building construction, and social environments.

In the year 2000, more Americans were over fifty than there were children enrolled in public school classes. In the United States, someone turned fifty-five years old about every eight seconds. These statistics leads one to believe that the American population as a whole is growing older very quickly. While many Americans spend their old age without the aid of mobility assistance, many others require the use of walkers and wheelchairs to move from place to place.

Disability is something that impacts everyone at all ages. It is especially common in older adults, women, and minorities. According to the CDC, one in four adults in the United States have some type of disability. It also affects two in five adults whom are 65 years or older. Disabilities, in general, still carry a stigma of being helpless or disease in the society. However, people living with disabilities are just like everyone else at all ages and can live a healthy life. Being healthy overall means the same for everyone, where they want to lead full lives, stay active, and be a part of a community. The type of disability we will be focusing on is mobility issues, where the disabled individual has immense difficulty walking or climbing stairs.

As the population grows older, there will be a definite higher demand for mobility-assistive devices such as wheelchairs. There are many types of wheelchairs that range from manual powered chairs that require pushing or rolling, electrically powered, standing chairs, scooters, and positioning wheelchairs. Motorized chairs are now available at relatively low prices. These chairs are truly liberating because they make it possible for the occupant to operate the vehicle without an aide. Motorized wheelchairs have baskets that can be attached so the occupant can move belongings from one place to another or can shop for many items at a grocery or department store. Various accessories, such as cup holders and shopping bags, are available for attachment to both motorized and manually operated chairs, making the use of the chair both more comfortable and more convenient. There are also many options of wheelchairs made with different types of material, and it is important for the wheelchair user to find the best fit for their lifestyle. Wheelchairs can be a costly investment that not everyone can afford. There are some organizations that provides wheelchairs for those in need such as the American Wheelchair Mission. Adults whom are 65 years and older can check with their primary care provider to see if they are qualified for a wheelchair provided by Medicare Plan B.

For someone who has mobility issues and cannot walk for short distances or get out of a chair, a wheelchair provides the user a sense of liberation and freedom. It allows them to re-engage in society by leaving their home and also re-gain some independence. Yet, there are still barriers that disabled individuals face in every day as a result of societal neglect. For example, some communities may not have adequate ramps or curb ramps for wheelchair users. Some businesses may not have convenient or enough accessibility entrances, which make it more difficult for wheelchair users to navigate around.

On the other hand, many businesses have worked towards increasing accessibility by providing motorized wheelchairs for the use by the disabled of all ages. They are often provided by large corporations such as Walmart, Target, BJs, or Costco. As the number of elderly who need wheelchairs to shop and conduct other business increases, so will the number of businesses that provide these chairs. A business that had one chair available in 1999 may find that in 2010, it must have two or three chairs available. Increasingly, such businesses will have to think about establishing rules and regulations relative to the use of motorized wheelchairs. For both businesses and individuals, there may be insurance issues related to the use of such chairs.

As more elderly people use wheelchairs, there will be modifications in home and building construction as well as employment of more people to assist wheelchair users. These modifications will include such things as lower curbs on showers and lower kitchen counters and range tops. Places of business will have to increase the space allocated for loading and unloading chairs so that several wheelchairs can be unloaded to sit side by side. As more elderly people use wheelchairs, the widths of wheelchair ramps and paths may have to be increased to at least 5 feet so that chairs moving in opposite directions can pass each other. Airports, restaurants, hotels, and motels are likely to employ more people who are trained to assist disabled elderly customers in wheelchairs.

—Annita Marie Ward
Updated by Shirley Kuan, RN

See also: Americans with Disabilities Act; Canes and walkers; Disabilities; Mobility problems

For Further Information

"Disability and Health Healthy Living." CDC, Centers for Disease Control and Prevention, 9 Aug. 2018. www.cdc.gov/ncbddd/disabilityandhealth/healthyliving.html. Discusses measures for disabled older adults to take to increase their quality of life.

"Disability Stigma and Your Patients." *Disability Stigma and Your Patients | Rehabilitation Research and Training Center on Aging with Physical Disabilities.* agerrtc.washington.edu/info/factsheets/stigma. Tips for caregivers on navigating around the stigmas and stereotypes of disability.

American Wheelchair Mission. amwheelchair.org/. The American Wheelchair Mission is a non-profit organization with a goal to deliver brand new, free wheelchairs and mobility aids to physically disabled children, teens and adults throughout the world who are without mobility or the means to acquire a wheelchair.

"Types of Wheelchairs—A Visual Tour." United Spinal Association, 15 Jan. 2019. www.unitedspinal.org/disability-products-services/types-of-wheelchairs/. Provides information, including images, on different kinds of wheelchairs.

WHEN I AM AN OLD WOMAN I SHALL WEAR PURPLE (BOOK)

Editor: Sandra Martz
Date: Published in 1987; 1991
Relevant Issues: Culture, family, friendship, play, psychology
Significance: This collection of prose and poetry deals with women's adjustments to and perceptions of the aging process.

When I Am an Old Woman I Shall Wear Purple is an anthology of well-written prose and poetry, by women and men, about women and their adjustments to and reflections on aging. The title of the book comes from the first line of a poem, *Warning*, by the Englishwoman Jenny Joseph (1932-2018). Her selection, like many of those included, reveals the emotional confidence of a woman who looks forward to using the opportunities of aging to appreciate the fullness of both the past and the present times of her life.

The majority of the authors are American, representing the high quality of writing on aging being done throughout the country. Brief biographies of each author are included at the end of the book. Selections are short to permit the widest variety of themes and writing styles. Representative themes include the influence of physical appearance on perceptions of aging ("The skin loosens; everything moves nearer the ground"), decision making in old age, mother-daughter relationships, caregiving ("I now mother my mother"), memories in time, women's roles, and cultivating aging. Many lines are likely to echo in the mind: "I watch my aging face...become yours"; "Memorizing the seasons, I touch things as if my fingers will learn them"; "Lipstick ran all over her face like a map of Chicago"; "I just sit and try to blend into the walls"; "...tending time more fragile than youth."

Women's attitudes toward the aging process have been associated traditionally with both their chronological age and the role in which they find themselves. The selections reflect the finely tuned individuality of the women described and their acute sensitivity to ordinary details from everyday experiences. The book and its signature poem have come to be associated with the popular Red Hat Society founded by Sue Ellen Cooper. As of 2019, it appears in at least 15 published formats.

—*Enid J. Portnoy*
Updated by Nancy A. Piotrowski, PhD

See also: Aging: Biological, psychological, and sociocultural perspectives; Aging process; Beauty; Caregiving; Cultural views of aging; Family relationships; Friendships; Social ties; Women and aging

WHITE HOUSE CONFERENCE ON AGING

Date: Every ten years; conferences held January 1961; November/December 1971; November/ December 1981; May 1995; December 2005; and July 2015

Relevant Issues: Law, sociology

Significance: The White House Conference on Aging is a national political and advocacy forum that addresses the issues of aging in the United States; decisions about policies and programs for older people are made from conference recommendations.

The White House Conference on Aging (WHCoA) is a political mechanism that allows for public participation in the development of national policies for older persons in the United States. In 1958, the U.S. Congress enacted legislation requesting the first WHCoA. This legislation was in response to three successful national aging conferences that were sponsored by the Federal Security Agency in 1950, 1952, and 1956. It was Congress's intention that a WHCoA be held every ten years.

Representatives, or delegates, from each state attend the WHCoA. These delegates are appointed by either the governor of each state or Congress members. Delegates represent the concerns of their geographical area at the WHCoA.

The WHCoA provides the opportunity to highlight the needs and interests of older persons and makes recommendations about what actions, programs, and services would meet those identified needs. Each WHCoA features preliminary meetings with older persons, professionals, private citizens, and state and local political leaders. These preliminary meetings are used to advance issues for the conference. Each conference forms a set of concrete conference recommendations. Follow-up procedures are developed to monitor progress on the recommendations.

Congress authorized the first conference to occur in 1961 during the final days of President Dwight D. Eisenhower's administration. The main focus of this conference was the medical problems of the elderly and how to finance medical costs. The work accomplished at this conference contributed to the enactment of Medicare, Medicaid, and the Older Americans Act of 1965.

The second WHCoA, which was held in 1971 during Richard M. Nixon's administration, recommended the development of a wide range of services for the elderly. It supported the establishment of a network of federal, state, and local planning and advocacy agencies, including the National Institute on Aging (NIA) and the House Select Committee on Aging. Delegates advocated for an expansion of programs under the Older Americans Act and the development of the Supplemental Security Income program.

The third WHCoA occurred in 1981 at the beginning of Ronald Reagan's administration. This conference recommended increases in government services for older Americans, including the maintenance of current Social Security benefits and the expansion of health insurance benefits for the elderly, which led to the Social Security Reform Amendments of 1983. It was influential in recommending amendments to the Older Americans Act and in supporting an emphasis on Alzheimer's disease research by the NIA.

Bill Clinton's administration hosted the fourth WHCoA in 1995. The focus of this conference was on economic security, health, and social wellbeing. Major recommendations from this conference included preservation of the Older Americans Act, Social Security, Medicaid, and Medicare. Delegates advocated for housing options, as well as health and social service programs that provide elders with a continuum of care.

The main agenda of the 2005 conference was to find solutions on how to accommodate 73 million baby boomers as they move into older age. By 2030, the number of adults over 65 years of age is expected to reach 19 percent of the population. A major focus of the conference was how to modernize aging policies to bring them into a twenty-first century system of coordinated services and networks to meet the future needs of baby boomers.

The themes of the 2015 conference were retirement security, long-term services, healthy aging, and putting an end to financial exploitation, neglect, and abuse. The Administration updated the conference to include "watch parties," where organizations like the American Association of Retired Persons (AARP) and the Diverse Elders Coalition, among others, could watch the conference remotely. The Administration launched Aging.gov, a one-stop resource for older adults and their families and caregivers.

—*Colleen Galambos*

See also: Advocacy; Housing; National Institute on Aging; Medicare; Older Americans Act of 1965; Social Security

WHY SURVIVE? BEING OLD IN AMERICA (BOOK)

Author: Robert N. Butler
Date: Published in 1975
Relevant Issues: Culture, sociology, values
Significance: Butler, who invented the term "ageism" to refer to the prejudicial stereotypes Americans assign to old people, wrote this book to show that the stereotypes are untrue and to reveal the extent of the neglect of the elderly.

As medical advances have steadily increased the life span of Americans, the aging population has grown, and their problems have increased. Among these problems are a growing number of misconceptions about the elderly, including the idea that most are infirm and live in rest homes, hospitals, or with their children; that they are emotionally disengaged and bored with life; that senility is inevitable and pervasive; and that they are unproductive and resistant to change. The elderly are often considered a burden to society and are shunted into retirement communities and nursing homes, where they are ignored and neglected.

In 1975, Robert N. Butler published *Why Survive? Being Old in America* to show the public that old people are not all the same and that many of them are not helpless; some even want to work. As a psychiatrist, he has confronted all the cultural problems of aging in his own patients. He maintains the view that most of the old can continue to make decisions regarding their lives, including the decision to let someone else decide matters for them. In great part, the problems of the aging are reparable if more social support systems are created to help people take care of themselves. The aged can remain in their own homes, for example, if help could come on a regular basis to perform chores that an infirm person cannot perform for themselves and to remind them to do things they might otherwise forget. This recourse is economically sound compared with consigning them to a nursing home.

Another theme of Butler's book is an examination of the economic reasons for the poverty of so many of the old. Pension plans may disappear during a person's lifetime if a business fails or business policy changes. The Social Security system provides inadequate support:

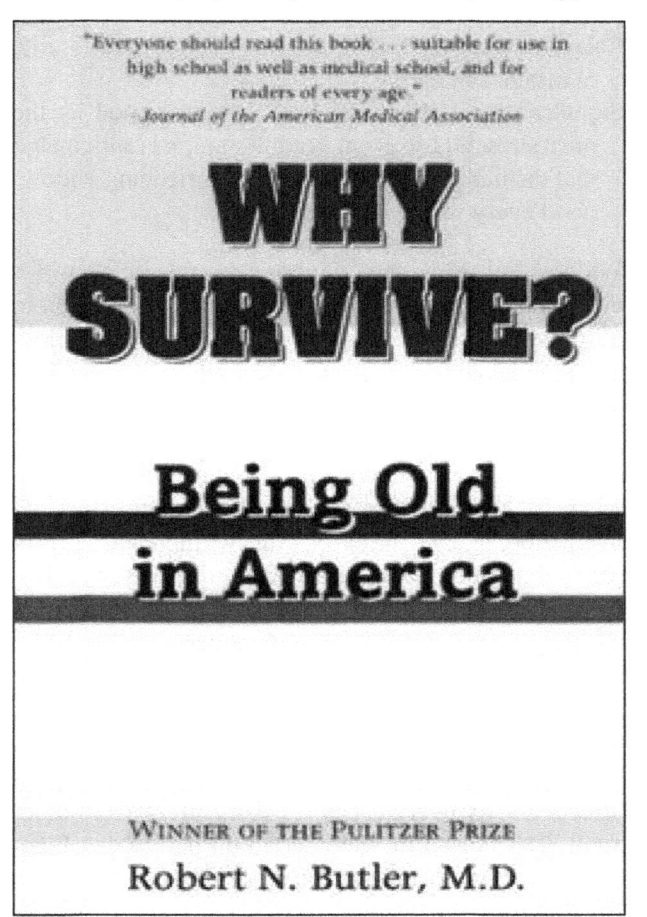

Payments have not increased at the same rate as inflation. Inflation reduces lifetime savings and investments below the expected standard of living for which the saver planned. In such circumstances, people often become destitute.

Butler's final point is that the issues he discusses belong to American culture as a whole and not just to the aged. Everyone lives side by side with those who are currently experiencing life as aged citizens, and everyone will eventually face these problems as they, too, age. As Butler predicted when he wrote the book in 1975, these problems have only worsened and become chronic with the passing of time.

—*Ann Stewart Balakier*

See also: Ageism; Poverty

WIDOWS AND WIDOWERS

Relevant Issues: Demographics, economics, family, marriage and dating

Significance: Widowhood has been identified as the most stressful life event in adulthood; it is anticipated that the number of older adults experiencing widowhood every year will increase.

Widowhood is a common, very stressful life event for older adults, particularly women; yet in comparison to loss of a spouse at a younger age, widowhood in older adulthood is considered a more "normal" life transition. Most older women are widows by age seventy and, as they do not tend to remarry, may experience two decades or more of widowhood. Men tend to remain widowers for a much shorter period of time because they are much more likely to remarry, often within the first eighteen months after the spouse's death. The impact of widowhood, particularly in the short term, is significant and multidimensional, regardless of gender.

THE IMPACT OF WIDOWHOOD

Widowhood has physical, emotional, social, and economic impacts on the spouse, regardless of gender, and affects almost every aspect of daily life for the older adult. The impact of widowhood on day-to-day functioning is particularly significant when it occurs in later life because that is the time when other physical, functional, and cognitive impairments are most likely to be experienced. The process of grieving the loss of a spouse is uniquely different for each individual and is influenced by a variety of factors, such as age at the time of the loss, length of the marriage, quality of the marriage, physical health status, socioeconomic status, and cultural mores and norms. However, some common adaptations are experienced, and some fundamental tasks must be accomplished.

The process of grief and mourning takes place over a period of one to three years rather than the six months that society has widely come to expect. In comparison to younger widows and widowers, older adults have been found to demonstrate a more prolonged grief reaction, extending beyond the "traditional" six-month grieving process. Additionally, older adults often experience other losses during the bereavement process, such as loss of a friend or even loss of personal health, which may further complicate the grieving process.

Resolution of grief includes acceptance of the loss and willingness to begin the transition to a different life without the deceased spouse. This may be particularly difficult for middle-aged or older adults, who are more likely to be in long-term marriages, which tend to be associated with a higher level of interdependence. As couples age together and experience the narrowing of support networks that often occurs, they tend to more exclusively meet each other's needs without the help of others.

Physical reactions to grief—such as gastrointestinal disturbances, shortness of breath, difficulty sleeping, and loss of energy—are common immediately after a death and generally diminish over time. When the loss of a spouse occurs during older age, the physical responses to grief may be worsened or exacerbated by preexisting or latent disease processes, and grief may exacerbate or precipitate an underlying disease pathology. During the grief process, the bereaved commonly experience vacillating emotional responses, including disbelief, numbness, anxiety, relief, guilt, and profound sorrow. Depression frequently occurs and, along with other symptoms, is found to lessen over time. Widowhood increases social isolation for both men and women, and loneliness is identified as a major problem by both widows and widowers, especially the aged.

The death of a spouse requires the development of a new social identity and social role: that of the widow or widower. Race and ethnicity compound the problem. Women in particular, especially if they were highly dependent upon their spouse, frequently encounter a drop-in status, both socially and economically. Middle-aged and young-old women often drop out of their familiar circle of social activities with married friends and experience both social and emotional loneliness. In contrast, women who are older when widowed are more likely to be able to join the ranks of friends who are also widows and to benefit from that support network. Men who become widowers are often the most isolated because they are less likely than women to have established close friendships and because they tend to grieve more in isolation. Widowed older men often encounter more difficulties in day-to-day functioning because they have relied heavily on their wives, particularly in domestic areas, and may have difficulty completing such basic tasks as cooking and washing clothes.

Older widows are more likely to suffer negative economic consequences, particularly if they were economically dependent on their husbands' earnings or were unfamiliar with the household finances. Often, the widow does not qualify for Social Security, there are inadequate or no pension benefits, and any insurance benefits are quickly exhausted. This situation is worsened if the woman had been caring for an ill husband for a long period of time before death.

ADJUSTMENT TO WIDOWHOOD

Despite the highly stressful nature of bereavement and the pain experienced during grieving, older adults usually cope quite well with the loss of a spouse. The experience of widowhood is often not entirely negative, and positive life transitions can even occur. For example, a woman who had been in a stable and successful marriage but who had been highly dependent upon her husband may, while grieving the loss of her spouse, achieve a sense of satisfaction and accomplishment from her new level of independence. Alternately, a spouse from a long-term but unhappy marriage may experience contentment for the first time, despite being alone and sometimes lonely. A husband or wife who has spent many years caring for a sick spouse may experience both a sense of relief and a sense of freedom, alternating with a sense of guilt, particularly early in the bereavement process, when those burdens are lifted. A widower may become active in a support group and gain new friendships and emotional experiences. Many younger widows continue in or return to work; this option is not available to women who are widowed at an older age, however. Women tend to be less interested in marrying again and are much less likely to remarry than are men; in contrast, more than one-half of widowed men will remarry.

Some factors that have been found to facilitate adjustment to widowhood include the quality of social support (including family and friends), the individual's ability to cope with stress, religion, health, and economic stability. Quality of relationships with family and friends is more important than quantity, and diversity of support networks is very important. Women are more likely than men to have had strong friendship relationships prior to widowhood, and these are often strengthened after the spouse's death. Friendships often provide more meaningful support than children in terms of reducing loneliness and providing recreational activities. Yet family relationships are extremely important, and children provide meaningful, tangible, and varied types of assistance. Men may have more difficulty maintaining family relationships than women and are less likely to have a confidant. Widows and widowers prefer to continue living away from their children as long as possible.

Past experience and abilities in coping with life stressors are important in coping with loss of a spouse. In general, individuals who have had prior major losses and have coped with them successfully are better able to adapt positively to widowhood. Some examples of positive coping strategies used by widows and widowers include staying busy, maintaining a regular routine, using distraction, expressing emotion, and owning pets. Religion is often important in coping during bereavement. Faith enhances coping in a variety of ways, including facilitating acceptance, offering support, promising continued relationship with the deceased, and combating loneliness.

The health status of the surviving spouse is an important contributor to adjustment to bereavement. Individuals with poor health are more likely to suffer worsening health status and additional health problems during the bereavement period. Health problems can often exacerbate or even trigger financial hardship in the bereaved person. Older widows are more likely to suffer from financial difficulties, and employment is generally not a reasonable option.

WAYS TO FACILITATE ADJUSTMENT TO WIDOWHOOD
Although most bereaved older adults cope successfully with the loss of their spouse, some experience a more intense, protracted, or "pathological" grief response and may benefit from professional assistance. Extensive feedback from widowed people themselves has generally demonstrated, however, that the bereaved benefit most from mutual help or support from other widowed people or peers. Numerous studies have shown that widows participating in these programs adapt quickly and positively. One of the first peer programs, the Widow-to-Widow Program, was developed by Phyllis Silverman. This program has been replicated numerous times throughout the United States, Canada, and Western Europe. AARP offers more than two hundred local programs for older widows and widowers. Numerous other mutual help programs also exist and are commonplace in collaboration with hospice organizations and funeral services.

—*Cynthia A. Padula*

See also: Death and dying; Depression; Grief; Loneliness; Marriage; Men and aging; Poverty; Religion; Relocation; Remarriage; Stress and coping skills; Women and aging

For Further Information
Filomena, Joann. *Widowed: Moving through the Pain of Widowhood to Find Meaning and Purpose in Your Life Again.* Morgan James Publishing in Partnership with Difference P, 2017. Filomena speaks widow to widow, having walked the path herself after the sudden loss of her husband.
Florian, Amy. "A Camp for Widows and Widowers Is Surprisingly Uplifting." Next Avenue, *Forbes*, 3 May 2017. www.forbes.com/sites/nextavenue/2017/05/03/a-camp-for-widows-and-widowers-is-surprisingly-uplifting/#93e890147953. Florian describes her positive experience at Camp Widow in Tampa, San Diego, and Toronto.
Holm, Anne Lise, et al. "Factors That Influence the Health of Older Widows and Widowers—A Systematic Review of Quantitative Research." *Nursing Open*, vol. 6, no. 2, 2019, pp. 591-611. doi:10.1002/nop2.243. A literature review to identify factors that influence the health of older widows and widowers.
Silverman, Phyllis. *Widow-to-Widow*. 2nd ed. Brunner-Routledge, 2004. Silverman provides an overview of the bereavement process, reports on the findings of the landmark Widow-to-Widow project, and illustrates how the program was of benefit to widows.
Stahl, Sarah T., and Richard Schulz. "The Effect of Widowhood on Husbands' and Wives' Physical Activity: The Cardiovascular Health Study." *Journal of Behavioral Medicine*, vol. 37, no. 4, 2013, pp. 806-17. doi:10.1007/s10865-013-9532-7. This prospective study examined the effect of widowhood on physical activity by comparing widowed elders to health status-, age-, and sex-matched married controls.
Wolfelt, Alan. *When Your Soulmate Dies: A Guide through Heroic Mourning*. Companion, 2016. In this compassionate guide by one of the world's most beloved grief counselors, readers will find empathetic affirmation and advice intermingled with real-life stories from other halved soulmates.

WILD STRAWBERRIES (FILM)

Director: Ingmar Bergman
Cast: Victor Sjöström, Bibi Andersson, Ingrid Thulin
Date: Released in 1957 as Smultronstället, released in the United States in 1959
Relevant Issues: Death, family, psychology, work
Significance: Bergman's most honored film is a meditative analysis of an old scientist's quest to come to terms with the inhumanity and lovelessness of his past life.

Like William Shakespeare's King Lear, Ingmar Bergman's *Wild Strawberries* is a study of an old man's need to discover painful truths about himself. Lear makes these discoveries through heart-wrenching sufferings leading to madness; Isak Borg (Victor Sjöström), the professor emeritus of medicine at the center of Bergman's film, finds out about his profound human failings through a succession of events and dreams during a trip to Lund, Sweden, where he is to receive an honorary degree. Borg, a bacteriologist and teacher, has sacrificed his humanity to his scientific work, leaving him an emotionally arid and spiritually adrift old man.

The film's story, which occurs during a single summer's day, focuses on the car trip that Borg makes to attend the ceremony with his daughter-in-law Marianne

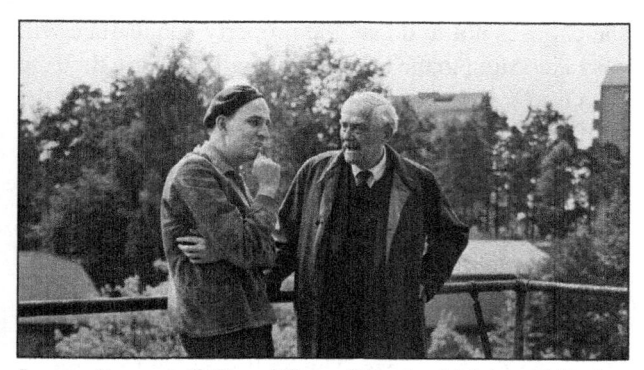

Ingmar Bergman (left) and Victor Sjöström (right) in 1957, during production of Wild Strawberries in the studios in Solna, Poland. (via Wikimedia Commons)

(Ingrid Thulin), who sees through his charming facade to his egocentric core. By the way Borg interacts with Marianne, his mother, and some hitchhikers, he is indeed revealed as cold-natured and authoritarian, and his dreams reveal him as fearful of death but also afraid of life. For example, he dreams of his former sweetheart Sara (Bibi Andersson) as she picks wild strawberries (Bergman's symbol for the fleeting happiness of youth), but she prefers his passionate brother to him, whom she regards as egotistical and aloof.

After these and other incidents in dream and reality, Borg emerges chastened by his confrontations with these repressed memories and hidden truths about himself. He receives his honorary degree, treats his son and daughter-in-law with a newly minted compassion, and retires to his bed, where he has another set of dreams. He again sees Sara, who takes him to an idyllic country setting where he waves to his young parents, whom he can now view with forgiveness and love. He has finally found a fulfilling meaning for his life, because he has been transformed into a human being with a growing awareness of the importance of emotional warmth and generosity.

—*Robert J. Paradowski*

See also: *King Lear*; Maturity; Old age

WILLS AND BEQUESTS

Relevant Issues: Death, family, law
Significance: A will is a legally enforceable document defining in writing how a person wishes his or her property distributed after death; bequests are specific gifts provided for by will.

A will takes effect on death and is revocable at the discretion of the maker, called a testator (testatrix, if female) during his or her lifetime. The validity and execution of a will requires certain legal formalities and may vary from one state to another according to state law. People who die without a will are said to die intestate, and their property will be distributed according to state intestacy laws under the state statute of descent and distribution. This scheme may be contrary to decedents' wishes.

People must have testamentary capacity in order to execute a will. That is, they must be adults (of legal age), mentally competent (of sound mind), and aware of the nature and extent of property owned and the natural "objects of their bounty" (recipients of property). They must also realize the implications and consequences of what they are doing.

TYPES OF WILLS

The "simple" will is the most widely utilized method of directing the administration and disposition of assets. It names an executor (executrix, if female) or personal representative to carry out the directions in the will. The executor may have special powers to sell property and settle claims. If one dies intestate, the probate court (also called orphan's court or surrogate's court) must appoint an administrator (administratrix, if female) to complete the same tasks as an executor.

Additionally, that person may have to post a security bond. In the United States, a will drawn up in one state will be good in another. If the testator dies owning property in more than one state, however, the will must be probated in more than one state. This second or ancillary administration requires proof of proper certification in the state of domicile. Generally, it is the laws of the state of domicile (where the testator has his or her primary residence) that govern probate of an estate.

While the formalities required in the execution of a will vary slightly from state to state, the most striking difference lies in the requirement of the witnesses. All wills must be signed by the testator, generally at the end of the document. Most states require that testators "publish" their wills (declaring it to be their will and the means by which they are directing disposition of their property) before witnesses who also sign the will. The purpose of witnesses is to establish that the will was voluntarily signed by the testator. Witnesses should be disinterested parties, not beneficiaries under the will. Some states, such as Pennsylvania, do not require wills to be witnessed. The practice, however, is advisable.

Certain property does not pass under a will: jointly held property; life insurance payable to a named beneficiary; trust property; retirement plans, including individual retirement accounts (IRAs), Keough accounts, and pensions; Totten trusts or pay-on-death bank accounts payable to a named beneficiary; deeds in which decedent held only a life estate with property going to a named beneficiary after death; and gifts in contemplation of death.

Statutory wills are available in California, Maine, Michigan, New Mexico, and Wisconsin. Created by state law, these are forms available in stationery stores that can be completed and witnessed. They are limited and cannot be changed, but they can be modified by adding codicils and specific bequests.

A joint will is a contract between two people requiring the consent of each to modify. Provisions generally state that each spouse's property will pass to the other and then specify what will happen to the property when the second person dies. In cases of simultaneous death, the heirs of the survivor even by one second will inherit the property of the other. Because this may have unintended consequences, the parties can specify by will who is to be the survivor. Property will pass accordingly. Divorce or annulment will revoke the entire will or at least those provisions in favor of the former spouse.

A testator may also place conditions on bequests received under a will, such as that the person receiving the bequest perform certain conditions in order to inherit. It is also permissible for a testator to disinherit anyone except a spouse. Under state law, a spouse is entitled to a portion of the estate even if the other spouse dies and makes no provision for the surviving spouse or conveys less than a certain percentage of decedent's assets. In that case, the surviving spouse can "take against the will" or choose to accept an amount allowed by law (usually one-third or one-half of the estate) instead of the amount bequeathed in the will. The surviving spouse is not required to take against the will. If he or she chooses not to do so, the property bequeathed will pass according to the terms of the will. This is called the "elective" or "forced share" provision. Revisions of the Uniform Probate Code have adopted a sliding scale for widows or widowers who take against the will: the longer the marriage, the higher the elective share.

A holographic will is a document entirely in decedent's handwriting, signed and dated. If executed with testamentary intent, it can be considered a valid, enforceable will. A nuncupative will is an oral will used by sailors on the high seas. This will is upheld if circumstances show that at the time of the oral will the decedent believed death to be imminent. A "pour-over" will accompanies a living (inter vivos) trust, stating in effect that any property not in trust will pass into the trust (pour over to it) through probate administration and the distribution provisions in a will. Living wills are not wills at all, but rather a signed and witnessed advance directive stating that, in the event of a catastrophic illness, the person does not wish to be kept alive by artificial means or heroic measures. Living wills can also specify which therapies the person does or does not wish to undergo in a terminal situation. All states recognize living wills.

PROBATE

The probate process consists of "proving" the decedent's last will (proper signature, validity, and the fact that it is the last will). This is also the court that deals with disputes concerning transfer of the property of decedents and claims against their estates. If the will is determined to be valid, the estate will be distributed according to the terms of the will. If it is invalid or if the decedent dies intestate, the estate will be distributed according to the state intestacy statute. If the original will is lost or destroyed, a certified copy is submitted to the court. The executor named in the will must petition (request) the court to probate the will. Notice of the petition is given to the decedent's heirs and other interested parties; some states require "publication" or placing a legal notice in a local newspaper listing death of the decedent, the name of the executor, and a date by which to object to the petition. From one to three months after appointment, the executor must file with the court an inventory of the estate's assets, including stocks, bonds, real estate, and jewelry owned by decedent at time of the death. Assets are not distributed until debts, fees, expenses, and federal and state taxes have been paid and accepted. "Small" estates are not required to file a federal tax return. Allowable amounts have been increased gradually through revisions in the tax code. State law governs amounts payable for state inheritance tax. When tax returns are accepted, the executor receives a "closing letter" stating that no further taxes are due in the estate.

After debts and expenses are paid and taxes are settled, the executor may prepare to distribute amounts remaining to beneficiaries according to the terms of the will. Beneficiaries must sign a release signifying acceptance of the distribution and releasing the executor from future claims. The executor must then file a final accounting with the court detailing all transactions made on behalf of the estate. When accepted by the court, the estate is closed, and the executor dismissed. The executor's fee is paid according to a sliding scale based on the size of the estate. The rate is fixed under state law.

CODICILS, REVOCATION, AND RULE OF ADEMPTION

A codicil is an addition or amendment to a preexisting will and must incorporate the preexisting will by reference. Otherwise, it may be considered a new will. The codicil must conform to the same requirements and formalities of the will. Codicils can also correct a deficiency or error in the original document.

Will revocation is necessary when the testator's intent changes with respect to the distribution of assets at death. When a new will is executed, all earlier wills are revoked and invalid. Even if a new will is not executed, the testator can revoke the old will by physically destroying it or doing some act with the intention of revoking the will. Marriage after the will is made revokes the will unless it was made in anticipation of marriage. A previously revoked will can also be revived if it was based on a material mistake. Divorce generally does not revoke a valid will. It does, however, revoke bequests to the former spouse or appointment of the former spouse as executor of the estate.

If a testator mentions a specific bequest of property in the will but disposes of the property during his or her lifetime, it will not be in the estate at death. The bequest, therefore, is said to be "adeemed," and the beneficiary gets nothing, regardless of the circumstances surrounding the disposal of the property. The subject of the bequest must exist and be owned by the testator at the time of death. Where the form of the bequest is altered, ademption also occurs because the property cannot be restored to its former state (for example, where wool is woven into cloth or cloth is made into a garment). If the original property is adeemed but a similar property exists at the time of death, the law presumes that the testator restored the adeemed property, and the bequest will be honored. The rule of ademption applies only to specific bequests or legacies other than money. Where a group of items is involved (a collection of objects), the bequest could be adeemed totally or partially if some of the articles are not part of the testator's estate.

ABATEMENT, LAPSE, AND INTESTACY

When the testator's estate does not contain sufficient assets to pay debts, expenses, and bequests in full, bequests are "abated," or reduced, according to certain rules unless the will specifies otherwise. The first to be reduced is the residuary bequest ("the rest, remainder, or residue of my estate"); some use personal property to pay costs before the sale of real estate, while others treat real estate and personal property alike for abatement purposes. Bequests will be abated proportionately.

Because a will "speaks at death," property cannot be transferred by will until the testator dies. An intended beneficiary under a will might predecease testator. If so, the intended gift to that person "lapses." In anticipation of this situation, the will can provide an alternate beneficiary. If lapse occurs and the state has an "anti-lapse" statute, a gift by substitution might occur, and a deceased beneficiary's children can accept the gift.

The scheme of distribution for a person who dies intestate (without a will) is generally the same in all states, although differences may occur under various state laws. If there are spouse and children, the estate passes one-half to the surviving spouse and one-half to the children. If a child is deceased but has offspring, the deceased child's share passes to his children. If there is a spouse but no children or grandchildren, one-half goes to spouse and one-half goes to blood relatives in the following order: parents, brothers and sisters, grandparents, aunts, uncles, cousins. If there are children or grandchildren but no spouse, the children will divide the entire estate equally. If one is deceased, his or her share passes to his or her children. Stepchildren are not considered next of kin, but children born after the decedent's death will inherit just as if they had been born during the decedent's lifetime. Adopted and natural children are treated the same for inheritance purposes. If no blood relatives survive the decedent, the estate will pass to the state of his or her principal residence at the time of death (escheat). Intestate succession may defeat the intent of the decedent and result in inheritance by certain unintended family members.

WILL SUBSTITUTES

An inter vivos, or living, trust is often called a will substitute because settlors or grantors (the person creating the trust document) can be their own primary beneficiaries and can also pass property to beneficiaries at their death. Inter vivos trusts can be structured so that settlors retain the right to change or terminate the trust during their lifetime and control the use of their property. Inter vivo trusts do not require probate. At the settlor's death, the property is immediately available for the use and benefit of the settlor's beneficiaries. Property held jointly with right of survivorship also does not require probate. During their lifetimes, each joint tenant owns an equal share of the property. At the death of the first tenant, the survivor retains his or her own interest and gets the interest of the decedent automatically by operation of law.

—*Marcia J. Weiss*

For Further Information

American Bar Association. *The ABA Guide to Wills and Estates*. 3rd ed. Random House, 2009. Written in plain language with practical situations and problems that most people are likely to encounter.

Lynn, Robert J. *An Introduction to Estate Planning*. 7th ed. West, 2019. Lynn's book is for lawyers and students with basic knowledge of property law.

Maple, Stephen M. *The Complete Idiot's Guide to Wills and Estates*. 4th ed. Alpha Books, 2009. Written in a humorous manner with charts and cartoons, this book contains helpful and easily understood information.

WISDOM

Relevant Issues: Culture, psychology, religion, values

Significance: Wisdom, the capacity to give meaning to one's experience, plays an important role for the elderly as they are challenged to consolidate a sense of meaning with which to face the future, the deaths of loved ones, and their own deaths. Wisdom is epitomized by sound action or decisions based on the application of good judgment, knowledge, and experience.

Erik Erikson proposed a series of eight stages through which all individuals pass during their life span. Each stage represents a particular challenge that must be met for the individual to adequately manage the demands of the specific period in development. The successful completion of each stage is accomplished through achieving a balance between two opposing forces.

The infant must balance a sense of trust and a sense of mistrust, the very young child must contend with the forces of autonomy and doubt, and the school-age child is faced with balancing initiative and guilt. The preadolescent is charged with coming to terms with the competing forces of industry and inferiority; the adolescent must contend with the pull of identity and identity diffusion; the young adult must find a way to navigate the draw of isolation and intimacy; and the middle-age person is challenged with balancing generativity and stagnation. The development task of old age, according to Erikson, is defined by the need to contend with forces of integrity and despair.

Successful completion of each stage not only readies the individual for the next stage but also produces, through the integration of opposing forces, a more adaptive approach toward life. Infants who pass successfully through the first stage of development are invested with an underlying sense of hope; toddlers are ideally equipped with a basic sense of their own will; and school-age children who have successfully balanced the opposing forces of industry and inferiority can face adolescence with a sense of competence. Adolescents who have successfully met the demands of their development stage are left with a sense of fidelity to certain values. Young adults who have found a way to manage the opposing pull of isolation and intimacy develop the capacity to love in a mature way. Middle-aged adults who have successfully integrated the desire to be productive and the pull of self-involvement are imbued with a fundamental sense of purpose. Successful completion of life's final stage requires coming to terms with feelings of despair and integrity. The integration of these two opposing forces in old age, according to Erikson, produces wisdom.

The culminating accomplishment of human development in this model of the life span is, therefore, wisdom. The achievement of wisdom, in the view of Erikson, requires not only the completion of a single, final developmental stage but also the reworking of all seven previous stages. The various physiological changes, which mark a general and often dramatic decline in physical and sometimes cognitive functioning, require the elderly to renegotiate all of life's developmental challenges, from the dialectic of trust-mistrust to the opposition of generativity-stagnation. In addition to this, the elderly are faced with accepting the imminence of their own deaths. Wisdom is thus a backward- and forward-looking developmental accomplishment entrusting the aged with a sense of meaning that situates them in the perspective of their own lives and the lives of others past, present, and future. As Erikson writes:

"The elderly are challenged to draw on a life cycle that is far more nearly completed than yet to be lived, to consolidate a sense of wisdom with which to live out the future, to place him-or herself in perspective among those generations now living, and to accept his or her place in an infinite historical progression. Applying wisdom gained from a life of trial, error, reflection and understanding is a gainful and rewarding end of life activity."

WISDOM, ACTIVE INVOLVEMENT, AND DISENGAGEMENT

Wisdom, as the culminating achievement of the life span, imparts upon the individual a capacity to live productively with the tension of integrity and despair. Wisdom also serves to allow the aged a way of managing the competing forces of active involvement and disengagement. As with all the earlier stages of development, individuals must invest themselves fully in the particular developmental challenge before them if they are to move forward. However, the aged are faced with the seemingly paradoxical task of actively involving themselves with life while at the same time disengaging from it. This happens because the waning physiological capacities of the aged make active involvement less possible and because the reality of death demands that they prepare for a future of total disengagement. "Wisdom," writes Erikson, is "truly involved disinvolvement."

The disengagement that wisdom makes possible in old age does not represent a form of apathy or nihilism. Instead, it involves the recognition that one's capacity to control the world, as well as one's ability to comprehend it, are fundamentally limited. Adaptation throughout life requires an acceptance of the potentialities and the limitations inherent in one's position along the developmental continuum. The elderly are faced with the task of accepting a greater level of reliance and dependence upon others while at the same time valuing their capacity to contribute greatly to their family and society at large. Wisdom imparts upon the elderly a dual awareness of how much is known and how much is still unknown and even unknowable. The wise share while the aspiring learn.

WISDOM AND RELIGION

Life span studies of the aged have found a uniform tendency among the elderly toward an increased appreciation of the importance of spirituality and religion. One theme that arises when speaking to seniors, irrespective of denominational affiliation, is the emphasis that they place on the importance of religious practice and faith for the next generation. In fact, even those in the older population who classify themselves as nonreligious often stress the value of spiritual and religious involvement for the world at large. Knowledge is gained, wisdom develops. Study, investigation, observation, and research leads to knowledge. The able wise use gained knowledge to discern applicable information in a right and lasting manner.

Among the classical Greeks, wisdom was understood to be the type of knowledge needed to discern the good and live the good life. It is a belief in the connection between wisdom and the good life, both for the society and for the individual, which appears to underlie the value that the elderly place upon religion. Psychologists have long appreciated the way in which religion functions as an adaptive force capable of reconnecting human fragmentation and providing the individual with a sense of wholeness and meaning. Religion also serves to restrain problematic drives and impulses. In facing the inevitability of death, religion may be seen by the aging as a confirmation of hope, a conservation of values, and a source of comfort.

The functional and adaptive role of spirituality and wisdom in the context of death and dying has been well researched by life span theorists. The concept of eternity has been found to be particularly salient to many older adults. Belief in an afterlife provides both the dying and those that survive them a shared frame of reference with which to give meaning to death. Loss of additional time on Earth is seen as being compensated for by the promise of life everlasting. Similarly, the deterioration in quality of life experienced by the dying appears less unfair when juxtaposed with the higher quality of existence in the life to come. Religion thus supplies the elderly and those who care for them with a sense that the limitations and suffering associated with death and dying are merely a prelude to a less restricted state of being.

Beyond its capacity to comfort the elderly as they approach their physical end, wisdom has traditionally provided the aged with a sense of importance and recognition as the bearers of tradition and culture. Religion has also served to strengthen bonds linking the elderly with those who will survive them. The intergenerational transmission of wisdom functions to preserve the "mind" of culture in the same way that the transmission of rituals, art forms, cuisine, and dress ensures the conservation of a culture's "body." By passing on wisdom, the elderly act as the linchpin of cultural continuity. In doing so, they may experience a sense of immortality, of transcending their own death through their generative contribution to future generations. Awareness of both the privilege and the profound responsibility inherent in this critical cultural role may lead the elderly to reevaluate their own constructions of wisdom. Erikson, in discussing the final task of the life cycle, writes:

"For perhaps the first time, the elder is a member of the omega generation, the oldest living generation in his or her family. There are no living elders to whom to look for guidance through the next stage. Members of the omega generation must be guided by ideological heroes and by their own wisdom and memories, as they themselves serve as guides for the generations that follow. It's a big responsibility and the thoughtful learn while the wise speak."

Although theorists have increasingly recognized the psychologically adaptive quality of religion, it should be noted that wisdom and spirituality are not identical or even necessarily congruent. The compensatory quality of religion, its capacity to provide hope and comfort in the face of suffering, renders it highly vulnerable to manipulation by those interested in the marginalization or exploitation of the elderly. Unscrupulous religious organizations have been known to prey upon the intense spiritual longings of the aged and the terminally ill. Religion may be used to divert older adults away from active participation in communal political institutions and causes. Spiritual veneration for the sagacity and wisdom of the elderly may go hand in hand with the removal of their decision-making power. Idealization of the moral and spiritual greatness of the aged can be used to deflect attention away from their need for social and economic resources.

CULMINATION OF A LIFE STORY

Some life span theorists consider the need to see one's life as a continuously evolving story bound together by a sense of connection, purpose, and direction to be a central and vital psychological need throughout development. However, it is believed that the impetus to draw together the events of a life history into a coherent whole has particular importance and salience for the aged. This perspective suggests that the fundamental tension of old age is not defined by the opposing forces of integrity and despair but is instead characterized by the dialectic of continuity and discontinuity. Wisdom, in this view, represents the threads of meaning and knowledge that weave together the various themes and events of a person's life into the tapestry of a narrative.

D. P. McAdams has argued that, from late adolescence, men and women in modern societies attempt to build a meaningful and coherent narrative of the self to provide them with a sense of direction and purpose. What seems to distinguish the creation of life stories in later life from narrative building during earlier stages of development is that older adults devote more space in their stories for generative and transcendent concerns. Unlike adolescents and younger adults who spend much of their time and energy accruing and developing "internalized" skills, talents, and knowledge, older adults tend to devote more of their life stories to "externalized" practices through which they invest their resources in wider, societal projects, causes, and movements.

During older adulthood, or mature adulthood, individuals tend to manifest their desire for generativity in the form of concrete assistance, whether this is accomplished through working within the existing power structure or by attempting to alter it. The elderly, because of their withdrawal from the public domain, tend to express their generative concerns less concretely. As the aged find themselves increasingly removed from participation in professional and political arenas, their life stories often begin to revolve around the passing on of knowledge and wisdom. Wisdom may, therefore, be understood as the final generative resource for the elderly as they find themselves concerned about the next generation but largely unable to act on this concern. In this way, wisdom helps the aged to continue to write a life story in which the need to maintain a prosocial identity is threatened by the loss of numerous capacities.

Recent efforts have looked more closely at the neurobiology of wisdom, involving imaging studies of activity between the limbic system of the brain and the prefrontal cortex of the brain. Neuroimaging and neurotransmitter studies have been correlated to wisdom characteristics including decision making/life knowledge, prosocial behaviors/attitudes, self-understanding, emotional balance, value insight, and effective management of uncertainty. Augmenting study of a primarily psychological and social entity like wisdom with biological inquiry and scientific measurement presents many challenges, but clinical investigators are approaching the problem. Neuroimaging combined with neurotransmitter analysis promises to better delineate biologic qualities of wisdom attainment and expression.

Study continues on the social and psychological aspects of wisdom development. The importance of society and social environments is explored in studies to better delineate ways effective social transactions generate a wise population. Difficult life events and their impact on wisdom development can be considered in an overall view related to the development of wisdom in society.

If wisdom helps to maintain a generative life narrative in the face of physical deterioration and societal marginalization, it also serves to make less painful the acceptance of death. That is, wisdom appears to be a basic ingredient both in lending vitality and purpose to the final chapter of a generative life story and in accepting the finality of life's end. Erikson proposed that the acceptance of death is only possible with the acquisition of wisdom. Wisdom makes possible this acceptance because it acknowledges the way in which one's own experience has been shaped by the intersection of an individual life cycle with cultural and political processes. Wisdom thus allows for an understanding of one's own life story as deeply embedded in a broader historical narrative and, in doing so, purportedly reduces the sting of death. As the final and culminating theme of a life story, wisdom makes possible what Erikson has characterized as a "post-narcissistic love of the human ego—not of the self—as an experience that conveys some world order and spiritual sense, no matter how dearly paid for."

—*Samuel Liebman and Steven Abell*
Updated by Richard P. Capriccioso, MD

See also: Creativity; Cultural views of aging; Death and dying; Erikson, Erik H.; Maturity; Mentoring; Middle age; Old age; Religion; Successful aging

For Further Information

Erikson, Erik H., Joan M. Erikson, and Helen Q. Kivnick. *Vital Involvement in Old Age.* W. W. Norton, 1986. Based upon the interviews of twenty-nine octogenarians, this book examines the final stage of Erikson's stage theory. Continual emphasis is given to the value of vital involvement throughout each stage of development, including the last one.

Handbook of the Psychology of Aging, 8th ed., edited by K Warner Schaie and Sherry Willis. Academic P, 2016. A basic reference source covering many behavioral aging processes and behavioral science perspectives on aging.

Igarashi, Heidi et al. "The Development of Wisdom: A Social Ecological Approach." *The Journals of Gerontology: Series B*, vol. 73, no 8, Nov. 2018, pp. 1,350-58. doi:10.1093/geronb/gby002. A consideration of the impact of society and environment on the development of wisdom.

Leland, John. "Wisdom of the Aged." *The New York Times*, 25 Dec. 2015. Six New Yorkers 85 years old or older are followed for a year with their reflections on life: sadness, happiness, and minimizing anger or worry.

Meeks T.W., and D. V. Jeste. "Neurobiology of Wisdom: A Literature Overview." *Arch. Gen. Psychiatry.* 2009, vol. 66, no. 4, pp. 355-65. doi:10.1001/archgenpsychiatry.

2009.8 A review of neurobiology studies related to the characteristics of wisdom.

Samuel, Lawrence R. "Are Older People Wiser?" *Psychology Today*, Aug. 2017. www.psychologytoday.com/us/blog/boomers-30/201708/are-older-people-wiser. A discussion related to wisdom as a form of compensation for an aging body.

Swarthmore College. "New Study Confirms Adage That with Age Comes Wisdom." *ScienceDaily*, 8 Aug. 2016. www.sciencedaily.com/releases/2016/08/160808163910.htm.

WOMAN'S TALE, A (FILM)

Director: Paul Cox

Cast: Sheila Florance, Gosia Dobrowolska, Norman Kaye, Chris Haywood

Date: Released in 1991

Relevant Issues: Death, family, health and medicine, media

Significance: This haunting Australian film depicts a woman's efforts to celebrate life despite her failing health and to live her last days fully.

In *A Woman's Tale*, seventy-two-year old Martha (Sheila Florance) lives alone in a walk-up apartment with her cat, canary, and mementos of a full life. The film follows her daily routine as she interacts with her home-care nurse, son, friends, and neighbors. She is dying of cancer but tries to live every day to the fullest.

Martha is visited daily by Anna (Gosia Dobrowolska), the young home-care nurse. They have developed a close, affectionate relationship. Martha loves life and romance. She supports Anna's affair with a married man by making her bedroom available for their lovemaking. When Anna reports that Martha's friend Billy (Norman Kaye), who is also Anna's patient, tried to fondle her breast, Martha suggests, "Why didn't you let him? He'll be dead soon. What's the difference?"

Billy provides a contrasting perspective on life and death. Whereas Martha celebrates the present and enjoys life, Billy lives in the past and slowly dies. His daughter is too busy to visit him. Martha helps him with toileting and other basics. In the end, Anna finds him alone in the darkness, dead in his chair.

Martha's son Jonathan (Chris Haywood) worries and checks up on her. The parent-child roles have reversed. When Martha is hospitalized after a fall and told that she has only one month to live, Jonathan tries to put her in a nursing home. She fights, with Anna's help, to return to her own home and maximize the quality of her last days of life. In the end, she tells Anna, "Life is so beautiful...."

Sheila Florance won the Australian Film Institute's Best Actress award for her portrayal of Martha. She died of cancer soon afterward.

—*John W. Engel*

See also: Cancer; Death and dying; Facility and institutional care; Family relationships; Friendship; Home services; Hospice; Sexuality; Women and aging

WOMEN AND AGING

Relevant Issues: Biology, culture, demographics, health and medicine, psychology, sociology, values

Significance: The rapid increase in the number of elderly persons in the United States, with women greatly outnumbering men, raises many social and economic issues that need to be addressed.

The unprecedented growth of the elderly as a proportion of the populations of all industrialized countries has political, economic, and social ramifications that require serious attention. The dimensions of the problem in the United States can be grasped by comparing statistics from the beginning of the twentieth century with those at its close and in current times.

In 1900, an informal social structure existed to care for the small number of elderly requiring care. In a generally rural economy, the elderly tended to be integrated into all aspects of family and social life and usually lived with relatives. Three million U.S. citizens, less than 4 percent of the population, were more than sixty-five years old; 44 percent were nineteen years of age or younger. The average life expectancy for women was about forty-eight years, or until about the time of the menopause. The lower life expectancy was largely a result of the high incidence of deaths in infancy and early adulthood; a woman who survived her childbearing years had a good chance of living into her sixties and beyond. Nevertheless, many women died in childbirth or from its complications, and so it was less common in the first decade of the twentieth century for women to live to see their grandchildren reach adulthood.

By contrast, the 1990 U.S. Census showed the following breakdown of older Americans: 18,218,481 persons sixty-five to seventy-four years of age, of whom 10,225,733 (about 56 percent) were women; and 12,976,794 persons seventy-five years and older, of whom 8,455,474 (about 65 percent) were women. Thus, more than 31 million persons were sixty-five years of age or older, or one-eighth the total U.S. population of 248.7 million; nearly 60 percent were female. Women also constituted 80 percent of the elderly living alone in the United States at that time, It was estimated that the aging of the so-called baby-boom generation (the result of the large number of births during and just after World War II) to create "senior boomers" early in the twenty-first century would result in one in five Americans being over the age of sixty-five. Furthermore, as a group, the oldest elderly, those over eighty-five years of age, was growing at six times the rate of the rest of the U.S. population. There has been a demographically significant rise in the median age: In 1970, it was twenty-eight years but in 2017, the median age was 38.1 years. According to Census Bureau predictions in 1986, by the middle of the twenty-first century, those nineteen years of age or younger will make up 23 percent of the population, and those over the age of sixty-five will constitute 22 percent, resulting from a decline in birthrates and a reduction in death rates. The ratio of retired persons to workers, was 1 to 5 in 1986.The worker to beneficiary ratio in the social security program was 1 to 2.9 in 2010 and is expected to reach 1 to 2.4 in 2030.

The proportion of elderly relatives to younger family members has increased. The cohort (a group of people who were born at about the same time and can be expected to share many common experiences) of frail elderly in the late twentieth century came of age around the time of the Great Depression and, as a group, typically had small families. In addition, there is a low birthrate of generations succeeding the elderly cohort in the 1990s, resulting in a high dependency rate, which is projected to continue climbing. The proportion of family caregivers to recipients had changed from 3:1 in 1910 to 1.2:1 by 1973. By 2010, about 39.8 million people, or 16.6 percent of the United States population, became caregivers to persons over 18 years old, averaging up to 20 hours of care per week.

SOCIAL ISSUES
Aging can be viewed from many perspectives: chronological, biological, psychological, and social. Old age as a category is partly a function of the relative age of the surrounding population and the vitality of the persons categorized as older. What was considered to be late middle age at the end of the twentieth century would have been considered elderly in primitive societies. Even in the 1970s, gerontologists typically referred to those fifty-five to seventy-five years old as the "young-old" and those over seventy-five as the "old-old". By the 1980s, in recognition of the growth of the elderly population, some gerontologists began using the term "young-old" to refer to those sixty-five to seventy-four years old, labeling persons seventy-five to eighty-five years old as the "old-old" and those over eighty-five as the "oldest-old."

The elderly, however defined, have been accorded different levels of status in different societies, ranging from reverence to hostility and abandonment. It appears that the status of a group advances and declines in a society as the ratio between the costs of maintaining it and the benefits it can provide changes. In societies in which the elderly control many resources or are seen as possessing special wisdom, their status is higher. However, even in societies in which the elderly are revered, aging women often are at a disadvantage because they seldom control a large number of resources. When a woman's value is based on physical attractiveness or the ability to bear and care for children, the end of youth and reproductive ability leaves her with little power. In the late twentieth century, activities open to the elderly, especially in work and community leadership, were limited in industrial societies.

In rural societies—even rural communities in industrialized nations—older citizens tend to be more integrated into the life of the community than in urbanized areas. *The Aging Experience: Diversity and Commonality Across Cultures* (1994), by Jennie Keith et al., provides a fascinating study of the different experiences of the aged and of how they are viewed by others in seven towns on four continents. The authors assert that "the attributes of social and cultural settings were not simply contexts that affected aging; they were part of the very meaning of age itself." For example, in the small town of Clifden, on the rugged, isolated west coast of Ireland, few people identified one another by relative age; rather, they noted traits such as the fact that a man was unable to shop without help or that a woman was being cared for by a niece.

As more women reach old age and continue to slip into poverty, several issues arise. Although the vast majority of elderly persons remain in the community and generally are cared for by family members when ill or infirm, about 70 percent of the residents of nursing homes are women, often with no living relatives. Several demographic trends related to this issue are expected to complicate it further, primarily the trend toward later childbearing and smaller families in the baby-boom generation, combined with the longer life expectancy of the same cohort. Another troubling demographic trend is the increase of childless women, which will result in an increasing number of isolated elderly women needing formal (that is, government-funded) help.

The picture for women is clouded by the fact that women, generally wives and daughters or daughters-in-law, have historically been expected to be the caregivers for elderly family members. Despite the increased participation of women in the workforce, this expectation seems stubbornly resistant to change. Women make up about 75 percent of the primary caregivers. In 1986, more than 60 percent of primary caregivers of the elderly were the wives of disabled, often-older husbands; 73 percent of these caregivers were over sixty-five years of age. At the same time, the average age of all such caregivers in the United States was fifty-seven years; more than 30 percent rated their health as fair or poor, and approximately 30 percent were classified as low income. As the population ages, the average age of these primary caregivers is likely to increase also, with the result that the oldest-old will increasingly be cared for by the merely elderly. Some women who have children in their thirties or later find themselves caring for toddlers and aging parents at the same time. Some women in their fifties and sixties must simultaneously cope with frail elderly parents and economically dependent adult children, creating the "sandwich generation."

A related issue of growing concern in the United States is the problem of elder abuse. The National Council on Aging (NCOA) provides sobering facts on elder abuse such as one in 10 Americans over the age of 60 has faced some form of elder abuse that equates to about 5 million older adults. Typically a family member, abusers are both women and men, In 2010, the Elder Justice Act was passed to protect seniors in some residential care settings from abuse, neglect, or exploitation. Staff are trained on reporting requirements if they suspect crimes against the elderly.

In most European countries, as well as Canada, old age pensions and medical care throughout life, not merely in old age, are considered to be appropriate functions of government. However, in the United States such social supports are reserved for the unemployed poor and the elderly. These services have institutionalized age and made the aged a class apart. Being marginalized, the elderly are thought of as a separate and distinct category of people. Critics of the U.S. system believe that treating the elderly as a distinct, homogeneous, dependent group creates a welfare program that increases isolation, dependency, and state control. When certain roles are restricted to certain ages, these age norms result in the increasing loss of roles the older one gets. Because senior citizens lack role models, they often try to maintain the standards of behavior and activity they had in middle age, hindering not only their socialization to old age but also that of society.

One sociological model used to describe the lowered status of elderly people posits that the decline in status results from a confluence of several factors. First, advances in health technology have resulted in longer lives, causing intergenerational competition for jobs. Retirement was developed to force the older generation to move aside. A second factor, the greater use of advanced technology in jobs, contributes to obsolescence of the skills of elderly people. The third factor—urbanization—caused younger family members to leave farms and rural areas for the greater opportunities of cities, which has led to generational isolation. Finally, literacy and mass education for the young meant that they had higher educational and professional status than did their elders in most cases. In the late twentieth century, elderly women were generally less educated, had less mastery of high-tech skills, and yet lived longer than men, adding an even greater degree of marginalization to their lives.

The experience of the elderly in the United States has been shaped by forces specific to the expansive nature of American society. The historical emphasis on individualism and independence and the advertising-driven emphasis on money, beauty, and sex appeal as important components of social success have created a society in which youth and vitality are prized more highly than age and wisdom. The cosmetic industry, pharmaceutical companies, and the medical specialty of cosmetic surgery profit from and reinforce the message that age will be honored mainly to the extent that one can achieve it without appearing to have been affected by it. Although men are not exempt from these appeals to vanity, the main targets and consumers of such products and services are women.

A society's social, political, and economic conditions affect how social issues, including aging, are treated and viewed. Unfortunately, many in society view the elderly as their least-able members. The variable and fluctuating nature of federal, state, and local governmental programs for the elderly have left many unmet needs. To fill these gaps, a vast web of private interests has grown up, often referred to as the "aging enterprise." Components of the aging enterprise include residential and health-care facilities, including nursing homes, insurance providers that specialize in policies that cover the gap in health-care payments left by Medicare, and manufacturers of products targeted toward the elderly. The aging enterprise has created a bureaucracy that further marginalizes the elderly to maintain the jobs and status of the members of the bureaucracy.

The United States pays a significantly higher percentage of its income maintenance programs to the elderly than do other countries. This does not mean that the U.S. elderly receive more generous old-age pensions than other countries—only that the U.S. government provides little assistance to the nonelderly. Some critics have referred to the United States as a Social Security welfare state. Because programs and policies related to old age support are based on preretirement income and work history, elderly women, the oldest-old, and elderly minorities are at the greatest financial disadvantage.

Pension plans may end benefits to the surviving spouse when the worker dies. A woman who relies on pension income from her husband's job may lose a major portion of her income if she loses her husband. Only limited government assistance is available for persons who cannot qualify for Social Security. All these factors contribute to the low economic status of elderly women as a group.

Retirement as a life stage with distinctive behaviors and expectations is a function of the creation of such social security programs. In earlier times, a person did not experience formal retirement. One farmed, baked, or sewed as long as one was able to do so, often in concert with family members. When frailty or disability precluded full participation in productive activities, one was cared for and supported by members of the extended family. Establishing retirement as a life stage in which certain roles and behaviors are predefined shapes people's ideas of what constitutes well-being. Categorizing seniors as a distinct group lessens the importance of seniority as the basis for prestige and community influence. Another factor is mobility. Younger family members move away from their aging parents, and seniors move away from established communities to be nearer to younger family members. When an elderly person moves to be near a child or other family member, he or she often moves into a community with a smaller elderly population and fewer resources for seniors to replace the social support systems he or she left behind. Research has demonstrated that communities in which residents are on the upper end of the social scale and in which there is a high level of residential mobility correlate with lower status and less social support for the elderly.

A happy marriage has been shown to provide both men and women with life-enhancing benefits of intimacy, interdependence, and a sense of belonging, although studies have shown men to be more satisfied with their marriages and the degree to which their needs are being met than are women. Women are less likely to die shortly after the death of a spouse than are men. However, after the death of a spouse, more than 25 percent of men over sixty-five years of age remarry, compared with less than 5 percent of women in that age group. Couples typically have twenty to forty years together after the last child leaves home, and retirement creates new challenges for both parties. Such long relationships are a new phenomenon. In 1900, the average length of marriage when the first partner died was twenty-eight years. In the 1990s, it had risen to more than forty-three years. Some marriages now last forty-five or more years before the death of a spouse. As more women engage in professional careers, issues of two-person retirement have arisen. Most men over the age of sixty-five are married, for several reasons. Men generally marry younger women, older men are more likely to remarry than are older women, and women have a longer life expectancy than men. Elderly women, conversely, are more likely to live alone. Often women have smaller Social Security checks and less income from private pensions. Women are already living in circumstances more disadvantaged than men and are at greater risk of impoverishment than are men.

HEALTH AND MEDICAL ISSUES

Women suffer more often from acute and chronic medical conditions than do men, although men have higher rates of cancer and heart disease. Despite the larger number of women in the population, women have been severely underrepresented in medical research as well as in studies of diseases in general. Fewer funds are allotted for the study of diseases that are most common in women. Many of the illnesses that most frequently affect women—arthritis, high blood pressure, strokes, diverticulitis, incontinence, and osteoporosis—are less likely to cause death and more likely to cause a woman to be bedridden for some time. In 2015, the leading causes of death in women were heart disease followed by cancer.

In the United States, the system of income maintenance for elderly citizens is newer, less comprehensive, and more bureaucratic than are related systems in European social democracies, partly because of different approaches to health care in different countries. The system in the United States is shaped by the U.S. medical orientation toward high-tech care for curable, acute conditions. Women suffer both from the lack of financial support when they are in the caregiver role and from being more prone to conditions requiring the long-term services of a caregiver.

As technological advances have compensated for physical decline, they have also undermined the social support and personal contact that were common in earlier times and that are more readily available in less advanced societies. The technology that makes aging a more positive experience does not create the true social security of continuing social participation. In the United States, the longer life expectancy brought about by high-tech medical treatments has little payoff for the woman doomed to spend her final years alone in a nursing home. As part of the work that must be done to deal with the aging population, society must ensure that cultural age barriers do not replace physical barriers in the future.

FEMINISM AND AGING

The women's movement in the United States that began in the 1960s often has been criticized for concentrating on the concerns of white, young and middle-aged, middle-class women. Increasingly, the movement is being urged to focus more closely on the needs of elderly women. One regular critic has been Barbara Macdonald, who, in her mid-seventies, wrote "Politics of Aging: I'm Not Your Mother" (Ms., July/August 1990), accusing feminists of seeing older women as mothers who should take care of them. Macdonald argued that ageism is a form of disempowerment for all women and that feminists should deal with it as such. As the movement's early leaders have aged, their concerns, mirroring their own experiences, have turned to issues such as the menopause and older women's health needs. Betty Friedan, generally considered to have ignited the late twentieth century women's movement with The Feminine Mystique (1963), began in her sixties to study aging, which culminated in The Fountain of Age (1993), a well-researched and provocative study of the aging in the late twentieth century.

—Irene Struthers-Rush
Updated by Marylane Wade Koch, MSN, RN

See also: All About Eve; Beauty; Breast cancer; Breast changes and disorders; Cosmetic surgery; Divorce; Dual-income couples; Estrogen replacement therapy; Face lifts; Family relationships; *Fountain of Age, The*; *Golden Girls, The*; In Full Flower: Aging Women, Power, and Sexuality; "Jilting of Granny Weatherall, The"; Kübler-Ross, Elisabeth; Kuhn, Maggie; *Look Me in the Eye: Old Women, Aging, and Ageism*; Marriage; Menopause; *Murder, She Wrote*; Neugarten, Bernice;

No Stone Unturned: The Life and Times of Maggie Kuhn; *Ourselves, Growing Older: A Book for Women over Forty*; Reproductive changes, disabilities, and dysfunctions; Sarton, May; Sexuality; Sheehy, Gail; *Sunset Boulevard*; *Tell Me a Riddle*; *Trip to Bountiful, The*; *When I Am an Old Woman I Shall Wear Purple*; Widows and widowers; *Woman's Tale, A*; "Worn Path, A"

For Further Information

Caregiver Statistics: Demographics. Family Caregiver Alliance, National Center on Caregiving. www.caregiver.org/caregiver-statistics-demographics Extensive demographic information on caregivers from the Family Caregiver Alliance (FCA), whose mission is to improve the quality of life for family caregivers and the people who receive their care.

Friedan, Betty. *The Fountain of Age*. Simon & Schuster, 1993/2006. A positive exploration of aging as a natural process, not a disease or pathology. Posits that social institutions and expectations negatively skew attitudes toward the aged, and that new social structures and attitudes can lead to a great improvement in the lives of older persons.

Holstein, Martha B. "On Being an Old Woman in Contemporary Society" American Society on Aging. www.asaging.org/blog/being-old-woman-contemporary-society This writer, speaker, and facilitator of women's groups pens her unique and personal reflections on what it is like to be as an old woman in contemporary society including a discussion of the gender factor which continues to frame women's lives.

Keith, Jennie, et al. *The Aging Experience: Diversity and Commonality Across Cultures*. Thousand Oaks, Calif.: Sage Publications, 1994. Presents results of field studies on aging and attitudes toward aging in Hong Kong; two towns in Botswana, Africa; a rural Irish town and a Dublin suburb; and a Midwestern farming community and an East Coast suburb in the United States. Accessible and informative.

Stibich, Mark. "How Is Aging Different for Men and Women?" *Verywell Health: Healthy Aging*. 5 Oct. 2018. www.verywellhealth.com/is-aging-different-for-men-and-women-2224332. Compares aging with men and women and highlights differences.

"Women, Ageing and Health: A Framework for Action Focus on Gender," World Health Organization. 2007. www.who.int/ageing/publications/Women-ageing-health-lowres.pdf. A 61-page report summarizing "the evidence about women, ageing and health from a gender perspective and provides a framework for developing action plans to improve the health and well-being of ageing women."

WORK. See EMPLOYMENT.

"WORN PATH, A" (SHORT STORY)

Author: Eudora Welty
Date: Published in 1941
Relevant Issues: Family, health and medicine, race and ethnicity, values
Significance: This short story exposes the cultural values and behavior of black and white folk in the rural South as an old black grandmother moves along a familiar path, struggling to adjust to the infirmities of aging.

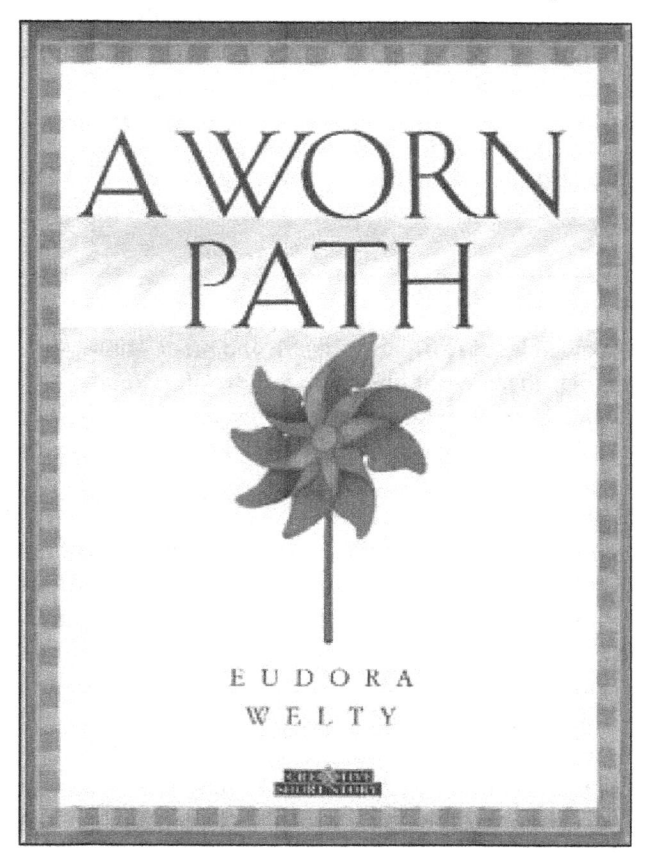

Eudora Welty's short story opens in winter against a sterile landscape that mirrors the fears of the main character, Phoenix Jackson. Phoenix is an impoverished African American grandmother completing a regular walking journey to a distant town to secure medical assistance for a family member. As she moves through wooded areas of the rural South, her vulnerability is exposed along with her fears of becoming dependent on others at this time in her life.

Phoenix represents the frail elderly who must continually readjust to changes in their aging condition. Mental and physical losses offer new challenges for an older person. When aging decreases sensory sharpness, the body cannot be trusted to complete routine tasks successfully. There is a growing need for support from others as well as more time and energy to complete simple activities.

Like the mythical bird that rose from ashes to begin a new life, however, Phoenix manages to find strength within herself to keep going. She finds satisfaction in reaching her destination and regains confidence after finding good fortune along the path.

In old age, each success can bring a renewed sense of well-being to an individual. Through a focus on both small and large accomplishments, the meaning of life is brought into focus as well. As Phoenix faces images of death, she realizes that, like life's journey, progress is made remembering past strengths and moving one step at a time. Phoenix's journey is imbued with a sense of endurance. Its completion becomes a celebration of life along one's aging course.

—*Enid J. Portnoy*

See also: African Americans; Aging process; Cultural views of aging; Death and dying; Old age; Wisdom

WRINKLES

Relevant Issues: Biology, health and medicine
Significance: Wrinkling is directly related to aging, as skin undergoes structural changes over time; the rate of the change can be reduced via dermatological processes.

Key Terms:

calcification: the hardening of tissue or other material by the deposition of or conversion into calcium carbonate or some other insoluble calcium compounds

collagen: the main structural protein found in skin and other connective tissues, widely used in purified form for cosmetic surgical treatments

copper peptides: naturally occurring complexes that have been used for a variety of purposes; the complexes are a combination of the element copper and three amino acids; in the human body, copper peptides are found in trace amounts in blood plasma, saliva, and urine

dermis: the thick layer of living tissue below the epidermis that forms the true skin, containing blood capillaries, nerve endings, sweat glands, hair follicles, and other structures

fibroblast: a cell in connective tissue that produces collagen and other fibers

All human body fibers are formed by specialized cells in the tissues and can be classified as inelastic or elastic. Inelastic fibers are rigid and provide support to the surrounding tissue, while elastic fibers are more malleable. With the passage of time, inelastic fibers tend to become even tougher because of structural changes that occur in collagen, the major protein found in skin, bones, and ligaments. The dermis, the inner layer of the skin, contains large amounts of collagen, which is responsible for the skin's mechanical characteristics, such as strength and texture. The skin cells that make and reproduce damaged collagen are called fibroblasts.

As a person ages, collagen tends to form cross-links between different parts of the molecule or between similar molecules that are near each other, thus creating a rigid nature that provokes skin to sag and wrinkle. Moreover, the recoiling ability of elastic fibers appears reduce, a condition that is often enhanced by calcification. Skin wrinkling is much more pronounced with prolonged exposure to wind and ultraviolet light. This effect appears to be cumulative along with collagen degeneration and epidermis thinning, as seen with people who do outdoor work. Other studies suggest that heavy cigarette smoking contributes to the risk of wrinkling.

Application of collagen-containing creams does not seem to reduce wrinkling because the collagen molecules are too large to penetrate the dermis. Such applications only temporarily cover wrinkles. Injecting collagen under the wrinkles in a way that pushes the groove up, causing it to become smooth, has some positive cosmetic effect but also serious drawbacks. The main problem comes from the animal source of the collagen, which may lead to serious allergic reactions by the immune system and may, in rare cases, trigger a long-lasting autoimmune disease. Moreover, the smoothing effect of the injections appears to be brief because of the inability of the animal collagen to integrate itself into the skin's collagen mesh. Better results are observed when biotechnology-synthesized collagen is used or when the patient's own fibroblasts are removed, grown in a laboratory, and re-injected into the body. The careful administration of vitamin C, collagen amino acids, or very small quantities of copper peptides may stimulate the skin to produce more collagen. In addition, topical application of growth factors and hormones that enhance the collagen-forming process of cells seems to give favorable results.

Chemical peels have been used to correct facial wrinkling in face-lift or eyelid surgeries. A mixture of chemicals is applied to the skin, leading to extreme swelling and consequent peeling of the old skin, thus providing a fresh skin in two weeks. Carbon dioxide lasers were first developed in 1964, but experiments that combined them with computer technology did not begin until the 1990s. This resurfacing technique, which affects an area of skin no more than one hair in thickness for no more than one thousandth of a second, works in a way similar to chemical peel. It is considered best for patients of fair to medium complexion who have good healing qualities and who have not used Accutane in the previous year.

—*Soraya Ghayourmanesh*
Updated by Bruce E. Johansen, PhD

See also: Anti-aging treatments; Beauty; Cosmetic surgery; Face lifts; Skin changes and disorders; Women and aging

For Further Information

Cole, Gary W. "Wrinkles: Facts on Treatments and Cosmetic Procedures." MedicineNet, 23 Oct. 2018. www.medicinenet.com/wrinkles/article.htm#wrinkles_facts. Basic reference article detailing the causes, risk factors, and treatment of wrinkles.

England, Kathryn, and Richard McFarland. *Grandfather's Wrinkles.* Flashlight P. 2007. In this children's book, a grandfather explains to his young granddaughter that his wrinkles are special because he got them from smiling so big on several important occasions. Contains beautiful illustrations of each life event.

Sibilla, Sara, and Maryam Borumand. "Effects of a Nutritional Supplement Containing Collagen Peptides on Skin Elasticity, Hydration and Wrinkles." *Journal of Medical Nutrition and Nutraceuticals*, vol. 4, no. 1, 5 Dec. 2014, pp. 47-53. doi:10.4103/2278-019x.146161. This study shows that the oral nutritional supplement consisting of hydrolyzed collagen, hyaluronic acid, and essential vitamins and minerals, leads to a significant improvement in wrinkle depth. It is also able to induce noticeable improvement in elasticity and hydration of the skin.

Zhang, Shoubing, and Enkui Duan. "Fighting against Skin Aging." *Cell Transplantation*, vol. 27, no. 5, 2018, pp. 729-38. doi:10.1177/0963689717725755. This review summarizes changes in skin aging, research advances of the molecular mechanisms leading to these changes, and the treatment strategies aimed at preventing or reversing skin aging.

YOU'RE ONLY OLD ONCE! (BOOK)

Author: Dr. Seuss (Theodor Seuss Geisel)
Date: Published in 1986
Relevant Issues: Health and medicine, psychology
Significance: In this Dr. Seuss book for "obsolete children," the central character, Everyman, who represents the aging population, presents a delightful defense against aging.

SUMMARY

Everyman has not been feeling his best. He checks into the Golden Years Clinic for a thorough checkup, even though he longs to be in the mountains with fresh air and no doctors. The book follows Everyman through a battery of tests, beginning with an eye test with a chart that reads, "Have you any idea how much money these tests are costing you?" The medical history includes questions about the ailments of parents, grandparents, and cousins. Did they have Bus Driver's Blight or Prune Picker's Plight? Did an uncle collapse from too much alphabet soup, or martinis perhaps?

The scenes are all true to life. The patient is stripped, and his clothes promptly lost. He is subjected to an ear test, an internal organs test, an allergy test, a stress test, and a "pill drill." Between tests, Everyman is seated in the hallway in an embarrassingly inadequate gown with a large back door that keeps flaring open. His companion in the hallway is a fish, Norval, who at first is quite sympathetic but quickly becomes bored with Everyman's tales of woe. Norval has heard them all before.

The doctors' names add charm to the story; Dr. Pollen is the allergy specialist. The nutrition doctor tests Everyman to be sure he gets nothing in his diet that he likes. The pill doctor gives him ten kinds of pills. Most important, the insurance forms must be filled out so Everyman can be billed—well, Everyman or his heirs. At last, Everyman finds his clothes, dresses, and bids Norval good-bye. The final upbeat diagnosis is that Everyman is in pretty good shape for the shape he is in.

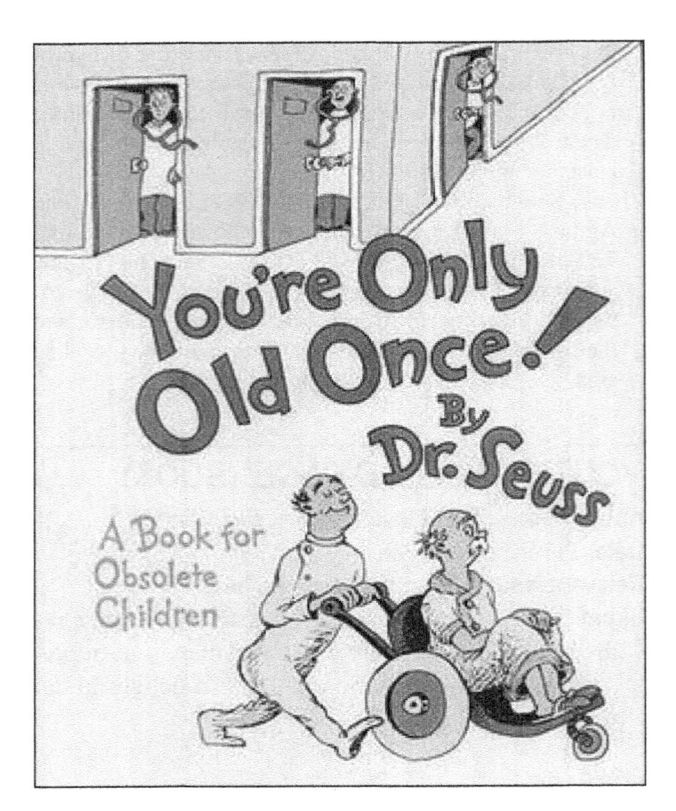

ANALYSIS

As his name suggests, Everyman is an archetype representing the entirety of the aging population. With humor, Seuss deals with serious issues facing older adults. As one gets older, they find themselves surrounded more often by doctors than by nature. Seuss drew on his own experiences of suffering through several illnesses and spending a lot of time in hospital waiting rooms. Readers laugh at the absurdity of the characters and illnesses, but the book stays grounded in real life: older adults must deal with a litany of health tests and screenings, a cornucopia of medications, the constant ping-ponging between a whole host of medical professionals, the high cost of medical services, and especially the excruciatingly long waits between visits. Older adults can feel out of control in these situations, handed over to "experts" who deem them either deficient in some way, or perfectly fine, which can be just as disheartening when one is looking for answers.

You're Only Old Once speaks to the aging population's anxiety over doctors, health tests, and medications. It makes the health-care system look like a conveyor belt, with patients having to navigate the endless waiting rooms and dealing with dispassionate doctors that are all too happy to throw some pills at a problem and call it a day. Everyman must endure these struggles, but Seuss leaves a glimmer of hope, however small, that this system may eventually come to an end. In the imagined future land of Fotta-fa-Zee:

> everybody feels fine
> at a hundred and three
> 'cause the air they breathe
> is potassium-free
> and because they chew nuts
> from the Tutt-a-Tutt Tree.
> This gives strength to their teeth,
> it gives length to their hair,
> and they live without doctors,
> with nary a care.

—Billie M. Taylor

See also: Health care; Health insurance; Humor; Middle age; Old age; Stereotypes

For Further Information

Bahrampour, Tara. "Dr. Seuss's Little-Known Book for Grown-Ups Is Just as Poignant 30 Years Later." *The Washington Post*, WP Company, 27 June 2016. www.washingtonpost.com/news/inspired-life/wp/2016/06/27/seuss/?utm_term= .929137c08c28. An article published on the 30th anniversary of the publication of You're Only Old Once! Bahrompour runs through the major themes found in the book and discusses the real-life experiences of Seuss at the time of writing the book, with input from Seuss' friends.

Levine, Carol. "What Dr. Seuss Saw at the Golden Years Clinic." The Hastings Center, 19 Feb. 2019. www.thehastingscenter. org/dr-seuss-saw-golden-years-clinic/. Discusses the themes of the book and how the medical industrial complex is much the same as it ever was.

Winakur, Jerald. "The Old Man Versus the Medical-Industrial Complex." *Caring for the Ages*, vol. 15, no. 7, July 2014, p. 15. doi:10.1016/j.carage.2014.06.017. Winakur uses "On Breaking One's Neck," by Arnold Relman to discuss the medical industrial complex and how it is deteriorating the patient-doctor relationship.

List of Entries by Category

CULTURAL ISSUES
African Americans
Ageism
Asian Americans
Baby boomers
Beauty
Communication
Cultural views of aging
Epidemiology and population statistics
Grandparenthood
Great-grandparenthood
Jewish services for the elderly
Latinx Americans
Leisure activities
LGBTQ+
Maturity
Men and aging
Middle age
National Asian Pacific Center on Aging
National Caucus and Center on Black Aged
National Hispanic Council on Aging
Native Americans
Old age
Over the hill
Parenthood
Religion
Stereotypes
Veterans
Women and aging

DEATH AND DYING
Acquired immunodeficiency syndrome (AIDS)
Breast cancer
Cancer
Cocoon
Cryonics
Death and dying
Death anxiety
Death of a child
Death of parents
Depression
Durable power of attorney
Estates and inheritance
Euthanasia
Funerals
Grief
Harold and Maude
Heart attacks
Hospice
I Never Sang for My Father
"Jilting of Granny Weatherall, The"
Kübler-Ross, Elisabeth
Last rites
Life expectancy
Living wills
Memento Mori
Palliative care
Pets
Prostate cancer
Psychiatry, geriatric
Remarriage
Robin and Marian
Shootist, The
Stress and coping skills
Strokes
Suicide
Tell Me a Riddle
Terminal illness
Trusts
Widows and widowers
Wills and bequests
Woman's Tale, A

EMPLOYMENT ISSUES
Adult education
Age discrimination
Age Discrimination Act of 1975
Age Discrimination in Employment Act of 1967
Americans with Disabilities Act
Caregiver absenteeism
Dual-income couples
Early retirement
Employment
Executive Order 11141
Johnson v. Mayor and City Council of Baltimore
Mandatory retirement
Massachusetts Board of Retirement v. Murgia
Matlock
Mentoring
Murder, She Wrote

Older Americans Act of 1965
Older Workers Benefit Protection Act
Retired Senior Volunteer Program (RSVP)
Retirement
Retirement planning
Vance v. Bradley
Volunteering

FAMILY ISSUES
Abandonment
Adopted grandparents
Biological clock
Caregiver absenteeism
Caregiving
Childlessness
Children of Aging Parents
Cohabitation
Death and dying
Death of a child
Death of parents
Divorce
Dual-income couples
Elder abuse Empty nest syndrome
Family relationships
Filial responsibility
Friendship
Full nest
Grandparenthood
Great-grandparenthood
Harry and Tonto
I Never Sang for My Father
King Lear
Leisure activities
Long-term Marriage
Neglect
Nursing and convalescent homes
On Golden Pond
Parenthood
Pets
Relocation
Remarriage
Sandwich generation
Sibling relationships
Singlehood
Skipped-generation parenting
Social ties
Tell Me a Riddle
Widows and widowers

FILMS
All About Eve
Best Exotic Marigold Hotel, The
Bucket List, The
Cocoon
Driving Miss Daisy
Grumpy Old Men
Harold and Maude
Harry and Tonto
I Never Sang for My Father
On Golden Pond
Robin and Marian
Shootist, The
Sunset Boulevard
Trip to Bountiful, The
Wild Strawberries
Woman's Tale, A

FINANCIAL ISSUES
Consumer issues
Discounts
Estates and inheritance
401(k) plans
Fraud against the elderly
Health insurance
Home ownership
Income sources
Individual retirement accounts (IRAs)
Life insurance
Pensions
Poverty
Retirement planning
Social Security
Trusts
Wills and bequests

HEALTH ISSUES
Acquired immunodeficiency syndrome (AIDS)
Affordable Care Act
Age spots
Aging process
Alcoholism
Alzheimer's disease
Antiaging treatments
Antioxidants
Arteriosclerosis
Arthritis
Back disorders

Balance disorders
Bone changes and disorders
Brain changes and disorders
Breast cancer
Breast changes and disorders
Bunions
Caloric intake
Cancer
Canes and walkers
Cardiovasclar disease
Cataracts
Cholesterol
Circadian rhythms
Corns and calluses
Cosmetic surgery
Cross-linkage theory of aging
Crowns and bridges
Cysts
Death and dying
Dementia
Dental disorders
Dentures
Depression
Diabetes
Disabilities
Emphysema
Estrogen replacement therapy
Euthanasia
Exercise and fitness
Face lifts
Fallen arches
Fat deposition
Foot disorders
Fractures and broken bones
Free radical theory of aging
Gastrointestinal changes and disorders
Genetics
Geriatrics and gerontology
Glaucoma
Gout
Gray hair
Hair loss and baldness
Hammertoes
Health care
Health insurance
Hearing aids
Hearing loss
Heart attacks

Heart changes and disorders
Hip replacement
Hospice
Hospitalization
Hypertension
Illnesses among older adults
Incontinence
Infertility
Influenza
Injuries among older adults
Kyphosis
Life expectancy
Long-term care
Longevity research
Macular degeneration
Malnutrition
Medicaid
Medicare
Medications
Memory loss
Menopause
Mobility problems
Multiple sclerosis
Nearsightedness
Nutrition
Obesity
Osteoporosis
Overmedication
Parkinson's disease
Pneumonia
Premature aging
Prostate cancer
Prostate enlargement
Reaction time
Reading glasses
Reproductive changes, disabilities, and dysfunctions
Respiratory changes and disorders
Rhinophyma
Sarcopenia
Sexual dysfunction
Skin cancer
Skin changes and disorders
Sleep changes and disturbances
Smoking
Stones
Strokes
Temperature regulation and sensitivity
Terminal illness

Thyroid disorders
Urinary disorders
Vaccines
Varicose veins
Vision changes and disorders
Vitamins and minerals
Weight loss and gain
Wheelchair use
Wrinkles

HOUSING ISSUES
Age discrimination
Empty nest syndrome
Facility and institutional care
Full nest
Home services
Homelessness
Housing
Laguna Woods, California
Long-term care
Home delivered meals program
Pets
Relocation
Retirement communities
Vacations and travel

LAWS AND COURT CASES
Age Discrimination Act of 1975
Age Discrimination in Employment Act of 1967
Americans with Disabilities Act
Darling v. Douglas
Executive Order 11141
Johnson v. Mayor and City Council of Baltimore
Massachusetts Board of Retirement v. Murgia
Older Americans Act of 1965
Older Workers Benefit Protection Act
Vance v. Bradley
White House Conference on Aging

LEGAL ISSUES
Age Discrimination Act of 1975
Age Discrimination in Employment Act of 1967
Americans with Disabilities Act
Durable power of attorney
Estates and inheritance
Fraud against the elderly
Living wills
Older Americans Act of 1965
Older Workers Benefit Protection Act
Trusts
Wills and bequests

LITERATURE
Fiction
Autobiography of Miss Jane Pittman, The
Bless Me, Ultima
"Dr. Heidegger's Experiment"
Driving Miss Daisy
Full Measure: Modern Short Stories About Aging
Gin Game, The
I Never Sang for My Father
"Jilting of Granny Weatherall, The"
King Lear
Memento Mori
Old Man and the Sea, The
On Golden Pond
Picture of Dorian Gray, The
"Roman Fever"
Tell Me a Riddle
When I Am an Old Woman I Shall Wear Purple
"Worn Path, A"
You're Only Old Once!

NONFICTION
Aging Experience: Diversity and Commonality Across Cultures, The
Change: Women, Aging, and the Menopause, The
Enjoy Old Age: A Program of Self-Management
Fountain of Age, The
Growing Old in America
Having Our Say: The Delany Sisters' First One Hundred Years
In Full Flower: Aging Women, Power, and Sexuality
Look Me in the Eye: Old Women, Aging, and Ageism
Measure of My Days, The
No Stone Unturned: The Life and Times of Maggie Kuhn
Ourselves, Growing Older: A Book for Women over Forty
This Chair Rocks: A Manifesto Against Ageism
Virtues of Aging, The
Why Survive? Being Old in America

MEDIA
Ageism
Communication

Social media
Stereotypes

MEN'S ISSUES
Divorce
Dual-income couples
Family relationships
Grumpy Old Men
Harry and Tonto
I Never Sang for My Father
King Lear
Marriage
Matlock
Men and aging
Old Man and the Sea, The
Prostate cancer
Prostate enlargement
Remarriage
Reproductive changes, disabilities, and dysfunctions
Sexual dysfunction
Sexuality
Widows and widowers
Wild Strawberries

ORGANIZATIONS AND PROGRAMS
AARP
Adult Protective Services
Affordable Care Act
Alzheimer's Association
American Society on Aging
Center for the Study of Aging and Human Development
Children of Aging Parents
Gerontological Society of America
Gray Panthers
Jewish services for the elderly
Little Brothers-Friends of the Elderly
Home delivered meals program
Medicaid
Medicare
National Asian Pacific Center on Aging
National Caucus and Center on Black Aged
National Council on the Aging
National Hispanic Council on Aging
National Institute on Aging
Retired and Senior Volunteer Program (RSVP)
Shepherd's Centers
Social Security

PEOPLE
Erikson, Erik H.
Kübler-Ross, Elisabeth
Kuhn, Maggie
Neugarten, Bernice
Sarton, May
Sheehy, Gail

PSYCHOLOGICAL ISSUES
Alzheimer's disease
Beauty
Behavioral and mental health
Biological clock
Creativity
Death and dying
Death anxiety
Death of a child
Death of parents
Dementia
Depression
Empty nest syndrome
Full nest
Grief
Hospice
Humor
Loneliness
Maturity
Memory loss
Midlife crisis
Over the hill
Personality changes
Psychiatry, geriatric
Sexuality
Stereotypes
Stress and coping skills
Suicide
Widows and widowers
Wisdom

SOCIAL ISSUES
Abandonment
Advocacy
African Americans
Age discrimination
Ageism
Aging: Biological, psychological, and sociocultural perspectives
Aging: Historical perspective

American Indians
Asian Americans
Baby boomers
Caregiver absenteeism
Caregiving
Centenarians
Communication
Consumer issues
Driving
Elder abuse
Facility and institutional care
Friendship
Funerals
Geriatrics and gerontology
Home services
Homelessness
Hospice
Housing
Humor
Laguna Woods, California
Latinx Americans
Leisure activities
Life expectancy
Long-term care
Longevity research
Men and aging
Middle age
Neglect
Old age
Pets
Relocation
Retirement communities
Senior citizen centers
Social media
Social ties
Sports participation
Townsend movement
Transportation issues
Vacations and travel
Women and aging

TELEVISION
Golden Girls, The
Grace and Frankie
Matlock
Murder, She Wrote

WOMEN'S ISSUES
Aging Experience: Diversity and Commonality Across Cultures, The
All About Eve
Beauty
Breast cancer
Breast changes and disorders
Cultural views of aging
Divorce
Dual-income couples
Estrogen replacement therapy
Family relationships
Fountain of Age, The
Golden Girls, The
In Full Flower: Aging Women, Power, and Sexuality
"Jilting of Granny Weatherall, The"
Kübler-Ross, Elisabeth
Kuhn, Maggie
Look Me in the Eye: Old Women, Aging, and Ageism
Marriage
Menopause
Murder, She Wrote
Neugarten, Bernice
No Stone Unturned: The Life and Times of Maggie Kuhn
Ourselves, Growing Older: A Book for Women over Forty
Reproductive changes, disabilities, and dysfunctions
"Roman Fever"
Sarton, May
Sexuality
Sheehy, Gail
Sunset Boulevard
Tell Me a Riddle
Trip to Bountiful, The
When I Am an Old Woman I Shall Wear Purple
Widows and widowers
Woman's Tale, A
Women and aging
"Worn Path, A"

Bibliography: Nonfiction

This bibliography of books and journals on aging offers guidance for further research. It is by no means an exhaustive list.

DATABASE

Abstracts in Social Gerontology. EBSCO database. This bibliographic database indexes essential age-related content for gerontology research. Those interested in the field of geriatrics will benefit from this resource, which includes records covering key areas relevant to geriatric studies. More than 120,000 records are catalogued dating back to 1966.

JOURNALS

Age and Ageing. Oxford U P. *Age and Ageing,* the journal of the British Geriatrics Society (BGS), is an international journal publishing refereed original articles and commissioned reviews on geriatric medicine and gerontology. Its range includes research on human ageing and clinical, epidemiological, and psychological aspects of later life.

Ageing and Society. Cambridge U P. *Ageing & Society* is an interdisciplinary and international journal devoted to the understanding of human ageing and the circumstances of older people in their social and cultural contexts. It draws from multiple contributions and has readers from many disciplines including gerontology, sociology, demography, psychology, economics, medicine, social policy, and the humanities. The journal promotes high-quality original research that is relevant to an international audience to encourage the exchange of ideas across the broad spectrum of multidisciplinary academics and practitioners working in the field of aging.

Ageing International. Springer Publishing. *Ageing International* is a quarterly, peer-reviewed journal dedicated to improving the quality of life of ageing populations worldwide. The Journal provides an intellectual forum for communicating common concerns, exchanging discoveries and analyses in scientific research, and crystallizing significant social and health policy issues.

Gerontology and Geriatrics Education. Taylor & Francis. Official journal of the Academy of Gerontology of Higher Education (AGHE), the educational unit of the Gerontological Society of America (GSA), beginning with Volume 26 (2005-2006). This quarterly journal looks to improve awareness of best practices and resources for gerontologists and gerontology and geriatrics educators.

Journal of Aging & Health Sage Publishing The *Journal of Aging & Health* explores the complex and dynamic relationship between gerontology and health; health is one of the fastest-growing areas in the field of gerontology. This academic journal provides comprehensive coverage of views and perspectives from a wide variety of scholarly disciplines.

Journal of Aging Research. Hindawi Publishing. The *Journal of Aging Research* is a peer-reviewed, open access (articles are available free of charge) journal that publishes original research articles, review articles, and clinical studies on all aspects of gerontology and geriatric medicine.

Journal of Applied Gerontology Sage Publishing. *Journal of Applied Gerontology,* the journal of The Southern Gerontological Society (SGS) provides an international forum for information that has clear and immediate applicability to the health, care, and quality of life of older persons. This monthly publication provides comprehensive coverage in all subdisciplines of gerontology whose findings, conclusions, or suggestions have clear and sometimes immediate applicability to the problems encountered by older persons as well as articles that inform research and the development of interventions.

Journal of the American Geriatrics Society. Wiley Publishing. *The Journal of the American Geriatrics Society (JAGS)* is the "go-to" journal for clinical aging research, providing a diverse, interprofessional community of health-care professionals with the latest insights on geriatrics education, clinical practice, and public policy. Since its first edition in 1953, The journal has remained one of the oldest and most impactful journals dedicated exclusively to gerontology and geriatrics.

Journal of Gerontological Social Work. Binghamton, N.Y.: Haworth P. This journal frequently publishes two volumes each year, with four issues per volume. Articles deal with social work theory, research, and practice in the field of aging. Examples of content include research on life after retirement, household composition, living arrangements, and minority issues.

MEMOIRS AND PERSONAL ESSAYS

Albom, Mitch. *Tuesdays with Morrie: An Old Man, a Young Man, and Life's Greatest Lesson.* Broadway Books, 1997. One of the more well-known memoirs of aging, *Tuesdays with Morrie* focuses on the relationship between a man around 40 and his former professor, who is dying of Amyotrophic Lateral Sclerosis (ALS), also known as Lou Gehrig's disease. Mitch Albom (1958-) met every Tuesday with Morrie Schwartz, his former sociology professor at Brandeis University and discussed life and death. A huge best-seller, *Tuesdays with Morrie* was made into a television movie in 1999, with Hank Azaria as Mitch and Jack Lemmon as Morrie.

Athill, Diana (1917-2019) Somewhere *Towards the End: A Memoir.* W.W. Norton, 2009 At the age of 91, Athill, an acclaimed editor and writer, candidly and sometimes with great humor, shared her observations on the condition of being old, the losses and occasionally the gains that age brings, and the wisdom and fortitude required to face death.

Bayley, John. *Elegy for Iris.* Picador, 1999. With remarkable tenderness, John Bayle (1925-2015), British literary critic and writer, recreates his passionate love affair with Iris Murdoch (1919-1999) —world-renowned writer and philosopher, and his wife of forty-two years—and poignantly describes the dimming of her brilliance due to Alzheimer's disease. *Elegy for Iris* is a story about the ephemeral beauty of youth and the sobering reality of what it means to grow old, but its ultimate power is that Bayley discovers great hope and joy in his celebration of Iris's life and their love.

Carter, Jimmy. *The Virtues of Aging.* Ballantine, 1998. A highly personal account of aging by Jimmy Carter (1924—) former president of the United States and winner of the Nobel Peace Prize, written when he was in his 70s. Carter emphasizes that the potential for self-fulfillment and service to others can be achieved by accepting challenges, continuing to seek opportunities for growth, living a simple life, and having faith and love.

Didion, Joan. *The Year of Magical Linking.* Vintage, 2006. Didion (1934—), acclaimed writer, shares an intensely personal, yet universal experience: a portrait of a marriage—and a life, in good times and bad—that will speak to anyone who has ever loved a husband or wife or child. Several days before Christmas 2003, Didion and her husband, writer John Gregory Dunne (1932-2003), saw their only daughter, Quintana, fall ill with what seemed at first flu, then pneumonia, then complete septic shock. She was put into an induced coma and placed on life support. Days later—the night before New Year's Eve—the Dunnes were just sitting down to dinner after visiting the hospital when John Gregory Dunne suffered a massive and fatal coronary. In a second, this close, symbiotic partnership of forty years was over. Didion shares her story of the year following Dunne's death.

Kinsley, Michael. *Old Age: A Beginner's Guide.* Tim Duggan Books, 2016. The baby boomers—the largest age cohort in history—are approaching the end and starting to plan their final moves in the game of life. Now they are asking: What was *that* all about? Was it about acquiring things or changing the world? Was it about keeping all your marbles? Or is the only thing that counts after you're gone the reputation you leave behind? In this series of essays, journalist Michael Kinsley (1951-) uses his own battle with Parkinson's disease to unearth answers to questions we are all at some time forced to confront. "Sometimes," he writes, "I feel like a scout from my generation, sent out ahead to experience in my fifties what even the healthiest Boomers are going to experience in their sixties, seventies, or eighties."

LeGuin, Ursula K. *No Time to Spare: Thinking About What Matters.* Houghton Mifflin Harcourt, 2017. Famed science fiction author LeGuin (1929-2018) put together a funny and incisive collection of essays taken from her blog—which she didn't start writing until she was past 80.

Mortimer, John. *The Summer of a Dormouse*. Viking, 2001. With his usual wit and style, acclaimed author John Mortimer (1923-2009) explores what it is like to be seventy-seven years of age but to feel like an eleven-year-old in his heart.

Veney, Loretta Anne Woodward. *Being My Mom's Mom: A Journey Through Dementia from a Daughter's Perspective*. Infinity Publishing, 2012. Veney shares her very personal journey of the years she took care of her aging mother as she slipped into dementia.

AGING RESOURCES

Aronson, Louise. *Elderhood: Redefining Aging, Transforming Medicine, Reimagining Life*. Bloomsbury, 2019. For more than 5,000 years, "old" has been defined as beginning between the ages of 60 and 70. That means most people alive today will spend more years in elderhood than in childhood, and many will be elders for 40 years or more. Yet at the very moment that humans are living longer than ever before, we've made old age into a disease, a condition to be dreaded, denigrated, neglected, and denied. Noted Harvard-trained geriatrician Louise Aronson uses stories from her quarter century of caring for patients, and draws from history, science, literature, popular culture, and her own life to weave a vision of old age that's neither nightmare nor utopian fantasy—a vision full of joy, wonder, frustration, outrage, and hope about aging, medicine, and humanity itself.

Bengtson, Vern L., and Richard A. Settersten Jr., Eds., *The Handbook of Theories of Aging*, 3rd Ed., Springer, 2016. This state-of-the art handbook will keep researchers and practitioners in gerontology abreast of the newest theories and models of aging. It addresses theories and concepts built on cumulative knowledge in four disciplines: biology, psychology, social sciences, and policy and practice, along with landmark advances in trans-disciplinary science. The handbook is unique in providing essential knowledge about primary explanations for aging. The 3rd edition also contains a new section, "Standing on the Shoulders of Giants," which includes personal essays by senior gerontologists who share their perspectives on the history of ideas in their fields, and on their experiences with the process and prospects of developing good theory.

Castel, Alan D. *Better with Age: The Psychology of Successful Aging*. Oxford UP, 2018. There is no single formula to successful aging, but UCLA psychology professor Alan D. Castel provides a comprehensive and practical guide for shaping a life that is joyful, productive, healthy, and meaningful. He debunks negative myths and self-defeating mind-sets about aging, and he reviews research studies that suggest that many people are happiest between the ages of 50 and 70.

Cavanaugh, John C., and Fredda Blanchard-Fields. *Adult Development and Aging*, 8th Ed. Cengage, 2019. Respected textbook. Chapters include the following: Neuroscience as a basis for adult development and aging; physical changes; longevity, health and functioning; attention and memory, and dying and bereavement.

Doyle, Kenneth O., and Larry K. Houk. *Peace of Mind for Your Aging Parents: A Financial, Legal, and Psychological Toolkit for Adult Children, Advisors, and Caregivers*. Santa Barbara, CA: Praeger, 2018. This book is aimed directly at the children and grandchildren of aging parents to prepare them for meaningful conversations with their parents and among themselves. It gives them the tools they need to communicate knowledgeably with caregivers and professional advisors and to make important decisions with, or on behalf of, those who depend on them. The authors provide legal and financial tools and techniques, including wills and trusts, cash management, and investment planning, approaching each from both a financial and a psychological perspective. They recognize that some of the challenges that people face during their last few years of life cannot be controlled and describe not only what these tools and techniques can do but also what they can't. Those that cannot be controlled, however, can still be managed, and the authors explain with clarity and compassion how to deal with them through psychological and spiritual engagement.

Freedman, Marc. *How to Live Forever: The Enduring Power of Connecting the Generations*. Public Affairs, 2018. In *How to Live Forever*, Encore.org founder and CEO Marc Freedman is a world expert on how to make your time—and your legacy—count. Freedman believes the best way to do that is by building bridges between generations. He suggests older adults can help younger generations as mentors, tutors, coaches, foster parents or foster grandparents, and describes programs around the country that match members of different generations in mutually beneficial ways.

Gawande, Atul. *Being Mortal: Medicine and What Matters in the End.* Metropolitan Books, 2014. Atul Gawande (1965-), a Boston-based surgeon and author, focuses on the medical side of aging and finds that sometimes the conflicts between what medicine can do and what it should do interfere with the quality of life. His focus is on ensuring people live good lives until the end and how the quality of life is important. He also acknowledges that many physicians are ill-trained to deal with end-of-life discussions and issues.

Geber, Sara Zeff. *Essential Retirement Planning for Solo Agers: A Retirement and Aging Roadmap for Single and Childless Adults.* Mango Publishing, 2018. This valuable book focuses on a significant segment of the 50-plus generation that is too often overlooked when it comes to retirement planning: the 15 million American men and women who are aging "solo," without benefit of the care-providing safety net so frequently supplied by adult children. Geber is a certified retirement coach who provides practical strategies and case histories with examples and possibilities.

Gratton, Lynda, and Andrew Scott. *The 100-Year Life: Living and Working in an Age of Longevity.* Bloomsbury, 2017. *The 100-Year Life* explores how living to 100 will have a profound effect on society and the economy and result in a complete restructuring of everyone's professional and personal lives.

Drawing on the unique pairing of their experience in psychology and economics, Lynda Gratton and Andrew Scott offer an analysis to help you rethink retirement, your finances, your education, your career, and your relationships to create a fulfilling 100-year life. The traditional notion of a three-stage approach to our working lives—education, followed by work and then retirement—is already beginning to collapse, as life expectancy is rising, final-salary pensions are vanishing, and increasing numbers of people are juggling multiple careers. Whether you are 18, 45, or 60, you will need to do things very differently from previous generations and learn to structure your life in completely new ways.

Gurian, Michael. *The Wonder of Aging: A New Approach to Embracing Life After Fifty.* Atria, 2013. Bestselling author and counselor Michael Gurian offers a comprehensive look at the emotional, spiritual, and cognitive dimensions of aging—and how to celebrate life after fifty.

Haber, David. *Health Promotion and Aging: Practical Applications for Health Professionals.* 8th Ed. Springer, 2019. This respected textbook champions healthy aging by demonstrating how to prevent or manage disease and make large-scale improvements toward health and wellness in the older adult population. The text synthesizes state-of-the-art research findings—providing convincing evidence that health promotion truly works—with practical, effective strategies and furnishes updated best practices and strategies to ensure the active participation of older adults in all aspects of life. The work features updated demographics and rankings for leading causes of death, new blood pressure screening guidelines and data on obesity and diabetes, updated exercise regimens, older-driver statistics and innovations such as the driverless car, cautions regarding ineffective brain-training programs, and more. In addition, it includes health-promoting tools, resource lists, assessment tools, illustrations, checklists, and tables.

Jenkins, JoAnn with Boe Workman. *Disrupt Aging: A Bold New Path to Living Your Best Life at Every Age.* Public Affairs, 2016. Jenkins, the CEO of AARP, focuses on three core areas—health, wealth, and self—to show how to embrace opportunities and change the way people look at getting older. Here, she chronicles her own journey and that of others who are making their mark as disruptors to show readers how they can be active, healthy, and happy as they get older. She touches on all the important issues facing people 50+ today, from caregiving and mindful living to building age-friendly communities and making money last.

Larson, Eric B., and Joan DeClaire. *Enlightened Aging: Building Resilience for a Long, Active Life.* Rowman & Littlefield, 2017. A leading expert in the science of healthy aging, Dr. Eric B. Larson offers practical advice for growing old with resilience and foresight. *Enlightened Aging* proposes a path to resilience—one that's proven to help many stave off disability until very old age. The steps on this path include pro-activity, acceptance, and building and maintaining good physical, mental, and social health. Using inspiring stories from Dr. Larson's experiences with study participants, patients, friends, and relatives, *Enlightened Aging* will help readers determine what their paths can look like given their own experiences and circumstances. It informs readers of the scientific evidence behind new perspectives on aging. It inspires readers with stories of people who are approaching aging with enlightened attitudes. It offers advice and resources for readers to build their own reserves for old age. It recommends ways for readers to work with their doctors to stay as healthy as possible for their age. And it offers ideas for building better communities for our aging population. Although especially relevant to the baby boomer generation, this work is really for people of all ages looking for encouragement and wise counsel to live a long, active life.

Levitin, Daniel J. *Successful Aging: A Neuroscientist Explores the Power and Potential of Our Lives.* Dutton Penguin, 2020. *Successful Aging* uses research from developmental neuroscience and the psychology of individual differences to show that sixty-plus years is a unique developmental stage that, like infancy or adolescence, has its own demands and distinct advantages. Levitin looks at the science behind what we all can learn from those who age joyously, as well as how to adapt our culture to take full advantage of older people's wisdom and experience. Throughout his exploration of what aging really means, Levitin reveals resilience strategies and practical, cognitive enhancing tricks everyone should do as they age.

Mehrotra, Chandra M., and Lisa S. Wagner. *Aging and Diversity: An Active Learning Experience.* 3rd Ed. Routledge, 2019. As the older population in the United States is becoming more racially and ethnically diverse, it is important to understand the characteristics, the potential, and the needs of this population. In *Aging and Diversity*, Chandra Mehrotra and Lisa Wagner address key topics in diversity and aging, discussing how the aging experience is affected by not only race and ethnicity but also gender, religious affiliation, social class, rural-urban community location, and sexual orientation and gender identity. Taking this broad view of human diversity allows the authors to convey some of the rich complexities facing our aging population—complexities that provide both challenges to meet the needs of a diverse population of elders and opportunities to learn how to live in a pluralistic society.

Merrill, Gary F. *Our Aging Bodies.* Rutgers UP, 2015. People in developed countries are living longer and, just as the aged population around the world is steadily growing, the number of adults eighty-five and older in the United States is projected to quadruple to twenty-one million people by 2050. The aging of our population has huge implications for baby boomers and their children and has generated a greater interest in the causes and effects of aging. Merrill, a Professor in the Department of Cell Biology and Neuroscience at Rutgers University, clearly explains what happens to all the major organ systems and bodily processes—such as the cardiovascular and digestive systems—as people age. The first section is an overview of secondary aging—changes that occur with age that are related to disease and the environment—and include the effect of such things as diet, humor, and exercise. Readers will also learn about primary aging—intrinsic changes that occur with the aging of specific organs and body systems (including the prostate, the heart, the digestive system, and the brain). Merrill weaves in personal anecdotes and stories that help clarify and reinforce the facts and principles of the underlying scientific processes and explanations. *Our Aging Bodies* is accessible to a general reader interested in the aging phenomenon, or baby boomers wanting to be more informed when seeing their doctor and discussing changes to their bodies as they age.

Miller, BJ, and Shoshana Berger. *A Beginner's Guide to the End: Practical Advice for Living Life and Facing Death.* Simon & Schuster, 2019. The first and only all-encompassing action plan for the end of life. Dr. BJ Miller, a hospital and palliative medicine physician who has worked in a wide variety of settings and has been interviewed by Oprah Winfrey, among others, and Shoshana Berger, who not only has extensive experience as a writer and editor, but also helped care for her father, who suffered from dementia, in the challenging years leading up to death, have created a guide to anything and everything that is involved in planning for and dealing with the inevitable future. They write in a clear and accessible way that makes it easy to understand and relate to the complexities of facing and dealing with death. Five sections, "Planning Ahead," "Dealing with Illness," "Help Along the Way," "When Death Is Close," and "After," offer advice and instructions for every problem that may arise, including writing a will; what to do with family heirlooms; preparing advance directives or living wills; dealing with the health-care system; coping with illness and all its symptoms and various manifestations; extensive information on planning funerals and various types of burial; dealing with grief and its many manifestations; and how to write a eulogy and an obituary and how to plan a funeral or memorial.

Moody, Harry R., and Jennifer R. Sasser. *Aging: Concepts and Controversies.* 9th Ed. Sage, 2018. This respected textbook on gerontology presents current research and encourages readers to get involved and take an informed stand on the major issues we face as a society about aging and older people. The authors focus on three broad domains of human aging: aging over the life course, health care, and the socioeconomic aspects of aging.

Morris, Virginia. *How to Care for Aging Parents: A One-Stop Resource for All Your Medical, Financial, Housing, and Emotional Issues.* 3rd Ed. Workman, 2014. An award-winning journalist, Virginia Morris has devoted her career to researching and writing about health care, medical research and related social and political issues. She also cared for her own parents during their final years. This work clearly and expertly covers all touchpoints of caring for aging parents.

Niles-Yokum, Kelly, and Donna L. Wagner. *The Aging Network: A Guide to Policy, Programs, and Services.* 9th Ed. Springer, 2019. This respected textbook offers comprehensive and up-to-date knowledge about aging services in the United States. Written for both students and practitioners of gerontology, along with all professionals involved in the well-being of older adults, this book provides a current and detailed description and analysis of local to global services for older people with or without cognitive, physical, or social needs. The Ninth Edition is updated to reflect critical changes to legislation, health care, and recent trends. It focuses on the strengths and diversity of older adults and the role our multilayered aging networks play in advocacy, community independence, and engagement. Commentary and critical thinking challenges from policymakers, program directors, and educators facilitate high-level reasoning and independent analysis of aging networks past, present, and future.

Novak, Mark. *Issues in Aging.* 4th Ed., Routledge, 2018. *Issues in Aging* combines social, psychological, biological, and philosophical perspectives to present a multifaceted picture of aging. Novak illustrates both the problems and the opportunities that accompany older age. This text helps students understand the tremendous variability in aging and introduces them to careers working with older adults. This fourth edition has been updated to include emerging issues in aging. These include the prevalence of HIV/AIDs in later life, current research on mental potential in old age, the creation of age-friendly cities, and new options for end-of-life care.

Orel, Nancy A., and Christine A. Fruhauf, eds. *The Lives of LGBT Older Adults: Understanding Challenges and Resilience.* American Psychological Association, 2015. Lesbian, gay, bisexual, and transgendered (LGBT) older adults have unique and varying physical and mental health needs. Yet their experiences have often been ignored in gerontological as well as LGBT studies. This book uses a life course perspective to investigate how LGBT older adults have been shaped by social stigma and systematic discrimination. The book explores not only the challenges and needs of this population but also their strengths and resilience. The intersection of cultural factors and personal attributes is emphasized.

Ramirez-Valles, Jesus. *Queer Aging: the Gayby Boomers and a New Frontier for Gerontology.* Oxford UP, 2016. As the first generation of gay men enters its autumn years, their responses to the physical and emotional tolls of aging promise to be as revolutionary as their advances in AIDS and civil rights activism. Older gay men's approaches to friendship, caregiving, romantic and sexual relationships, illness, and bereavement is upending conventional wisdom regarding the aging process, LGBTQ communities, and the entire field of gerontology.

Rosenblatt, Carolyn. *The Family Guide to Aging Parents: Answers to Your Legal, Financial, and Healthcare Questions.* Sanger, CA: Familius, 2015. Carolyn Rosenblatt, RN, an elder law attorney, offers expert advice to competently handle the legal, financial, and health-care issues that lie ahead with aging parents, including how to find the right words to approach parents regarding their finances; how to get past any resistance from them; how to best protect aging loves ones from financial predators; and how to competently choose a home care worker, assisted living or nursing home.

Scardamalia, Robert L., ed. *Aging in America* 3rd Ed. Bernan P, 2018. Today, concerns about the financial stability of Social Security, trends in disability, health care costs, and the supply of caregivers are all driven by the coming explosion in the number of people over the age of 65. *Aging in America* focuses on the economic and demographic portrait of the senior population and can provide a context for analysis of broader population issues. It provides a wide range of characteristics of the older population including: age composition, race and Hispanic origin, educational attainment, living arrangements, veteran status, employment and income, health insurance, disability and housing characteristics.

Skinner, B. F., and M.E. Vaughan. *Enjoy Old Age: A Practical Guide.* Norton, 1997 (originally published in 1983). Noted behavioral psychologist Skinner joins Vaughan, an expert on aging, to examine the emotional life of the aging and some of the challenges these individuals face. Believing that people can live well by planning well, the authors give advice to older adults on ways to enjoy themselves, to keep in touch with the world and their own past, to think more clearly, to stay busy, to feel good, to enjoy good days, to get along with other people, to keep from letting the fear of death ruin present joy of living, and to reconcile themselves to the inevitable characteristics of old age.

Stearns, Ann Kaiser. *Redefining Aging: A Caregiver's Guide to Living Your Best Life.* Johns Hopkins UP, 2017. Caring for an elderly family member can be overwhelming. But fulfilling life experiences are still possible for both caregivers and their loved ones, despite the stress and fatigue of caregiving. Stearns explores the practical and personal challenges of both caregiving and successful aging. She couples findings from the latest research with powerful insights and problem-solving tips to help caregivers achieve the best life possible for those they care for and for themselves as they age.

Terkel, Studs. *Coming of Age: Growing Up in the Twentieth Century.* The New P, 2007. Studs Terkel (1912-2008) was the bestselling author of twelve books on oral history. A *New York Times* bestseller when this was first published in 1995, (as *Coming of Age: The Story of Our Century by Those Who've Lived It*). *Coming of Age* presents a portrait of American life and the experience of aging in the twentieth century by seventy-four very different people, the youngest of whom is seventy and the oldest ninety-nine. Inspiring in the honesty of their voices and their lack of nostalgia or illusions, these are people with the widest range of experiences from all around the country; many were at the vanguard of their movements, whether of trade unions, gay liberation, or the arts. They remind us what we once were, what we have lost, and the extraordinary extent to which we've been transformed as a society over the span of the twentieth century.

Wacker, Robbyn R., and Karen A. Roberto. *Community Resources for Older Adults: Programs and Services in an Era of Change.* 5th Ed., Sage, 2019. *Community Resources for Older Adults: Programs and Services in an Era of Change* provides comprehensive, up-to-date information on programs, services, and policies pertaining to older adults. Wacker and Roberto build reader awareness of programs and discuss how to better understand help-seeking behavior, as well as explain ways to take advantage of the resources available to older adults.

Whitbourne, Susan Krauss, ed. *The Encyclopedia of Adulthood and Aging.* 3-volume set. Wiley-Blackwell, 2016. This authoritative reference work contains more than 300 entries covering all aspects of the multi-disciplinary field of adult development and aging. Under the general editorship of Susan Krauss Whitbourne, a noted pioneer in the field, the entries bring together summaries of classic topics as well as the most recent thinking and research in new areas. They educate readers on the most important facts, theories, research, practice, and contemporary trends. The *Enyclopedia* covers a broad range of issues, from biological and physiological changes in the body to changes in cognition, personality, and social roles to applied areas, such as psychotherapy, long-term care, and end-of-life issues.

—*Compiled by Claire B. Joseph, MS, MA, AHIP*

Mediagraphy: Film, Fiction, Television & Music

The following compiles media portrayals of the complex issues of aging. Media includes movies, TV, books of fiction, plays, and music. Some delve into aging as just another normal process of life, while others focus on how elders see themselves or are seen by society, both positively and negatively. Critical aspects and themes related to aging are explored in the context of relationships-whether between spouses, parents and children, or grandparents and children-and of memories. Some of these materials also explore key roles for elders in society. This list is by no means comprehensive but rather meant to be representative of the many portrayals of elders in popular media.

FILMS

About Schmidt (2002), Jack Nicholson, playing against type, portrays Warren Schmidt, a retired actuary, unhappily married to Helen and living a humdrum existence. When Helen suddenly dies, Schmidt decides to visit his daughter and try to stop her wedding to a man he disapproves. But standing in his way is Randall's feisty mother, and slowly he realizes he must make the most of his remaining life.

Age of Miracles (1996), directed by Peter Chan. This Chinese film tells the story of a devoted mother who decides to sacrifice her life to save one of her sons from an early death. However, her effort is not totally appreciated by the son, causing the family to experience a complex tragedy that forces them all into a better understanding of their familial bonds. Originally in Chinese and Cantonese, the film is available with English subtitles. Performers include Alan Tam, Anita Yuen, Eric Tsang, Jordan Chan, Teresa Carpio, Christina Ng, and Roy Chiao.

Age Old Friends (1989), directed by Allan Kroeker. This film, starring Hume Cronyn, Vincent Gardenia, Esther Rolle, and Tandy Cronyn, is about a man who turns down a chance to live with his daughter in favor of residing at a retirement home. Once at the home, he enjoys a close friendship with another resident, only to find that his friend is beginning to experience senility. The main character's struggle to decide whether to stay in the home to help his friend or to go to his daughter's home becomes the crux of this film whose primary themes are loyalty, friendship, personal meaning, and the decisions elders make later in life.

All About Eve (1950), directed by Joseph L. Mankiewicz. Acclaimed actor Bette Davis plays an aging actress who faces unexpected competition from a younger, ambitious actress, played by Anne Baxter, who dupes Davis's character into taking her under her wing and ultimately betrays her.

All of Me (1984), directed by Carl Reiner. This comedy is about a dying woman who gets a second chance at life. However, her soul takes over only one-half of another person, who just happens to be a rather odd lawyer. Steve Martin stars in this film, along with Lily Tomlin, Madolyn Smith, Victoria Tennant, and Basil Hoffman.

Arsenic and Old Lace (1944), directed by Frank Capra. Starring Cary Grant, Priscilla Lane, Raymond Massey, and Peter Lorre, this film focuses on how looks can be deceiving. Two little old ladies who, on the surface, seem as gentle as can be to their young nephew are actually poisoning older gentlemen who come to visit and burying them in the cellar.

Autumn Spring (2001), Czech with English subtitles. Fanta refuses to "act his age"; instead, he squanders the savings that his wife has put away for their eventual funerals and burials by playing pranks and running up large food and other tabs with his friend Eda, much to his wife's increasing frustration. Meanwhile Fanta's son is pressuring his parents to move into a retirement home so he can have their apartment. A funny, tender, and poignant look at aging.

Away from Her (2006), Julie Christie (1940-) plays Fiona who has been happily married for many years to Grant (Gordon Pinsent). When Fiona's Alzheimer's worsens, she goes to a nursing home. When Grant visits her, he finds that she barely knows him and has grown attached to another man, a fellow resident at the home.

Battling for Baby (1992), directed by Art Wolff. Suzanne Pleshette and Debbie Reynolds each play a grandmother who competes with the other for time to baby-sit their grandchild. The film uses humor to show how important it is for grandparents to have time with a grandchild and how simple chores can take on greater meaning and purpose in the life of an elder.

Black or White (2014), when his wife dies in a car crash, Elliott Anderson (Kevin Costner) fields another blow: the realization that he must raise his biracial granddaughter, Eloise (Jillian Estell), alone. However, the child's paternal grandmother, Rowena (Octavia Spencer) feels that she is better equipped to take care of the child and sues for custody. With Eloise caught in the middle, both Elliott and Rowena are forced to confront their true feelings about race, forgiveness, and understanding.

Bucket List, The (2007), Billionaire Edward Cole (Jack Nicholson) and car mechanic Carter Chambers (Morgan Freeman) are complete strangers, until fate lands them in the same hospital room. The men find they have two things in common: a need to come to terms with who they are and what they have done with their lives, and a desire to complete a list of things they want to see and do before they die. Against their doctor's advice, the men leave the hospital and set out on the adventure of a lifetime.

Captiva Island (1995), directed by John Biffar. This comedic and poignant film portrays the life of retirees in Florida as perceived by a teenager who becomes friends with some senior citizens. Ernest Borgnine, Arte Johnson, Bill Cobbs, George Blair, Jesse Zeigler, and Amy Bush star.

Cemetery Club, The (1992), directed by Bill Duke. This comedy, which stars Ellen Burstyn, Danny Aiello, Olympia Dukakis, and Diane Ladd, focuses on the weekly meetings of three friends. As each is widowed, they share their difficulties in trying to date as senior citizens, bonding together as they learn what it is like to look for a new husband.

Cocoon (1985), directed by Ron Howard. This inspiring film, starring veteran actor Don Ameche, is about a group of elders whose quiet life in a senior citizens' home is disrupted when they are given a chance at eternal youth by extraterrestrial visitors. A 1988 sequel, *Cocoon 2: The Return*, was directed by Daniel Petrie and featured the return of the seniors to Earth to see their families.

Cold Comfort Farm (1995), directed by John Schlesinger. This comedic film stars Kate Beckinsale, Joanna Lumley, Rufus Sewell, Ian McKellen, Eileen Atkins, Sheila Burrell, Stephen Fry, Freddie Jones, and Miriam Margolyes. In it, a young, orphaned woman must live with a group of odd relatives on a farm in the country. The strong wishes of the matriarchal grandmother regarding how the house should be run clash with the desires of the young orphan.

Country Life (1984), directed by Michael Blakemore. This film celebrates the age-old theme of an older man finding love with a younger woman. In bringing his young love to his small town, however, the older man experiences not only social tension from the townspeople but also competition from younger men. Sam Neill, Greta Scacchi, Michael Blakemore, John Hargreaves, Kerry Fox, and Robyn Cruze star.

Dad (1989), directed by Gary David Goldberg. This film tells the story of a son who comes home to be reunited with his aging father. As they struggle through a family illness together, the son tries to connect with his father after a distant, two-year separation. The film emphasizes the value of parent-child relationships in later life. Jack Lemmon and Ted Danson star.

Dennis the Menace (1993), directed by Nick Castle. This classic story of a young boy who innocently drives his grouchy old neighbor crazy stars Walter Matthau and Mason Gamble. Although the film exemplifies how young people often try to cause mischief for the unsuspecting, it also shows how elders, even when duped, are never too far from appreciating the spirit of youth.

Don Juan de Marco (1995), directed by Jeremy Leven. In this film, an older psychologist (Marlon Brando) who is nearing retirement becomes involved in the unusual case of a young man (Johnny Depp) who believes he is the fabled romancer Don Juan de Marco. Through his study of the young man, the psychologist is forced to reexamine his own ideas of what it means to love throughout life, especially during the later years.

Dream a Little Dream (1989), directed by Marc Rocco. One of many films that allow the old to become young again, *Dream a Little Dream* shows the pros and cons of such a situation when the souls of an elderly couple are placed into the bodies of two teenagers. Jason Robards and Corey Feldman star.

Driving Miss Daisy (1989), this film, based on the play by Alfred Uhry, who wrote the screenplay, shows the complex relationship that develops between an elderly southern woman and the African American chauffeur that the woman's son demands that she use to make her way around town. The film excels in highlighting issues not only about race relations in southern United States, including generational ones, but also about the struggles that can occur between older parents and their children. Veteran actress Jessica Tandy (1909-1994) played Miss Daisy, for which she won an Oscar as Best Actress, and acclaimed actor Morgan Freeman (1937-) played her chauffer, reprising his role from the original Off-Broadway production.

Eighteen Again! (1988), directed by Paul Flaherty. In this comedy-which stars George Burns, Charlie Schlatter, Tony Roberts, Red Buttons, and Jennifer Runyon-an accident causes a lively eighty-year-old bachelor to switch souls with his grandson for a period of time.

End, The (1978), directed by Burt Reynolds. This comedy focuses on a middle-aged man's desire to end his life and his inability to do so. The film captures moments during which the man gets close to death, reflects on his life, and finally goes through the common process of bargaining with God to stay alive. Burt Reynolds, Sally Field, Dom DeLuise, and Joanne Woodward star.

Everybody's Fine (2009), eight months after the death of his wife, Frank Goode (Robert DeNiro) looks forward to a reunion with his four adult children. When all of them cancel their visits at the last minute, Frank, against the advice of his doctor, sets out on a road trip to reconnect with his offsprings. As he visits each one in turn, Frank finds that his children's lives are not quite as perfect as he's been led to believe. Frank and his children reconnect in a meaningful way.

Family Business (1989), directed by Sidney Lumet. Sean Connery, Matthew Broderick, Dustin Hoffman, and Rosana De Soto star in this film about three generations of men in a family. The family traits of cleverness, a desire for excitement, pride, and criminal skill combine to bring these three men together to face a difficult choice when a risky robbery runs into trouble. Though subtle, the film portrays the important cultural theme of elders sacrificing for their children and the costs and benefits of such gestures of love between generations.

Family Reunion (1981), directed by Fielder Cook. This film stars Bette Davis as an old schoolteacher who feels displaced after retiring. In her efforts to reconnect with her roots and with her family, she becomes aware of some untidy business and must decide how to intervene.

Family Reunion (1987), directed by Vic Sarin. A grandfather's birthday celebration draws a family together for a reunion and spawns a humorous situation based on misunderstandings about a grandson's love life. This film stars David Eisner, Rebecca Jenkins, and Linda Sorensen.

Father of the Bride II (1995), directed by Charles Shyer. Shyer revisits the story of *Father of the Bride* in a film that announces the coming of a grandchild. Steve Martin and Diane Keaton star as expectant grandparents who are struggling with what it means to have a grandchild. Martin Short, Kimberly Williams, George Newbern, and Kieran Culkin also star.

Four Seasons, The (1981), directed by Alan Alda. This film focuses on three couples of different ages whose lives come together in complex relationships. The story shows how maturity does not always come with age and how wisdom can sometimes be found in unexpected places. The film stars Alan Alda, Carol Burnett, Rita Moreno, Sandy Dennis, Len Cariou, and Jack Weston.

The Ghost and Mrs. Muir (1947), directed by Joseph L. Mankiewicz. This film tells the story of a widow who is romanced through her loneliness by the ghost of a mariner who visits her home. The ghost helps her write a novel that brings a potential husband to her life, forcing her to choose between the ghost of the captain and the new friend. Though the film is not specifically about aging, it does deal with the difficult and complex feelings that come when one loses a spouse to death at a later age in life. Gene Tierney,

Rex Harrison, George Sanders, Edna Best, Anna Lee, Robert Coote, and Natalie Wood appear.

The Farewell (2019). Billi's family returns to China under the guise of a fake wedding to stealthily say goodbye to their beloved matriarch-the only person that doesn't know she only has a few weeks to live.

45 Years, (2015), famed British actors Charlotte Rampling (1946-) and Tom Courtenay (1937-) portray a happily married couple about to celebrate their 45th wedding anniversary. By chance, the wife discovers startling information about her husband's deceased former girlfriend that not only shakes her to her core, but makes her question all she has assumed about her marriage.

Going in Style (1979), directed by Martin Brest. This comedy, starring George Burns, Art Carney, and Lee Strasberg, features three retirees who decide to rob a bank to make their retirement a little more lucrative and a little less boring. However, the robbery involves some unexpected turns of events. The film does well to highlight the issue of boredom during retirement in a humorous way.

Goodbye People, The (1986), directed by Herb Gardner. An elderly gentleman decides to revisit his past by reopening a hot dog stand he once had on the beach. A daughter with whom he has had a distant relationship and an artist friend help him as he embarks on his effort to recapture the past and enliven the present. The film stars Judd Hirsch, Martin Balsam, Pamela Reed, and Ron Silver.

Gran Torino (2008). Retired auto worker and Korean War vet Walt Kowalski (Clint Eastwood) is lonely, but keeps up his car and home, and despises the many Asian, Latino, and black families in his neighborhood. Walt becomes a reluctant hero when he stands up to the gangbangers who tried to force his Korean teen neighbor to steal Walt's treasured car. An unlikely friendship and grudging respect develops between Walt and the teen and changes Walt's life forever.

Grumpy Old Men (1993), directed by Donald Petrie. This film-which stars Walter Matthau, Jack Lemmon, Ann-Margret, Burgess Meredith, Daryl Hannah, Ossie Davis, Buck Henry, and Kevin Pollack-focuses on the feud that develops between two elderly men who vie for the attentions of a young female neighbor. A sequel, *Grumpier Old Men* (1995), was directed by Howard Deutch and continues the theme of the two men feuding over yet another woman, despite her probable deleterious effect on their neighborhood. See entry in *Aging.*

Guarding Tess (1994), directed by Hugh Wilson. Nicolas Cage, Shirley MacLaine, Austin Pendleton, Edward Albert, James Rebhorn, and Richard Griffiths star in this film about a spirited former First Lady and her relationship with her younger, male bodyguard. This film portrays the off-balance, odd friendship that the two share, sometimes showing the unexpected weakness of the younger man and strengths of the older woman.

Harold and Maude (1971), directed by Hal Ashby. This dark comedy-starring Ruth Gordon, Bud Cort, Vivian Pickles, and Cyril Cusack-follows a fond relationship that blossoms between two unlikely people: a young man named Harold who is obsessed with death, and Maude, a woman sixty years his senior who loves to attend funerals in her celebration of life. See entry in *Aging.*

Harry and Son (1984), directed by Paul Newman. Newman wrote, directed, and starred in this film about a father and son who face numerous interpersonal battles as they confront their different views of life. Robby Benson, Joanne Woodward, and Ellen Barkin also star.

Heaven Can Wait (1943), directed by Ernst Lubitsch. This film stars Don Ameche, Laird Cregar, Charles Coburn, Marjorie Main, Lewis Calhern, and Gene Tierney. The struggle of dying, final judgment, and atoning for the mistakes of a lifetime are the themes of this film about a man who, after his death, recounts his relationships with his wife and other women.

I'm Not Rappaport (1996), directed by Herb Gardner. In this humorous film, two elders (portrayed by Walter Matthau and Ossie Davis) become friends in Central Park in New York City, despite obvious differences in their backgrounds and lifestyles.

The Intern (2015). Looking to get back into the game, 70-year-old widower Ben Whittaker (Robert De Niro) seizes the opportunity to become a senior intern at an online fashion site. Ben soon becomes popular with his younger co-workers, including Jules Ostin (Anne Hathaway), the boss and founder of the company. Each generation has something to learn from the other.

Make Way for Tomorrow (1937), a retired married couple, played by Victor Moore and Beulah Bondi, are loving parents to their five grown children. When they lose their home to foreclosure, which one of their children will step up and offer their parents a home, one where they will not be "in the way"? A problem that plagues families to this day. Poignant look at aging.

A Man Called Ove (2015). Swedish with English subtitles. Based on the 2012 novel by Fredrik Backman (see novels), Ove is a 59-year-old curmudgeon who is extremely set in his grumpy ways. He is also depressed and lonely; his beloved wife succumbed to cancer 6 months earlier, and he is forced to retire from his job of 43 years. Ove is ready to "check out" of life, but life just won't let him. A funny, sweet, and poignant look at aging.

The Mule (2018). Broke, alone and facing foreclosure on his business, 90-year-old horticulturist Earl Stone (Clint Eastwood) takes a job as a drug courier for a Mexican cartel. His immediate success leads to easy money and a larger shipment that soon draws the attention of the DEA. When Earl's past mistakes start to weigh heavily on his conscience, he must decide whether to right those wrongs before law enforcement and cartel thugs catch up to him. Based on a true story.

Nebraska (2013). Cranky Woody Grant (Bruce Dern) can barely walk down the street of his home in Billings, Montana, without stopping for a drink. So when Woody receives a sweepstakes notice in the mail and insists on making a 750-mile trip to Lincoln, Nebraska, to collect his prize, it falls to baffled son David (Will Forte) to accompany him. During a stop in their Nebraska hometown, word gets out about Woody's fortune, first making him a hero, then later, the target of predatory people.

The Old Man and the Gun (2018), at the age of 70, Forrest Tucker makes an audacious escape from San Quentin, conducting an unprecedented string of heists that confound authorities and enchant the public. Wrapped up in the pursuit are detective John Hunt, who becomes captivated with Forrest's commitment to his craft, and a woman who loves him in spite of his chosen profession.

On Borrowed Time (1939). Veteran actor Lionel Barrymore (Drew's great-uncle) plays Gramps, who looks after his orphaned grandson and tries to protect him from his conniving aunt. When death, in the form of the debonair Mr. Brink, (played by Cedric Hardwicke), comes to claim him, Gramps tricks him into climbing his magic apple tree where he is trapped. Gramps is delighted, but soon learns the cost of postponing his death and the death of others.

On Golden Pond (1981), acclaimed film version of Ernest Thompson's play, (see drama) with screenplay by Thompson. Starred veteran actors Henry Fonda (1905-1982) and Katharine Hepburn (1907-2003) as an aging couple; their daughter was played by Fonda's real-life daughter, actress Jane Fonda, who accepted Fonda's Best Actor Oscar posthumously on his behalf.

The Straight Story (1999). The film is based on the true story of Alvin Straight's 1994 journey across Iowa and Wisconsin on a lawn mower. Alvin (Richard Farnsworth) is an elderly World War II veteran who lives with his daughter Rose (Sissy Spacek), a kind woman with an intellectual disability. When he hears that his estranged brother Lyle (Harry Dean Stanton) has suffered a stroke, Alvin makes up his mind to go visit him and hopefully make amends before he dies. But Alvin doesn't have a driver's license or a car, so, determined to visit his brother one last time, he makes the trip by his John Deere lawn Tractor, crossing 240 miles at 5 miles per hour.

Two Weeks (2006). North Carolina matriarch Anita Bergman (Sally Field) enters the final stage of her battle with cancer, and her four adult children gather at her bedside. As the siblings face their mother's imminent demise, home movies provide insight into family relationships.

An Unfinished Life (2005). Einar (Robert Redford), a recovering alcoholic rancher who lives with his loyal pal Mitch (Morgan Freeman), gets an unexpected visit from his daughter-in-law, Jean (Jennifer Lopez), and granddaughter, Griff (Becca Gardner). Einar holds a grudge against Jean because he feels she's responsible for his son's accidental death, but he reluctantly lets her stay at the farm when he learns that she's trapped in a violent relationship. Over time, they grow closer and try to heal their emotional wounds.

WRITTEN WORKS & DRAMA

The Autobiography of Miss Jane Pittman (1971), by Ernest J. Gaines. In this novel, a black woman who is more than one century old shares her lifetime recollections, both as an individual who has grown old and as an elderly black woman. Her life experiences include firsthand observation of such disturbing historical trends as slavery and other social and racial tensions. The narrative reveals this character to have a complex understanding of human relations, and it provides a good example of the wisdom and value of elderly people's perspectives on history. See entry in *Aging*.

Bless Me, Ultima (1972), by Rudolfo A. Anaya. Set in the period immediately following World War II, this story focuses on the awakening process that a young boy goes through in his relationship with a woman named Ultima. Ultima is a *curandera,* or woman who uses herbs, magic, and the wisdom of ancestors for healing and guidance in spiritual and other matters. The boy matures throughout the course of the story, calling into question traditional beliefs, his guides and elders, and God. The rich relationship between the boy and the *curandera* emphasizes the value of mentorship, guidance from elders, and self-discovery. It also provides a stirring example of how a person can live on through others in lessons and memories, even after death. See entry in *Aging*.

"Dr. Heidegger's Experiment" (1837), by Nathaniel Hawthorne. This short story focuses on four elderly friends who gather at the laboratory of their friend, Dr. Heidegger, to participate in an experiment. They all agree to drink a special liquid, rumored to come from the fountain of youth. What ensues is a mix of expectations and wishes, as well as a temporary willingness to let go of the perception of oneself as being old. The story amplifies both the wish that many people have to return to their youth and the power of the mind to accomplish such a task. See entry in *Aging*.

Death of a Salesman (1949). Acclaimed Pulitzer Prize and Tony Award winning drama by Arthur Miller, debuted on Broadway in 1949, with actor Lee J. Cobb as Willy Loman, an aging, tired, unsuccessful and unstable travelling salesman and his relationship with his wife and sons, Biff and Happy. It was made into a 1951 movie with Fredric March as Willy Loman, and again in a 1985 made-for-TV version with Dustin Hoffman as Loman. *Death of a Salesman* was revived on Broadway four times; and has been performed across the world.

Driving Miss Daisy (1987), by Alfred Uhry, won the 1988 Pulitzer Prize for Drama. This play shows the complex relationship that evolves over time between a woman and her chauffeur in the southern United States. The value of this long-term relationship overrides the obvious cultural and ethnic tensions that define the context of the story. *Driving Miss Daisy* was made into an acclaimed film in 1989. See entry in *Films*.

Fried Green Tomatoes at the Whistle Stop Cafe (1987), by Fannie Flagg. This story focuses on four women in a small town in Alabama in the 1930s who reminisce about their life experiences at the Whistle Stop Cafe fifty years earlier. Touches on relationships between women, individuals of different racial backgrounds, and rich and poor. The main theme of the novel, however, is the value of friendships for women in later life. The novel was the basis for the film *Fried Green Tomatoes* (1991), directed by Jon Avnet and starring Kathy Bates, Mary Stuart Masterson, Mary-Louise Parker, Jessica Tandy, and Cicely Tyson.

Full Measure: Modern Short Stories on Aging (1988), by Dorothy Sennett. This collection of short stories features a variety of elders as main characters, explores many of the concerns that elders deal with on a daily basis and provides a unique elderly perspective on these issues. Though each story is unique, the overriding theme of the collection is that elders come in all forms and dispositions, have all the same desires and wants that younger people have, and definitely are not to be taken for granted. Physical and mental ailments do affect many of the characters, but each deals with them in a different way. Fears of aging, of being feeble-minded, of being unwanted, of being left alone, and of being taken advantage of are addressed in several stories. See entry in *Aging*.

The Gin Game (1976), by D. L. Coburn, is a two-person, two-act play that won Coburn the 1978 Pulitzer Prize for Drama. Weller Martin and Fonsia Dorsey, two elderly residents at a nursing home for senior citizens, strike up an acquaintance. Neither seems to have any other friends, and they start to enjoy each other's company. Weller offers to teach Fonsia how to play gin rummy, and they begin playing a series of games that Fonsia always wins. Weller's inability to win a single hand becomes increasingly frustrating to him, while Fonsia becomes increasingly confident. While playing their games of gin, they engage in lengthy conversations about their families and their lives in the outside world. Gradually, each conversation becomes a battle, much like the ongoing gin games, as each player tries to expose the other's weaknesses, to belittle the other's life, and to humiliate the other thoroughly.

Golden Years Golden Words (1993), by Michael Ryan. This is a collection of quotes, phrases, and stories of life lessons and of the wisdom offered by elders.

I Never Sang for My Father (1968), by Robert Anderson. This play tells the story of a son who commits his life to winning the love of his father. This is not an easy task, however, as the father is set in his ways and is highly opinionated. Through perseverance, the son is able to break through his father's hostility and rejection and establish an emotional, father-son connection. Made into a 1970 film with Melvyn Douglas and Gene Hackman as father and son.

"The Jilting of Granny Weatherall" (1930), by Katherine Anne Porter. This short story is about an older woman who is on her death bed, recounting her life and the people in her life. What is most profound about this story is its message of how losses, disappointments, and the emotional trauma attached to unexpected events in life can stay with a person to the end of life and even into the process of dying. See entry in *Aging*.

King Lear, by William Shakespeare. "How sharper than a serpent's tooth it is / to have a thankless child" (Act 1, Scene 4). King *Lear* is a tragedy written by William Shakespeare. It tells the tale of a king who bequeaths his power and land to two of his three daughters, after they declare their love for him in an extremely fawning and obsequious manner. His third daughter gets nothing, because she will not flatter him as her sisters had done. When he feels disrespected by the two daughters who now have his wealth and power, he becomes furious to the point of madness. He eventually becomes tenderly reconciled to his third daughter, just before tragedy strikes her and then the king. The play has been widely adapted for the stage and motion pictures, with the title role coveted by many of the world's most accomplished actors.

Memento Mori (1959), by Muriel Spark. The phrase *memento mori* is Latin for "reminder of death." Along these lines, this novel is a dark story about old age that offers both seriousness and humor. See entry in *Aging*.

Old Man and the Sea, The (1952), by Ernest Hemingway. This novel is about an old Cuban fisherman who encounters a huge marlin and goes on a journey of discovery as he pursues the catch of a lifetime. As with many fishing tales, what goes on in the mind of the fisherman influences what he catches. The fisherman learns the lessons of persistence in the face of loss; another major theme is the sense of courage necessary to go into battle with the unknown and to face oneself later in life. The novel was made into a film in 1958. See entry in *Films*.

On Golden Pond (1979), by Ernest Thompson. This play shows how the experience of a family retreat can quell long-standing disagreements and friction among different generations of family members. It also shows the value of not letting such disagreements get in the way of having a relationship, as well as the value of developing and nurturing family relationships, even in later life. The play was made into a film in 1981. See entry in *Films*.

The Picture of Dorian Gray (1890), by Oscar Wilde, is a classic novel telling the story of a handsome young man named Dorian Gray who so desperately desires eternal youth that he is willing to pay for it with his soul. While he remains young and handsome, his portrait instead ages and shows every hint of the decadent life Dorian ultimately follows.

"Rabbi Ben Ezra" (1864), by Robert Browning. This poem, which begins with the line, "Grow old along with me/ the best is yet to be," tells the story of how old age is a time of appreciation for life. Old age, rather than being feared, is seen as a time of great wealth.

"Roman Fever" (1933), by Edith Wharton. This story follows a conversation between two elderly, lifelong acquaintances who loved the same man (who has long since passed away). It focuses on issues of self-exploration and social restrictions both in general and among the elderly. The passing of a day is used as a backdrop to symbolize the passing of a lifetime and to show how delicate social issues may present themselves in unexpected ways throughout life. See entry in *Aging*.

The Stone Angel (1964), by Margaret Laurence Chicago: Chicago UP. In this novel, ninety-year-old Hagar Shipley tells her life story. Her complex narrative focuses on the double nature of most things in life, particularly one's way of handing people and situations. The story does well to show how elders work hard to maintain a cohesive, competent social facade and how most people of age struggle to compose coherent narratives of their experiences. Key life events that occur around the beginnings and ends of relationships are also central to this work, once again emphasizing the importance of memories to everyone, but particularly to the elderly.

Tell Me a Riddle (1976), by Tillie Olsen. This novella, set in the early twentieth century, is about a Jewish woman who reaches old age and decides that it is time for her to assert her wishes. As a grandmother, many of her assertions challenge traditions and social behaviors that are important to her husband and family. See entry in *Aging*.

When I Am an Old Woman I Shall Wear Purple (1987), by Sandra K. Martz. This book is a collection of poems, stories, and photographs created by more than sixty individuals. As a whole, the book honors the process of aging and reveals the daring and power that the process can inspire. Wisdom, life experiences, and the many colors and textures of what it means to be old, particularly an older woman, are described in rich detail. The same title is also connected to a poem, written by Jenny Joseph, that is included in this book and that exemplifies the wisdom of daring to live fully throughout life. See entry in *Aging*.

"When You Are Old" (1893), by William Butler Yeats. This beautiful poem from the collection *The Rose* tells of how to cope with the last years of life. Yeats compares life to a book and reminds the reader to re-read the pages written and to remember connections with those closest to the heart who were there to see the changes over the course of one's life.

"Worn Path, A" (1941), by Eudora Welty. This short story is about an elderly black woman named Phoenix Jackson. Like her first name, she is not kept down for long and seems to be able to find the good in just about any situation. An analogy for life, "A Worn Path" tells the story of a walk that Phoenix takes and the frightening, annoying, and helpful encounters she has along the way. Her journey culminates in a self-realization that prompts her to make a gift to the youth in her life. Welty touches upon the themes of being ignored, of coping with physical limitations, and of being perceived as a sick elder. See entry in *Aging*.

You're Only Old Once! (1986), by Dr. Seuss. In this humorous and lighthearted book, Dr. Seuss takes on some difficult topics in a nonthreatening way. Such issues as the process of growing old and coping with doctors are presented sensitively and with humor. See entry in *Aging*.

"Youth and Age" (1834), by Samuel Taylor Coleridge. This poem focuses on seeing life experiences as growth experiences, even to the end of life. It also emphasizes the importance of maintaining hope and a positive perspective to continue enjoying life.

SONGS

Beatles, The "When I'm Sixty-Four" (1967). Written by John Lennon and Paul McCartney, this humorous, classic song from the album *Sgt. Pepper's Lonely Hearts Club Band* playfully asks whether there is any need or love for a person later in life, after the body and mind start to break down during the process of aging.

Bergman, Alan, Marilyn Bergman, and Marvin Hamlisch. "Way We Were" (1974). The theme song to the popular 1973 film of the same name, and originally recorded by the star of the film, Barbra Streisand. This song dramatically conveys the power of memories and photographs to evoke strong feelings and how, even when strong, memories can be called into question as one struggles to make sense out of how events did or did not happen in life.

Blood, Sweat, and Tears. "When I Die" (1972). Despite the ominous title, this song is upbeat and features the band singing about a natural, unencumbered death that leaves a legacy to the next generation of people. The song is available on the remastered compact disc.

Brock, Jerry and Sheldon Harnick. "Sunrise, Sunset" (1964) From the musical, "Fiddler on the Roof." At his daughter's wedding, a father reflects poignantly on how "swiftly flow the years."

Chapman, Tracy. "At This Point in My Life" (1995). This song, from the album *New Beginning,* is about the process of reflecting on one's life.

Denver, John. "Grandma's Feather Bed" (1974). From the album *John Denver, Home Again,* this song captures the youthful sense of adventure that comes from being at a grandmother's home with other young family members.

Durante, Jimmy. "Look Ahead Little Girl" (1963). From the album *September Song*, this song features an older man singing some bedtime advice to a little girl about what is to come in life as she grows older.

———. "September Song" (1963). Originally written in 1938 for the play *Knickerbocker Holiday,* this song from Durante's album *September Song* conveys the preciousness of time, particularly in relationships, as one ages. The last months of the year are used to represent the latter years of life.

———. "Young at Heart" (1963). This song tells of the magic and importance of always keeping youth within one's mind no matter how old one gets. From the album *September Song,* "Young at Heart" maintains that a youthful outlook is more valuable than any material possession.

Dylan, Bob. "Forever Young" (1974). This song by Bob Dylan first appeared on his album "Planet Waves" In 1988 Rod Stewart wrote and performed a very similar song on his album "Out of Order." Dylan and Stewart agreed to split the royalties on this song, in which a father offers his hopes with his child, including that they remain "Forever Young."

Eberhardt, Cliff. "My Father's Shoes" (1989). Taken from the album *Legacy: A Collection of New Folk Music,* this poignant and cutting song gives voice to a son's turmoil as he struggles with what he has inherited from his father, both materially and as a person.

Five for Fighting. "*One Hundred Years*" (2003). Originally released by Five for Fighting, the pseudonym of John Ondrasik, this song depicts the musings of a young man as he ages, noting the years 15, 40, and 99.

Fogelberg, Dan. "In the Passage" (1980). From the album *The Age of Innocence,* this rather solemn song tells of the process of looking back on life through the eyes of wisdom and noticing decisions made, paths taken or not taken, and how, in reflection, there can be only acceptance for how one has lived.

Grateful Dead, The "Attics of My Life" (1970). This somewhat somber song uses many metaphors to reflect on memories from a rich life and relationship. The lyrics compare memories to articles one might find in an attic, and compares the days of life to pages in a book. This song is from the album *American Beauty.*

———. "Touch of Grey" (1987). This playful song from *In the Dark* features Jerry Garcia singing about surviving as time passes and how his touch of grey, or wisdom from life lessons and experiences, helps him on a daily basis.

Haggard, Merle, and Willie Nelson. "My Life's Been a Pleasure" (1982). In this song from *Poncho and Lefty*, Haggard and Nelson sing about how a man has had a good life because of his lasting relationship with his wife. The lyrics go on to compare the month of May to youth, a time when the relationship began and when outer beauty was noticeable in the woman for whom the song is sung.

Jennings, Waylon, Willie Nelson, Jessi Colter, and Tompall Glaser. "Yesterday's Wine" (1977). These four artists perform a stirring rendition of this song, from the album *The Outlaws*, in which each sip of wine is a metaphor for a memory. The song suggests that some memories become finer with age and are nearly intoxicating.

Kane, Daniel. "Remember When" (1982). This earlier instrumental piece from *On the Street Where You Live* (1992) was written to commemorate the value of exploring and reminiscing about memories of close personal relationships.

Mayer, John. "Stop This Train" (2006). This song first appeared on Mayer's album "Continuum." A young man reflects on how time truly "flies."

Mitchell, Joni. "The Circle Game" (1966). In her soulful voice, Mitchell sings of how time passes quickly for all, of teaching people to become more realistic, and of recognizing the seasons of life. The song is from the album *Ladies of the Canyon*.

Morrison, Van. "A Sense of Wonder" (1984). Morrison sings of the seasons of life, of the value of gaining experience through life, and of how the same things can take on different meaning through the eyes of wisdom and aging in this rich and hearty song from the album *A Sense of Wonder*.

Nash, Graham. "Teach Your Children" (1970). This first appeared on the 1970 Crosby, Stills, Nash & Young album "Harvest." A sensitive understanding of how the generations can learn from each other.

Nelson, Willie. "Funny How Time Slips Away" (1976). In this reflective and light song from *The Sound in Your Mind,* Nelson sings about how quickly time passes when one does not attend to it and how this can surprise people later when they finally do stop to observe their surroundings.

Nelson, Willie, and Waylon Jennings. "Old Friends" (1983). This country-western song, from the album *Take It to the Limit*, is about recollecting the experiences that old friends share after many years of knowing each other and the special value of such relationships across a lifetime.

———. "Would You Lay with Me (In a Field of Stone)" (1983). This ballad from *Take It to the Limit* is about a love that lasts a lifetime, through thick and thin, and through all eternity.

Nelson, Willie, and Leon Russell. "Danny Boy" (1979). From the album, *One for the Road,* this song is about the love felt for a friend remembered.

"Old and in the Way" (1975). From the signature album *Old and in the Way*, this bluegrass song explores the fear that when one ages and youth fades, one may be left alone, uncared for, ignored, and unnoticed.

Pettis, Pierce. "Legacy" (1989). This song from *Legacy: A Collection of New Folk Music* captures the complex feelings that come with all the thoughts, feelings, physical attributes, relationships, and possessions that one can inherit through one's family legacy.

Pink Floyd. "Time" (1973). This song from the classic album *Dark Side of the Moon* captures, in its words and tempo, how time is elusive, is always one step ahead, can be full of surprises, and is leading everyone through the journey of life to the grave.

Presley, Elvis. "Memories" (1990). Available on the compact disc *Elvis: The Great Performances*, this song features Presley singing poignantly about the ability of memories to evoke strong feelings, no matter how brief. As in other songs, memories are said to age like fine wine and to be like pages in the book of one's life.

Richards, Johnny, and Carolyn Leigh. "Young at Heart" (1953). A lighthearted pop standard that advocates for remaining "young at heart."

Ryan, Irene. "No Time at All" (1972). From the musical *Pippin*, this song advises people to live to the fullest and to stay young.

Schmidt, Harvey, and Tom Jones. "Try to Remember" (1960). This poignant song about nostalgia was written for the off-Broadway musical "The Fantasticks." It was the world's longest running musical; running from 1960-2002, with 17,162 performances.

Shocked, Michelle. "When I Grow Up" (1986). This humorous song from the album *Short, Sharp, Shocked* is about a woman who wants to grow up to be very old, find an old man, and live a simple life.

Simon, Paul, and Art Garfunkel. "Bookends Theme" (1967). The importance of preserving memories is poignantly conveyed in this song from the album *Bookends*.

———. "A Hazy Shade of Winter" (1967). The sadder side of being old is conveyed in this song of advice offered by an old man who tells the tales of being old and lonely, filled with despair, and in need. The song also touches on the themes of the importance of memory to elders and the value of being remembered by others.

———. "Voices of Old People" (1967). In this song from *Bookends*, Simon and Garfunkel attempt to capture what it sounds like to listen to the voices of the old from a distance. It artfully captures some interesting snippets of elderly concerns in voice samples of older people recorded in New York City and Los Angeles.

Sinatra, Frank. "You Make Me Feel So Young" (1956). This song, available on the compact disc *Songs for Swingin' Lovers* (1987), features Sinatra singing about how love makes one feel good and how feeling good means feeling young.

Sonia Dada. "The River Runs Slow" (1995). *A Day at the Beach*, a relaxing and reflective album, offers this song that has the singer comparing life to a slow-running river. Transitions in life are also compared to bends in a long, winding road as a singer thinks about his growing child.

Stern, Isaac. "Sunrise, Sunset" (1971). The lyrics of this song describe how the passing of a lifetime is like the passing of a day and how elders, with a sense of both joy and sadness, watch their children grow and assume the role of adulthood. Sung by the entire cast, this soulful song comes from the musical and album *Fiddler on the Roof*.

Stevens, Cat. "Father and Son" (1970). This song of life advice from a father to a son from the album *Tea for the Tillerman* focuses on the importance of patience, judicious decision making, self-expression, valuing one's dreams, finding satisfying relationships, and accepting the impermanence of life.

Vereen, Ben. "Simple Joys" (1972). From the 1970s musical and album *Pippin*, this song proclaims that the best things in life are the simple things, that life is to be lived in the present, and that this kind of freedom is best learned before one reaches the end of life.

Weill, Kurt, and Maxwell Anderson. "September Song" (1938) Written for a 1938 musical, "Knickerbocker Holiday," this song was sung by an older man contemplating a May-December romance and conveys how fleeting and precious time is.

Young, Neil. "Comes a Time" (1978). In this song from the album *Comes a Time,* Young sings about how recognizing that time is passing can cause a person to make changes in his or her life.

———. "My Boy" (1985). This song from the album *Old Ways* features a father who notices his son growing up fast and who makes efforts to give advice to his son about how time passes quickly. As with other songs touching on the theme of aging, the metaphor of summer is used to represent the prime of life.

———. "Old Man" (1972). In this song from the album *Harvest,* Young provides the voice of a son singing about his recognition of how he is like his father, about the process of growing older, and about gaining wisdom and insight during the course of aging.

———. "Old Ways" (1985). Found on the album *Old Ways,* Young sings this self-reflective, humorous song about how it is hard to change the habits that one has acquired over a lifetime, even when one recognizes them and wants to change.

TELEVISION PROGRAMS

Blackish (2014-). Combines humor with social consciousness, this series is about a successful African American family, the Johnsons, consisting of Dad Dre, an advertising executive, Mom Rainbow ("Bo") a physician, and their five children. The family is multigenerational, with Dre's divorced parents living with the family and offering their insights and wisdom.

Blue Bloods (2010-). A police drama whose main characters are members of the multigenerational police family the Reagans, headed by patriarch played by actor Tom Selleck (1945-) as the NYC Police Commissioner.

Frasier (1993-2004). This comedy series, primarily about middle-aged radio psychologist Frasier Crane, has the unique feature of showing an elder parent living with his son. Played by John Mahoney, the character of Martin Crane regularly pushes the envelope of what it means to be an old, widowed man. He strives for time alone from his son and regularly puts an end to any notion that he is lonely, useless, or unable to have fun.

The Goldbergs (2013-). Set in the 1980s, the show depicts a middle-class Jewish family, including businessman father, stay-at-home mother, and three children. Also living with the family is the beloved grandfather, played by veteran actor George Segal (1934-).

The Golden Girls (1985-1992). This television comedy series featured the day-to-day lives of four women-Blanche (Rue McClanahan), Rose (Betty White), Dorothy (Bea Arthur), and Dorothy's mother Sophia (Estelle Getty)-who are all over the age of forty. The show portrayed the caring, strong, and complex relationships among these four women and dealt with such issues as jealousy, teamwork, dating, dealing with children, and coping with decisions and fears about health.

The Last of Summer Wine, (1972). This long-running British television show is set in the small town of Yorkshire and tells many stories about the characters who live there. The focus is on three old friends-Compo, Clegg, and Foggy-and the adventures they have with neighbors and with one another. The characters are lively and shatter many elderly stereotypes.

Matlock (1986-1995). This television series starred Andy Griffith as Ben Matlock, an older, clever, small-town lawyer. The character was also featured in a series of television films.

Modern Family (2009-). This comedy series follows the Pritchetts, the patriarch, Jay Pritchett, played by actor Ed O'Neill (1946-) and his younger second wife, Gloria, their son and Gloria's son; Jay's daughter Claire and her husband and three children; and Jay's son Mitchell, his husband Cameron and their adopted children. A funny and realistic portrait of this loving multigenerational family.

Murder, She Wrote (1984-1996). Very popular series starring Angela Lansbury as the older, amateur super sleuth Jessica Fletcher, who was skilled at solving mysteries and intervening in crimes.

Waiting for God (1990-1994). This British comedy series showed the daily absurdities and humor involved in the lives of a group of slightly off-kilter elders living in the Day View Retirement Home. Power of attorney, physical operations, and dealing with relatives were some of the topics of this series.

—*Compiled by Claire B. Joseph, MS, MA, AHIP*

Organizational Resources

AARP
601 E Street, NW
Washington, DC 20049
Toll Free Nationwide: 1-888-OUR-AARP
 (1-888-687- 2277)
Toll Free Spanish: 1-877-342-2277
www.aarp.org

Formerly the American Association of Retired Persons, AARP is a nonprofit, nonpartisan organization whose mission is to empower people to choose how they live as they age. Founded in 1958, they strive to remain true to their founding principles: to promote independence, dignity and purpose for older persons; to enhance the quality of life for older persons; and to encourage older people "To serve, not be served." With a nominal fee ($15/year as of August, 2019, with free membership for spouse/partner), members, who must be fifty years of age or older, receive valuable information on a wide variety of topics of interest to older people, from Medicare, Social Security, taxes, prescriptions, keeping healthy, job searching, and volunteer opportunities, to movie and book reviews; members also are eligible for a wide variety of discounts, including on auto insurance, life insurance, travel, and at a variety of stores and restaurants. Membership also includes the bi-monthly journal, *AARP: The Magazine* (formerly *Modern Maturity*).

Academy for Gerontology in Higher Education (formerly the Association for Gerontology in Higher Education)
1220 L Street NW, Suite 901
Washington, DC 20005
Ph: (202): 289-9806
www.aghe.org

Established in 1974, Academy for Gerontology in Higher Education (AGHE) is a membership organization of colleges and universities that offers education, training, and research programs in the field of aging. Their mission is two-fold: (1) to advance gerontology and geriatrics education in academic institutions, and (2) to provide leadership support of gerontology and geriatrics educating faculty and students at scholastic institutions. Their publications include their official scholarly Journal, *Journal of Gerontology & Geriatrics Education; Gerontology Competencies for Undergraduate & Graduate Education,* and a list of fiction books for K-Primary students.

Administration for Community Living (ACL)
330 C Street SW
Washington, DC 20201
Ph: (202) 401-4634
acl.gov

All Americans—including people with disabilities and older adults—should be able to live at home with the supports they need, participating in communities that value their contributions. To help meet these needs, the US Department of Health and Human Services (HHS) created the Administration for Community Living (ACL) in 2012. ACL brings together the efforts and achievements of the Administration on Aging (AoA), the Administration on Intellectual and Developmental Disabilities (AIDD), and the HHS Office on Disability to serve as the Federal agency responsible for increasing access to community supports, while focusing attention and resources on the unique needs of older Americans and people with disabilities across the lifespan.

ADvancing States
241 18th Street S, Suite 403
Arlington, VA 22202
Ph: (202) 898-2578
Fax: (202) 898-2583
info@advancingstates.org
www.advancingstates.org

ADvancing States, formerly the National Association of State Units on Aging (NASUA)'s mission is to design, improve, and sustain state systems delivering long-term services and supports for older adults, people with disabilities, and their caregivers. They represent 56 officially designated state and territorial agencies on aging and disabilities. They advocate for the advancement and sustainability of federal legislation, policies, and regulation that address the needs of state agencies, the individuals they serve, and the communities in which they live. They offer a list of jobs, grants, and events in the aging and disability networks. The ADvancing States iQ Online Learning Center offers courses including "Introduction to the Independent Living Movement," and "Adult Protective Services." Their Home- and Community-Based Services (HCBS) Clearinghouse offers resources and tools for research, policymaking, and program development in a one-stop online library, including the outstanding "Directory of ACL National Resource Centers," current as of April 30, 2019 (*Note:* ACL is the Administration for Community Living).

Alzheimer's Association
225 N. Michigan Avenue, Floor 17
Chicago, IL 60601
24/7 Helpline: 800-272-3900
www.alz.org
Founded in 1980, the Alzheimer's Association is the leading voluntary health organization in Alzheimer's care, support, and research. Their mission is to eliminate Alzheimer's disease through the advancement of research; to provide and enhance care and support for all affected; and to reduce the risk of dementia through the promotion of brain health. Offers wide variety of help, information, and resources for researchers, patients, and caregivers, including how to locate local chapters.

American Bar Association Commission on Law & Aging
1050 Connecticut Avenue NW
Suite 400
Washington, DC 20036
Ph: (202) 662-8690
Fax: (202) 662-8698
aging@americanbar.org
www.americanbar.org/aging
As stated on its website: "The ABA Commission on Law and Aging leads the Association in strengthening and securing the legal rights, dignity, autonomy, quality of life and quality of care of older adults. The Commission accomplishes its work through research, policy development, advocacy, education, training and through assistance to lawyers, bar associations and others working on aging issues."

BIFOCAL: The Journal of the Commission on Law and Aging is available on their website. Recent issues covered topics including screening for elder fraud and abuse; older immigrants and public benefits; bridging the lawyer-clinician gap in advance care planning, and examining Medicare and oral health coverage.

American Council of the Blind (ACB)
1703 N. Beauregard Street
Suite 420
Alexandria, VA 22311
Ph: 202-467-5081
Toll Free: 800-424-8666
Fax: 703-465-5085
info@acb.org
www.acb.org
The American Council of the Blind (ACB) is a national membership organization of blind and visually impaired people; it was founded in 1961, but many of its state affiliates and local chapters can be traced back to the 1880s. The ACB's mission is to increase the independence, security, equality of opportunity, and quality of life for all blind and visually impaired people. Their national advocacy efforts have included collaborating with other disability organizations on the passage and protection of the Americans with Disabilities Act (ADA); working closely with the Federal Communications Commission (FCC) and industry leaders following the passage of the twenty-first century Communications and Video Accessibility Act (CVAA); and working with the Rehabilitation Services Administration (RSA) to ensure that services provided to blind and visually impaired American by each state and territory are appropriate and effective. The ACB offers a wide variety of programs and services; resources, including a list of publications and training sites, and contacts for peer support groups for, among others, people with low vision, people who are blind, people who are deaf-blind, guide dog users, seniors, students, the LGBT community, women and families experiencing vision loss. Many of these groups host regular meetings by conference call. In addition, *ACB Radio* has been broadcasting across multiple streams since 1999.

American Foundation for the Blind (AFB)
1401 South Clark Street
Suite 730
Arlington, VA 22202
Phone: 212-502-7600
www.afb.org
A national nonprofit, the American Foundation for the Blind (AFB) was founded in 1921; their mission is to

create a world of no limits for people who are blind or visually impaired. AFB champions access and equality and is at the forefront of new technologies and evidence-based advocacy. Formed through the support of philanthropist MC Migel, AFB's profile was raised when Helen Keller, the world-famous author, activist, and advocate, began working with the organization in 1924. [Helen Keller (1880-1968) was left blind and deaf after a childhood illness; her early life was dramatized in the acclaimed play (and later movie) *The Miracle Worker.*] AFB expands and shares knowledge, including original research, in their peer-reviewed journal for professionals, *Journal of Visual Impairment & Blindness* (available by subscription). Their monthly publication, *Access World Magazine,* which offers informed commentary, cutting-edge news, product reviews, and trends concerning information technology and visual impairment is available on their website. Their work devoted to aging, *No Limits Aging,* (afb.org/research-and-initiatives/aging) addresses the fact that an aging population means increases in age-related vision issues (e.g., macular degeneration, cataracts, and glaucoma). Through their *Twenty-First Century Agenda on Aging and Vision Loss* they are joining with other advocates to protect and promote the rights of seniors with vision loss to live lives of enjoyment, inclusion, and independence. In addition, the AFB houses the Helen Keller Archive, the world's largest repository of letters, speeches, audio-visual materials, and other items, relating to Helen Keller. This archival collection is now available to researchers and the general public as the first ever fully accessible *Helen Keller Digital Archives. (afb.org/HelenKellerArchive).*

American Geriatrics Society (AGS)
40 Fulton Street
18th Floor
New York, NY 10038
Ph: (212) 308-1414
Fax: (212) 832-8648
info.amger@americangeriatrics.org
www.americangeriatrics.org
The American Geriatrics Society (AGS), founded in 1942, is a nationwide, not-for-profit society of geriatrics health-care professionals dedicated to improving the health, independence, and quality of life of older people, and ensure that older people have access to high-quality, person-centered care informed by geriatrics principles. They offer education to professionals, including a list of their "Position Statements," and meetings. The "For the Public" section takes the user to their site "HealthinAging.org" (healthinaging.org/) that features educational materials for older people and caregivers, and a directory of geriatrics health-care professionals. The AGS also publishes four professional journals: *Journal of the American Geriatrics Society; Journal of Gerontological Nursing; Geriatric Nursing; and Annals of Long-Term Care.*

American Macular Degeneration Foundation (AMDF)
PO Box 515
Northampton, MA 01061-0515
Ph: (413) 268-7660
Toll Free: 1-888-MACULAR (1-888-622-8527)
www.macular.org
Macular degeneration is the leading cause of vision loss in Americans 60 and older. There are two types, dry and wet; wet occurs in about 10% of people with macular degeneration and causes most of the vision loss associated with the condition.

The American Macular Degeneration Foundation (AMDF) site includes "About Macular Degeneration," "Treatment," "Research and Cases," and "Service Providers," where one can find a professional by area and specialty across the United States.

American Society on Aging (ASA)
575 Market Street, Suite 2100
San Francisco, CA 94105-2869
Ph: (415) 974-9600 OR (800)-537-9728
Fax: (415) 974-0300
www.asaging.org
The American Society on Aging (ASA), founded in 1954 as the Western Gerontological Society, is an association of diverse individuals bound by a common goal: to support the commitment and enhance the knowledge and skills of those who seek to improve the quality of life of older adults and their families. Their membership is multidisciplinary and inclusive of professionals who are concerned with the physical, emotional, social, economic and spiritual aspects of aging. ASA offers professional education, publications, and online information and training resources. ASA's annual conference, *Aging in America* (www.asaging.org/aia) is the nation's largest gathering of professionals in health care, govern-

ment, business and philanthropy with expertise in providing services and products for older adults. *Aging Today,* ASA's bimonthly newspaper, covers news, advances and controversies in research, practice, and policy; *Generations* is their scholarly quarterly journal with in-depth articles. Both publications are available by subscription.

Asociacion Nacional por Personas Mayores / National Association for Hispanic Elderly (ANPPM/NAHE)
234 East Colorado Boulevard, Suite 300
Pasadena, CA 91101
Ph: (626) 564-1988
Fax: (626) 564-2659
www.anppm.org
The Asociacion Nacional por Personas Mayores/National Association for Hispanic Elderly (ANPPM/NAHE) was founded in 1975 to serve the needs of Hispanic elderly and other low income persons. It is recognized as the pioneer and leading organization in the field of Hispanic Aging. The scope of the Association's work includes employment programs, services for the elderly, and economic development projects that include low-income housing and neighborhood development programs, research and data collection, and training and technical assistance. They also offer free bilingual educational materials in a fotonovela format.

Association of Jewish Aging Services (AJAS)
2519 Connecticut Avenue NW
Washington, DC 20008
Ph: (202) 543-7500
www.ajas.org
Founded in 1960, the Association of Jewish Aging Services (AJAS) is a unique association of not-for-profit community-based organizations, rooted in Jewish values, which promotes and supports the delivery of services to an aging population. There are over 95 member communities in the United States and Canada, and members as far away as Israel and Australia. A searchable map allows users to find one nearest to them. In addition, there are "Resources on Jewish Aging," a link to "Find an Elder Abuse Shelter," and "Useful Links for Caregivers." There are also job postings in the field under "Careers."

B'nai B'rith Center for Senior Services (part of B'nai Brith International)
1120 20th Street NW
Suite 300N
Washington, DC 20036
Ph: (202) 857-6600
www.bnaibrith.org/seniors.htttml
B'nai B'rith International (www.bnaibrith.org) is a highly respected organization that has been dedicated to improving the quality of life for those around the globe since 1843. As advocates, B'nai Brith Center for Senior Services works in Washington, DC to inform elected officials how seniors feel regarding various legislation, including housing, health care and Medicare, and Social Security. The mission of B'nai B'rith Senior Housing is to provide seniors with quality, affordable housing in a secure, supportive community environment, without regard to religion, race or national origin to maximize their independent and dignified lifestyle. Their *"Seniority Report"* newsletter is available on their website and also will be sent to individuals on request.

Centers for Medicare & Medicaid Services
7500 Security Boulevard
Baltimore, MD 21244
Ph: (410) 786-0727
Toll Free: 866-226-1819
TTY (410) 786-3000
TTY Toll-Free: 877-267-2323
www.cms.gov
The place for information on Medicare, Medicaid, and the Health Insurance Exchanges. Offers helpful links to all Centers for Medicare & Medicaid Services (CMS) & US Department of Health & Human Services (HHS) (websites. Under "Contacts" drop-down menus allows locating contacts by location and type of service.

Center for the Study of Aging & Human Development
Duke University Medical Center
Box 3003 DUMC
Room 352
Brusse Bldg, Blue Zone, Duke South
Durham, NC 27710
Ph: (919) 668-7500
Fax: (919) 668-0453
sites.duke.edu/centerforaging

The Center for the Study of Aging and Human Development was one of five centers for aging research established by the Surgeon General of the United States in 1955. It is the only continuously funded member of the original group. With more than 126 Faculty (Senior Fellows) and core staff, and more than $20 million in age-related research funding, it remains a vital national resource for the study of aging. Duke researchers understand that the growing number of older adults will have a significant impact on our society's arrangements for income maintenance, health care, social services, housing and transportation. Studies being conducted at Duke today already are addressing the complex health problems of a longer-lived population, and developing programs that will enable the elderly to receive care while maintaining their independence for as long as possible.

Children of Aging Parents (CAPS)
PO Box167
Richboro, PA 18954
Ph: (800) 227-7294
info@caps4caregivers.org
www.caps4caregivers.org
Children of Aging Parents (CAPS) is a nonprofit, charitable organization whose mission is to assist the nation's caregivers of the elderly or chronically ill with reliable information, referrals and support, and to heighten public awareness that the health of family caregivers is essential to ensure quality care of the nation's growing elderly population.

Experience Works
4401 Wilson Boulevard, Suite 220
Arlington, VA 22203
Ph: (703) 522-7272
Toll Free: (866) 397-9757
www.experienceworks.org
Experience Works is a national, nonprofit organization dedicated to helping people age with dignity and purpose through training, community service, and employment.

First started in 1965 when the National Farmers Union piloted a jobs program for older displaced farmers called Green Thumb, Experience Works focuses in three main areas: (1) "Ticket to Work," a free and voluntary program that can help Social Security beneficiaries with disabilities access meaningful employment and become financially independent; (2) Retired Senior Volunteer Program (RSVP), which provides the opportunity for people age 55 or older to share their time and talent in a wide variety of volunteer activities, and (3) Senior Community Service Employment (SCSEP), a community service and work-based job training program for older adults that serves as a bridge to securing unsubsidized jobs with local employees.

Gerontological Society of America (GSA)
1220 L Street NW, Suite 901
Washington, DC 20005
Ph: (202) 842-1275
www.geron.org
Founded in 1945, the Gerontological Society of America (GSA) is the nation's oldest and largest interdisciplinary organization devoted to research, education, and practice in the field of aging. The principal mission of GSA is to advance the study of aging and disseminate information among scientists, decision makers, and the general public. The GSA consists of four professional sections: Biological Sciences, Behavioral and Social Sciences, Health Sciences, and Social Research, Policy, and Practice. GSA publishes the longest-running and most widely cited peer-reviewed journals in its field: *The Gerontologist; The Journals of Gerontology Series A: Biological Sciences and Medical Sciences,* and *The Journals of Gerontology Series B: Psychological Sciences Social Sciences.* In 2017, GSA launched *Innovation in Aging,* its first interdisciplinary open access journal. The Academy for Gerontology in Higher Education (AGHE) (*see separate entry*) is GSA's educational organization, and the National Academy on an Aging Society, conducts and compiles research on issues related to population aging and provides information to the public, the press, policymakers, and the academic community.

Gray Panthers
733 15th Street, NW
Suite 437
Washington, DC 20005
Ph: (202) 737-6637
Toll Free: (800) 280-5362
Fax: (202) 737-1160
info@graypanthers.org
www.graypanthers.org/home.htm
The Gray Panthers is a national organization of intergenerational activists—young, old, and everyone

in between—dedicated to social change. Founded in 1970 by social activist Maggie Kuhn, the organization consists of more than fifty local networks that work for peace, employment, housing, antidiscrimination legislation, greater rights for the disabled, family security, environmental issues, and campaign reform. The Gray Panthers has helped fight forced retirement at age sixty-five, has exposed nursing home abuse, and has worked for the adoption of universal health care. Members of the Gray Panthers mobilize voters on a variety of issues; testify before legislative bodies, at utility board hearings, and in various forums; and take part in demonstrations, either alone or in coalitions, to bring certain problems to the attention of the public and the media. See entry in *Aging*.

HealthinAging.org
40 Fulton St., 18th Floor
New York, NY 11038
Ph: (212) 308-1414
Fax: (212) 832-8646

Created by the American Geriatrics Society (AGS) and accessible via their website, HealthinAging.org features educational materials for older people and caregivers, and a directory of geriatrics health-care professionals.

Hospice Association of America (HAA)
228 Seventh Street, SE
Washington, DC 20003
Ph: (202) 547-7424
hospice.nahc.org

The Hospice Association of America (HAA) is an affiliate of the National Association for Home Care & Hospice (NAHC) that represents thousands of hospice organizations, caregivers, and volunteers who serve terminally ill patients and their families. HAA advocates on behalf of the industry's interests before Congress and regulatory agencies, as well as other national organizations, the courts, the media, and the public. The site includes regulatory resources, regulatory policy positions, legislative resources, and legislative policy positions. A twice-monthly newsletter, *Hospice Notes*, and a Home Care & Hospice Members Email Listserv are available to members.

LeadingAge
2519 Connecticut Avenue NW
Washington, DC 20008
Ph: (202) 783-2242
info@leadingage.org
www.leadingage.org

In 2008, the American Association of Homes and Services for the Aging (AAHSA) decided to change its name to LeadingAge to better reflect their work and give them a redefined identity that reflected their future aspirations. LeadingAge is a non-profit association whose membership spans the entire field of aging services and includes 38 state partners, and many businesses, consumer groups, foundations and research partners. Their focus is education, advocacy, and applied research.

Little Brothers—Friends of the Elderly
954 W. Washington Blvd.
5th Floor
Chicago, IL 60607
Ph: (312) 829-3055
Fax: (312) 829-3077
national@little-brothers.org
www.little-brothers.org

The U.S. national headquarters of Little Brothers is located in Chicago, and sites within the United States are located in Boston, Chicago, Cincinnati, Minneapolis-St. Paul, Philadelphia, San Francisco, and the Upper Peninsula of Michigan. Specific addresses for local sites can be obtained from the website or through the national office. Little Brothers-Friends of the Elderly is a national, nonprofit organization committed to relieving isolation and loneliness among the elderly. They offer to people of good will the opportunity to join the elderly in friendship and the celebration of life. The organization was founded in 1946 by French nobleman Armand Marquiset, who devoted himself to alleviating what he termed "the greatest poverty of all—the poverty of love." After witnessing the suffering and hardships of the elderly after World War II, Marquiset began visiting and delivering hot meals with flowers to the elderly poor in Paris. Chartered in 1959 in the United States (one of eight member countries, including Canada, France, Germany, Ireland, Mexico, Morocco, and Spain), Little Brothers is a founding member of the Fédération Internationale des petits frères des Pauvres (International Federation of Little Brothers of the Poor).

National Adult Protective Services Association (NAPSA)
1612 K Street NW, #200
Washington, DC 20006
Ph: (202) 370-6292
www.napsa-now.org

The National Adult Protective Services Association (NAPSA) is a non-profit organization with members in all fifty states. Formed in 1989, the goal of NAPSA is to provide Adult Protective Services (APS) programs a forum for sharing information, solving problems, and improving the quality of services for victims of elder and vulnerable adult mistreatment. Its mission is to strengthen the capacity of APS at the national, state, and local levels, to effectively and efficiently recognize, report, and respond to the needs of elders and adults with disabilities who are the victims of abuse, neglect, or exploitation, and to prevent such abuse whenever possible. NAPSA conducts research and works to increase national awareness of elder and vulnerable adult mistreatment through education, advocacy, and congressional testimony.

National Asian Pacific Center on Aging (NAPCA)
1511 Third Avenue
Suite 914
Seattle, WA 98101-1626
Ph: (206) 624-1221
Fax: (206) 624-1023
www.napca.org

NAPCA envisions a society in which all Asian Americanand Pacific Islanders (AAPI) age with dignity and well-being. The relationships NAPCA has developed with AAPI communities and their extensive direct service to AAPI older adults has allowed them to identify their unique needs and focus on areas to improve their quality of life. Under each "Impact Areas," Dementia, Elder Abuse Prevention, Family Caregiving, Healthy Aging and Mature Workers, the site explains "the Challenge, What They Do, the Impact, and Resources." In another section of the site are "Programs and Special Projects." Their National Resource Center on AAPI Aging, established in 2015, is the nation's first and only technical assistance dedicated to building the capacity of long-term service and support systems to equitably serve AAPI seniors and their caregivers. This section includes information on Medicare Information and Assistance and how to help stop Medicare fraud; AAPI population counts and identifying AAPI languages.

National Association for Home Care & Hospice (NAHC)
228 7th Street, SE
Washington, DC 20003
Ph: (202) 547-7427
Fax: (202) 547-3540
www.nahc.org

The National Association for Home Care & Hospice (NAHC) is the largest professional organization representing the interests of chronically ill, disabled, and dying Americans of all ages and the caregivers who provide them with in-home health and hospice services. NAHC is a trade association that represents the nation's 33,000 home care and hospice organizations. Consumer information includes a "Home Care and Hospice Agency Locator," "Home Care & Hospice Basics" information, and "What Are the Standard Billing and Payment Practices?"

National Association of Area Agencies on Aging (n4a)
1100 New Jersey Avenue, SE, Suite 350
Washington, DC 20003
Ph: (202) 872.0888
Fax: (202) 872-0057
info@n4a.org
www.n4a.org

The primary mission of the National Association of Area Agencies (n4a) is to build the capacity of their members so they can help older adults and people with disabilities live with dignity and choices in their homes and communities for as long as possible. They help Washington set priorities, raise the visibility of AAAs and their programs nationwide, and offer training and educational events. Several consumer brochures are available in English and Spanish for download; some may be ordered for postal delivery.

National Association of Nutrition and Aging Services Programs (NANASP)
1612 K Street, NW
Suite 200
Washington, DC 20006
Ph: (202)-682-6899
Fax: (202)-223-2099

nanasp.org

Founded in 1977, the National Association of Nutrition and Aging Services Programs (NANASP) is a leading organization advocating for community-based senior nutrition programs and staff. Their member programs represent a wide range of essential services providers who support the nutrition, health and quality of life of seniors. NANASP is an active member of the aging network and works collaboratively with key coalitions on issues including nutrition, Medicare and Medicaid, elder justice, Social Security, transportation, and older workers' issues.

The National Caucus and Center on Black Aging, Inc. (NCBA)
1220 L Street NW
Suite 800
Washington, DC 20005
Ph: (202) 637-8400
Fax: (202) 347-0895
www.ncba-aging.org

The National Caucus and Center on Black Aging, Inc. (NCBA) was founded in 1970 to ensure that the particular concerns of elderly minorities would be addressed in the then-upcoming 1971 White House Conference on Aging (WHCoA). Since then, NCBA has helped protect and improve the quality of life for elderly populations, making certain that legislators, policymakers, philanthropists, advocacy groups, service organizations, thought leaders and the public-at-large include minority seniors in their programs, policy and law making, and giving. NCBA is one of the country's oldest organizations dedicated to aging issues and the only national organization devoted to minority and low-income aging. Services include employment, health and wellness, and affordable housing. In addition, there is a list of "Helpful Links," including "Caregiving and Caring for Self," "Exercise," and "Finances."

National Center for Creative Aging (NCCA)
2519 Connecticut Avenue NW
Washington, DC 20016-2105
Ph: (202) 895-9456
Fax: (202) 895-9483
info@creativeaging.org
www.creativeaging.org

It's projected that by 2030 more than 70 million people, or 28% of Americans, will be 65 or older, and between 2000 and 2040, the number of Americans age 85 or older will grow from 4.3 million to 19.4 million. As biomedicine has eliminated some of the more debilitating conditions of old age, we can expect people to live longer, healthier, and more productive lives than ever before. Therefore, professionals in many disciplines are keenly interested in the theory and practice of creative work by, and for, older people—whether fully active or frail. Those in creative fields are finding an extraordinary opportunity: to transform the experience of being old in America by giving meaning and purpose, not only to aging, but to the community at large. The National Center for Creative Aging (NCCA) was established in 2001 as a program within Elders Share the Arts (ESTA) through a Partnership with the National Council on Aging (NCOA) and the National Endowment for the Arts (NEA). NCCA is the "go-to" resource for creative consulting and training.

National Committee to Preserve Social Security and Medicare (NCPSSM)
111 K Street NW, Suite 700
Washington, DC 20002
Ph: 1-800-966-1935
www.ncpssm.org

The National Committee to Preserve Social Security and Medicare (NCPSSM) was founded in 1982 to serve as an advocate for the landmark federal programs of Social Security and Medicare for all Americans who seek a healthy, productive, and secure retirement. A membership organization, NCPSSM is the second-largest grassroots citizens' organization devoted to the retirement future of all citizens, both current and future generations. Volunteer opportunities run the gamut from displaying a bumper sticker to joining a Capitol Action Team. Site resources include "Ask our Social Security Experts," "Equal Time," which fact-checks the politically charged myths and misleading media statements about Social Security and Medicare, and "The 115th Congress," which tracks bills as they move through Congress.

National Council on Aging (NCOA)
251 18th Street S, Suite 500
Arlington, VA 22202
Ph: (571) 527-3900
www.ncoa.org

Founded in 1950 in response to concerns about rising health costs and mandatory retirement, the National Council on Aging (NCOA) continues to champion important issues and create innovative programs that reflect our core values and that make life better for all older adults, especially those who are struggling. NCOA is a respected national leader and trusted partner to nonprofit organizations, government, and business to provide innovative community programs and services, online help, and advocacy. Their purview includes the National Institute of Senior Citizens, the Center for Benefits Access, and the Center for Healthy Aging. Website sections include "Economic Security," "Healthy Living," and "Public Policy," and resources are available for "Professionals," "Older Adults & Caregivers," and "Advocates."

National Federation of the Blind (NFB)
200 East Wells Street at Jernigan Place
Baltimore, MD 21230
Ph: (410) 659-9314
nfb@nfb.org
www.nfb.org
Founded in 1940, the National Federation of the Blind (NFB) was founded on the guiding principles that blind people have an inalienable right to independence, have equal capacity, and that only blind people themselves can legitimately speak for the blind community. The NFB is the largest organization of blind people in the United States, with affiliates in all 50 states and Puerto Rico. Along with services to all blind people, the NFB provides many resources for seniors, (seniors.nfb.org/). By contacting a state affiliate one can learn about area programs. In addition, there is a link to find libraries that provide services to the blind, visually impaired, and a link to find information to join a series of telephone conference calls discussing specific issues of blindness and life.

National Hispanic Council on Aging (NHCOA)
"Casa Iris" NHCOA's Housing Facility
2201 12th Street NW, Suite 101
Washington, DC 20009
Ph: (202) 347-9733
Fax: (202) 347-9735
www.nhcoa.org
The National Hispanic Council on Aging (NHCOA) is the leading national organization working to improve the lives of Hispanic older adults, their families, and their caregivers. In light of the rapid growth of the Latinx aging population, NHCOA also empowers Hispanic older adults and families through leadership development to enable them to age with dignity and become their own best advocates. NHCOA has developed a Hispanic Aging Network of community-based organizations across the United States and Puerto Rico. It also works to ensure the Hispanic community is better understood and fairly represented in US policies. They focus on health, economic security, leadership development and empowerment, and housing. Hispanic older adults are the fastest-growing aging segment of the US population, yet the amount of research related to Latinx seniors is limited. NHCOA has been working to increase and find opportunities for new research related to Hispanic older adults. NHCOA has been working to learn about Alzheimer's disease within the Hispanic community, and has recently conducted research to provide the basis for interventions to ensure early detection of Alzheimer's. In addition, they have conducted one of the first studies of its kind focused specifically on LGTBG Latinx seniors.

National Hospice and Palliative Care Organization (NHPCO)
1731 King Street
Alexandria, VA 22314
Ph: (703) 837-1500
Fax: (703) 837-1223
www.nhpco.org
Founded in 1978, the National Hospice and Palliative Care Organization (NHPCO) is the nation's largest membership organization for providers and professionals who care for people affected by serious and life-limiting illness. Its broad community of members includes local hospice and palliative care providers, networks serving large regions of the United States, and individual professionals. NHPCO gives ongoing inspiration, practical guidance, and legislative representation to hospice and palliative care providers so they can enrich experiences for patients and ease caregiving responsibilities and emotional stress for families. For consumers there is extensive information on hospice and palliative care, including FAQs, and information on how to choose a hospice and a section on "Help me find a provider," based on geographical location.

National Institute on Aging (NIA)
Building 31, Room 5C27
31 Center Drive, MSC 2292
Bethesda, MD 20892
Ph: 1-800-222-2225
TTY: 1-800-222-4225
niaic@nih.gov
www.nia.nih.gov
The National Institute on Aging (NIA), is one of 27 Institutes and Centers of the National Institutes of Health (NIH), which in turn, is part of the US Department of Health & Human Services (HHS). The NIA leads a broad scientific effort to understand the nature of aging and to extend the healthy, active years of life. In addition, the NIA is the primary Federal agency supporting and conducting Alzheimer's disease research. The site contains a wealth of user-friendly health information of interest to older adults, including a browsable A-Z Health Topics list.

National Osteoporosis Foundation (NOF)
251 18th Street S, Suite 630
Arlington, VA 22202
Ph: 1-800-231-4222
info@nof.org
www.nof.org
Founded in 1984, the National Osteoporosis Foundation (NOF) is the leading health organization dedicated to preventing osteoporosis and broken bones, promoting strong bones for life and reducing human suffering through programs of public and clinician awareness, education, advocacy and research. The NOF is, in fact, the nation's only health organization solely dedicated to osteoporosis and bone health. Studies show that one in two women and up to one in four men over age 50 will break a bone due to osteoporosis in their lifetime. Along with information for professionals, there is extensive information for consumers, including educational resources in the NOF Resource Library.

Senior Service America, Inc. (SSAI)
8403 Colesville Road
Suite 200
Silver Spring, MD 20910
Ph: (301) 578-9800
contact@ssa-i.org
www.seniorserviceamerica.org
Senior Service America, Inc. (SSAI) is the only national entity dedicated exclusively to the employment of workers over 50, connecting experienced Americans, especially low income and disadvantaged adults, including veterans and formerly incarcerated workers, with employers in all 50 states, in both rural areas and cities (and everything in between), to ensure a vibrant, diverse, and productive workforce. Their headquarters are in Silver Spring, MD, but they operate offices in California, Maryland, Michigan, and Wyoming.

Stanford Letter Project
Stanford University School of Medicine
291 Campus Drive
Li Ka Shing Building
Stanford, CS 94305-5101
Ph: (650) 493-5000 x65039
periyakoil@stanford.edu
med.stanford.edu/letter/html
This initiative of the Medical School of Stanford University, a prestigious private university in California, was started in 2015 and has as its goal "to help, empower and support all adults to prepare for their future and take the initiative to talk to their doctors and their friends and family about what matters most to them at life's end." Americans don't like to talk about and prepare for the last phase of life, and find it extremely difficult to discuss this important issue with their doctors and with their friends and family. Stanford Medicine created the Letter Project tools to help people write letters about their wishes for care in the future. The website supplies letter templates specifically designed to help voice key information. Templates are free and include "What Matters Most," one for those currently in good health and one for those with chronic illness, both available in eight languages; the "Life Review Letter," which covers seven vital tasks, including acknowledging the important people in one's life, remembering treasured moments, and apologizing to loved ones that the letter writer may have hurt; and even a "Bucket List" template, an itemized list of goals people want to accomplish before they "kick the bucket," or die. AARP has featured the Stanford Letter Project in their *AARP Bulletin*.

United Auto Workers (UAW) Retired and Older Workers Department
8731 E. Jefferson Avenue
Detroit, MI 48214
Ph: (313) 926-5231
Fax: (313) 926-5666
www.uaw.org/members/retirees

The United Auto Workers (UAW) Retired and Older Workers Department was established in 1957 to develop programs and provide services to UAW retirees. The UAW constitution mandates each local union with twenty-five or more retirees to establish a retiree chapter. In 1999, there were 791 chartered chapters. The constitution also requires the establishment of regional councils, as well as area and international area councils. A retiree regional council has been set up in each UAW region. The regional director establishes area councils where there are too few local unions or too few retired members to organize chapters. International area councils are established by the Retired and Older Workers Department to provide services to retirees who live in those parts of the country where there are no local unions but where retirees now live. In 1999, there were a total of thirty-three international area councils. The organization also provides UAW retirees with counseling services and other problem-solving matters at drop-in centers located throughout the United States.

—Compiled by Claire B. Joseph, MS, MA, AHIP

Notable People in the Study or Image of Aging

Angelou, Maya (1928-2014). Celebrated African American poet, singer, memoirist and civil rights activist. Known for her memoirs, especially her first, *I Know Why the Caged Bird Sings* (1969). In 1981 she was appointed to the lifetime Reynolds Professorship of American Studies at Wake Forest University in Winston-Salem, North Carolina. Her poem *On Aging* expressed her positive outlook on getting older in spite of the negative stereotypes associated with it. She began lecturing in 1990 and continued well into her 80s.

Arthur, Beatrice (1923-2009). American actress, most noted for TV, Arthur exemplified the independent middle-aged or older woman in situation comedies, first on the *All in the Family* spinoff *Maude* (1972-1978), and then as Dorothy on *The Golden Girls* (1985-1992).

Atchley, Robert C. (1939-2018). Leader in social gerontology. Professor at Miami University in Oxford, Ohio, and Director of their Scripps Gerontology Center; later Chair of the Gerontology Department at Naropa University in Colorado. He played leadership roles in the American Society on Aging, the Gerontological Society of America, and the Association for Gerontology in Higher Education. His book *The Social Forces in Later Life* (1972), revised as *Social Forces and Aging* (9th ed., 1999) is a standard.

Ball, Lucille (1911-1989). American television and film actress. She starred in the beloved series *I Love Lucy* (1951-1957), with husband Desi Arnaz, as a middle-aged wife and mother trying to enter show business. After their divorce, Ball played an independent older woman in the series *The Lucy Show* (1962-1968) and *Here's Lucy* (1968-1974).

Baltes, Paul B. (1939-). German American psychologist. Baltes built upon the work of Erik H. Erikson in the study of wisdom and successful aging from a cognitive prospective. Baltes taught and conducted research in both the United States and Germany. His work in life span developmental psychology and gerontology produced important books and papers, such as *Successful Aging* (1990), edited with wife Margret.

Bengtson, Vern L. (1941-). American sociologist. Professor at the University of Southern California (USC) Edward R. Royal Institute on Aging. Also holds the title of AARP Professor of Gerontology, University Professor Emeritus. Past President of the Gerontological Society of America. Bengston has conducted a number of studies and written several books as well as many journal articles.

Bismarck, Otto von (1815-1898). German chancellor (1871-1890). In 1880, Bismarck instituted the first program of old-age pensions, which were made available at sixty-five. This became the official age for retirement, and a marker for old age, in most Western countries.

Bourgeois, Louise (1911-2010). Famed French American artist best known for her large-scale sculpture and installation art. She continued working and exhibiting into the last year of her life.

Brennan, William J., Jr. (1906-1997). U.S. Supreme Court justice. Appointed to the Court in 1956, Brennan continued to hear cases until 1990, when he retired at the age of eighty-four.

Burns, George (1896-1996; b. Nathan Birnbaum). American vaudevillian and film actor. Burns gained fame for his act with wife Gracie Allen, who died in 1964. He made a comeback at the age of seventy-nine with the film *The Sunshine Boys* (1975) and went on to star in *Oh, God!* (1977), *Going in Style* (1979), and *Eighteen Again!* (1988). Burns became a symbol for successful aging. He performed stand-up comedy routines, usually about old age, until his death at one hundred.

Butler, Robert N. (1927-2010). Butler was a scholar, psychiatrist, and Pulitzer Prize-winning author who revolutionized the way the world thinks about aging and the elderly. One of the first psychiatrists to engage with older men and women outside of institutional settings, Butler coined the term "ageism" to draw attention to discrimination against older adults and spent a lifetime working to improve their status, medical treatment, and care.

Calment, Jeanne (1875-1997). Frenchwoman. For many years, Calment was officially the world's oldest person. She took up fencing at eighty-five and continued to ride a bicycle at one hundred. She attributed her longevity to port wine, olive oil, and chocolate. She gave up smoking in 1995 only because she could no longer light her own cigarettes. Calment gave many interviews and became a popular media figure.

Camp, Cameron J. (1952-). With over three decades of dedication to the applied and translational research of gerontology, dementia intervention, and cognitive intervention, Dr. Camp has earned international renown for his work to improve the quality of life for persons with dementia and memory disorders. Director of Research and Development at the Center for Applied Research in Dementia in Ohio.

Campisi, Judith, PhD (1952-). Campisi is director of the Campisi Lab at the Buck Institute for Research on Aging, part of the School of Gerontology at the University of Southern California, Davis. Her research focuses on taming cellular senescence, the source of chronic inflammation in major age-related diseases. Co-editor of the respected textbook *The Molecular and Cellular Biology of Aging* (2016).

Castel, Alan, PhD Castel is a Professor in the Department of Psychology at the University of California, Los Angeles (UCLA), where he is the Director of the Castel Memory & Lifespan Cognition Lab. He studies learning, memory, and aging and is interested in how younger and older adults can selectively remember important information. Author of *Better with Age: The Psychology of Successful Aging* (2018).

Coleman, Paul D. (1927-). American neuroscientist. With Steve Buell, Coleman demonstrated that the dendrites of neurons grow in normal aging brains. Until this work, it was assumed that no brain development occurs in later years. Coleman taught in the neurobiology and anatomy department at the University of Rochester.

Costa Jr. Paul T. (1942-) and **Robert R. McCrae** (1949-). American psychologists. Costa and McCrae both worked at the Laboratory of Personality and Cognition at the National Institute on Aging. They developed the Revised NEO Personality Inventory and wrote *Personality in Adulthood* (1990). Costa and McCrae found that personality is quite stable in adulthood, findings that challenge the idea of a midlife crisis.

Cotman, Carl W. (1940-). Cotman is a professor of neurology at the University of California, Irvine School of Medicine, where he is also the founding director of the Institute for Brain Aging and Dementia and the Institute for Memory Impairments and Neurological Disorders (UCI MIND). He is known for researching the neurochemistry of Alzheimer's disease and other forms of dementia.

Cronyn, Hume (1911-). American film and theater actor. Cronyn often worked with his wife, Jessica Tandy. In their later years, they starred in plays and films addressing aging, such as *The Gin Game* (1984) and *Cocoon* (1985). Cronyn co-wrote the play *Foxfire* (1982), for which Tandy won a Tony Award.

Dalí, Salvador (1904-1989). Spanish surrealist painter and writer. The eccentric Dalí was known for his distinctive moustache and his dream imagery, such as melting clocks. His prolific career spanned six decades.

Delany, Sadie (1889-1999; b. Sarah Louise) and **Bessie Delany** (1891-1995; b. Annie Elizabeth). African American sisters. Sadie was a teacher, and Bessie was a dentist. In 1993, they wrote *Having Our Say: The Delany Sisters' First One Hundred Years*, which described their extraordinary lives and made them celebrities.

Dole, Bob (1923-). U.S. senator from Kansas. Dole won the Republican Party's presidential nomination in 1996, at seventy-three. Some critics and humorists focused on his age as a liability. After losing the election to Bill Clinton, Dole stayed in the public eye by speaking out, from personal experience, about prostate cancer screening and treatments for erectile dysfunction, such as the drug Viagra.

Eastwood, Clint (1930-). Popular TV and movie actor and film director. Starting with his role as Rowdy Yates in TV's popular Western *Wagon Train* (1959-1965), Eastwood went on to star in a number of films. Perhaps his two most iconic roles were as "The Man With No Name" in Sergio Leone's "spaghetti westerns" trilogy: *A Fistful of Dollars* (1964), *For a Few Dollars More* (1965) and *The Good, the Bad and* *the Ugly* (1966), and as antihero cop Harry Callahan in five *Dirty Harry* films in the 1970s and 1980s. While continuing to act, Eastwood also began directing. The western *The Unforgiven* (1992) won Eastwood an Oscar as Best Director, and the movie won as Best Picture; he also starred in the film. In 2004 the dark sports film, *Million Dollar Baby* won as Best Picture; again, Eastwood starred in the film. Eastwood's Oscar as Best Director at the age of 74 made him the oldest winner in that category in Oscar history. Eastwood remains active; in his latest film *The Mule* (2018), Eastwood both starred and directed.

Elizabeth, the Queen Mother (1900-2002). Queen of Great Britain as the wife of George VI, she became known as the Queen Mother after the accession of her daughter Queen Elizabeth II to the throne. Immensely popular with the public, in her advanced years she remained active in the traditions of her prominent but troubled family.

Elizabeth II (1926-). Queen of Great Britain. Ascended to the throne in 1953 after the death of her father, George VI (1895-1952); longest reigning British monarch.

Erikson, Erik H. (1902-1994). German psychologist. Erikson was famous for his eight stages of psychosocial development, which included three stages in adulthood. His stages of generativity (in middle age) and ego integrity (in old age) are included in every aging textbook and are cited in most works on understanding the self and relationships in adulthood. See entry in *Aging*.

Fonda, Henry (1905-1982). American film actor. After a long and celebrated career, Fonda won his first Academy Award as Best Actor at age seventy-seven for his role as an aging father in *On Golden Pond* (1981). Because he was too ill to take the stage, daughter and costar Jane Fonda accepted for him.

Franklin, Benjamin (1706-1790). American diplomat, inventor, scientist, businessman, and writer. Franklin spent his seventies as a diplomat at the court of Louis XVI in France and served as an important member of the Constitutional Convention of 1787. He was active in politics and social issues until his death at age eighty-four.

Friedan, Betty (1921-; b. Betty Goldstein). American feminist. Friedan gained fame for her book *The Feminine Mystique* (1963), which addressed the lack of fulfillment among white, middle-class housewives. She tackled the social perceptions of older people in *The Fountain of Age* (1993).

Fry, Christine L. (1943-). Fry has specialized in the anthropology of age by first living in a retirement community and then investigating the cognitive organization of the life-course in the United States. Most recently she has directed Project AGE, a cross-cultural research endeavor to examine the meaning of age and how different communities shape the experience of aging.

Ginsburg, Ruth Bader (1933-). Appointed as Supreme Court Justice in 1993, Ginsburg had a long and celebrated career as an attorney who was devoted to gender equality and women's rights. In 2018 a documentary of Ginsburg *RBG* was released, and in 2019 a feature film *On the Basis of Sex* with Felicity Jones as Ginsburg focused on her early career.

Glenn, John (1921-2016). American astronaut and U.S. senator from Ohio. In 1962, as one of the original NASA astronauts, he became the first American to orbit the earth. Glenn was elected to the U.S. Senate from Ohio in 1975. In 1998, at the age of seventy-seven, he returned to space as a member of a shuttle crew, this time to test the effects of zero gravity on the aged body. He became the oldest person to travel into space.

Gordon, Ruth (1896-1985). American film and theater actress, playwright, and screenwriter. Gordon won an Academy Award as Best Supporting Actress for *Rosemary's Baby* (1968). She earned a cult-like following for her starring role as a vivacious, eccentric woman turning eighty in *Harold and Maude* (1971).

Graham, Martha (1893-1991). American dancer, choreographer, and teacher. Graham had the greatest influence on modern dance in the twentieth century. She retired from dancing in 1970, at seventy-seven. Graham continued to choreograph, arranging Igor Stravinsky's *Rite of Spring* at the age of ninety.

Griffith, Andy (1926-2012). American film and television actor. Best known for his television series, *The*

Andy Griffith Show (1960-1968) and *"Matlock"* (1986-1995).

Hayflick, Leonard (1928-). Leonard Hayflick is a Professor of Anatomy at the University of California, San Francisco (UCSF) School of Medicine, and was Professor of Medical Microbiology at Stanford University School of Medicine. He is a past president of the Gerontological Society of America and was a founding member of the council of the National Institute on Aging. Books include *How and Why We Age* (1996).

Hepburn, Katharine (1907-2003). American film actress. Hepburn won four Academy Awards as Best Actress, three of them in her later years for her roles in *Guess Who's Coming to Dinner?* (1967), *The Lion in Winter* (1968), and *On Golden Pond* (1981). She remained active and independent throughout her life.

Hope, Bob (1903-2003). American comedian and actor whose career spanned vaudeville, radio, movies, and television. Best remembered for his series of "Road" movies with Bing Crosby (1903-1977) and for entertaining US troops with a USO (United Service Organization) show from 1941-1991.

Hopper, Grace Murray (1906-1992). American mathematician and computer pioneer. In the 1950s, as a member of the U.S. Navy, she worked on such computer languages as FLOW-MATIC and COBOL. Rear Admiral Hopper retired in 1986, at age eighty, as the oldest active Navy officer.

Jackson, James S. (1944-). American sociologist. Jackson is known for his psychological work on the African American family, particularly the elderly. He is the author of *Life in Black America* (1991).

Kalish, Richard A. (1930-). American sociologist. A behavioral scientist in the field of death and dying, Kalish coined the term "new ageism." He theorized that at least three factors contribute to diminished death anxiety in the old. Kalish is the author of *The Psychology of Human Behavior* (1969) and *Death, Grief* and *Caring Relationships* (1981).

Keith, Jennie (1942-). A leading authority on aging and professor emeritus of Anthropology at Swarthmore, she is co-author of *The Aging Experience: Diversity and Commonality Across Cultures* (Sage Publications, 1994), which presents findings of a decade-long cross-cultural study of growing old in the United States and several other countries. Because of the value this society places on independence, and because care for the elderly often emphasizes institutionalization over community and home settings, Keith finds that older people in America face a unique set of challenges. Among several dozen other books and articles, she is the author of *Old People, New Lives: Community Creation in a Retirement Residence* (U of Chicago P, 1977).

Kennedy, Rose Fitzgerald (1890-1995). American matriarch. As the wife of Joseph Kennedy, Sr., U.S. ambassador to Great Britain, and the mother of President John F. Kennedy and Senators Robert F. and Edward (Ted) Kennedy, Rose Kennedy helped shape the foremost political dynasty in the United States until her death at 105.

Kevorkian, Jack (1928-2011). American pathologist and euthanasia proponent, Kevorkian provided the medical means for over a hundred people to end their lives by voluntary euthanasia. In 1998 he was convicted of second-degree murder and served 8 years of a 10-25-year sentence. The publicity surrounding his cases helped focus the national debate about physician-assisted suicide.

Kleemeier, Robert W. (1915-). American sociologist. Kleemeier, a former president of the Gerontological Society of America, made exemplary contributions to the quality of life through research in aging.

Kübler-Ross, Elizabeth (1926-2004). Swiss American psychiatrist. Kübler-Ross described five distinct stages through which many terminally ill patients pass: denial, anger, bargaining, depression, and acceptance. She wrote in *On Death and Dying* (1969) that each stage acts as a defense mechanism against the fear of death. See entry in *Aging*.

Kuhn, Maggie (1905-1995). American social activist. In 1971, Kuhn founded the Consultation of Older and Younger Adults for Social Change, which was soon renamed the Gray Panthers. She worked for nursing home reform, fought ageism, and claimed that "old people constitute America's biggest untapped and undervalued human energy source." See entry in *Aging*.

Kurosawa, Akira (1910-1998). Japanese director. Kurosawa continued to make critically acclaimed films in his eighties, even after he became blind.

La Lanne, Jack (1914-2011). American fitness guru. Known as the Godfather of Physical Fitness, La Lanne began in the fitness business in 1936 and was still going strong in his eighties thanks to a vegetarian diet and an intense exercise regimen. Throughout his career, he encouraged seniors to become more active to lead healthier, longer lives.

Lansbury, Angela (1925-). American film, actor, and television actress. After a long career on stage and screen, Lansbury played the role of older mystery writer and amateur detective Jessica Fletcher on the popular series *Murder, She Wrote* (1984-1996).

Lawton, M. Powell (1923-2001). American sociologist. Lawton became known for his studies on the fit between person and environment and how that fit affects competence in the elderly. His work shows that, as with other groups, the optimal environment for the elderly involves challenge.

Lemmon, Jack (1925-). American film actor. Lemmon's later roles, often opposite Walter Matthau, appealed to older audiences. They starred in *Grumpy Old Men* (1993), *Grumpier Old Men* (1995), *Out to Sea* (1997), and *The Odd Couple II* (1998). Lemmon also starred in *My Fellow Americans* (1996) as a former U.S. president.

Levinson, Daniel (1920-1994). American psychologist. Levinson is known for *The Seasons of a Man's Life* (1978), the first book to address the concept of midlife crisis. He outlined the stages that men may go through in adulthood, and his later research provided information on women's stages as well.

Lloyd, Norman (1914-). Noted veteran actor of the stage, screen, and TV, and TV producer. What happens to his character (the saboteur) in Alfred Hitchcock's *The Saboteur* (1942) after he is chased to the torch of the Statue of Liberty is an iconic image in film history. Later starred as Dr. Daniel Auschlander in the popular TV medical series *St. Elsewhere* (1982-1988). Latest film role was in Amy Schumer's film *Trainwreck* (2015).

Lopata, Helena Znaniecki (1925-2003). Polish American sociologist, author, and researcher. Lopata studied lives of women and wrote, among other works, *Widowhood in an American City* (1973) and *Women as Widows: Support Systems* (1979).

Marshall, Thurgood (1908-1993). First African American Supreme Court Justice. A former attorney with a long and respected history of fighting for equality, it was Marshall who successfully argued the landmark case *Brown v. the Board of Education* in 1954 before the Supreme Court. Continued as Supreme Court Justice until 1991 when he retired at the age of 83.

Matthau, Walter (1920-; b. Walter Matuschanskayasky). American film actor. Matthau's later roles, often opposite Jack Lemmon, appealed to older audiences. They starred in *Grumpy Old Men* (1993), *Grumpier Old Men* (1995), *Out to Sea* (1997), and *The Odd Couple II* (1998). Matthau also starred in *I'm Not Rappaport* (1996) and as Albert Einstein in *I.Q.* (1994).

Moreno, Rita (1931-). Puerto Rican actress/singer/dance of film, Broadway, and TV. Began her career playing stereotypical Latinas in movies, went on to become one of a small number of performers who have won all four major performing awards: the Oscar, Emmy, Grammy, and Tony. Her performance as Anita in 1961's film version of *West Side Story* won her a Best Supporting Actress Oscar. Moreno plays the matriarch of a Cuban American family in *"One Day at a Time"* (2017-), a reboot of the series that first ran from 1975-1984.

Morgenthau, Robert (1919-2019). Served as District Attorney of Manhattan (NYC) from 1975-2009, retiring at the age of 90.

Morrison, Toni (1931-2019) Acclaimed African American author and teacher. Morrison's first novel, *The Bluest Eye*, was published in 1970. Her 1987 novel *Beloved* won the Pulitzer Prize and was made into a 1998 film with Oprah Winfrey and Danny Glover. In 1993 Morrison was awarded the Nobel Prize in Literature. She held the Robert F. Goheen Chair in the Humanities at Princeton University from her appointment in 1989 to her retirement in 2006. Her last novel, *God Help the Child,* was released in 2015.

Moses, Grandma (1860-1961; b. Anna Mary Robertson). American folk artist. Moses took up painting in her seventies after the death of her husband. She became known for primitive paintings depicting rural life in the nineteenth and twentieth century United States.

Myerhoff, Barbara G. (1936? -1985). American anthropologist. Myerhoff became known for her work with the urban elderly, especially the elderly Jews of Los Angeles, as depicted in the book and Academy Award-winning documentary *Number Our Days*. With Myerhoff's work, the anthropological study of the urban elderly grew tremendously.

Neugarten, Bernice (1916-2001). Neugarten was an American psychologist who specialized in adult development and the psychology of ageing.

Newman, Paul (1925-2008). American film actor and businessman. A longtime favorite with critics and audiences, Newman won his first Academy Award at age sixty-one for *The Color of Money* (1986) for a reprisal of his character Fast Eddie Felson from *The Hustler* (1961). In the 1980s, he started a successful nonprofit food company called Newman's Own, and he continued his hobby of car racing into his seventies.

O'Keeffe, Georgia (1887-1986). Famed American painter, "Mother of American Modernism." She is known for her paintings of New Mexico landscapes and close-up large-scale flowers. Remained active into her 90s.

Palmer, Arnold (1929-2016). American golfer. Palmer won four Master championships in the 1950s and 1960s. In the 1980s, he became a popular fixture on the Senior PGA Tour, winning ten tournaments. In 1998, he played in his forty-fourth Masters but was sidelined briefly for treatment of prostate cancer.

Pauling, Linus (1901-1994). American chemist and pacifist. Pauling won Nobel Prizes in Chemistry (1954) and in Peace (1962). By the time of his death at age ninety-three, however, he was probably better known for his work on nutrition. He made talk-show appearances, published papers, and made presentations about a nutritional healing specialty he named "orthomolecular medicine." Pauling wrote best-selling books on vitamin C, the common cold, and cancer.

Pepper, Claude (1900-1989). U.S. representative from Florida. Pepper became known nationwide for his advocacy of the rights of older Americans. He was first elected to the House of Representatives in 1962 and served until his death at age eighty-nine. As the oldest member of Congress in his last years, he defended Social Security and opposed retirement restrictions.

Poon, Leonard (1942-). American psychologist. Poon became known for his work on memory and aging. He headed the Georgia Centenarian Study, one of the largest studies on centenarians in the United States.

Quadagno, Judith S., PhD (1942-). Dr. Quadagno is the Mildred and Claude Pepper Institute on Public Aging and Policy Emerita Scholar at Florida State University (FSU), where she was a Professor in the Department of Sociology. Author of *Aging and the Life Course: An Introduction to Social Gerontology*, 7th ed. (2018).

Randall, Tony (1920-; b. Leonard Rosenberg). American film and television actor. Randall became best known as the fussy Felix Unger on the series *The Odd Couple* (1970-1975). He founded the National Actors Theatre in 1992 and made headlines in 1997 by becoming a first-time father at the age of seventy-seven.

Reagan, Ronald (1911-2004). U.S. president (1981-1989). Reagan was first elected president at the age of seventy. When he left office, at seventy-eight, he was the oldest person to serve as president. In 1994, Reagan announced that he was suffering from Alzheimer's disease, thus raising awareness of this debilitating condition.

Redford, Robert (1936-) Popular and acclaimed actor and director, Redford has appeared in a number of popular films, including two with Paul Newman, 1969's. *Butch Cassidy and the Sundance Kid* and 1973's *The Sting*. His first film as Director was in 1981 with *Ordinary People* that won him the Oscar for Best Director. Redford founded the Sundance Institute in 1981 in Utah, a non-profit organization committed to the growth of independent artists. One of its programs is the annual Sundance Film Institute. In 2018, Redford starred in *The Old Man and the Gun* about an aging bank robber; he announced that he is now retiring from film.

Rowe, John W. (1944-). Julius B. Richmond Professor of Health Policy and Aging at the Columbia University Mailman School of Public Health. Dr. Rowe was a Professor of Medicine and the founding Director of the Division on Aging at the Harvard Medical School and Director of the MacArthur Foundation Research Network on Successful Aging; currently he leads the MacArthur Foundation's Network on An Aging Society. He is the co-author with Robert L. Kahn, PhD (1918-2019) of the book *Successful Aging* (1998).

Salthouse, Timothy (1947-). Salthouse is Brown-Forman Professor of Psychology at the University of Virginia; he was previously Professor of Psychology at the University of Missouri-Columbia and the Georgia Institute of Technology. A former editor of the journal *Psychology and Aging,* Salthouse is known for his work on cognitive research on aging.

Sanders, Harland (1890-1980). American businessman. Known as Colonel Sanders, he opened his first restaurant in 1939. In 1952, at the age of sixty-two, he granted the first franchise in what became the international chain Kentucky Fried Chicken. In 1964, Sanders sold the company for two million dollars but stayed on as spokesperson.

Sarton, May (1912-1995). Belgian American writer. Sarton examined the experience of aging in her poetry and novels and in her journals, including *At Seventy: A Journal* (1984), *Endgame: A Journal of the Seventy-ninth Year* (1992), *Encore: A Journal of the Eightieth Year* (1993), and *At Eighty-two: A Journal* (1996).

Schaie, K. Warner (1928-). Schaie is an American social gerontologist and psychologist best known for founding the Seattle Longitudinal Study in 1956. The Seattle Study took a 'life span' approach to aging and cognition, studying subjects from birth through the life course.

Serra, Richard (1938-). One of the preeminent American sculptors of our era, Richard Serra has long been acclaimed for his challenging and innovative work, which emphasizes materiality and an engagement between the viewer, the site, and the work. In the early 1960s, Serra turned to unconventional, industrial materials and began to accentuate the physical properties of their art. Over the years, Serra has expanded his spatial and temporal approach to sculpture and has focused primarily on large-scale work, including many site-specific works that engage with a particular architectural, urban, or landscape setting. Serra continues to work and exhibit.

Sheehy, Gail (1937-). American writer. Sheehy wrote the popular books *Passages: Predictable Crises of Adult Life* (1976) and *The Silent Passage: Menopause* (1992). Some claim that Sheehy stole Daniel Levinson's theories to serve as the backbone for *Passages*. See entry in *Aging.*

Shock, Nathan (1906-1989). Nathan W. Shock was known as the "father of gerontology" and head of the Gerontology Research Center of the National Institutes of Health (NIH) for nearly 35 years-until 1976. He then became scientist emeritus at the center.

Skinner, B. F. (1904-1990). American behavioral psychologist. Skinner was the foremost authority in his field for several decades. An incredibly productive scholar, he published hundreds of books and articles during his career as professor at Harvard University. As he aged, Skinner developed lifestyle strategies to continue doing the work that he loved, a process he described in *Enjoy Old Age* (1983).

Stuart, Gloria (1910-2010). American film actress of the 1930s, Stuart retired from filmmaking, but began to return to the screen in the late 1970s. She played the 101-year-old Rose in *Titanic* (1997). At the age of eighty-seven, she received an Academy Award nomination as Best Supporting Actress for that performance.

Tandy, Jessica (1909-1994). American film and theater actress. Tandy often worked with her husband, Hume Cronyn. In their later years, they starred in plays and films about the experience of aging, such as *The Gin Game* (1984) and *Cocoon* (1985). Tandy won a Tony for the play *Foxfire* (1982), co-written by Cronyn, and an Academy Award as Best Actress for *Driving Miss Daisy* (1989) at the age of eighty.

Teresa, Mother (1910-1997; b. Agnes Gonxha Bejaxhiu). Albanian nun. Mother Teresa founded the Missionaries of Charity in 1950 in Calcutta, India. She spent the rest of her life tending to the "poorest of the poor" and was awarded the 1979 Nobel Peace Prize for her work. Soon after death at age eighty-seven, the Catholic Church began an investigation into naming her a saint.

Thurmond, Strom (1902-). U.S. senator from South Carolina. Thurmond began his first term in 1954, and his reelection in 1996 at the age of ninety-four made him the oldest person ever to serve in Congress.

Townsend, Francis Everett (1867-1960). American physician. His campaign for federally funded old-age pensions became known as the Townsend Plan and influenced the administration of Franklin D. Roosevelt to found the Social Security system.

Van Dyke, Dick (1925-). Actor/comedian, star of popular *"The Dick Van Dyke Show"* which ran on TV from 1961-1966, and later *"Diagnosis Murder" (1993-2001) and "Murder 101"* (2006-2008). In 1964, he co-starred with Julie Andrews (1935-) in the hit movie *"Mary Poppins"*; remarkably, he performed a dance routine in *"Mary Poppins Returns"* in 2018.

Walford, Roy (1924-). American physician. Walford gained fame for his work on life extension through low-calorie, nutrient-rich diet and exercise. He became particularly known for his work with the experiments Biosphere 1 and 2.

Wellin, Christopher, PhD. Doctor Wellin is a professor at the Department of Sociology and Gerontology Program Coordinator at Illinois State University. He is the editor of the well-received text *Critical Gerontology Comes of Age: Advances in Research for a New Century* (2018).

White, Betty (1922-). Popular actress known primarily for television, especially her roles as catty Sue Ann Nivens in the *Mary Tyler Moore Show* (1973-1977), sweet, often befuddled Rose Nylund in *Golden Girls* (1985-1992) and Elka in *Hot in Cleveland* (2010-2015). White hosted *Saturday Night Live* in 2010 at the age of 88.

Winkler, Henry (1945-). Yale-trained versatile actor, best known for his portrayal of greaser Arthur "Fonzie/The Fonz" Fonzarelli in the popular TV show set in the 1950s, *Happy Days* (1984-1994); won his first Emmy in 2019 for his role as Gene in the dark comedy *Barry* (2018-).

Wood, Beatrice (1893-1998). American potter, ceramist, artist, and photographer. Wood was known as the "Mama of Dada" for her association with painter Marcel Duchamp during World War I, Wood continued to work until her death at age 105. The inspiration for the 101-year-old character of Rose in the film *Titanic* (1997), she cited "chocolate and young men" as the keys to her longevity.

—Compiled by Claire B. Joseph, MS, MA, AHIP

Glossary

acetabulum: the socket of the hipbone, into which the head of the femur fits

acetylcholine: serves as a transmitter substance of nerve impulses within the central and peripheral nervous systems

adiposity: a condition of being severely overweight, or obese

agnosia: inability to interpret sensations and hence to recognize things

alveolar sac: tiny air-filled chambers within the lungs that allow oxygen and carbon dioxide to move between the lungs and bloodstream

alveolar walls: walls of the alveoli, membranous sacs in the lungs; it is through these membranes that dissolved gasses pass during respiration

ampulla: a sac-like enlargement of a canal or duct

amygdala: a roughly almond-shaped mass of gray matter inside each cerebral hemisphere, involved with the experiencing of emotions

analgesic: a pain-killing drug

anemia: a condition marked by a deficiency of red blood cells or of hemoglobin in the blood, resulting in pallor and weariness; results from a lack of certain vitamins and minerals

anthropometry: is the study of human body measurements. Measures the body weight, height, subscapular skinfold, triceps skinfold, mid arm muscle circumference, elbow breadth, abdominal circumference and calf circumference.

anticholinergics: inhibit the transmission of parasympathetic nerve impulses, thereby reducing spasms of smooth muscles

antioxidant: a substance that reduces damage due to oxygen, such as that caused by free radicals

aphasia: loss of ability to understand or express speech

apraxia: inability to perform particular purposive actions

arrhythmic: lacking rhythm or regularity

artery: any of the muscular-walled tubes forming part of the circulation system by which blood (mainly that which has been oxygenated) is conveyed from the heart to all parts of the body

arthroplasty: the surgical reconstruction or replacement of a joint

basal ganglia: a group of structures linked to the thalamus in the base of the brain and involved in coordination of movement

beneficiary: a person who derives advantage from something, especially a trust, will, or life insurance policy

benign: a tumor that does not invade nearby tissue or spread to other parts of the body the way cancer can; can be serious if they press on vital structures such as blood vessels or nerves

Bioelectrical Impedance Analysis (BIA): estimates total body muscle and water composition by measuring resistance to electrical flow.

biologic response modifiers: substances that stimulate the body's response to infection and disease; biologics work by interrupting immune system signals involved in the damage of joint tissue

biopsy: a procedure to remove a small sample of breast tissue for laboratory testing; a breast biopsy is a way to evaluate a suspicious area in the breast to determine whether it is breast cancer

body mass index (BMI): a person's weight in kilograms (kg) divided by his or her height in meters squared

butyrophenones: any of a class of antipsychotics, as haloperidol, used to relieve symptoms of schizophrenia, acute psychosis, or other severe psychiatric disorders

calcification: the hardening of tissue or other material by the deposition of or conversion into calcium carbonate or some other insoluble calcium compounds

calorie: the energy people get from the food and drink they consume, and the energy they use in physical activity

carcinogen: a substance capable of causing cancer in living tissue

cartilage: firm, whitish, flexible connective tissue found in various forms in the larynx and respiratory tract, in structures such as the external ear, and in the articulating surfaces of joints; the wearing down of cartilage can cause bones to rub together, potentially resulting in arthritis

cavity: permanently damaged areas in the hard surface of teeth that develop into tiny openings or holes

cemented prosthesis: uses fast-drying bone cement to help affix prosthetic to the bone

cementless prosthesis: sometimes called a press-fit prosthesis, is specially textured to allow the bone to grow onto it and adhere to it over time

cerebral cortex: the most highly developed part of the human brain and is responsible for thinking, perceiving, producing and understanding language

cervical: seven vertebral bodies that make up the upper most part of the spine and connect the spine to the skull

chemical peeling: a skin-resurfacing procedure in which a chemical solution is applied to the skin to remove the top layers; the skin that grows back after a chemical peel is smoother and younger looking

chromosome: a threadlike structure of nucleic acids and protein found in the nucleus of most living cells, carrying genetic information in the form of genes

chronobiology: the branch of biology concerned with natural physiological rhythms and other cyclical phenomena

chronological (biological) age: number of years a person has lived at a particular measurement point

coccygeal: refers to the coccyx, the small tail-like bone at the bottom of the spine, which is made up of 3-5 (average of 4) rudimentary vertebrae

collagen: the most abundant protein in the human body, found in the bones, muscles, skin, and tendons

comorbidity: the simultaneous presence of two chronic diseases or conditions in a patient

conductive hearing loss: occurs when there is a problem transferring sound waves anywhere along the pathway through the outer ear, eardrum, or middle ear; if a conductive hearing loss occurs in conjunction with a sensorineural hearing loss, it is referred to as a mixed hearing loss

contracture: a condition of shortening and hardening of muscles, tendons, or other tissue, often leading to deformity and rigidity of joints

copper peptides: naturally occurring complexes that have been used for a variety of purposes; the complexes are a combination of the element copper and three amino acids; in the human body, copper peptides are found in trace amounts in blood plasma, saliva, and urine

cornea: the transparent layer forming the front of the eye

corns and calluses: thick, hardened layers of skin that develop when your skin tries to protect itself against friction and pressure

corticosteroids: can be used to treat inflammation of small areas of the body, such as inflammation of a specific joint or tendon

creative potential: ability to raise expression of individual creative abilities and creative performance through creativity training

creative productivity: the value of creative work produced in a day

cryotherapy: This procedure involves using a cotton-tipped swab to apply liquid nitrogen or another freezing agent to the age spots to destroy the extra pigment

cued recall: the retrieval of memory with the help of cues

cystoscopy: procedure in which a lighted optical instrument called a cystoscope is inserted through the urethra to look at the bladder

deferred income: a portion of an employee's compensation that is set aside to be received after the period in which it was earned

demographics: the number and characteristics of people who live in a particular area or form a particular group, especially in relation to their age, economic status, and race

dentin: hard dense bony tissue forming the bulk of a tooth, beneath the enamel

dependency ratio: the number of dependents in a population divided by the number of working age people; dependents are defined as those aged zero to 14 and those aged 65 and older; working age is from 15 to 64

dermabrasion: the removal of superficial layers of skin with a rapidly revolving abrasive tool, as a technique in cosmetic surgery

dermis: the thick layer of living tissue below the epidermis that forms the true skin, containing blood capillaries, nerve endings, sweat glands, hair follicles, and other structures

desynchronization: the relation that exists when things occur at unrelated times

diaphysis: the shaft or central part of a long bone

diastolic: relating to the phase of the heartbeat when the heart muscle relaxes and allows the chambers to fill with blood

diploid cells: cells that contain two sets of chromosomes

disease-modifying antirheumatic drugs (DMARDs): a group of medications that work to suppress the body's overactive immune and/or inflammatory systems

disinhibition: unrestrained behavior resulting from a lessening or loss of inhibitions or a disregard of cultural constraints

diverticulitis: inflammation of a diverticulum, especially in the colon, causing pain and disturbance of bowel function

dopamine: helps regulate movement, attention, learning, and emotional responses

dual energy X-ray absorptiometry (DEXA scan): is used to measure skeletal mass and bone density.

dynamic bone remodeling: a lifelong process where mature bone tissue is removed from the skeleton and new bone tissue is formed

dyspnea: difficult or labored breathing

elastic recoil: the rebound of the lungs after having been stretched by inhalation or the ease with which the lung rebounds

embolic stroke: when a blood clot that forms elsewhere in the body breaks loose and travels to the brain via the bloodstream

enamel: the hard, outer surface layer of teeth that serves to protect against tooth decay; it is the hardest mineral substance in your body, even stronger than bone

endometrium: the innermost lining layer of the uterus, and functions to prevent adhesions between the opposed walls of the myometrium, thereby maintaining the patency of the uterine cavity; during the menstrual cycle, the endometrium grows to a thick, blood vessel-rich, glandular tissue layer

endovenous thermal ablation: a newer technique that uses a laser or high-frequency radio waves to create intense local heat in the varicose vein or incompetent vein

epidermis: the outermost of the three layers that make up the skin, the inner layers being the dermis and hypodermis

epiphyses: the end part of a long bone, initially growing separately from the shaft

episodic memory: a type of long-term memory that involves conscious recollection of earlier experiences together with their context in terms of time, place, associated emotions, and so on

estradiol: an estrogen steroid hormone and the major female sex hormone; it is involved in the regulation of the female reproductive cycles and is responsible for the development of female secondary sexual characteristics such as the breasts, widening of the hips, and a feminine pattern of fat distribution in women

estrogen: any of a group of steroid hormones that promote the development and maintenance of female characteristics of the body

estrone: the major postmenopausal estrogen derived from the conversion of androgens, mainly androstenedione, produced by the ovaries and adrenal glands

fascia: a band or sheet of connective tissue, primarily collagen, beneath the skin that attaches, stabilizes, encloses, and separates muscles and other internal organs

femoral head: the highest, globular part of the femur; it participates in the hip joint

fibroblast: a cell in connective tissue that produces collagen and other fibers

free-recall test: participants study a list of items on each trial, and then are prompted to recall the items in any order

functional age: measure of functional capabilities indexed to a chronological age standard that considers physiological, psychological and social factors; this is generally applied to individuals

gait cycle: the time period or sequence of events or movements during locomotion in which one-foot contacts the ground to when that same foot again contacts the ground, and involves propulsion of the center of gravity in the direction of motion

generativity: a concern for establishing and guiding the next generation

get-up-and-go test: measures the time a person takes to rise from a chair, walk 10 feet, turn around, walk back to the chair, and sit down

globus pallidus: a structure in the brain involved in the regulation of voluntary movement

group annuity: an employer establishes a group annuity on behalf of its employees by signing a master contract with an insurer; this contract details the agreement between the insurer and employer, such as plan type, contribution requirements and administrative fees

handgrip strength: measures the muscular strength in the hands and forearm.

haploid cells: cells that have half the usual number of chromosomes

hemorrhagic stroke: when a weakened blood vessel ruptures and spills blood into brain tissue

highly active antiretroviral therapy (HAART): the use of a combination of three or four anti-HIV drugs in an HIV positive individual to suppress replication of new HIV particles and slow the progression to full-blown AIDS

hippocampus: the elongated ridges on the floor of each lateral ventricle of the brain, thought to be the center of emotion, memory, and the autonomic nervous system

hormone therapy: treatment of disease or symptoms with synthetic or naturally derived hormones

hypertrophy: the enlargement of an organ or tissue from the increase in size of its cells; cells increase in size as we age

hypothalamus: a region of the forebrain below the thalamus that coordinates both the autonomic nervous system and the activity of the pituitary, controlling body temperature, thirst, hunger, and other homeostatic systems, and involved in sleep and emotional activity

incentives: money that a person, company, or organization offers to encourage certain behaviors or actions, like joining a pension plan

interdigital: between the fingers or toes

interphalangeal joints: between the phalanges (bones) of the toes; each toe has two interphalangeal joints, except the big toe, which has one

intestacy: referring to a situation where a person dies without leaving a valid will

intrapleural pressure: the pressure within the pleural cavity, a narrow, fluid-filled space covering the lungs and lining the chest cavity

intrinsic factor: a substance secreted by the stomach that enables the body to absorb vitamin B_{12}

Kaposi's sarcoma: a form of blood vessel tumor that produces pink to purple splotches or plaques on the skin in about 25 percent of persons with AIDS and may also affect internal organs; caused by sexual transmission of human herpes virus 8 (HHV8)

keratin: protein found in the upper layer of the skin, hair, and nails

keratosis: an area of skin marked by overgrowth of horny tissue

kyphotic curve: normally present in the thoracic; looks like the letter "C" with the opening of the C pointing towards the front

lactation: the secretion of milk by the mammary glands

life expectancy at birth (LEB): mean number (statistically) of years of life remaining at a given age for a person from a particular demographic; this is influenced by gender, infant mortality rate, medical advancements, and demographic factors (e.g. AIDS epidemic in Africa)

lifespan: A general term that designates a life

lipoprotein: any of a group of soluble proteins that combine with and transport fat or other lipids in the blood plasma

liquid nitrogen: nitrogen in a liquid state, about 200° C (320° F) below zero

lobules: a breast lobule is a gland that makes milk

longevity: a long duration of individual life

lordotic curve: convex curvature of the cervical and lumbar regions of the spine

lumbar: five vertebral bodies that extend from the chest to the bottom of the spine

macerate: the softening and breaking down of skin resulting from prolonged exposure to moisture

macula: an irregularly oval, yellow-pigmented area on the central retina, containing color-sensitive rods and the central point of sharpest vision

malignant: tumors can invade and destroy nearby tissue and spread to other parts of the body

malocclusion: imperfect positioning of the teeth when the jaws are closed

mammary gland: the milk-producing gland of women or other female mammals

mammography: a technique using X-rays to diagnose and locate tumors of the breasts

mastalgia: a medical term used to describe breast pain

medial longitudinal arch: the inner part of the longitudinal arch of the foot

meiosis: a type of cell division that results in four daughter cells each with half the number of chromosomes of the parent cell, as in the production of gametes

melanin: a dark brown to black pigment occurring in the hair, skin, and iris of the eye in people and animals; it is responsible for tanning of skin exposed to sunlight

melanoblast: a cell that originates from the neural crest and differentiates into a pigment cell

melanocyte: a mature melanin-forming cell, especially in the skin

metastasize: the spread of a disease-producing agency, like cancer cells, from the initial or primary site of disease to another part of the body

metatarsal bones: a group of five long bones in the foot, located between the tarsal bones of the hind- and mid-foot and the phalanges of the toes

mutual fund: a professionally managed investment fund that pools money from many investors to purchase securities

neurodegenerative: resulting in or characterized by degeneration of the nervous system, especially the neurons in the brain

neurogenesis: the growth and development of nervous tissue

neurotransmitter: a chemical substance that is released at the end of a nerve fiber by the arrival of a nerve impulse and, by diffusing across the synapse or junction, causes the transfer of the impulse to another nerve fiber, a muscle fiber, or some other structure

nonsteroidal anti-inflammatory drugs (NSAIDs): a class of analgesic medication that reduces pain, fever, and inflammation

obesity: a condition characterized by the excessive accumulation and storage of fat in the body

oncogene: a gene that in certain circumstances can transform a cell into a tumor cell.

oogenesis: the production or development of an ovum

optic disc: the raised disk on the retina at the point of entry of the optic nerve, lacking visual receptors and so creating a blind spot

ossification: the process of laying down new bone material by cells called osteoblasts

osteoblasts: cells that secrete the matrix for bone formation

osteocytes: bone cells, formed when an osteoblast becomes embedded in the matrix it has secreted

otosclerosis: a hereditary disorder causing progressive deafness due to overgrowth of bone in the inner ear

oxygenation: the process of adding oxygen to the body system

p53: a gene that is thought to play a role in regulating cell death or apoptosis, in suppressing tumors, in regulating the cell cycle, and in stopping the cell from dividing when the DNA is damaged

parenchyma: the essential and distinctive tissue of an organ or an abnormal growth as distinguished from its supportive framework

peripheral vision: side vision; what is seen on the side by the eye when looking straight ahead

phenothiazines: medications used to treat schizophrenia and manifestations of psychotic disorders

plantar: the sole of the foot

pleiotropy: the production by a single gene of two or more apparently unrelated effects

procedural memory: a type of long-term memory involving how to perform different actions and skills

progeroid syndromes: a group of rare genetic disorders that mimic physiological aging, making affected individuals appear to be older than they are

progesterone: a steroid hormone released by the corpus luteum that stimulates the uterus to prepare for pregnancy

pronation: when the foot rolls inward (about 15 percent) as weight is placed on it

prostate enlargement: a common condition as men get older; can cause uncomfortable urinary symptoms, such as blocking the flow of urine out of the bladder; can also cause bladder, urinary tract or kidney problems

prostatectomy: a surgical operation to remove all or part of the prostate gland

protease-antiprotease imbalance: smoking increases the level of proteases while inhibiting antiproteases; the imbalance can cause the destruction of the walls of the lungs

punctum: a tip or small point, often dark colored; the punctum is the opening of the cyst

purine: a natural substance found in some foods; as the body digests purine, it produces a waste product called uric acid

recognition memory: the ability to recognize earlier encountered events, objects, or people

retina: a layer at the back of the eyeball containing cells that are sensitive to light and that trigger nerve impulses that pass via the optic nerve to the brain, where a visual image is formed

sacrum: a triangular bone in the lower back formed from fused vertebrae and situated between the two hipbones of the pelvis; supports the weight of the upper body as it is spread across the pelvis and into the leg

saturated fat: a type of fat containing a high proportion of fatty acid molecules without double bonds, considered to be less healthy in the diet than unsaturated fat

sclerotherapy: the treatment of varicose blood vessels by the injection of an irritant that causes inflammation, coagulation of blood, and narrowing of the blood vessel wall

sebaceous: relating to a small gland in the skin that secretes a lubricating oily matter (sebum) into the hair follicles to lubricate the skin and hair

senescence: the condition or process of deterioration with age

sensorineural: hearing loss caused by a lesion or disease of the inner ear or the auditory nerve

Short Physical Performance Battery (SPPB) evaluates lower extremity function in older adults.

source memory: recalling the source of learned information, such as knowledge of when or where something was learned

spatial memory: part of the memory responsible for the recording of information about one's environment and spatial orientation

spermatogenesis: the production or development of mature spermatozoa *stagnation*: a refusal to grow, an acquiescence to old methods and perspectives

stapes: a bone in the middle ear of humans and other mammals which is involved in the conduction of sound vibrations to the inner ear

striatum: coordinates multiple aspects of cognition, including both motor and action planning, decision-making, motivation, reinforcement, and reward perception

substantia nigra: an important player in brain function, in particular, in eye movement, motor planning, reward-seeking, learning, and addiction

syndrome: a collection of symptoms associated with a disease state; an individual patient may show some, but not necessarily all, of these symptoms

synovial fluid: produced in the spaces between certain joints to help reduce friction and facilitate movement between articular cartilages

synovial membrane: a layer of connective tissue that lines the cavities of joints, tendon sheaths, and bursae and makes synovial fluid, which has a lubricating function

systolic: relating to the phase of the heartbeat when the heart muscle contracts and pumps blood from the chambers into the arteries

T4 cells: also called CD4 cells or T-helper cells; a specific type of white blood cell (lymphocyte) that regulates the entire immune system and is the preferred target for HIV infection, resulting in immunodeficiency

tear duct: a passage through which tears pass from the lachrymal glands to the eye or from the eye to the nose

telomere: a region of repetitive nucleotide sequences at each end of a chromosome, which protects the end of the chromosome from deterioration or from fusion with neighboring chromosomes

tenancy: a holding of an estate or a mode of holding an estate

testator: a person who has made a will or given a legacy

therapeutic hypothermia: deliberate reduction of the core body temperature, typically to a range of about 32° to 34° C (89.6° to 93.2° F) in patients who don't regain consciousness after return of spontaneous circulation following a cardiac arrest

thoracic vertebrae: twelve vertebral bodies that make up the mid-region of the spine; this section of the spine has a kyphotic curve

thrombotic stroke: when a blood clot forms and blocks blood flow through the artery in which it formed

trans fat: a type of fat that is usually found in processed foods such as baked goods, snack foods, fried foods, shortening, margarine, and certain vegetable oils; eating trans fat increases blood cholesterol levels and the risk of heart disease

trust corpus: the sum of money or property that is set aside to produce income for a named beneficiary

tunnel vision: defective sight in which objects cannot be properly seen if not close to the center of the field of view

uric acid: a chemical created when the body breaks down substances called purines

urinalysis: analysis of urine by physical, chemical, and microscopic testing for the presence of disease, drugs, etc.

urinary tract infection: an infection of the kidney, ureter, bladder, or urethra; common symptoms include a frequent urge to urinate and pain or burning when urinating

usual gait speed: measures the walking speed on normal pace for a determined distance (usually 10-8 feet).

vein stripping: a surgical procedure done under general or local anesthetic to aid in the treatment of varicose veins; the surgery involves making incisions (usually the groin and medial thigh), followed by insertion of a special metal or plastic wire into the vein; the vein is attached to the wire and then pulled out from the body

ventilation: the act or process of inhaling and exhaling

viral load: a measurement of the amount of HIV present in the blood; often used to monitor the effectiveness of anti-HIV therapy

visual acuity: sharpness of vision, measured by the ability to discern letters or numbers at a given distance according to a fixed standard

vitrification: an ice-free process in which more than 60% of the water inside cells is replaced with protective chemicals; this completely prevents freezing during deep cooling

Index

AARP, 1-3
Abandonment, 3-4
Abdominal fat, 547, 548
Abkhazia, 1561, 152
Abscessed tooth, 208
Absenteeism. *See* Caregiver absenteeism
Abuse. *See* Elder abuse
Accelerated aging, 307
Acceptance, 4, 163, 193, 230, 262, 434, 437, 453, 697, 700
Accidents, 22, 58, 59, 98, 119, 132, 184, 189, 198, 214, 235, 511, 595, 601
Acetaminophen, 85, 500
Acetylcholine, 115, 507, 569
Achilles tendon, 296
Acquired immunodeficiency syndrome (AIDS), 4-7
Acrochordons, 663
Acting, 5, 6, 11, 18, 35, 75, 87, 499, 505, 525, 554, 566, 571, 575, 599
Actinic keratoses, 658, 663
Active euthanasia, 194, 270, 272
Active involvement. *See* Vital involvement
Activism, 12, 88
Activities of daily living, 54, 64, 69, 117, 146, 155, 204, 221, 237, 274, 277, 284, 285, 399, 411, 445, 449, 472
Activity theory of aging, 185
Acute care, 213, 245, 283, 284, 360, 362, 363, 367, 395, 396, 397
Acute illness, 367, 398, 399, 720
ADA. *See* Age Discrimination Act of 1975
Americans with Disabilities Act, 71-74
ADEA. *See* Age Discrimination in Employment Act of 1967
Adler, Felix, 181
Administration on Aging, 13, 23, 89, 233, 533, 554
Adopted grandparents, 7
Adult children. *See* Children
Adult day care, 2, 43, 67, 148, 206, 472, 492, 605, 619, 640
Adult education, 7-10
Adult-onset diabetes. *See* Type II diabetes
Adult Protective Services, 10-11
Advance directives, 157, 194, 203, 270, 271, 272, 292, 400-401

Adverse drug reactions, 399, 499, 560-563
Advertising, 175, 303, 345, 490, 755
Advisory Committee on Older Americans, 554
Advocacy, 11-15
Aerobic exercise, 97, 114, 141, 274, 275, 276
Aerobic fitness, 274, 275, 280, 637
Affordable Care Act, 15-18
African Americans, 18-22
Afterlife, 126, 197, 318, 434, 759
AGE. *See* Americans for Generational Equity (AGE) Age discrimination
Age Discrimination Act of 1975, 27-28
Age Discrimination in Employment Act of 1967, 28-29
Age Game, The, 45, 46
Age-integrated societies, 48
Age-related diseases, 74, 76, 114, 129, 589, 590
Age-related macular degeneration, 476, 477, 478, 728, 730
Age spots, 29-30
Age stratification model of aging, 185
Age wars, 293
Aged, 4, 7, 11, 12, 13, 54, 63, 66, 274, 609, 621, 633
Ageism, 22, 27, 28, 30-33
Aging: fear of, 101, 182, 185
Aging: Biological, psychological, and sociocultural perspectives, 34-45
Aging Experience: Diversity and Commonality Across Cultures, The (Keith), 45, 753
Aging: Historical perspective, 46-50
Aging process, 183, 222, 234, 273, 275, 291, 294, 308, 316, 317, 318, 324, 325, 327, 330, 331, 332, 333, 344, 353, 355, 406, 407, 408, 414, 431, 436, 448, 466, 467, 508, 528, 536, 541
Agricultural societies AIDS. *See* Acquired immunodeficiency syndrome (AIDS)
Alcohol use disorder, 57-61
Alendronate, 557
All About Eve, 61-62
Allopurinol, 338
ALLY. *See* Alternative Living in Later Years
Almshouses, 12, 49

Alopecia, 354
Alveoli Alzheimer, Alois, 69, 204
Alzheimer's Association, 62-63
Alzheimer's disease, 63-70
Amabile, Theresa, 174
Ambrosia, 467
American Association for Old-Age Security, 12
American Association of Retired Persons. *See* AARP
American Red Cross, 706
American Society on Aging, 70-71
Americans for Generational Equity (AGE), 623
Americans with Disabilities Act, 71-74
Amputation, 198, 217, 414, 670
Amyloid precursor protein, 69
Androgenetic alopecia, 354
Androgens, 40, 468, 512, 514, 592
Andrus, Ethel Percy, 1, 13
Anemia, 103, 320, 344, 413, 414, 478, 481, 732
Aneurysms, 416, 692
Anger, 9, 68, 144, 164, 190, 201, 596
Angina, 39, 139, 376, 398, 732
Angiography, 478
Angiomas, 663
Animals. *See* Pets
Ankylosing spondylitis, 84
Annuities, 572
Antacids, 500
Antagonistic pleiotropy Anthropology, 327
Anti-aging treatments, 74-77
Antibiotics, 10, 124, 132, 172, 187, 251, 321, 413, 414
Antidepressants, 207, 431, 613, 614, 646, 671, 691
Antidiuretic hormone, 712
Antiproteases, 250
Antipsychotics, 431, 614, 643
Anxiety, 57, 58, 59, 93, 102, 103, 104, 117, 420, 426, 434
AoA. *See* Administration on Aging
Aphasia, 58, 64, 204, 416, 694
Apoptosis, 327
Arcus senilis, 728
Area Agencies on Aging, 148, 157
Aristotle, 48, 181, 406
Arteries, 39, 52, 79, 81, 123, 139, 140, 142, 176, 217, 267, 374, 380, 408

Arthritis Foundation, 392
ASA. *See* American Society on Aging
Ascorbic acid. *See* Vitamin C
Asian Americans, 86-89
Assault, 246, 660
Assets, 20, 162, 163, 186, 253, 264
Assimilation, 88, 183, 492, 536
Assisted living, 64, 67, 146, 157, 192, 552, 579
Assisted suicide, 270, 271, 272, 273
Ataxia telangiectasia, 326
Atchley, Robert C., 18
Atherosclerosis, 39, 53, 79, 80, 81, 117, 139, 158, 217, 267, 268, 325, 413, 414
Atria, 378
Atrophic gastritis, 320
Attention span, 55, 56, 207, 415, 506, 669
Auditory system, 36, 371
Autobiography, 89
Autobiography of Miss Jane Pittman, The (Gaines), 90
Autoimmune disorders, 40, 427
Automobile insurance, 2, 235
Automobiles, 233, 235, 265

Baby boomers, 90-94
and elderly dependency burden, 14
and Medicare, 1
and Social Security, 1
Back disorders, 94-98
Bacon, Francis, 331
Bad breath, 210
Bad cholesterol. *See* Low-density lipoproteins (LDLs)
Balance, 1, 14, 36, 40, 42, 50, 51, 58, 66, 75, 98
Balance disorders, 98-99
Balanced Budget Act of 1997, 1, 496, 497
Baldness. *See* Hair loss and baldness
Baltes, Paul, 41
Baltimore Longitudinal Study on Aging, 184, 736
Banner, Lois W., 418
Barbiturates, 499, 561, 613
Bargaining, 190, 417, 437, 700
Barja, Gustavo, 468
Basal cell carcinoma, 657, 658, 659, 660, 664
Basal ganglia, 113, 115, 116
Basal metabolic rate, 35, 55
Beard, Belle Boone, 152
Beard, George Miller, 180

Beauty, 2, 30, 61, 99-102, 755
Bed sores, 399, 440, 480, 662
Behavioral and mental health, 102-105
Behavioral and Social Research Program, 535
Beneficiaries, 200, 264, 265, 293, 367, 397, 398, 399, 400
Benefits, 403, 404, 406, 407, 408, 422, 445, 446, 449, 453, 455, 457, 458, 459, 460, 462, 468, 485, 488, 494, 501, 519
Benign prostatic hyperplasia, 593
Bequests. *See* Wills and bequests
Bereavement counseling, 351, 394
Bergman, Ingmar, 262, 744
Bernarducci, Marc, 468
Best Exotic Marigold Hotel, The, 105-106
Beta-blockers, 287, 377
Beta carotene, 77, 78, 111, 450, 561, 731
BFOQ. *See* Bona fide occupational qualification (BFOQ)
Bible, 47, 151, 152, 406
Bifocals, 728
Bile, 40, 81, 158, 159, 319, 406, 414, 688, 689
Biofeedback, 372, 421
Bioflavonoids, 731
Biological clock. *See also* Circadian rhythms
Biological perspective on aging. *See* Aging: Biological, psychological, and sociocultural perspectives
Biology of Aging Program, 535
Biosphere 2, 128, 130
Birren, James E., 184
Bismarck, Otto von, 240, 509, 621
Blacks. *See* African Americans
Bladder
Bladder stones, 420, 594, 686, 688, 689
Blended families. *See* Stepfamilies
Blepharoplasty, 172, 282
Bless Me, Ultima (Anaya), 107-108
Blind spot, 335, 476, 520
Blindness, 217, 218, 335, 345
Block Nurse Program. *See* Living at Home/Block Nurse Program
Blood clots, 375, 377, 382, 577, 723, 724
Blood pressure, 278, 280, 301, 356, 374, 375, 376, 378, 379, 380, 408, 409, 410, 411, 464, 465, 500, 506, 508, 521, 549, 550, 561
Blood transfusions, 4
Blue bloaters, 248

Blue Cross, 364
Blue Shield, 364
Blurred vision, 217, 477, 561, 570, 693, 729
BMI. *See* Body mass index (BMI)
BMR. *See* Basal metabolic rate
Body composition, 143, 274, 294, 374, 399, 499, 543, 547, 549, 636, 735, 736, 737
Body image, 165, 559, 614, 641, 642, 643, 647
Body mass index (BMI), 547
Body shape, 100
Bombeck, Erma, 407
Bona fide occupational qualification (BFOQ), 435
Bone changes and disorders, 108-113
Bone cysts, 187
Bone loss, 36, 37, 75, 76, 94, 111, 112, 129, 211, 325, 416, 481, 515, 544, 556, 557, 636
Boosters. *See* Vaccines
Borg, Isak, 262, 744
Boston Women's Health Book Collective, 559
Bowel movements, 322, 689, 725
Bradley, Holbrook, 721
Bradycardia, 275, 380, 413
Brain, 5, 37, 39, 40, 691, 692, 693, 694, 699, 704, 720, 727, 729, 751
Brain changes and disorders, 44, 113-118
Brain damage, 116, 271, 380, 693
Brain waves, 667, 668
Breast cancer, 118-122
and estrogen, 40
screening, 123
Breast changes and disorders, 122-125
Breast cysts, 187
Breast implants, 124
Breasts, 40, 122, 123, 267, 662
Breathing, 52, 53, 71, 84, 209, 132, 250, 260, 274, 319, 407, 436, 439, 461, 464, 561, 565, 582, 583, 617, 668, 672
Breathing difficulty. *See* Respiratory changes and disorders
Bridge jobs, 622
Bridges. *See* Crowns and bridges
Brim, Orville Gilbert, 524
Bronchioles, 248, 250
Bronchitis, 248, 250, 260, 617, 618, 670
Brothers, 461, 486, 653, 654, 747
Brow lifts, 172
Brown bag days, 500

Brown-Sequard, Charles Edouard, 468
Bruises, 664
Bucket List, The, 125-127
Bunions, 127-128
Burial, 313, 317
Burns, 407, 408, 540, 658, 662
Burns, George, 407
Buses, 605, 708, 717
  discounts, 225-228
Butler, Robert N., 537, 741
Bypass, 398, 466

Cachexia, 635
Caffeine, 420, 630, 668
Calcitonin, 110
Calcium, 470, 480, 500, 516, 544, 556, 557, 686, 688, 731
Calculi, 415, 686, 713
California, 129, 188, 194, 242, 262, 265, 271, 285, 334, 412, 440, 444
Calluses. *See* Corns and calluses
Caloric restriction, 128-131, 467, 468
Cancer, 131-136
  cells, 169
Candidiasis, oral, 210
Canes and walkers, 137-138
Capillaries, 135, 319, 379, 571, 662, 711
Capital gains tax, 162, 243, 388, 710
CAPS. *See* Children of Aging Parents
Car accidents. *See* Traffic accidents
Carbohydrates, 143, 217, 320, 470, 736
Carcinogens, 134, 136, 546, 732
Carcinoma. *See* Basal cell carcinoma
Cardiac arrest, 374
Cardiac catheterization, 546
Cardiac output, 8, 52, 275, 276, 499, 712
Cardiac rehabilitation, 377, 378
Cardiovascular disease, 139-143
  and estrogen, 40
  and vitamins, 111
Cardiovascular system, 39, 52, 139, 141, 152, 276, 410, 413
Cards, greeting. *See* Greeting cards
Careers, 87, 106, 144, 147, 226, 228, 237, 237, 238, 296, 350, 486, 488, 492, 624, 633, 656, 756
Caregiver absenteeism, 143-145
Caregiving, 145-149
  and Alzheimer's disease, 113, 115
  and communication, 165
  by friends, 312
  by spouses, 566
Caries. *See* Cavities
Carney, Art, 358

Carotenoids, 543, 544, 546
Cars. *See* Automobiles, Driving
Carter, Jimmy, 726
Cartilage, 52, 54, 82
Cartoons, 92, 407
Casa Iris, 535
Case management, 390, 470, 475, 596
Cataracts, 476, 481, 511, 589
Catecholamines, 141, 142
Catholic Church, 394, 441
Cavities, 113, 208, 210
CCRCs. *See* Continuing care retirement communities (CCRCs)
Cellular aging, 77, 184, 329
Center for the Study of Aging and Human Development, 154-155
Central adiposity, 548
Cerumen, 372
Change: Women, Aging, and the Menopause, The (Greer), 154-155
Charity, 49, 351, 395, 710
Cheilitis, 210
Chemotherapy, 121, 135, 172
Cherokees, 536
Cherry angiomas, 663
Cheyenne, 289
Chicanos. *See* Latinx Americans
Child care, 295, 465, 634
  by grandparents, 342
Child rearing, 347, 608, 624, 656, 665
Childbearing, 106, 154, 156, 559, 607, 633, 752
Childlessness, 155-157
Children, 157, 163, 166, 183, 191, 198
  as caregivers, 203
  death of, 203
Children of Aging Parents, 157-157
Chinese Americans. *See* Asian Americans
Chlamydia, 426
Choking, 432
Cholecystitis, 414
Cholesterol, 158-159
Choline, 505
Cholinesterase inhibitors, 66, 207
Chromosomes, 77, 324, 424, 425, 466
Chronic bronchitis, 248, 250, 260, 670
Chronic conditions, 71, 192, 360, 542, 545, 560
Chronic illness, 103, 135, 147, 154, 260, 362, 384, 398, 429, 465, 470, 480, 485, 493, 564, 584, 600, 603
  and suicide, 695

Chronic obstructive pulmonary disease, 190, 248, 260, 415, 511, 617, 670
Chronological age, 34, 142, 183, 186, 537, 670
Churches, 12, 148, 352, 390, 402, 442, 551, 552, 640, 668, 685
Cicero, 48
Cimetadine, 499
Circadian rhythms, 159-161
Circulatory problems, 414, 664, 731
Cirrhosis, 40, 190, 688
Citrus, 111, 731
Civil Rights Act of 1964, 24, 25, 26, 27
Climacteric, 40, 41, 200
Clinton, Bill, 14, 28, 469, 740
Clitoris, 610, 641
Clothing, 64, 100, 101, 136, 168, 265, 342, 348, 422, 427, 432, 660, 662, 664, 699, 725, 736
Clots. *See* Blood clots
Cochlea, 371, 372
Cockayne syndrome, 326
Cocoon, 161-162
Cod-liver oil, 111, 467
Codicils, 746, 747
Coffins, 317
Cognitive impairment, 205, 399, 400, 421, 742
Cognitive skills, 64, 673
Cohabitation, 162-165
Cohen, Wilbur, 495
Cohort, 551, 577, 589, 599, 633, 655
Collagen, 628, 758, 759
Colon, 133, 134
Colon cancer, 134, 267, 322, 414,
  screening, 59, 81, 760, 112, 123, 134, 158
Color vision, 728
Commission on Civil Rights, 27
Common-law marriage, 163
Communal living, 403
Communication, 165-167
  with children, 289
  about death, 701
Community property states, 265
Comorbidity, 36, 120, 397
Companion animals. *See also* Pets
Companionship, 147, 148, 163, 192, 291, 456, 461, 463
Compassionate Friends, 199
Compensation benefits, 254
Competency, 30, 32, 67, 117, 239, 271
Compulsory retirement. *See* Mandatory retirement

818 • Index

Computers, 8, 479, 622, 672, 681
Con artists, 246, 306
Condom catheters, 422
Conductive hearing loss, 368, 369, 372
Confusion, 382, 399, 417, 474, 523, 561, 570, 583
Congestive heart failure, 39, 79, 408
Conservators, 11, 293
Constipation, 53, 704, 725
Constitution, U.S., 24, 188
Consumer issues, 167-169
Contact dermatitis, 662
Contests, 304, 305
Continuing care retirement communities (CCRCs), 472, 626
Convalescent homes. *See* Facility and institutional care
Coordination, 8, 97, 113, 277, 297, 360, 361, 391, 415, 450, 470, 484, 508, 530, 531, 557, 569, 671, 683
COPD. *See* Chronic obstructive pulmonary disease
Coping skills. *See* Stress and coping skills
Cornea, 149, 150, 335, 336, 538, 539, 727, 728
Corns and calluses, 169-171
Coronary artery disease, 139, 158, 374, 376, 380, 408, 411, 589, 671
Corpus luteum, 267, 513
Cortese, Ross, 440, 441
Corticosteroids, 82, 84, 112, 150, 251, 337, 338
Corticotropin, 531
Cosmetic surgery, 171-173
Costa, Paul T., 523
Coughing, 248, 515, 582, 720
Coumadin, 499
Cox inhibitors, 85
Creativity, 173-176
Cremation, 157, 180, 317
Crime against the elderly, 246
Crohn's disease, 414
Cross-cultural attitudes. *See* Cultural views of aging
Cross-linkage theory of aging, 176-177
Cross-sectional studies, 184, 636
Crowns and bridges, 177-178
Cruzan, Nancy, 271
Cryopreservation, 180
Crystallized intelligence, 42, 184
Cuban Americans, 410, 443, 444, 445, 446
Cued recall, 503, 504, 506

Cultural views of aging. *See also* Aging: Biological, psychological, and sociocultural perspectives
Curve of productivity, 180
Cutaneous horns, 663
CVA. *See* Cerebrovascular accident (CVA)
Cyanosis, 248, 250
Cysts, 187

Darling v. Douglas, 188-189, 527, 530, 531
Davis, Leonard, 2
Dawkins, Richard, 466
Daytime serials, 32
Deafness, 368, 369
Death and dying, 189-195
Death anxiety, 195-198
Death of a child, 192-193
Death of a spouse. *See* Widows and widowers
Death of parents, 190-191
Death of siblings, 654-55
Death rates. *See* Mortality rates
Decay theory of memory loss, 505
Decubital ulcers, 399
Deductibles, 362, 366
Deferred annuities, 572
Defined benefit pension plans, 254
Dehydration, 52, 58, 206, 540, 699
Dehydroepiandrosterone (DHEA), 468
Delayed retirement, 20
Delirium, 65, 66, 205, 399
Delirium tremens, 65, 66, 205, 399
Delivery of goods, 391
Dementia, 5, 6, 35, 36, 39, 41, 58, 62, 515, 566, 595
Democratic Party, 13
Demographics, 11, 15, 18, 46, 90, 117, 118, 145, 151, 155, 259, 603, 607
Demyelination, 520, 531
Denial, 17, 25, 190, 197, 202, 231, 298, 316, 351, 434
Dental disorders, 207-210
Dentin, 53, 207, 208, 209
Dentures, 210-212
Dependency burden ratio, 253
Depression, 212-216
Dermatitis, 630, 662, 664
Dermatoheliosis, 661
Dermis, 29, 39, 55, 171
Derogatory terms, 32
Designer estrogens, 516

Despair, 42, 43, 60, 165, 181, 182, 184, 190, 230, 231, 262, 317, 349, 351, 599, 601
Detached retina, 151
DHEA. *See* Dehydroepiandrosterone (DHEA)
DHT. *See* Dihydrotestosterone (DHT)
Diabetes, 216-221
Diabetes insipidus, 217, 712
Diabetic retinopathy, 729
Diagnosis-related groups, 362
Dialysis, 217, 362, 409
Diastolic pressure, 52, 375, 379, 410
Diazepam, 104, 561
Diet. *See* Nutrition
Dietary restriction, 129, 130, 307, 467
Dietary supplements, 75, 112, 468
Dieting, 549
Digestive system, 136, 318
Digit span, 505
Digital rectal examination (DRE), 591
Dihydrotestosterone (DHT), 355
Diphtheria, 507, 718, 720
Disability insurance, 365, 367, 674
Discounts, 225-228
Discretionary income, 622
Diseases, age-related, 74, 76, 114, 129, 589, 590
Disengagement, 185, 213, 749
Disinhibition, 174, 175
Disks, 54, 94, 95, 96, 97
Disorientation, 59, 98, 370, 474, 606, 701
Disposable soma theory, 327, 328
Diuretics, 58, 251, 372, 431, 500, 643
Diverticulitis, 319, 321, 414, 420, 756
Diverticulosis, 320, 321, 414
Divorce, 228-232
Dizziness, 98, 99, 103, 139, 356, 378, 431, 643, 692, 714
DNA. *See* Deoxyribonucleic acid (DNA)
DNR status. *See* "Do not resuscitate" status
"Dr. Heidegger's Experiment," 232-233
Dr. Seuss, 759
Domestic violence, 224, 245, 246, 386, 540
Dopamine, 103, 115, 116, 569, 570
Doress-Worters, Paula, 559
Double standard of aging, 100
Double vision, 530, 729
Dowager's hump. *See* Kyphosis
Down syndrome, 69, 185, 325
Downsizing, 23, 93, 240, 241

Dramas. *See* Plays
DRE. *See* Digital rectal examination (DRE)
DRGs. *See* Diagnosis-related groups
Driving 233-35
Driving Miss Daisy (Uhry), 21, 235-36
Drug interactions, 58, 205, 501
Drugs. *See* Medications
Dry mouth, 210, 319, 570
Dry skin, 171
Dual-income couples, 236-239
Duke Longitudinal Studies, 154, 291
Duke University, 154, 599
Durable power of attorney, 11, 67, 163, 205, 239-240
Dying. *See* Death and dying
Dyspareunia, 613, 642

E-mail, 304, 306, 407, 566, 606, 673, 681, 717
Eardrum, 38, 368, 371
Ears, 4, 5, 6, 7, 8, 11, 12, 296, 298, 303, 663
Ebbinghaus, Hermann, 505
ECG. *See* Electrocardiography
Echo housing, 405
Eczema, gravitational, 664
Edema, 248, 398, 664, 719
Educational institutions, 241, 510
EEG. *See* Electroencephalography
EEOC. *See* Equal Employment Opportunity Commission
Eggs, 40, 111, 130, 238, 376, 425, 426, 428, 513, 543, 719
Ego development, 263
Ejaculation, 53, 427, 593, 612, 614, 641, 642, 643, 644, 648
EKG. *See* Electrocardiography
Elastin, 37, 40, 55, 250
Elder care. *See* Caregiving
Elderhostel, 37, 40, 55, 250
Elderly dependency burden, 253
Elections, 496, 498, 739
Electrocardiography, 377
Electroencephalography, 205
Electronic mail, 407, 717
Embolus, 116, 692
Emphysema, 248-251
Employee Retirement Income Security Act of 1974, 23, 423, 573, 574
Empty nest syndrome, 182, 222, 256-258
Enamel, 207, 208
End-of-life issues, 239, 522

Endocrine system, 40, 267, 645, 704
Endometrium, 54, 267, 426, 512, 513, 515, 516
Endoscopy, 398
Endurance training, 527
Engagement theory, 213
Enjoy Old Age: A Program of Self-Management (Skinner and Vaughan), 258-259
Enlarged heart, 52, 409
Entitlements, 14, 25, 537
Enzymes, 40, 53, 77, 83, 176, 249, 250, 307, 308, 319, 320, 321, 344, 377
Epidemics, 429
Epidemiology, 249, 259, 261
Epidermis, 29, 171, 281, 543, 657, 659, 661
Epididymis, 427
Episodic memory, 41, 503, 506
Equal Credit Opportunity Act, 26
Equal Employment Opportunity Commission, 25, 28, 73, 93
Equity, 387, 388, 402, 404, 424, 488
Erectile dysfunction, 97, 427, 428, 614, 643
Erection, 41, 53, 425, 427, 611, 612, 614
Erikson, Erik H., 44, 184
ERISA. *See* Employee Retirement Income Security Act of 1974
Esophageal cancer, 546
Esophagus, 53, 318
Estradiol, 266, 267, 268, 514
Ethnic minorities. *See* Minority groups
Euthanasia, 269-273
Evolution, 263
Executive Order 11141, 273
Executors, 702
Experience, 2, 5, 7, 274, 275, 712, 713
Extended care for the elderly. *See* Long-term care for the elderly
Extended families, 49, 181, 183, 240, 288, 566, 610
Extracorporeal shock wave lithotripsy, 687
Eye disease. *See* Vision changes and disorders
Eye examinations, 477, 478, 729
Eyeglasses. *See* Reading glasses
Eyes, 37, 38, 354, 373, 538
Eyesight. *See* Vision changes and disorders

Face lifts, 172, 280-283
Factories, 323, 507, 620

Faith, 14, 21, 87, 231, 394, 599, 601, 602, 603, 749
Fallen arches, 287-288
Falls, 1, 8, 36, 58, 59, 98, 103, 138, 193, 198, 219, 249, 300, 301, 431
Familial adenomatous polyposis, 133
Family relationships, 148, 321, 257
and caregiving, 312
and divorce, 340
and grandparents, 86
and hospice, 194
and neglect, 179
Family violence. *See* Domestic violence
Farsightedness, 37, 54, 470
Fascia, 96, 97, 296, 297
Fashion, 41, 83, 100, 101, 166, 168, 645, 657, 685
Fat deposition, 294
and medications, 301
Fat-soluble medications, 499
Fatty streaks, 79, 81
Fear of aging, 101, 182, 185
Fear of death. *See* Death anxiety
Fear of pain, 195, 393, 644
Feces, 320, 322, 420
Federal Council on Aging, 554
Feet. *See* Foot disorders
Feminism, 756-757
Feminization of poverty, 485
Fertility rates, 655
Fever, 5, 82, 97, 124, 321, 412, 413, 414, 421, 428, 430
Fiber, 38, 54, 55, 66, 78, 335, 336, 546, 616
Fibroadenomas, 123, 124
Fibrocystic disease, 123
Fiction. *See* Novels; Plays; Poems; Short stories
Fictive kinship relations, 289
Fictive siblings, 653
Fight-or-flight response, 141
Filial responsibility, 294-295
Filipino Americans. *See* Asian Americans
Films, 63, 101, 407, 433, 512, 622
Final expenses, 457, 459, 460
Financial assets, 286, 609
Financial planning, 458, 459, 460, 628
Fires, 66, 432, 607, 671
Fischer, David Hackett, 47, 352
Fitness. *See* Exercise and fitness
Flatfeet, 287, 296
Floaters, 728

Florida, 232, 242, 259, 299, 336, 409, 604
Flu. *See* Influenza
Fluid intelligence, 42, 152, 184
Fluoride, 208
Flurazepam, 561
Folic acid, 731
Follicles, hair, 123, 187, 344, 657
Follicles, ovarian, 513, 514
Fonda, Henry, 555
Food, 36, 39, 53, 85, 103, 110, 129, 130, 314, 318, 319, 467, 482
Foot disorders, 170, 295-298
Forand Bill, 495
Forced retirement. *See* Mandatory retirement
Foreign travel, 715-716
Forgetfulness. *See* Memory loss
Foster Grandparent Program, 465, 618
Fountain of Age, The (Friedan), 298, 299, 456
Fountain of youth, 75, 161, 173, 232
401(k) plans, 299-300
Fourteenth Amendment, 24, 489
Fowler, James, 601
Fractured tooth, 208
Fractures and broken bones, 300-302
Frail elderly, 12, 15, 200, 312, 404, 422, 480, 493, 637, 753
Framingham Heart Study, 79, 467
Franklin, Benjamin, 331, 619, 688
Fraternal Order of the Eagles, 12
Fraud against older adults, 303-306
Free radical theory of aging, 307-309
Free radicals, 77, 115, 129, 136, 307
Free recall, 504
Freud, Sigmund, 261, 576
Freudian psychology, 261
Friedan, Betty, 298, 756
Friends of Little Brothers, 461
Friendship, 309-313
and death, 328
Frostbite, 662
Fry, William F., 406
Full dentures. *See* Dentures
Full Measure: Modern Short Stories on Aging (Sennett, ed.), 313
Full nest, 313-316
Functional age, 34, 484
Functional incontinence, 421
Funerals, 316-318

Gait, 51, 82, 98, 127, 128, 137, 277, 416, 431, 531, 561, 569, 671

Gallbladder, 40, 318, 319, 320, 398, 414, 688, 681
Gallstones, 40, 53, 320, 686, 688-689
Gamete intrafallopian transfer, 428
Gastritis, atrophic, 320
Gastrointestinal changes and disorders, 318-323
Gay men. *See* LGBTQ+
Gene therapy, 74, 76-77
Generation gap, 521
Generativity, 42, 191, 262, 491, 522, 524, 550, 567, 748, 749
Genetic engineering, 75, 509
Genetic predisposition, 374, 457, 538, 594
Genetic testing, 76
Genital herpes, 426
Genitals, 100, 610, 612
Georgia, Republic of, 151, 295
Geriatric Depression Scale, 104, 214, 696
Geriatrics and gerontology, 330-333
Geriatrics Program, 536
Germ-cell dysplasia, 427
Gerontological Society of America, 333-334
Gerontologist, 30, 31, 33, 34, 235, 244, 326, 331, 332, 333, 385
Gerontology. *See also* Geriatrics and gerontology
Gerontophobia, 22
Gift taxes, 710
Gingival hyperplasia, 209
Gingivitis, 209
Ginkgo, 505
Glass ceiling, 254
Glaucoma, 37, 217, 335-336
Glucagon, 40, 219
Glucophage, 219
Glucose, 53, 55, 115, 141, 142, 216, 217, 219, 278, 527, 711, 713, 732
Glucosuria, 217
Golden Girls, The, 32, 336, 403
Golden handshake, 23
Gonorrhea, 426, 427
Good cholesterol. *See* High-density lipoproteins (HDLs)
Gordon, Ruth, 357
Gout, 83-84
Government-subsidized housing, 404
Grace and Frankie, 338, 339
Graduated retirement, 510
Grandfathers, 290, 343, 348, 566
Grandmother hypothesis, 517

Grandmothers, 289, 290, 341, 342, 343
Grandparenthood, 340-3444
adopted, 7, 24, 26, 90, 101, 144, 341
Grandparents raising grandchildren. *See* Skipped-generation parenting
Graves' disease, 705
Gravitational eczema, 664
Gray barrier, 518
Gray hair, 344
Gray lobby, 13, 345
Gray Panthers, 345-346
Great Depression, 12, 23, 49, 92, 185, 240, 577, 621, 705, 753
Great-grandparenthood, 346-348
Great Society, 23, 496, 554
Greece, 9, 181, 406, 507, 639
Greer, Germaine, 154
Grief, 2, 43, 58, 68, 126, 148, 195, 200, 350, 742
Griffith, Andy, 490
Group travel, 716
Growing Old in America (Fischer), 352-353
Growth hormone, 75, 110, 468, 527
Grumpy Old Men, 353
GSA. *See* Gerontological Society of America
Guardians, 11, 67, 264, 293, 666

Hair, 8, 26, 33, 37, 39, 52, 53, 55, 98, 344, 353, 354, 647, 657
Hair color, 171, 344
Hair growth, 172, 356, 663
Hair loss and baldness, 353-356
Hair transplantation, 172, 355
Halitosis, 210
Hall, David, 183
Hall, G. Stanley, 182
Hallucinations, 57, 65, 570
Hammertoes, 356-357
Handicaps. *See* Disabilities
Happiness, 183, 223, 238, 257, 282, 290, 485, 486, 488, 567, 568, 656
Harman, Denham, 307
Harold and Maude, 357-358
Harris, Mary B., 100
Harry and Tonto, 358
Hashimoto's disease, 704
Havighurst, Robert, 184
Having Our Say: The Delany Sisters' First One Hundred Years (Delany and Delany), 358-359
Hawthorne, Nathaniel, 232
Hayflick, Leonard, 184, 323, 466

Hayflick limit, 324, 327, 466
HDLs. *See* High-density lipoproteins (HDLs)
Head trauma, 204, 569
Health and Human Services, Department of, 25, 88
Health benefits, 16, 25, 144, 251, 274
Health care, 2, 5, 15, 17, 46, 60, 63, 65, 67, 71, 516, 522, 532, 533
Health care benefits of retirees, 574
Health care decisions, 163, 239, 463
Health Care Financing Agency, 496
Health care reform, 534
Health, Education, and Welfare, Department of, 25, 554
Health fraud, 303
Health insurance, 364-368
Health maintenance organizations (HMOs), 364, 365, 391, 496, 508
Healthy Block program, 345
Healthy Seniors Project, 389, 390
Hearing, 2, 12, 38, 222, 234
Hearing aids, 56, 303, 361, 367
Hearing loss, 38, 54
Heart attacks, 374-378
 and estrogen, 40
 and menopause, 154
Heart changes and disorders, 378-380
Heart disease. *See* Cardiovascular disease
Heart failure, 39, 52, 75, 76, 399
Heartbeat, 219, 356, 380, 408, 596
Heartburn, 321, 557
Heat loss, 699
Heat stroke, 416, 662
Heel lifts, 297
Heels, 138, 148, 297, 357, 383, 385, 391, 431
Heirs, 100, 250, 264, 609, 746, 760
Helplessness, 102, 213, 476
Hemingway, Ernest, 553
Hemoglobin, 140, 217, 480, 732
Hemorrhoids, 415
Hemosiderosis, 664
Hepburn, Katharine, 555
Herbal remedies, 500
Herniated disk, 95
Herpes, 4, 426, 427, 664
Herpes zoster, 664
HEW. *See* Health, Education, and Welfare, Department of
High blood pressure. *See* Hypertension
High-density lipoproteins (HDLs), 140, 375, 544

Higher Education Amendments of 1998, 28
Hinduism, 600
Hip fractures, 300, 302, 431, 526, 556, 561
Hip replacement, 381-383
Hiring practices, discriminatory. *See* Age discrimination
Hispanic Americans. *See* Latinx Americans
Historical perspective on aging. *See* Aging: Historical perspective
HIV. *See* Human immunodeficiency virus (HIV)
HMOs. *See* Health maintenance organizations (HMOs)
Holistic care, 393
Home care, 2, 43, 88, 146, 157, 162, 221, 224, 284, 286, 492, 493, 494
Home-delivered meals programs, 383-385
Home equity schemes, 402, 587, 588
Home exchanges, 717
Home health agencies, 390, 564, 701
Home health aides, 554
Home ownership, 387-389
Home services, 389-392
Homelessness, 385-387
 among Native Americans, 536-538
Homeostasis, 50, 110, 112
Homosexuality, 71, 451, 542
Hormone replacement therapy, 119, 123, 124, 155, 266
Hormone therapy, 119, 121
Hormones, 37, 40, 103, 111, 119, 267, 416, 425, 428, 464
 and infertility, 4205, 426, 427
 and longevity, 33, 129, 327, 467, 468
Hospice, 392-396
Hospital Advantage, 2
Hospitalization, 396-401
Hostels, 9, 716
Hot flashes, 9, 716
House Select Committee on Aging, 740
Housing, 46, 163, 168, 222, 223, 245, 247, 345, 385, 386, 388
 and Native Americans, 536-538
 and homelessness, 385-387
HRT. *See* Hormone replacement therapy
Human Genome Project, 509
Human growth hormone, 75, 468
Human immunodeficiency virus (HIV), 71, 205, 457
Hunchback. *See* Kyphosis

Hundred-year-olds. *See* Centenarians
Huntington's disease, 205, 325, 695
Hutchinson-Gilford progeria, 325, 589
Hydrocephalus, 204, 205, 415
Hydrochloric acid, 40, 53, 320, 543
Hydroxyl radical, 307
Hygiene, 39, 64, 208, 209, 210, 331, 391, 540, 613, 632, 668
Hypercholesterolemia, 140, 141
Hyperglycemia, 217, 220
Hyperopia. *See* Farsightedness
Hyperparathyroidism, 112
Hyperplasia, 123, 124, 209, 593, 663, 664
Hypertension, 408-411
 and exercise, 75, 158, 219, 251, 275, 276, 279, 283, 320, 521, 590, 618
Hyperthyroidism, 112, 205, 344, 704, 705
Hypoglycemia, 219, 220, 561, 596
Hypothalamus, 113, 116, 267, 426, 464
Hypothermia, 178, 432, 662, 699
Hypothyroidism, 112, 205, 704
Hysterectomy, 268, 422, 515, 516, 559, 613

I Never Sang for My Father (Anderson), 412
Ibuprofen, 75, 85, 500
Identity and aging, 166
Images of aging. *See* Films; Literature; Television
Immune system, 4, 5, 36, 40, 84, 427, 466, 515
Immunizations and boosters. *See* Vaccines
Immunosuppression, 658, 659
Impotence. *See* Sexual dysfunction
In Full Flower: Aging Women, Power, and Sexuality (Banner), 418-419
In vitro fertilization, 428
Incapacitation, 194, 234, 696
Indian Health Service, 183, 537
Indian Self-Determination Act of 1975, 536
Indigestion, 53, 376, 690
Individual retirement accounts (IRAs), 423-424
Industrial Revolution, 620-21
Industrialization, 49, 185, 585, 620, 679
Infertility, 424-428
Infidelity, 229
Inflation, 52, 93, 241, 484, 496
Influenza, 428-430

Inheritance. *See* Estates and inheritance
Inner ear, 38, 54, 368, 369, 371
Insomnia, 36, 59, 234, 469, 471, 561
Instrumental activities of daily living, 445, 472
Insulin, 40, 55, 218, 379
Insulin-dependent diabetes. *See* Type I diabetes
Insurance, 2, 17, 137, 225, 361, 390, 457
Insurance schemes, 246
Integrity, 42, 56, 262, 491
Intelligence, 8, 184
Intensive care, 251, 360, 552, 564
Inter vivos trusts. *See* Living trusts
Intercourse: pain during, 515, 644
Interfaith Volunteer Caregivers, 389, 390
Intergenerational relations, 288, 289, 353, 412
Intermediate care facility, 285
Intermittent claudication, 414, 732
International Congress of Gerontology, 332
Intestate, 264, 745, 746
Intrinsic factor, 480, 543, 661
Ionizing radiation, 307
IRAs. *See* Individual retirement accounts (IRAs)
Iris, 149, 317, 318, 336, 388, 395, 727
Iron-deficiency anemia, 481, 732
Islets of Langerhans, 111, 217
Isolated systolic hypertension, 76, 378
Isolation, 3, 34, 35, 233, 394, 452, 470, 673

Jackson, Hobart C., 533
Jacques, Elliott, 522
Japanese Americans. *See* Asian Americans
Jaundice, 414, 688
Jaw, 96, 177, 207, 208, 558, 662
Jet lag, 160
Jewish Community Center, 433
Jewish Family Services, 433
Jewish services for the elderly, 433
Jilting of Granny Weatherall, The, (Porter), 433-434
Jobs, 20, 22, 23, 24, 28, 45, 49, 91, 92, 93, 144, 147, 228, 233, 237, 238, 252, 253, 254, 255, 273, 350, 445, 446
Johnson, Lyndon B., 93, 273
Johnson v. Mayor and City Council of Baltimore, 435
Joint ownership of property, 265
Joints, 54, 82, 356, 380

Joseph, Jenny, 739
Journal of Gerontology, 333
Journals, 196, 227, 334, 407
Just Friends, 312

Kegel exercises, 421, 422
Kennedy, John F., 93, 273, 495
Kenyon, Cynthia, 466
Keratin, 170, 187, 354, 661, 663
Keratoacanthoma, 663
Keratoses, 658, 663
Kerr-Mills Bill, 495
Ketone bodies, 217
Ketosis, 217
Kevorkian, Jack, 270
Kidney disease, 190, 337, 367, 386, 481, 549, 589, 713
Kidney failure, 217, 408
Kidney stones, 78, 337, 338, 415, 686, 688, 689
Kidneys, 40, 52, 53, 121, 141, 187, 217, 337, 409, 415, 687, 699
Kinase, 326, 377
King Lear (Shakespeare), 435-437
Kivnick, Helen Q., 263, 289, 551
Koenig, Harold, 599
Kohlberg, Lawrence, 601
Korean Americans. *See* Asian Americans
Kübler-Ross, Elisabeth, 190, 194, 392, 437, 700
Kuhn, Maggie, 438-439
Kyphosis, 439-440

L-dopa, 116
Labor force participation, 238, 252, 254, 256, 588, 676
Labor unions, 71, 495, 573, 626
Lactic acid, 276
Language skills, 63, 715
Lansbury, Angela, 532, 581
Large intestine, 53, 318, 319, 711
Last rites, 441-443
Latinx Americans, 443-447
Laughterk, 318, 406, 407
Laxatives, 103, 321, 322, 383, 500, 561
Layoffs, 483, 623
LDLs. *See* Low-density lipoproteins (LDLs)
Leadership of Aging Organizations, 534
Learned helplessness, 213
Learning, 7, 9, 56, 113, 292, 383, 545, 596
Lecithin, 7, 10, 71, 349, 545, 551, 596

Lee, I-Min, 467
Leflunomide, 85
Legal issues. *See* Durable power of attorney; Estates and inheritance; Living wills; Trusts; Wills and bequests
Legionnaires' disease, 413
Legs, 29, 37, 51, 248, 268, 723
Leisure activities, 447-451
Leisure World, 441
Lemmon, Jack, 353
Lens, 37, 149, 335, 511, 539, 598, 727
Lentigo, 29, 659, 663
  maligna, 29, 53, 120, 134, 659
Lesbians. *See* LGBTQ+
Levinson, Daniel, 523
Levodopa, 569, 570
Lewy bodies, 116, 569
LGBTQ+, 451-454
  and discrimination, 453
  and marriage, 152, 153, 228, 343
Life care facilities, 403, 472
Life expectancy, 6, 18, 23, 34, 47, 134, 145, 147, 182, 340, 455
  and African Americans, 18-22
  and women, 20, 32, 57, 83, 182, 252
Life experience, 9, 36, 174, 175, 184
Life insurance, 457-460
Life review, 42, 174, 175, 181, 206, 491
Life satisfaction, 238-239
Life span, 31, 34, 55, 74, 117, 129, 153, 185, 278, 308
Life support, 67, 180, 270
Ligaments, 82, 95, 127
Light-headedness, 376
Lighthouse for the Blind, 392
Likert scale, 196
Limbic system, 115, 751
Lipids, 77, 81, 140, 379, 544
Lipofuscin, 732
Lipoproteins, 79, 140, 278, 375, 544
Liposuction, 171, 282
Literature, 9, 36, 48, 94, 523
Little Brothers-Friends of the Elderly, 460-461
Litwak, Eugene, 291
Liver, 29, 40, 53, 318, 319, 338
Liver spots, 29, 732
Living at Home/Block Nurse Program, 389, 390
Living together. *See* Cohabitation
Living trusts, 203, 264, 303
Living wills, 461-463
Lobbying, 1, 13, 345

Long-term care, 469-475
Long-term memory, 8, 41, 503
Longevity, 33, 34, 151, 308, 340
Longevity research, 465-469
Longitudinal studies, 154, 184, 254, 291
Look Me in the Eye: Old Women, Aging, and Ageism (Macdonald with Rich), 475-476
Love, Susan M., 123
Low-density lipoproteins (LDLs), 79, 140, 278, 544
Lowenthal, David, 468
Lumbago, 96
Lung cancer, 322, 416, 591
Lung disease, 144, 248, 393, 399, 517, 581, 582, 584
Lupus, 84, 557

McCay, Clive, 129
Macdonald, Barbara, 475, 756
Macrophages, 250
Macular degeneration, 476-479
Magnesium, 500, 731, 732
Major medical insurance, 364
Male pattern baldness, 354, 356
Malignant melanoma, 657, 659, 660
Malnutrition, 129, 209, 210, 319, 321
Malocclusion, 208, 209
Mammograms, 17, 123, 124
Managed care, 2, 284, 360, 362, 366, 404
Mandatory retirement, 482-484
Manganese, 732
MAO inhibitors. *See* Monoamine oxidase (MAO) inhibitors
Marital satisfaction, 156, 290, 488, 521
Marquiset, Armand, 461
Marriage, 4, 7, 88, 152, 162, 228, 236, 290, 458
Marshall, Thurgood, 435, 489, 722
Marx, Karl, 185
Mass media. *See* Media *Massachusetts Board of Retirement v. Murgia*
Mastalgia, 122, 123
Mastitis, 124
Matlock, 490
Matriarchs, 21
Matthau, Walter, 353
Maturity, 490-491
Maturity-onset diabetes. *See* Type II diabetes
Meals-on-wheels programs. *See* Home-delivered meals programs

Measure of My Days, The (Scott-Maxwell), 491-492
Media, 11, 12, 161, 285, 477, 622
Median age, 256, 725, 753
Medicaid, 14, 15, 291, 492
Medical care. *See* Health care
Medical directives. *See* Advance directives
Medical insurance. *See* Health insurance.
Medical Payment Advisory Commission (MedPAC), 496
Medicare, 1, 137, 285, 291, 360, 367
 and early retirement, 510
 and hospice, 194, 367
 and marriage, 152, 228
 reform, 1, 345, 423
Medicare Catastrophic Coverage Act of 1988, 367
Medications, 498-502
 and body fat, 278
 and exercise, 75, 158, 219, 251, 275, 276, 283, 320, 407, 75, 158, 219
 and falls, 138, 399
 and impotence, 592, 685
 and sexual dysfunction, 641-646
 and smoking, 80, 139, 171, 209, 544
Medigap, 2, 286, 494
MedPAC. *See* Medical Payment Advisory Commission (MedPAC)
Megadosing, 468
Melanin, 29, 37, 171, 344, 657, 661
Melanoblasts, 657, 658, 659
Melanocytes, 29, 55, 344, 657, 661, 663
Melanoma, 657, 658, 659
Melatonin, 40, 469, 669
Memento Mori (Spark), 502-503
Memorial service, 317
Memory loss, 503-507
Men and aging, 507-512
 African American, 18-22
 and reproductive changes, 610-615
 and suicide, 271, 695, 701
 and widowhood, 484, 653
Menopause, 512-517
Menstruation, 106, 111, 123, 182, 425, 512, 513, 520, 646
Mental health, 16, 42, 49, 76, 102, 204, 485, 545, 595, 600, 696
Mental illness, 35, 71, 88, 89, 247, 386, 483
Mentoring, 519-520
Mercy killing. *See* Euthanasia
Metabolism, 36, 40, 54, 77, 110, 111, 216, 500, 560, 595

Methylprednisolone, 531
Mexican Americans. *See* Latinx Americans.
Micronutrients, 77, 78, 730
Middle adulthood, 189, 228, 262, 656, 657
Middle age, 19-20
Middle Ages, 181, 406
Middle ear, 98, 368, 369, 371
Middle-old, 360, 551, 624
Midlife crisis, 522-525
Midlife Development in the United States (MIDUS) survey, 524
Milk, 4, 109, 119, 123, 481
Mineral deficiencies, 321
Minerals, 95, 109, 110, 129, 309, 355, 470, 479, 500, 544, 636
Minority groups, 11, 15, 456
Minoxidil, 172, 356
Mitochondria, 307, 308, 323, 329
Mobile homes, 2
Mobility problems, 525-529
Modernization theory, 185
Monoamine oxidase (MAO) inhibitors, 561
Monounsaturated fats, 141
Morse, Donald, 466
Mortality rates, 191, 200, 399
Mortgages, 226, 388, 404
Motherhood, 21, 106, 107, 455
Motor skills, 22, 234, 277, 505, 683
Motorized wheelchairs, 738, 739
Mourning, 203, 230, 316, 350, 523, 742
Mouth cancer, 209
Mouth disorders, 209
Movies. *See* Films
Multiple sclerosis, 529-532
Murder, 32, 90, 436, 490, 532
Murder, She Wrote, 532
Murgia, Robert, 489
Murray-Wagner-Dingell Bill, 495
Muscle loss, 76, 637
Muscles; 40, 51, 52, 382, 414, 510, 725
Musculoskeletal system, 54
Mutations, 69, 77, 119, 132, 323
Mutual funds, 2, 241, 424, 458
Myelin, 39, 530, 531
Myocardial infarctions. *See* Heart attacks
Myocardium, 139
Myopia. *See* Nearsightedness

Nails, 170, 659, 661

824 • Index

NAPCA. *See* National Asian Pacific Center on Aging
Narcotics, 393, 395, 415
National Academy on Aging, 334
National Asian Pacific Center on Aging, 532-533
National Caucus and Center on Black Aged, 533-534
National Cholesterol Education Program, 141, 544
National Conference on Aging, 13
National Council on the Aging, 534
National Fraud Information Center, 305
National Hispanic Council on Aging, 535
National Hospice Organization, 391, 396
National Institute on Aging, 13, 117, 331
National Institutes of Health (NIH), 62, 79, 251, 331, 535, 544, 731
National Media Watch Project, 345
National Museum of the American Indian, 537
National Senior Service Corps, 618
Native Americans, 536-538
Natural selection, 327, 328
Naturally occurring retirement communities, 43, 605
NCBA. *See* National Caucus and Center on Black Aged
NCOA. *See* National Council on the Aging
NCSC. *See* National Council of Senior Citizens
Nearsightedness, 538-539
Neglect, 540-541
Nephritis, 190, 415, 713
Nephrons, 711, 712
Nerve deafness, 369
Nerves, 39, 79, 94, 95, 96, 712, 727, 731
Nervous system, 40, 54, 275, 378, 398, 416
Neugarten, Bernice, 541
Neuritic plaques, 117
Neurofibrillary tangles, 65, 69, 325
Neuromas, 295, 296
Neurons, 40, 42, 114, 160, 505, 570
Neurotransmitters, 66, 114, 481
Neutrophils, 40, 250
Never-married, 655, 656
New Passages: Mapping Your Life Across Time (Sheehy), 650
Newspapers, 289, 359, 479, 512, 598
NHCoA. *See* National Hispanic Council on Aging

NLA. *See* National Institute on Aging
Niacin, 480, 481, 731
Night blindness, 37, 728
Night vision, 431
NIH. *See* National Institutes of Health (NIH)
NIMH. *See* National Institute of Mental Health (NIMH)
Nipples, 123, 124
Nitroglycerin, 377
No Stone Unturned: The Life and Times of Maggie Kuhn (Kuhn), 542
Nocturnal myoclonus, 668
Nolen, Granville, 467
Non-insulin-dependent diabetes. *See* Type II diabetes
Nonsteroidal anti-inflammatory drugs (NSAIDs), 75, 84, 97
NORCs. *See* Naturally occurring retirement communities
Normal aging, 36, 39, 40, 41, 543, 544, 550
North American Securities Administrators Association, 305
Nose, 37, 55, 282, 630
Novels, 30, 638
Nurses, 147, 284, 285, 471, 493
Nutrients, 77, 81, 129, 139, 320, 378, 736
Nutrition; 39, 75, 78, 129, 141, 142, 345, 383, 407, 691
Nutritional deficiencies. *See* Mineral deficiencies; Vitamin deficiencies

OAA. *See* Older Americans Act of 1965
OASDI. Social Security, 674, 675, 676
Obergefell v. Hodges, 453
Obesity, 547-550
OBRA. *See* Omnibus Reconciliation Act (OBRA)
Occupational therapy, 76, 206, 285, 302, 390
Occupations. *See* Employment
Ohio v. Betts, 555
Old age, 550-553
Old-age homes. *See* Facility and institutional care
Old-age pensions. *See* Pensions
Old-Age, Survivors, and Disability Insurance. *See* Social Security
Old Man and the Sea, The (Hemingway), 553
Old-old, 47, 146, 147, 186, 360, 363, 541, 551, 624, 685, 753

Old Testament, 47, 406
Older Americans Act of 1965, 554
Older Americans Resources and Services Program, 154
Older Workers Benefit Protection Act, 554-555
Oldest-old, 12, 186, 385, 753, 754, 755
Olsen, Tillie, 698
Omaha tribe, 289
Omega generation, 750
Omega fatty acids, 75, 81
Omnibus Reconciliation Act (OBRA), 283
On Death and Dying (Kübler-Ross), 190, 194, 395, 437
On Golden Pond (Thompson), 555
Oncogenes, 132, 325
Ontogenetic diseases. *See* Age-related diseases
Oocyte, 513
Opioids, 36, 84, 103, 455, 643
Orchiectomy, 592
Oregon Death with Dignity Act, 194
Organ of Corti, 371, 372
Orgasm, 123, 610, 611, 612, 613, 614, 641, 642, 643, 644, 645, 646, 647, 648, 650
Orthotic devices, 97
Osteoarthritis, 76, 82, 83, 85, 86, 96, 112, 210, 381, 416, 481, 549, 561, 613, 643
Osteomalacia, 112
Osteopenia, 78, 112, 636
Osteoporosis, 556-558
Otosclerosis, 38, 368, 369, 372
Oubre v. Entergy, 555
Ourselves, Growing Older: A Book for Women over Forty (Doress-Worters and Siegal), 559
Ovaries, 54, 106, 111, 120, 121, 187, 267, 425, 426, 428, 512, 513, 514, 515, 556, 610, 611, 613
Over-the-counter medications, 2, 614, 643, 696
Over the hill, 559-560
Overbite, 209
Overflow incontinence, 420, 422
Overmedication, 560-563
Over nutrition, 480, 481
Ovulation, 154, 425, 426, 513, 514
Ovum, 267, 424, 513
OWBPA. *See* Older Workers Benefit Protection Act
Owens, Norma

Oxygen, 39, 51, 97, 115, 378, 391, 406, 409, 415, 466, 480, 527, 583, 615, 617, 692
Oysters, 467

Pacific Islanders, 604, 695, 735
Paffenbarger, Ralph, 467
Page, Geraldine, 708
Paget's disease, 112
Pain:
 abdominal, 321, 557
 back, 95, 96, 97, 98,
 breast, 122, 123
 fear of, 195, 393, 644
 hip, 381, 382
 management, 393, 558
 spinal, 96
Painkillers, 84, 407, 416, 671, 700
Palliative care, 564-565
Palmore, Erdman, 291
Pancreas, 55, 141, 217, 218, 219, 220, 260, 318, 319, 320, 327, 414
Pantothenic acid, 731
PAP test. *See* Prostate acid phosphatase (PAP) test
Paralysis, 234, 409, 480, 529, 530, 531, 692, 694
Paranoia, 60, 66, 470, 471, 503, 596
Parasympathetic nervous system, 275
Parathyroid hormone, 110
Parenthood, 565-568
 and death of a child, 192, 198-201
 and grandparents, 566
Parkes, Colin Murray, 349
Parkinson, James, 115, 570
Parkinson's disease, 568-571
Part-time employment, 252, 484, 533
Partial dentures, 208, 212
Passages: Predictable Crises of Adult Life (Sheehy), 650
Passive euthanasia, 194, 270, 271
Passports, 716
Patient Self-Determination Act, 271, 400, 701
Patients' Rights Act of 1980, 486
Patronizing speech, 166, 167
Pattison, E. Mansell, 700
Pauling, Linus, 468
Peace Corps, 734
Pedestrians, 432
Pelvic inflammatory disease, 425, 426
Pelvic prolapse, 422
PEM. *See* Protein energy malnutrition (PEM)

Penile clamp, 422
Penis, 5, 425, 427, 590, 593, 611, 613, 614, 641, 687
Pension Benefit Guaranty Corporation, 253, 573
Pensions, 571-575
 and women, 572, 573
Pepper, Claude, 14
Pepsin, 53, 320
Peptic ulcers, 320, 321
Pericardium, 378
Perimenopause, 103, 267, 426, 513, 515, 516, 517
Periodic leg movement during sleep, 668
Periodontal disease, 37, 53, 208, 209, 210, 319, 320, 321
Peripheral vision, 38, 234, 258, 335, 727
Peroxide, 307, 308, 372, 468
Personality changes, 575-577
Pessary, 422
Petits Frères des Pauvres, Les, 461
Pets, 577-580
Pharmacists, 366, 399
Phenomenology, 186
Phobias, 102, 540, 595
Phosphorus, 731, 732
Photoreceptors, 38, 727, 728
Photosensitivity, 326, 662
Physical disabilities. *See* Disabilities
Physical therapy, 76, 97, 381, 382, 383, 389, 390, 417, 648, 691, 694
Physician-assisted suicide, 271, 272, 696
Phytoestrogens, 516
Piaget, Jean, 601
Picture of Dorian Gray, The, 580-581
Pierpaoli, Walter, 469
Pink puffers, 248
Pituitary gland, 52, 55, 111, 267, 425, 426, 427, 464, 513, 515, 704, 712
Plantar fasciitis, 295, 296
Plaque, dental, 209, 321
Plaques, 4, 65, 69, 79, 117, 118, 140, 204, 325, 374, 379, 413, 515, 658
Plastic surgery, 171, 173, 281
Plato, 181, 406
Pleiotropy, 323, 327
Pneumococcal infections, 412, 581
Pneumonia, 190, 398, 581-585
Poems, 181, 638
Poetry, 175, 638, 739
Point-of-service plans, 366
Poisoning, 432, 499, 569, 695
Polypharmacy, 399, 500
Polyps, 414

Polyunsaturated fats, 141
Poor farms, 49
Population. *See* Demographics
Population aging, 36, 88, 98, 117, 134, 168, 188, 207, 219, 251, 252, 293, 317, 331, 333, 360, 385, 433, 480, 481, 529, 533, 536, 541, 547, 602, 652, 658, 707, 708, 725, 726, 741, 756, 759, 760
Porter, Katherine Anne, 433, 434
Postindustrialization, 22, 679
Postmenopausal osteoporosis, 95, 556
Posture, 33, 37, 51, 96, 234, 279, 297, 431, 439, 469, 508, 570, 646
Potassium, 547, 561, 732, 760
Poverty, 585-589
 among African American workers, 255
 and health care, 586
 among Latino workers, 255
 and women, 588
Poverty line, 367, 451, 485, 586, 587, 588
Power of attorney. *See* Durable power of attorney
PPOs. *See* Preferred provider organizations (PPOs)
PPS. *See* Prospective payment system
Precancerous, 122, 134, 209, 663
Prednisone, 561
Preferred provider organizations (PPOs), 364
Preferred providers, 365
Premature aging, 589-590
Premature ejaculation, 614
Premiums, 362, 366, 457, 458, 459, 494, 495, 497, 528
Prenuptial agreement, 290, 609
Preretirement. *See* Retirement; Retirement planning
Presbycusis, 38, 54, 369, 370, 372
Presbyopia, 37, 38, 54, 150, 598, 728
Prescription drugs. *See* Medications
Pressure sores, 440
Pressure ulcers, 399, 431, 600, 662
Preventive care, 361, 446, 457
Primary aging, 185
Primitive societies, 47, 154, 753
Probate, 11, 264, 265, 266, 293, 709, 710, 745, 746, 748
Procedural memory, 41, 42, 503, 505, 506

Productivity, 22, 30, 76, 144, 145, 174, 175, 180, 223, 331, 550, 595, 684, 685, 722
Professional organizations, 81, 227, 519
Progeria, 307, 325, 589
Progeroid syndromes, 323, 325, 326
Progesterone, 55, 103, 119, 120, 121, 267, 268, 426, 513, 610, 611, 613
Programmed senescence, 327
Project Rescue, 386
Prolapsed disk, 95
Pronation, 295, 296, 297
Property: joint ownership of, 265
Prosorba, 85
Prospective payment system, 292, 362, 397, 496
Prostate cancer, 590-593
Prostate enlargement, 593-594
Prostate gland, 41, 427, 511, 590, 591, 592, 593, 594, 714
Prostate-specific antigen (PSA) test, 134, 415, 511, 591, 593
Prostatectomy, 590, 592, 593, 594
Prostatitis, 593, 594, 732
Proteases, 248, 250
Protein, 37, 40, 65, 69, 74, 77, 79, 81, 82, 84, 85, 109, 110, 111, 114, 117, 120, 127, 132, 133, 140, 150, 543, 589, 591, 611, 636, 637, 686, 713, 719, 728, 736, 758
Protein energy malnutrition (PEM), 480
Proto-oncogenes, 132, 324, 325
PSA test. *See* Prostate-specific antigen (PSA) test
Pseudodementia, 205, 216
Psychiatric nursing care, 390
Psychiatry, geriatric, 594-597
Psychological perspective on aging. *See* Aging: Biological, psychological, and sociocultural perspectives; Aging process
Psychosis, 65, 206, 569, 614
Public education about aging, 49, 536
Public housing, 404, 626
Public transportation, 73, 146, 235, 403, 432, 528, 529, 706, 707, 717, 736
Pueblo tribe, 289
Puerto Ricans, 183, 410, 444, 445
Pulmonary disease. *See* Chronic obstructive pulmonary disease; Lung disease
Pulmonary edema, 398
Pulmonary embolism, 723, 724
Pulmonary function, 249, 250, 251, 415, 616
Pulmonary system. *See* Respiratory system
Pulse, 52, 57, 378, 413
Pupil, 37, 149, 336, 478, 727, 728
Puritans, 48, 181
Pyelonephritis, 415, 713
Pyorrhea, 209

Q-TIP. *See* Qualified terminable interest property trust
Qualified terminable interest property trust, 265
Quality of life, 34, 64, 66, 75, 76, 122, 125, 194, 207, 211, 213, 222, 223, 224, 234, 246, 260, 272, 287, 293, 301, 332, 618, 667, 702, 707, 726, 730, 750
Quetelet, Adolphe, 331
Quinlan, Karen, 271

Rabinowitz, Harold, 466
Radiation, 35, 77, 120, 121, 132, 135, 136, 307
Radiation therapy, 35, 135, 322, 427, 592, 660, 704
Rail passes, 716
Raloxifene, 268, 516, 557
Rapid eye movement (REM) sleep, 36, 667
Reaction time, 8, 40, 51, 184, 222, 234, 597-598
Reading glasses, 598
Reagan, Ronald, 14, 26, 423, 496, 740
Receding gums, 208, 209
Receding hairline, 354, 355
Reconstructive surgery, 171
Recreation, 1, 7, 10, 157, 166, 199, 222, 225, 233, 240, 715, 733, 738
Recreational therapy, 285
Recreational vehicles (RVs), 717
Red Cross, 226, 706, 734
Reductions, 25, 40, 54, 115, 116, 130, 213, 234, 268, 276, 496, 669
Reflexes, 54, 97, 431
Refractory period, 641, 642
Rehabilitation, 56, 97, 222, 281, 284, 286, 297, 302, 360, 448, 471, 581, 596, 640, 693, 694, 706
Rehabilitation Act of 1973, 26, 27, 71, 223
Religion; 598-603
Relocation; 603-607

REM sleep. *See* Rapid eye movement (REM) sleep
Remarriage, 607-610
 and parenthood, 607
 and Social Security benefits, 609
Remission, 83, 135, 441, 530, 531
Renaissance, 180, 181
Renal pelvis, 686, 687
Repair services, 169
Reproductive changes, disabilities, and dysfunctions, 610-615
Reproductive tract, 425, 426, 427
Republican Party, 13, 236, 495, 496
Research Network on Successful Midlife Development, 524
Resilience, 8, 57, 349, 550, 552, 638, 648, 690, 696
Resistance training, 76, 280, 527, 637
Respect for the elderly, 21, 346
Respiration, 176, 239, 248, 269, 307, 323, 328, 561, 617, 641, 668
Respiratory changes and disorders, 615-618
Respiratory system, 40, 51, 52, 274, 322, 615, 617, 720, 731
Respite care, 66, 68, 157, 390, 391, 640, 666
Rest homes. *See* Facility and institutional care
Resting heart rate, 275
Resuscitation. *See* "Do not resuscitate" status
Retin A, 29, 283, 664
Retina, 38, 149, 151, 335, 409, 476, 477, 478, 520, 598, 727, 728, 729
Retinal detachment, 416, 729
Retinol. *See* Vitamin A
Retired and Senior Volunteer Program (RSVP), 618-619
Retirement, 619-625. *See also* Delayed retirement; Early retirement; Graduated retirement
Retirement age, 625
Retirement benefits, 13, 25, 46, 93, 162, 226, 367, 445, 488, 572, 625, 656, 676
Retirement communities, 625-628
Retirement Equity Act of 1984, 573
Retirement housing, 441, 472
Retirement planning, 628-630
Reverse mortgage, 388, 402, 404
Revolving door syndrome, 521
Rheumatoid arthritis, 83, 84, 85, 86, 96, 372, 373, 381, 557, 613
Rhinophyma, 630-631

Rhytidectomy. *See* Face lifts
Rhytids, 281
Riboflavin, 481, 731
Right to die, 272, 461
Ringing in the ears, 38, 372
Rivers, Joan, 407
Robin and Marian, 631-632
Rogaine. *See* Minoxidil
Role reversal, 148, 566, 568
"Roman Fever" (Wharton), 632
Rome, 507, 632
Roosevelt, Franklin D., 23, 706
Root canal, 177, 208
Rosacea, 630
Rose, Michael, 509
Ross, Morris, 129
Roth IRAs, 243, 424
RSVP. *See* Retired and Senior Volunteer Program (RSVP)
Rudeness, 175
RVs. *See* Recreational vehicles (RVs)

Saarela, Seppo, 469
Safe Return Program, 63
Safety measures, 136
SAGE. *See* Senior Aging in a Gay Environment (SAGE)
Sagging skin, 171
Saliva, 4, 53, 208, 209, 210, 211, 318, 319, 758
Salmon, Michael, 461
Salt, 39, 53, 82, 85, 117, 152, 217, 267, 327, 376, 384, 408, 410, 481, 545, 704, 712, 713, 730
Sandwich generation, 632-635
Sarcopenia, 635-638
Sarton, May, 638-639
Satisfaction. *See* Job satisfaction; Life satisfaction; Marital satisfaction
Saturated fat, 141, 152, 158, 219, 376, 380, 478, 480, 481, 544, 737
Saunders, Cicely, 395
Savings, 20, 241, 359, 404, 423, 424, 474, 496, 498, 509, 588, 621, 627, 628, 629, 675, 685, 710, 742
Scalds, 432
Scalp reduction, 355
Schaie, K. Warner, 182, 332
Schools:
 funding of, 92
 volunteering in, 682
Schroots, Johannes J. F., 184
Sclerosing adenosis, 124
Sclerotherapy, 722, 724

Scoliosis, 95, 440
Scott-Maxwell, Florida, 491, 492
Scrotum, 187, 427
Seasons of a Man's Life, The (Levinson), 523-524
Sebaceous cysts, 187
Sebaceous glands, 123, 657, 661, 662
Seborrheic keratosis, 663
Secondary aging, 185
Sedation, 561
Sedentary lifestyle, 141, 692, 699
Segregation by age, 24, 448
Selective estrogen receptor modulators (SERMs), 516
Selegiline, 75
Selenium, 77, 732
Self-esteem, 3, 30, 55, 165, 173, 213, 214, 226, 277, 285, 349, 420, 432, 448, 450, 483, 488, 519, 555, 630, 641, 644, 649, 685
Semantic memory, 41, 505, 506
Semen, 4, 420, 427, 593
Senescence, 41, 74, 182, 183, 261, 308, 323, 324, 327, 328, 329, 520, 589
Senile, 69, 180, 204, 271, 325, 481, 556, 662, 663, 728, 732
Senile dementia. *See* Alzheimer's disease; Dementia
Senile osteoporosis, 556
Senile plaques, 69, 325
Senile purpura, 662, 732
Senility, 8, 87, 88, 313, 412, 555, 741
Senior apartments, 472
Senior citizen centers, 639-640
Senior citizen discounts. *See* Discounts
Senior citizens. *See* Elderly
Senior Citizens' Equity Act, 573
Senior Citizens for Kennedy, 13
Senior Community Service Employment Program, 533
Senior Companion Program, 618
Senior discount days, 226
Senior Environmental Employment Program, 533, 534
Senior movement, 13
Senior Olympics, 683
Senior Reach Program, 386
Senior rights, 13, 14
Sensorineural hearing loss, 368, 369, 372
Sequential studies, 332, 519
Serial monogamy, 608
SERMs. *See* Selective estrogen receptor modulators (SERMs)

Serotonin, 66, 103, 104, 114, 115, 116, 481, 669
Servicemen's and Veteran's Survivor Benefits Act of 1957, 573
Sexual dysfunction, 641-646
 and prostate cancer, 590-593
 and smoking, 670-672
Sexual relationships, 257, 449, 610, 666
Sexuality, 646-650
 and men; 647, 648
 and women, 646, 647, 648
Sexually transmitted diseases, 425, 426, 427
Shakespeare, William, 181, 435, 744
Share the Care, 312
Shared housing, 472, 542
Sheehy, Gail, 650
Shelters, 92, 361, 385, 386, 401, 572, 579, 733
Shepherd's Centers, 651-652
Shingles, 664, 718, 720
Shivering, 699
Shock, 95, 104, 146, 190, 191, 202, 219, 296, 298, 301, 349, 395, 508, 571, 687, 700
Shoes, 127, 128, 170, 296, 297, 357, 431, 716
Shootist, The, 652-653
Short stories, 313
Short-term memory, 8, 41, 222, 481, 505, 530
Shortness of breath, 102, 139, 202, 248, 250, 376, 413, 414, 582, 584, 612, 617, 719, 724, 742
Sibling relationships, 653-655
Siegal, Diana Laskin, 559
Sight. *See* Vision changes and disorders
Silent Passage: Menopause, The (Sheehy), 650
Silicone, 125, 150, 422
Silverman, Phyllis, 744
Singlehood, 655-657
Sinus node, 378, 380
Sisters, 359, 395, 653, 654, 747
Situation comedies, 407
Skilled nursing facility, 283, 286, 472, 492
Skin cancer, 657-661
Skin changes and disorders, 661-665
Skin resurfacing, 280, 281, 282
Skin tags, 663
Skinfolds, 547
Skinner, B. F., 258
Skipped-generation parenting, 665-667

Slavery, 21, 289, 619
Sleep apnea, 549, 668
Sleep changes and disturbances, 667-670
Sleeping pills, 561
Small intestine, 111, 318, 319, 320, 321, 414
Smell, 39, 54, 103, 416, 432, 470, 482, 506, 544, 561
Smoking, 670-672
 and impotence, 671
 and macular degeneration, 671
 and wrinkles, 670
Soap operas. *See* Daytime serials
Social competence, 185, 577
Social exchange theory of aging, 185
Social media, 672-674
 benefits of, 673
 platforms, 673
 risks of, 673
Social Security, 674-677
 amendments to, 675
 and baby boomers, 675
 benefits, 675
 and marriage, 676
 reform, 677
 and women, 674, 675
Social Security Act of 1935, 12, 49, 367, 509, 622, 675
Social Security Reform Amendments of 1983, 740
Social ties, 677-682
 and singlehood, 655-657
 and volunteering, 733-735
Societal influence, 31, 44, 106, 106, 200
Sociocultural perspective on aging. *See* Aging: Biological, psychological, and sociocultural perspectives; Cultural views of aging
Sodium, 152, 219, 376, 384, 410, 411, 481, 737
Soft tissue injuries, 96
Solar keratosis, 663
Soup kitchens, 246
Source forgetting, 504
Spark, Muriel, 502
Speaking, 12, 19, 41, 71, 108, 159, 164, 175, 215, 303, 338, 351, 372, 377, 417, 474, 478, 533, 562, 583, 584, 606, 619, 681, 692, 730, 749
Special-interest groups, 392
Speech problems, 209
Sperm, 41, 425, 426, 427, 428, 593, 612, 714
Spinal problems. *See* Back disorders

Spine, 84, 94, 95, 96, 97, 98, 101, 111, 300, 439, 558, 646, 711, 720
Spirituality, 43, 44, 197, 418, 551, 599, 603, 727, 749, 750
Spondylosis, 95
Spontaneous life review. *See* Life review
Sports participation, 682-684
Spouses as caregivers, 146
Squamous cell carcinoma, 657, 658, 659, 660, 663, 664
SRAs. *See* Supplemental savings accounts (SRAs)
SSI *See* Supplemental Security Income
Stagnation, 42, 191, 213, 257, 262, 455, 522, 524, 601, 602, 748, 749
Stasis dermatitis, 664
State Agencies on Aging, 245
State and Local Fiscal Act of 1972, 26
State Long-Term Care Ombudsman program, 245
State unit on aging, 554
Statins, 81, 159
Statutory wills, 746
Stereotypes, 684-686
Steroids, 85, 172, 214, 287, 321, 531, 557, 729
Stock market, 241, 458
Stocks, 241, 265, 299, 424, 458, 493, 623, 624, 746
Stomach, 40, 58, 85, 134, 260, 318, 319, 320, 321, 322, 349, 414, 499, 543, 546, 557, 560, 561, 569, 653, 689
Stomach cancer, 260, 653
Stones, 686-689
 kidney, 78, 337, 338, 415, 420
Strength, 21, 25, 35, 37, 40, 48, 51, 52, 54, 74, 75, 76
Strength training, 141, 275, 277, 278, 280, 449, 526, 527
Streptococcal pneumonia, 581, 583, 584
Streptokinase, 377
Stress and coping skills, 689-691
Stress incontinence, 53, 420, 421, 422, 515, 714
Stroke volume, 52, 275
Strokes; 691-695
 and menopause; 692
SUA. *See* State unit on aging Subculture theory of aging
Substance abuse. *See* Alcohol use disorder; Medications; Overmedication
Substandard housing, 404, 405, 446
Suburbs, 91, 527

Successful aging, 43, 185, 186, 273, 449, 491, 599
Suicide, 695-697
Sulfonylureas, 219
Sun damage, 171, 281, 282, 664, 699
Sun exposure, 29, 184, 481, 543, 557, 658, 661, 663, 664
Sunburn, 659, 660
Sundowning, 206
Sunset Boulevard, 697-698
Superoxide radical, 307, 308
Supplemental savings accounts (SRAs), 621
Supplemental Security Income, 14, 46, 162, 223, 445, 674, 676, 740
Support groups, 67, 148, 157, 199, 203, 207, 231, 290, 291, 312, 394, 433, 465, 487, 512, 652, 666
Supported employment, 223
Supreme Court decisions, 435
Surrogate parenthood, 342
Survivor benefits, 162, 574, 575, 676
Survivor status, 20
Survivorship, right of, 265, 455, 748
Sweat glands, 36, 55, 171, 657, 661, 662, 758
Sweating, 5, 57, 102, 139, 276, 376, 399
Sweepstakes, 304, 305
Swindles, 246
Sympathetic nervous system, 278, 464
Sympathy, 313, 700
Synapses, 114
Syncope, 431
Synovial membrane, 82, 83
Systemic lupus erythematosus, 84
Systolic pressure, 374, 379, 409

Tachycardia, 52, 380
Tagamet, 499
Tagliacozzi, Gaspare, 171, 281
Tamoxifen, 121, 136, 268
Tandy, Jessica, 161, 235, 236
Tartar, 209
Taste, 39, 53, 54, 103, 142, 258, 319, 432, 470, 481, 482, 544, 561, 670, 732
Taste buds, 39, 53, 54, 210, 319
Tax rates, 162, 710
Tax Reform Act of 1986, 423, 573, 710
Taxes:
 on estates, 264
 on gifts, 710
Teeth, 53, 177, 178, 207, 208, 209, 211, 318, 320, 321, 557, 662, 670
Telangiectasias, 663, 664

Telemarketing fraud, 304, 305, 306
Telephone Consumer Protection Act, 305
Television, 20, 30, 32, 33, 90, 101, 126, 149, 166, 336, 337, 339, 353, 359, 403, 407, 412, 465, 490, 504, 512, 532, 552, 581, 622, 627, 729
Tell Me a Riddle (Olsen), 698-699
Telomerase, 77, 135, 324, 466
Telomeres, 77, 324, 326, 327, 329, 466
Temperature regulation and sensitivity, 699-700
Temporomandibular (TMJ) syndrome, 210
Tendinitis, 295, 296
Tendons, 54, 82, 96, 127, 128, 170, 295, 296, 356, 357
Tennis, 112, 138, 277, 296, 383, 431, 509, 683
Term-life policies, 457, 459
Terminal illness, 700-703
  and suicide, 701
Tertiary aging, 185
Testamentary trusts, 710
Testators, 264, 710, 745
Testicles, 425, 427, 592
Testosterone, 55, 103, 134, 158, 354, 355, 427, 468, 469, 511, 514, 520, 527, 538, 591, 592, 611, 612, 614, 637, 644, 647, 735
Tetanus, 55, 718, 719, 720
Theater, 61, 101, 226
Theft, 245, 246, 490, 673, 674
Theories of aging. *See* Cellular clock theory of aging; Cross-linkage theory of aging; Free radical theory of aging; Genetic design theory of aging; Neuroendocrine theory of aging; Wear-and-tear theory of aging
Thermoregulation, 699
Thiamine, 481, 731
This Chair Rocks: A Manifesto Against Ageism, 703
Thompson, Ernest, 555
Thrombolytic therapy, 377
Thrush, 210
Thymus gland, 40
Thyroid disorders, 703-705
Thyroid gland, 55, 110, 703, 704, 705
Thyroxine, 704
TIAs. *See* Transient ischemic attacks (TIAs)
Time share resort, 717
Tinnitus, 38, 98, 372

TMJ syndrome. *See* Temporomandibular (TMJ) syndrome
Tobacco, 36, 136, 152, 153, 209, 251, 374, 375, 376, 427, 508, 561
Toes, 82, 169, 170, 295, 296, 297, 356, 357, 416, 570
Tongue, 53, 209, 210, 319, 343, 504, 570
Tooth decay, 207, 208, 211
Tooth loss, 37, 53, 208, 209, 210
  and smoking, 209
Tophi, 337, 338
Torticollis, 96
Totten trusts, 710, 746
Touch, 37, 39, 123, 149, 172, 183, 442, 470, 523, 534, 578, 627, 647, 648, 661, 673, 693, 739
Toupees, 355
Tours, 2, 716
Townsend, Francis Everett, 23, 705
Townsend movement, 705-706
TPA, 377, 694
Track and field, 683
Traffic accidents, 233, 235, 432
Trail of Tears, 536
Tranquilizers, 301, 499, 561
Transfusions, 4
Transient ischemic attacks (TIAs), 116, 413
Transportation issues, 706-708
Travel. *See also* Foreign travel; Vacations and travel
Tremors, 54, 57, 59, 234, 416, 511, 569, 571, 704
Tretinoin. *See* Retin A Triglycerides
Triiodothyronine, 704
Trip to Bountiful, The, 708-709
Trisomy 21, 69, 325
Trustees, 264, 651, 677, 709, 710
Trusts, 709-711
Tryptophan, 467, 481
Tuberculosis, 55, 72, 84, 95, 124, 386, 413
Tumor necrosis factor, 85
Tumor suppressor genes, 132, 133, 325, 659
Tunnel vision, 335, 336
Tylenol, 84, 85, 500
Tympanic membrane, 371
Type I diabetes, 218, 219
Type II diabetes, 218, 219, 379, 445, 481, 546, 549

Uhry, Alfred, 235, 236
Ulcerative colitis, 414

Ulcers, 85, 315, 320, 321, 357, 399, 414, 420, 431, 600, 662, 664
Ultraviolet rays, 136, 150, 661
Underbite, 209
Under nutrition, 129, 480
Unemployment, 24, 28, 252, 253, 292, 464, 623
Unions, 28, 71, 365, 495, 573, 626
United Nations, 345, 438, 534
Universal health care, 17, 345, 362, 498
Universal life policies, 458
Unmarried couples, 162, 192
Ureters, 420, 687, 711, 713
Urethra, 420, 421, 427, 590, 593, 687, 688, 711, 713, 714
Urge incontinence, 420, 421, 422
Uric acid, 83, 84, 337, 338, 686
Urinary disorders, 711-715
Urinary incontinence. *See* Incontinence
Urinary system, 39, 687, 711, 713, 714
Urinary tract infections, 714
Urine:
  blood in the, 594, 688, 713
  protein in the, 415
  sugar in the, 217
Uterine cancer, 267, 268, 516
Uterus, 40, 54, 119, 267, 426, 428, 512, 513, 515, 516, 613
Utopian communities, 403
UV rays. *See* Ultraviolet rays

Vacation homes, 717
Vacations and travel, 715-718
Vaccination, 55, 429, 584, 718, 719, 721
Vaccines, 5, 55, 135, 189, 412, 413, 718-721
Vagina, 5, 40, 267, 422, 426, 515, 516, 610, 611, 613, 641, 646
Vaginal dryness, 515, 613, 644
Vaginismus, 613
Valium, 104, 561
Vance v. Bradley, 721-722
Varicose veins, 722-725
Vas deferens, 427
Veins, 123, 173, 378, 415, 670, 722, 723, 724
Venous insufficiency, 664
Ventilation. *See* Breathing Ventricles
Ventricular fibrillation, 374
Vertebrae, 52, 54, 84, 94, 95, 97, 110, 111, 112, 416, 419, 439, 440, 556
Vertigo, 98, 431
Very low-density lipoproteins (VLDLs), 79, 140

Very-old, 680
Vested pensions, 574
Veterans, 725-726
   and homelessness, 726
Viagra, 428, 645, 646, 647
Violence. *See* Domestic violence; Elder abuse
Viral infections, 5, 132, 569, 583
Virtues of Aging, The (Carter), 726-727
Vision changes and disorders, 727-730
Visitation rights of grandparents, 290, 343
Vital involvement, 262, 263, 551
Vitamin A, 77, 111, 112, 543, 544, 731
Vitamin B_1. *See* Thiamine
Vitamin B_2. *See* Riboflavin
Vitamin B_3. *See* Niacin
Vitamin B_5. *See* Pantothenic acid
Vitamin B_6, 480, 543, 731
Vitamin B_{12}, 205, 321, 344, 480, 481, 506, 543, 731
Vitamin C, 77, 78, 111, 468, 479, 480, 481, 546, 731, 759
Vitamin D, 76, 110, 111, 112, 481, 516, 543, 544, 556, 557, 558, 660, 661, 731
Vitamin deficiencies, 204, 209, 210, 731
Vitamin E, 75, 77, 78, 468, 479, 732
Vitamins and fat-soluble medications, 499
Vitamins and minerals, 730-733
Vitreous humor, 728
VLDLs. *See* Very low-density lipoproteins (VLDLs)
Volunteering, 733-735

Waist-hip ratio, 548
Walford, Roy, 128
Walkers. *See* Canes and walkers
Walking, 67, 71, 76, 97, 112, 128, 137, 141, 269, 274, 357, 376, 381, 431, 605, 626, 636, 683, 694, 722, 725, 738, 757
Walking pneumonia, 581
Wandering, 63, 66, 206, 540
War on Poverty, 586
Warfarin, 499, 694
Wasting, 69, 85, 277, 480, 556, 635, 637, 735
Water pills, 500
Water-soluble medications, 499
Wax in the ear, 369, 372
Wayne, John, 652
We Are Age and Youth in Action, 345
Wear-and-tear theory of aging, 551
Websites, 304, 392, 683, 717
Weight loss and gain, 735-738
Welfare state, 619, 621, 624, 755
Wellness Promotion and Disease Prevention Program, 534
Welty, Eudora, 757
Werner, Huber, 467
Werner's syndrome, 323, 325, 467, 589
Western Gerontological Society, 70
WGS. *See* Western Gerontological Society Wharton, Edith
WHCoA. *See* White House Conference on Aging
Wheelchair use, 738-739
When I Am an Old Woman I Shall Wear Purple (Martz, ed.), 739-740
White House Conference on Aging, 740-741
Whole-life policies, 457, 458, 459, 460
Why Survive? Being Old in America (Butler), 741-742
Widow-to-Widow Program, 744

Widows and widowers, 742-744
Wild Strawberries, 262, 744-745
Wills and bequests, 745-748
Wisdom, 748-752
Witch's chin, 281
Woman's Tale, A, 752
Women and aging, 752-757
   and poverty, 754
   and retirement, 754, 755, 756
Women's movement, 298, 756
Woopies, 586
Work. *See* Employment
Working memory, 41, 42, 506
World Masters Championships, 683
World Veterans Games, 683
"Worn Path, A" (Welty), 757-758
Wounds, 40, 198, 199, 217, 284, 300, 580, 662, 719, 720, 732
Wright, Woodring, 466
Wrinkles, 8, 30, 55, 100, 476, 661, 758-759

Xeroderma pigmentosum, 134, 328
Xerosis, 662
Xerostomia, 210, 319

Yen, Samuel, 468
Yogurt, 130, 467
Young-old, 12, 47, 147, 186, 360, 541, 551, 624, 684, 743, 753
You're Only Old Once! (Seuss), 759-760
Youth bias, 100
Youth culture, 30, 483
Youth hostels, 716

Zinc, 77, 320, 370, 478, 479, 480, 481, 544, 732